Natural Products and Drug Discovery

Natural Products and Drug Discovery

Special Issue Editor

Pinarosa Avato

MDPI • Basel • Beijing • Wuhan • Barcelona • Belgrade • Manchester • Tokyo • Cluj • Tianjin

Special Issue Editor
Pinarosa Avato
Università degli Studi di Bari Aldo Moro
Italy

Editorial Office
MDPI
St. Alban-Anlage 66
4052 Basel, Switzerland

This is a reprint of articles from the Special Issue published online in the open access journal *Molecules* (ISSN 1420-3049) (available at: https://www.mdpi.com/journal/molecules/special_issues/molecules_NPDD).

For citation purposes, cite each article independently as indicated on the article page online and as indicated below:

LastName, A.A.; LastName, B.B.; LastName, C.C. Article Title. *Journal Name* **Year**, *Article Number*, Page Range.

ISBN 978-3-03928-746-8 (Pbk)
ISBN 978-3-03928-747-5 (PDF)

Contents

About the Special Issue Editor

Pinarosa Avato graduated with a degree in biological sciences. In 2004, she was appointed Full Professor of Pharmacognosy for the Faculty of Pharmacy, now the Department of Pharmacy-Drug Sciences, of the University of Bari (Italy). Since 2004 she has been president of the degree classes in "Pharmaceutical Science and Technologies". She holds a degree in Science and Technology of Herbal and Health Products and a degree in Herbal Techniques. Since 1987 she has been a teacher of phytochemistry, medical botany and pharmacognosy. Since 1999 she has been a member of the research doctorate program Chemical and Molecular Sciences. From 2014 to 2015 she was a member of the teaching board of the Master (II level) in Biotechnology for Medicinal and Aromatic Plants, in Partnership with UNESCO. She is presently a member of the Master (II level) in Science of Cosmetics (Univ. of Bari), and teaches phytocosmetics. She has been member of various committees (teaching activities, Student's Welcome, tutoring, and the library committee) of the Department of Drug Sciences. Presently she is a delegate for the Socrates/Erasmus Programme and member of the University Research Center for Collaboration to Development. During 1989, 1990, and 1991, she was part of a joint Research Programme and a Visiting Professor at the Danish Royal School of Pharmacy of Copenhagen (Denmark), Department of Medicinal Chemistry, Section of Pharmacognosy/Section of Natural Product Chemistry. In 2003, she was an Invited Scientist at the 5° EPSA Summer University, Phytotherapy, Orhid, FYR Macedonia. In 2006 she was a Visiting Professor at the Institute of Biology, University of Latvia, Riga, Lettonia, and in 2007 a Visiting Professor at the Henan Normal University of Xinxiang, China. In 2015, she was a Visiting Professor of the Faculty of Pharmacy of Gdansk, Poland. In 2018 she was a Visiting Professor of the Faculty of Pharmacy of the University of Seville, Spain. She has had scientific cooperation with national and international research institutions. Her research activity mainly concerns lipid chemistry, chemical and bioactivity of specialized metabolites, plant biodiversity, and biocidal compounds from natural sources. She has been a research leader and associate researcher of several research projects, as well as a regional representative of the Phytochemical Society of Europe, PSE (2007–2010); a member of the Executive Board of the Italian Society of Phytochemistry, SIF (2013–2015; 2016–2018); a member of the Executive Board of the Phytochemical Society of Europe, PSE—Meetings Secretary PSE (2012-2017); and a member of the Executive Board of "Sezione Pugliese" of the Italian Society of Botany, SBI (2015–2017; 2017–2020). She is a Review Editor of "Frontiers in Pharmacology-Ethnopharmacology" (2015–present), and, in 2017, was a Guest Editor of a SI of *Molecules* (section Natural Products): *Selected papers from 2nd International Symposium on Phytochemicals in Medicine and Food (2-ISPMF, Fuzhou, 2017)*. She is a member of the following organizations: Società Italiana di Fitochimica; Società Italiana di Farmacognosia; Società Italiana di Farmacologia; Società Botanica italiana; Società Italiana Ricerca Olii Essenziali; Phytochemical Society of Europe; Society for Medicinal Plant Research. She is currently a reviewer of several ISI Journals (e.g., *Phytochemistry*, *Phytochemistry Review*, *Journal of Agricultural and Food Chemistry*, *Molecules*, *Industrial Crops and Products*, *Journal of Pharmaceutical and Biomedical Analysis*, *Journal of Natural Products*, *Applied Soil Ecology*, *Frontiers*, *Natural Product Communications*, and *Journal of Essential Oil Research*). She authored book chapters and numerous publications in ISI Journals (e.g., *Phytochemistry*; *Phytochemistry Reviews*; *Lipids*; *Journal of Agricultural and Food Chemistry*; *European Journal of Plant Pathology*; *Journal of Pest Sciences*; *Molecules*; *Plant Science*; *Plants*; *Planta*; *Flavour and Fragrance Journal*; *Planta Medica*; *Journal of Natural Products*; and *Phytotherapy Research*). She is a member of the Scientific/Organizing Committee of several national and international Symposia (most recently: "Biodiversità e intensificazione ecosostenibile", Matera, Italy, 2016; "Plant Omics for Biotechnology and Human Health", Gent, Belgium, 2016; the International Symposium "Trends in Natural Product Research", Pulawy, Poland, 2016; Workshop "Essenze Aromatiche: Vizi e Virtù del loro Uso in Terapia", Bari, Italy, 2016; the "9th Joint Natural Products Conference", Copenhagen, Denmark, 2016; "New & Old Phytochemicals: Their Role in Ecology, Veterinary & Welfare", Francavilla al Mare, Italy, 2017; "Natural Products in Health, Agro Food and Cosmetics", Lille, France, 2017; "Phytochemicals in Food and Medicine" Fuzhou, China, 2017; "Advances in Phytochemical Analysis—Trends in Natural Products Research", Liverpool, UK, 2018; "Natural Products in Cancer Prevention and Therapy—Third Edition", Napoli, Italy, 2018.

molecules

MDPI

Editorial

Editorial to the Special Issue–"Natural Products and Drug Discovery"

Pinarosa Avato

Dipartimento di Farmacia-Scienze del Farmaco, Università degli Studi di Bari Aldo Moro, Via Orabona 4, 70125 Bari, Italy; pinarosa.avato@uniba.it

Received: 28 February 2020; Accepted: 2 March 2020; Published: 3 March 2020

Natural products hold a prominent position in the discovery and development of many drugs used nowadays, with diverse indications for human and animal health. Especially, plants have played a leading role as source of specialized metabolites with medical effects, while other organisms such as marine and terrestrial animals and microorganisms produce very important drug candidate molecules. Specialized metabolites from all these natural sources can be used directly as bioactive compounds, or as drug precursors. Due to their wide chemical diversity they can act as drug prototypes and/or be used as pharmacological tools for different targets.

Many scientists have contributed to this Special Issue-SI which includes 21 papers, among them original articles as well as survey articles, that give the readers of *Molecules* updated and new perspectives about natural products in drug discovery.

Trabace et al. [1] reported the impact of celastrol, a pentacyclic terpene produced by the medicinal plant *Tripterygium wilfordii*, on behavioural dysfunctions observed in adult mice exposed to subanesthetic doses of the N-methyl-D-aspartate receptor antagonist ketamine at PNDs. This study suggested that the NOX inhibition by the early administration of celastrol can prevent ketamine-induced psychotic-like behavioural dysfunctions, as well as the increase of cerebellar oxidative stress and the reduction of anti-inflammatory cytokines. Results open up new pharmacological insights into the possible use of this phytochemical for neuroprotection during brain development.

The current production of artemisinin, the antimalarial drug from *Artemisia annua*, is still mainly based on the use of cultivated plants. Various alternative strategies have been explored to improve its production in the plant. In their paper, Simonsen et al. [2] describe the heterologous expression of artemisinin biosynthetic pathway in *Physcomitrella patens*, showing novel insights into the potential of this model organism for artemisinin production. The moss was shown to express endogenous enzymes with similar activity to that for artemisinin biosynthesis in *A. annua*, suggesting the possibility of engineering artemisinin biosynthesis and that of other related high-value terpenoids in *P. patens*.

Recent data highlight that glucosinolates, the sulfur compounds produced in the Brassicaceae plant family, have pain-relieving efficacy. Mannelli and coworkers [3] describe the anti-hyperalgesic efficacy of a defatted seed meal of *Eruca sativa* along with glucoerucin, its main glucosinolate, on streptozotocin induced diabetic neuropathic pain in mice. Both myrosinase bio-activated *E. sativa* meal and glucoerucin showed a dose-dependent pain relief effect in diabetic mice, with the meal being more active. Co-administration of the meal and glucoerucin with H_2S scavengers abolished the induced pain relief. The authors also showed that repeated treatments did not induce tolerance to the anti-hypersensitive effect. The paper nicely indicates a potential of *E. sativa* seed meal to treat patients with diabetic neuropathy.

Wolfender et al. [4] propose a new approach to discover new bioactive natural products. They make use of a metabolomic strategy in combination with multivariate data analysis and multi-informative molecular maps to profile extracts of *Bacopa* species (*B. monnieri, B. caroliniana,* and *B. floribunda*) and screen for anti-lipid peroxidation activity. This approach allowed the identification of six inhibitors of lipid peroxidation from the three *Bacopa* species. Three of them were novel molecules. Data obtained by this method permitted to discover the potential bioactivity for each compound directly from the crude plant extracts prior to any physical separation process.

The genus *Phyllantus* includes some Cuban endemic species traditionally used for the treatment of different diseases. Wessjohann et al. [5] report on the chemical characterization of the aqueous extract from *Phyllantus,* known to have in vitro antiviral activity and protective effect against UV-light induced DNA damage and genotoxicity. The chemical structure of a novel C-glycosylated flavonol, named fideloside, with a promising anti-inflammatory capacity in human explanted monocytes is described.

Tran et al. [6] describe the anti-tumor effect of 2′,4′-dihydroxy-6′-methoxy-3′,5′- dimethylchalcone (DMC) against some human pancreatic cancer cell lines. In a cell proliferation assay, the compound, isolated from buds of *Cleistocalyx operculatus,* was shown to be cytotoxic against PANC-1 and MIA PACA2 cells in a dose-dependent manner. In addition, treatment with DMC led to apoptosis of PANC-1 cells inducing proteolytic activation of caspase-3. A possible use of this natural product as chemotherapeutic agent to fight human pancreatic cancer is suggested.

The paper by Avato and Argentieri [7] describes for the first time the chemical profile of a commercial spagyric tincture prepared from the dried roots of devil's claw. Compositional consistence of this preparation over time was investigated by comparison with an already expired devil's claw spagyric tincture from the same producer. The two preparations had no significant compositional variations. In addition, their antioxidant potential based on the DPPH assay showed similar IC50. From this investigation, it could be demonstrated that the two spgayric tinctures maintain good stability and biological activity for at least four years after production.

While several species of *Astragalus* have been extensively investigated, phytochemical and pharmacological information on *A. boeticus* is very limited. Scognamiglio et al. [8] report on the chemical characterization of acylatd cycloartane glycosides from this species and on their cytoxicity towards human colorectal cancer cell lines. The authors show that, among the five isolated cycloartane-type glycosides, 6-*O*-acetyl-3-*O*-β-d-xylopyranosylcycloastragenol, with acylation at C-3 and C-6 and the C-25 free hydroxyl function, had the highest activity, thus confirming some structural requirements for the cytotoxicity of cycloartane derivatives.

The study by Rivière et al. [9] reports on the antimicrobial effect of hop extracts and their main prenylated phenolics (xanthoumol, desmethylxanthohumol and lupulone) against MRSA strains, and on their antiparasitic activity against *Trypanosoma brucei* and *Leishmania mexicana.* Besides considering the antibacterial effect of single hop components, the authors also describe the positive effect obtained by different combinations of xanthoumol with desmethylxanthohumol or with lupulone. They also investigated post-antibiotic effects and found that xanthoumol and desmethylxanthohumol cause a significant delay of bacterial re-growth. Among hops active principles, lupulone was shown as the most active against *T. brucei* and *L. mexicana,* while humulone was the less active.

The paper by Koh et al. [10] represents an extensive phytochemical investigation of *Lee indica,* an evergreen perennial shrub/small tree distributed in Southeast Asia, traditionally used as medicinal plant with various indications. A total of 31 compounds belonging to different chemical groups (flavonoids, coumarins, oxylipins, etc.) have been identified. Three of them are novel dihydrochalcones: 4′,6′-dihydroxy-4-methoxydihydrochalcone 2′-*O*-rutinoside, 4′,6′-dihydroxy-4-methoxydihydro chalcone 2′-*O*-glucosylpentoside and 4′,6′-dihydroxy-4-methoxydihydrochalcone 2′-*O*-(3″-*O*-galloyl)-β-D-glucopyranoside.

Tava et al. [11] illustrate the chemical and biological diversity in terms of phenolics content and antioxidant capacity of leaves and flowers extracts from a set of *Trifolium* species originating from contrasting growing environments. Variations in the distribution of total phenolics were found between lowland and mountain germplasm rising some considerations on the different adaptive strategies. Accordingly, differences in the scavenging capacity of clove extracts from lowland and mountain germplasm and/or plant part were observed. Based on these results, the authors also discuss the possible link between environmental factors, chemical composition, and content of phenolics in *Trifolium.*

Marine organisms are an important resource of peptides which due to their unique structure may have several physiological functions. Pang et al. [12] designed the synthesis of seven new tripeptide derivatives of the marine cyclopeptide xyloallenoide A to investigate their capacity to promote cellular proliferation in human endotelial cells and zebrafish embryos. With their study, the authors gain interesting Structural-Activity-Relationships. For example, it was shown that tripeptides containing L-Tyr or D-Pro fragments have a higher potency to promote the cellular proliferation of human endotelial cells.

The hypoglycemic effect and the mechanism of action of an ethanolic extract of *Sennae folium* on L6 rat skeletal muscle cells are described by Yang et al. [13]. The drug shows a strong effect in promoting glucose uptake, GLUT4 expression and translocation and promotes cytosolic Ca^{2+} levels. It is thus suggested that *Sennae folium* might have a role for the treatment of insulin resistance.

Hartmann et al. [14] describe the composition of sulfated metabolites from the siphonous green alga *Dasycladus vermicularis*, widely distributed throughout tropical to temperate regions. The phytochemical analysis led to the isolation of two sulfated phenolic acids and four sulfated coumarins including two novel compounds, 5,8′-di-(6(6′),7(7′)-tetrahydroxy-3-sulfoxy-3′-sulfoxycoumarin), named dasycladin A and 7-hydroxycoumarin-3,6-disulfate, named dasycladin B. In addition, for the first time, a validated HPLC method for the separation and quantification of sulfated coumarins is presented.

The work by Sulaiman et al. [15] aims to study the analgesic effect of cardamonin, isolated from *Boesenbergia rotunda*. Its antinociceptive activity was examined using chemical and thermal mice models of nociception. The authors show that cardamonin is able to produce significant analgesia in formalin-, capsaicin- and glutamate-induced paw licking tests. In addition, they demonstrated that the phytochemical induces a significant increase in the response latency time of animals subjected to hot-plate thermal stimuli. In conclusion, this study shows that cardamonin exerts significant peripheral and central antinociception in mice through the involvement of TRPV1, glutamate and opioid receptors.

Ho et al. [16] investigated the chemical profile of *Imperata cylindrica* and the growth inhibitory effects of each identified constituent on different cancer cell lines. They achieved the isolation of 2-methoxysterone, 11,16-dihydroxypregn-4-ene-3,20-dione, and tricin, which were found to inhibit the growth of some breast and colon cancer cell lines.

The study by Chang et al. [17] aimed to further characterize the cytotoxic constituents from *Dryopteris fragrans*, a valuable medicinal plant with anti-cancer activity. Isolation of six known compounds plus two new bioactive phenolics, namely dryofragone and dryofracoumarin B, was achieved by a cytotoxicity-guided tracking. The immunomodulatory capacity of these compounds has also been described and results showed that some of them may activate the LPS signaling pathway thus affecting the growth of tumor cells through immuno-regulation.

Lai et al. [18] review the activity of natural terpenes and their derivatives against pathogenic bacteria with particular attention to terpenes effective in the treatment of microbial resistance. They also discuss future prospects, such as new natural sources, drug delivery systems to be used in clinical trials, possible structural modification, either synthetically or via biotransformation, to increase the bioactivity, and the development of combination drugs with fewer side effects.

Marine organisms are a potential sustainable source of peptides that act as ACE inhibitors and are considered as therapeutic agent to combat hypertension. The review by Pujiastuti et al. [19] summarizes information on their distribution among marine organisms, their production, chemical characterization, and bioactivity.

The role of carotenoids to counteract oxidative stress and promote healthy aging is discussed by Tan and Norhalzan [20]. As many studies have shown an inverse relationship between carotenoids and age-related diseases by reducing oxidative stress, carotenoids are potential candidates to counteract age-associated pathologies. Besides a description of the chemical types of carotenoids and their natural sources, the authors review the underlying mechanisms of action to understand their role on human health.

The review by Scharenberg and Zidorn [21] illustrates the phytochemistry of the holoparasitic genus *Orobanche*. Both genuine metabolites produced by *Orobanche* species as well as natural products sequestered from their host plants are reviewed. In addition, an overview of the biological activity of extracts and pure compounds from different species of *Orobanche* is also given. Information was retrieved from SciFinder and ISI Web of Knowledge databases, taking into account reports until the end of 2017.

Overall, this special issue contributes to highlighting new biological activities for known plants and natural compounds. In addition, some of the studies have disclosed novel plant molecules with promising pharmacological applications.

Conflicts of Interest: The author declares no conflict of interest.

References

1. Schiavone, S.; Tucci, P.; Trabace, L.; Morgese, M. Early Celastrol Administration Prevents Ketamine-Induced Psychotic-Like Behavioral Dysfunctions, Oxidative Stress and IL-10 Reduction in The Cerebellum of Adult Mice. *Molecules* **2019**, *24*, 3993. [CrossRef] [PubMed]
2. Ikram, N.; Kashkooli, A.; Peramuna, A.; Krol, A.; Bouwmeester, H.; Simonsen, H. Insights into Heterologous Biosynthesis of Arteannuin B and Artemisinin in Physcomitrella patens. *Molecules* **2019**, *24*, 3822. [CrossRef] [PubMed]
3. Lucarini, E.; Pagnotta, E.; Micheli, L.; Parisio, C.; Testai, L.; Martelli, A.; Calderone, V.; Matteo, R.; Lazzeri, L.; Di Cesare Mannelli, L.; et al. *Eruca sativa* Meal against Diabetic Neuropathic Pain: An H2S-Mediated Effect of Glucoerucin. *Molecules* **2019**, *24*, 3006. [CrossRef] [PubMed]
4. Saesong, T.; Allard, P.; Ferreira Queiroz, E.; Marcourt, L.; Nuengchamnong, N.; Temkitthawon, P.; Khorana, N.; Wolfender, J.; Ingkaninan, K. Discovery of Lipid Peroxidation Inhibitors from Bacopa Species Prioritized through Multivariate Data Analysis and Multi-Informative Molecular Networking. *Molecules* **2019**, *24*, 2989. [CrossRef]
5. Francioso, A.; Franke, K.; Villani, C.; Mosca, L.; D'Erme, M.; Frischbutter, S.; Brandt, W.; Sanchez-Lamar, A.; Wessjohann, L. Insights into the Phytochemistry of the Cuban Endemic Medicinal Plant *Phyllanthus orbicularis*: Fideloside, a Novel Bioactive 8-C-glycosyl 2,3-Dihydroflavonol. *Molecules* **2019**, *24*, 2855. [CrossRef] [PubMed]
6. Tuan, H.; Minh, B.; Tran, P.; Lee, J.; Oanh, H.; Ngo, Q.; Nguyen, Y.; Lien, P.; Tran, M. The Effects of 2′,4′-Dihydroxy-6′-methoxy-3′,5′- dimethylchalcone from *Cleistocalyx operculatus* Buds on Human Pancreatic Cancer Cell Lines. *Molecules* **2019**, *24*, 2538. [CrossRef] [PubMed]
7. Avato, P.; Argentieri, M. Quality Assessment of Commercial Spagyric Tinctures of *Harpagophytum procumbens* and Their Antioxidant Properties. *Molecules* **2019**, *24*, 2251. [CrossRef]
8. Graziani, V.; Esposito, A.; Scognamiglio, M.; Chambery, A.; Russo, R.; Ciardiello, F.; Troiani, T.; Potenza, N.; Fiorentino, A.; D'Abrosca, B. Spectroscopic Characterization and Cytotoxicity Assessment towards Human Colon Cancer Cell Lines of Acylated Cycloartane Glycosides from *Astragalus boeticus* L. *Molecules* **2019**, *24*, 1725. [CrossRef]
9. Bocquet, L.; Sahpaz, S.; Bonneau, N.; Beaufay, C.; Mahieux, S.; Samaillie, J.; Roumy, V.; Jacquin, J.; Bordage, S.; Hennebelle, T.; et al. Phenolic Compounds from *Humulus lupulus* as Natural Antimicrobial Products: New Weapons in the Fight against Methicillin Resistant *Staphylococcus aureus*, *Leishmania mexicana* and *Trypanosoma brucei* Strains. *Molecules* **2019**, *24*, 1024. [CrossRef]
10. Singh, D.; Siew, Y.; Chong, T.; Yew, H.; Ho, S.; Lim, C.; Tan, W.; Neo, S.; Koh, H. Identification of Phytoconstituents in *Leea indica* (Burm. F.) Merr. Leaves by High Performance Liquid Chromatography Micro Time-of-Flight Mass Spectrometry. *Molecules* **2019**, *24*, 714. [CrossRef]
11. Tava, A.; Pecetti, L.; Lo Scalzo, R.; Stochmal, A.; Pecetti, L. Phenolic Content and Antioxidant Activity in *Trifolium* Germplasm from Different Environments. *Molecules* **2019**, *24*, 298. [CrossRef] [PubMed]
12. Zheng, Y.; Tong, Y.; Wang, X.; Zhou, J.; Pang, J. Studies on the Design and Synthesis of Marine Peptide Analogues and Their Ability to Promote Proliferation in HUVECs and Zebrafish. *Molecules* **2019**, *24*, 66. [CrossRef] [PubMed]

13. Zhao, P.; Ming, Q.; Qiu, J.; Tian, D.; Liu, J.; Shen, J.; Liu, Q.; Yang, X. Ethanolic Extract of *Folium Sennae* Mediates the Glucose Uptake of L6 Cells by GLUT4 and Ca2+. *Molecules* **2018**, *23*, 2934. [CrossRef] [PubMed]
14. Hartmann, A.; Ganzera, M.; Karsten, U.; Skhirtladze, A.; Stuppner, H. Phytochemical and Analytical Characterization of Novel Sulfated Coumarins in the Marine Green Macroalga *Dasycladus vermicularis* (Scopoli) Krasser. *Molecules* **2018**, *23*, 2735. [CrossRef]
15. Ping, C.; Tengku Mohamad, T.; Akhtar, M.; Perimal, E.; Akira, A.; Israf Ali, D.; Sulaiman, M. Antinociceptive Effects of Cardamonin in Mice: Possible Involvement of TRPV1, Glutamate, and Opioid Receptors. *Molecules* **2018**, *23*, 2237. [CrossRef]
16. Wang, Y.; Shen, J.; Chan, Y.; Ho, W. Identification and Growth Inhibitory Activity of the Chemical Constituents from *Imperata Cylindrica* Aerial Part Ethyl Acetate Extract. *Molecules* **2018**, *23*, 1807. [CrossRef]
17. Zhang, T.; Wang, L.; Duan, D.; Zhang, Y.; Huang, S.; Chang, Y. Cytotoxicity-Guided Isolation of Two New Phenolic Derivatives from *Dryopteris fragrans* (L.) Schott. *Molecules* **2018**, *23*, 1652. [CrossRef]
18. Mahizan, N.; Yang, S.; Moo, C.; Song, A.; Chong, C.; Chong, C.; Abushelaibi, A.; Lim, S.; Lai, K. Terpene Derivatives as a Potential Agent against Antimicrobial Resistance (AMR) Pathogens. *Molecules* **2019**, *24*, 2631. [CrossRef]
19. Pujiastuti, D.; Ghoyatul Amin, M.; Alamsjah, M.; Hsu, J. Marine Organisms as Potential Sources of Bioactive Peptides that Inhibit the Activity of Angiotensin I-Converting Enzyme: A Review. *Molecules* **2019**, *24*, 2541. [CrossRef]
20. Tan, B.; Norhaizan, M. Carotenoids: How Effective Are They to Prevent Age-Related Diseases? *Molecules* **2019**, *24*, 1801. [CrossRef]
21. Scharenberg, F.; Zidorn, C. Genuine and Sequestered Natural Products from the Genus *Orobanche* (Orobanchaceae, Lamiales). *Molecules* **2018**, *23*, 2821. [CrossRef] [PubMed]

molecules

MDPI

Article

Early Celastrol Administration Prevents Ketamine-Induced Psychotic-Like Behavioral Dysfunctions, Oxidative Stress and IL-10 Reduction in The Cerebellum of Adult Mice

Stefania Schiavone, Paolo Tucci, Luigia Trabace * and Maria Grazia Morgese

Department of Clinical and Experimental Medicine, University of Foggia, Viale Pinto, 1 71122 Foggia, Italy; stefania.schiavone@unifg.it (S.S.); paolo.tucci@unifg.it (P.T.); mariagrazia.morgese@unifg.it (M.G.M.)

* Correspondence: luigia.trabace@unifg.it; Tel.: +39-0881-588056

Academic Editor: Pinarosa Avato

Received: 19 July 2019; Accepted: 25 October 2019; Published: 5 November 2019

Abstract: Administration of subanesthetic doses of ketamine during brain maturation represents a tool to mimic an early insult to the central nervous system (CNS). The cerebellum is a key player in psychosis pathogenesis, to which oxidative stress also contributes. Here, we investigated the impact of early celastrol administration on behavioral dysfunctions in adult mice that had received ketamine (30 mg/kg i.p.) at postnatal days (PNDs) 7, 9, and 11. Cerebellar levels of 8-hydroxydeoxyguanosine (8-OHdG), NADPH oxidase (NOX) 1 and NOX2, as well as of the calcium-binding protein parvalbumin (PV), were also assessed. Furthermore, celastrol effects on ketamine-induced alterations of proinflammatory (TNF-α, IL-6 and IL-1β) and anti-inflammatory (IL-10) cytokines in this brain region were evaluated. Early celastrol administration prevented ketamine-induced discrimination index decrease at adulthood. The same was found for locomotor activity elevations and increased close following and allogrooming, whereas no beneficial effects on sniffing impairment were detected. Ketamine increased 8-OHdG in the cerebellum of adult mice, which was also prevented by early celastrol injection. Cerebellar NOX1 levels were enhanced at adulthood following postnatal ketamine exposure. Celastrol *per se* induced NOX1 decrease in the cerebellum. This effect was more significant in animals that were early administered with ketamine. NOX2 levels did not change. Ketamine administration did not affect PV amount in the cerebellum. TNF-α levels were enhanced in ketamine-treated animals; however, this was not prevented by early celastrol administration. While no changes were observed for IL-6 and IL-1β levels, ketamine determined a reduction of cerebellar IL-10 expression, which was prevented by early celastrol treatment. Our results suggest that NOX inhibition during brain maturation prevents the development of psychotic-like behavioral dysfunctions, as well as the increased cerebellar oxidative stress and the reduction of IL-10 in the same brain region following ketamine exposure in postnatal life. This opens novel neuroprotective opportunities against early detrimental insults occurring during brain development.

Keywords: ketamine; psychosis; cerebellum; celastrol; oxidative stress; NADPH oxidases

1. Introduction

The recreational use of the N-methyl-D-aspartate receptor (NMDA-R) antagonist ketamine, at subanesthetic doses, has been widely reported to cause psychedelic effects in humans [1]. Moreover, the development of a psychotic-like state has also been described following prolonged assumption of this psychoactive compound [2,3]. Despite an increasing scientific interest in ketamine's psychotogenic effects, the mechanisms underlying the pathological contribution of this NMDA-R antagonist in psychosis development need to be further elucidated. In this context, the administration of subanesthetic doses of ketamine to rodents represents a reliable tool to mimic neuropathological alterations reminiscent of those observed in psychotic patients, in terms of biomolecular alterations, neurochemical dysfunctions and behavioral impairment [4]. Indeed, in rodents, increased locomotor activity and decreased discrimination abilities have been respectively associated with the agitation and disorganized behavior, as well as with the cognitive impairment observed in subjects suffering from psychosis [5–7]. Moreover, abnormalities in social behavior, such as withdrawal and decreased interactions, have been related to negative symptoms observed in psychotic patients [8].

Numerous lines of evidence have considered the psychotic disease to be the final result of a series of events occurring during the early stages of brain development [9]. Hence, animal models obtained by administering ketamine during a crucial period of central nervous system (CNS) maturation, such as the second postnatal week of life [10], might provide information on the possible pathogenetic contribution of an early insult to an enduring psychotic state in adulthood.

Together with the widely known role of the prefrontal cortex in the pathogenesis of psychosis, in recent years, an emerging interest has been directed towards a possible implication of cerebellum in the development of this mental disorder [11,12]. Indeed, preclinical, clinical, neuroanatomical and neuroimaging reports began to highlight its important role not only in motor function regulation but also in the modulation of emotional and cognitive processes [13–16]. Structural cerebellar abnormalities, such as deficits in its gray matter volume, have also been described in antipsychotic-naive schizophrenic patients [17]. Moreover, vascular insults occurring in this brain region resulted in the onset of unremitting psychosis [18].

Administration of subanesthetic doses of ketamine in both early life stages and adult life has been widely reported to reduce the amount of the calcium-binding protein parvalbumin (PV) in different brain regions, such as prefrontal cortex and hippocampus [19–22]. However, poor evidence is available on the effects of early ketamine administration on cerebellar amount of PV, which has been shown to play a key role in regulating several physiological processes in this brain region [23], such as cell firing, synaptic transmission, as well as the resistance to neuronal degeneration following a variety of acute or chronic insults [24,25].

Oxidative stress, defined as an imbalance between reactive oxygen species (ROS) production and the antioxidant defenses of the cells, has been described as a key player in the pathogenesis of several CNS diseases, going from neurodegenerative to neuropsychiatric disorders [26], including psychosis [27]. The family of the Nicotinamide Adenine Dinucleotide Phosphate (NADPH) oxidase (NOX) enzymes represents one of the major ROS sources in the CNS, where it is involved in several physiological functions [28]. In particular, enhanced levels of NOX1 enzyme have been reported in neuropsychiatric diseases characterized by psychotic symptoms [29,30], and increased NOX2 expression was observed in specific brain regions, such as the prefrontal cortex and nucleus accumbens of environmental [19,31,32] and pharmacologic rodent models of psychosis, including the one obtained by ketamine administration in adult mice [33–35]. NOX1 and NOX2 mRNA and proteins have been detected in rodent cerebellum starting from postnatal day (PND) 4, meaning that the developing cerebellum is able to actively produce ROS. Moreover, administration of antioxidant/NOX inhibitor compounds, such as apocynin, has been demonstrated to decrease ROS levels in Purkinje cells [36]. However, so far, little is known about possible changes of NOX1 and NOX2 enzymes in this brain area following an early CNS insult leading to a later psychotic disease. Together with oxidative stress, increased inflammatory states and/or reduced anti-inflammatory pathways have been reported following ketamine administration [37–39]. Furthermore, the developing CNS has been described as being particularly vulnerable to enhanced peripheral and central inflammation following an external insult [40].

Together with its anti-inflammatory actions [41], celastrol, extracted from the medicinal plant *Tripterygium wilfordii*, has been described to have significant benefits in preventing neuropathological alterations observed in animal models of neurodegenerative diseases [42–44], through numerous mechanisms, including ROS level decrease [45]. In particular, celastrol has been characterized as an effective NOX enzyme inhibitor, with an increased potency against NOX1 and NOX2, acting via the suppression of the association between the enzymatic subunits, located in the cytosol, and the membrane flavocytochrome [46]. Importantly, no available reports investigate the effects of celastrol administration in animal models of psychosis. Moreover, no evidence has been previously published on the possible impact of celastrol administration during a crucial period of brain maturation, or on the development of a psychotic state following an early CNS insult.

A major challenge in the field of oxidative stress in the CNS is represented by the possibility to directly measure ROS production and release in this body district. Therefore, different indirect approaches have been used to quantify free radical amount in the CNS, including the analysis of 8-hydroxydeoxyguanosine (8-OHdG), a reliable marker of DNA oxidation levels [47,48].

Here, we investigated the impact of early celastrol administration on behavioral dysfunctions observed in adult mice exposed to subanesthetic doses of ketamine at PNDs 7, 9 and 11. The effects of this compound on ketamine-induced oxidative stress, as well as on NADPH oxidase expression alterations and PV levels in the cerebellum, were also assessed. Moreover, we also evaluated early celastrol effects on possible ketamine-induced changes of proinflammatory (Tumor Necrosis Factor alpha (TNF-α), interleukin-6 (IL-6) and interleukin-1 beta (IL-1β)), as well as anti-inflammatory [interleukin-10 (IL-10)] cytokines in the same brain region.

2. Results

2.1. *Early Celastrol Administration Prevented Cognitive Dysfunctions in Adult Mice Exposed to Ketamine in Postnatal Life*

To evaluate the possible effects of early celastrol administration on cognitive dysfunctions induced by ketamine exposure in postnatal life, we performed the Novel Object Recognition (NOR) test in 10 weeks mice. While no differences were detected in the discrimination index among saline, dimethyl sulfoxide (DMSO) and celastrol-treated mice, a significant decrease of this parameter was observed in adult mice who had received ketamine in postnatal life. Early celastrol administration to ketamine-treated mice was able to prevent this cognitive dysfunction (Figure 1, One Way Analysis of variance-ANOVA, followed by Tukey's post hoc test F = 7.387, $p < 0.01$ ketamine vs. saline; $p < 0.05$ ketamine vs. DMSO and vs. ketamine + celastrol; $p < 0.001$ ketamine vs. celastrol; $p > 0.05$ saline vs. DMSO, celastrol and ketamine + celastrol; $p > 0.05$ DMSO vs. celastrol and ketamine + celastrol; $p > 0.05$ celastrol vs. ketamine + celastrol).

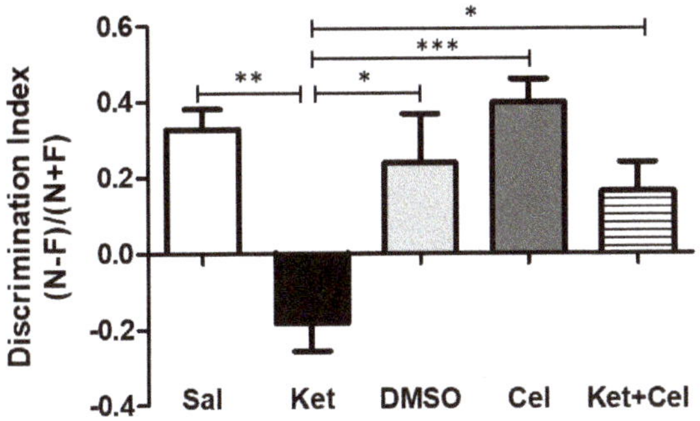

Figure 1. Celastrol administration in postnatal life prevented ketamine-induced cognitive dysfunctions, evaluated at adulthood. Discrimination index (N − F)/(N + F) (*N* = time spent in exploration of the novel object during the T2; F = time spent in exploration of the familiar object in the T2) in adult mice receiving saline (Sal, $n = 6$) or ketamine (Ket, $n = 13$) or a 50% DMSO in phosphate-buffered saline (PBS) (DMSO, $n = 7$) or celastrol (Cel, $n = 6$) or ketamine + celastrol (Ket + Cel, $n = 14$) at PNDs 7, 9 and 11. One Way ANOVA, followed by Tukey's post hoc test F = 7.387, *** $p < 0.001$; ** $p < 0.01$; * $p < 0.05$.

2.2. Early Celastrol Administration Prevented Locomotor Dysfunctions in Adult Mice Exposed to Ketamine in Postnatal Life

To assess the possible impact of early celastrol administration on ketamine-induced locomotor alterations, we performed the Open Field (OF) test in adult mice. Ketamine administration in postnatal life significantly enhanced locomotor activity at 10 weeks of age, with respect to the saline, DMSO and celastrol-treated groups, within which no differences were observed. Celastrol co-administered with ketamine at PNDs 7, 9 and 11 was able to prevent the observed hyperlocomotion (Figure 2, One Way ANOVA, followed by Tukey's post hoc test, F = 10.34, $p < 0.001$ ketamine vs. saline, DMSO, celastrol and ketamine + celastrol; $p > 0.05$ saline vs. DMSO, celastrol and ketamine + celastrol; $p > 0.05$ DMSO vs. celastrol and ketamine + celastrol; $p > 0.05$ celastrol vs. ketamine + celastrol).

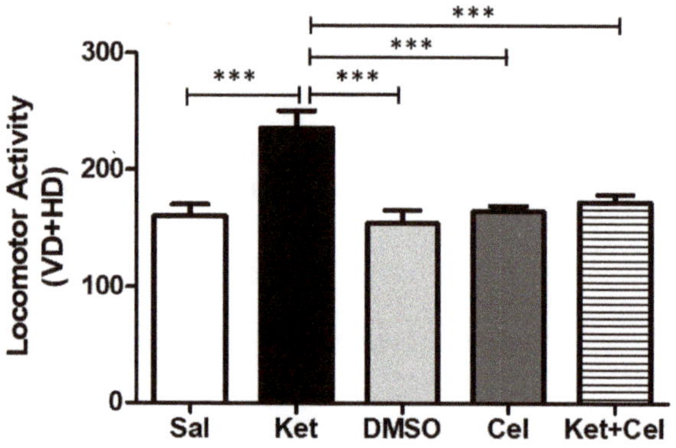

Figure 2. Celastrol administration in postnatal life prevented ketamine-induced increased in locomotor activity in later adulthood. Locomotor activity (VD = vertical displacements; HD = horizontal displacements) in adult mice receiving saline (Sal, $n = 7$) or ketamine (Ket, $n = 13$) or a 50% DMSO in PBS (DMSO, $n = 7$) or celastrol (Cel, $n = 8$) or ketamine + celastrol (Ket + Cel, $n = 14$) at PNDs 7, 9 and 11. One Way ANOVA, followed by Tukey's post hoc test F = 10.34, *** $p < 0.001$.

2.3. Early Celastrol Administration Prevented Social Behavior Dysfunctions in Adult Mice Exposed to Ketamine in Postnatal Life

To investigate the effects of early celastrol administration on ketamine-induced social behavior impairments, we performed the Social Interaction (SI) test in adult mice. Animals receiving ketamine at PNDs 7, 9 and 11 showed a decrease in the sniffing time with respect to saline, DMSO- and celastrol-treated mice. A significant difference in this parameter was also observed in ketamine-treated mice who had also received celastrol in postnatal life compared to the saline group (Figure 3A, One Way ANOVA, followed by Tukey's post hoc test, F = 6.856, $p < 0.01$ ketamine vs. saline; $p < 0.05$ ketamine vs. DMSO and celastrol; $p < 0.05$ ketamine + celastrol vs. saline; $p > 0.05$ saline vs. DMSO and celastrol; $p > 0.05$ DMSO vs. celastrol; $p > 0.05$ ketamine vs. ketamine + celastrol). Postnatal ketamine exposure caused a significant increase in the close following time, which was prevented by the concomitant treatment with celastrol (Figure 3B, One Way ANOVA, followed by Tukey's post hoc test, F = 13.10, $p < 0.05$ ketamine vs. saline; $p < 0.001$ ketamine vs. DMSO, celastrol and ketamine + celastrol; $p > 0.05$ saline vs. DMSO, celastrol and ketamine + celastrol; $p > 0.05$ DMSO vs. celastrol and ketamine + celastrol; $p > 0.05$ celastrol vs. ketamine + celastrol). The same pattern was observed for the celastrol effects on ketamine-induced elevation of time spent in allogroming (Figure 3C, One Way ANOVA, followed by Tukey's post hoc test, F = 12.50, $p < 0.001$ ketamine vs. saline and DMSO; $p < 0.01$ ketamine vs. celastrol and ketamine + celastrol; $p > 0.05$ saline vs. DMSO, celastrol and ketamine + celastrol; $p > 0.05$ DMSO vs. celastrol and ketamine + celastrol; $p > 0.05$ celastrol vs. ketamine + celastrol).

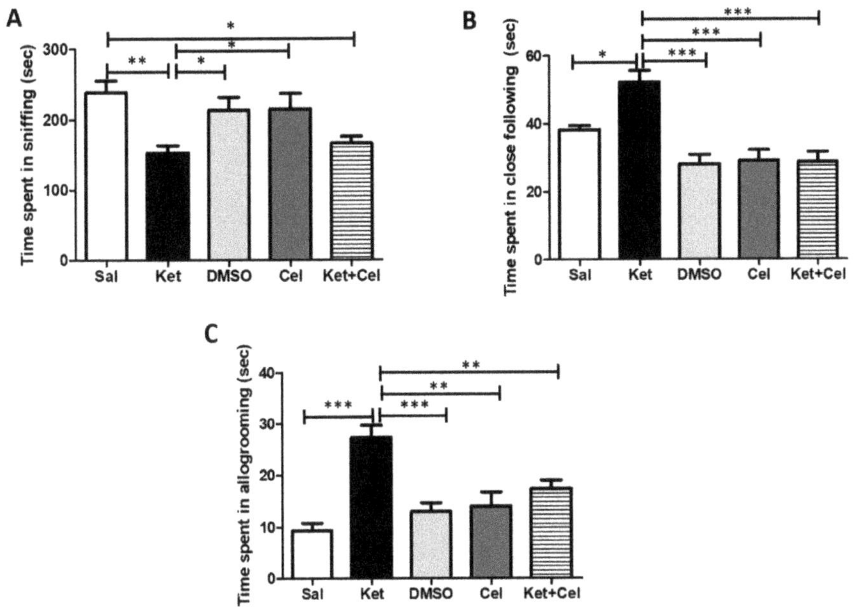

Figure 3. Celastrol administration in postnatal life prevented ketamine-induced social behavior dysfunctions in later adulthood. (**A**). Time spent in sniffing (seconds, sec) in adult mice receiving saline (Sal, $n = 4$) or ketamine (Ket, $n = 8$) or a 50% DMSO in PBS (DMSO, $n = 4$) or celastrol (Cel, $n = 4$) or ketamine + celastrol (Ket + Cel, $n = 7$) at PNDs 7, 9 and 11. One Way ANOVA, followed by Tukey's post hoc test F = 6.856, ** $p < 0.01$; * $p < 0.05$. (**B**). Time spent in close following (seconds, sec) in adult mice receiving saline (Sal, $n = 4$) or ketamine (Ket, $n = 7$) or a 50% DMSO in PBS (DMSO, $n = 4$) or celastrol (Cel, $n = 4$) or ketamine + celastrol (Ket + Cel, $n = 7$) at PNDs 7, 9 and 11. One Way ANOVA, followed by Tukey's post hoc test F = 13.10, *** $p < 0.001$; * $p < 0.05$. (**C**). Time spent in allogroming (seconds, sec) in adult mice receiving saline (Sal, $n = 5$) or ketamine (Ket, $n = 6$) or a 50% DMSO in PBS (DMSO, $n = 4$) or celastrol (Cel, $n = 4$) or ketamine + celastrol (Ket + Cel, $n = 6$) at PNDs 7, 9 and 11. One Way ANOVA, followed by Tukey's post hoc test F = 12.50, *** $p < 0.001$; ** $p < 0.01$.

2.4. Early Celastrol Administration Prevented Oxidative Stress Increase in the Cerebellum of Adult Mice Exposed to Ketamine in Postnatal Life

To assess the effects of early celastrol administration on ketamine-induced oxidative stress in the cerebellum of adult mice, we quantified 8-OHdG levels in this brain region. Mice receiving ketamine at PNDs 7, 9 and 11 showed a significant elevation of this biomarker of oxidative stress with respect to saline-treated animals whose 8-OHdG amount was comparable to the one of the DMSO and celastrol-treated animals. Early celastrol administration was able to prevent ketamine-induced enhancement of this biomarker (Figure 4, One Way ANOVA, followed by Tukey's post hoc test, F = 6.361, $p < 0.05$ ketamine vs. saline; $p < 0.01$ ketamine vs. ketamine + celastrol; $p > 0.05$ saline vs. DMSO, celastrol and ketamine + celastrol; $p > 0.05$ DMSO vs. celastrol and ketamine + celastrol; $p > 0.05$ celastrol vs. ketamine + celastrol).

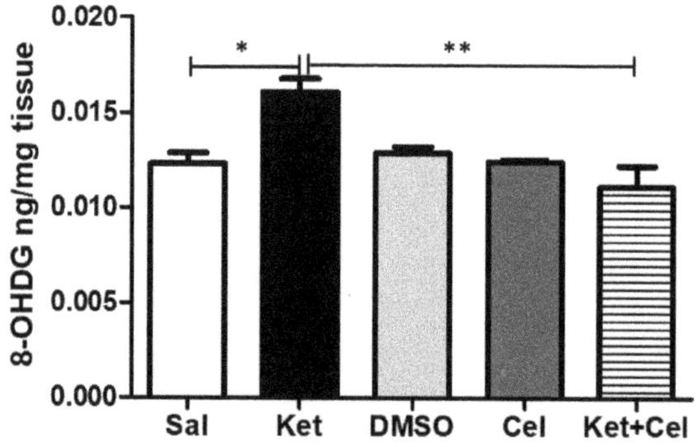

Figure 4. Celastrol administration in postnatal life prevented ketamine-induced oxidative stress in the cerebellum in later adulthood. 8-OHdG levels (ng/mg tissue) in the cerebellum of adult mice receiving saline (Sal, $n = 3$) or ketamine (Ket, $n = 5$) or a 50% DMSO in PBS (DMSO, $n = 3$) or celastrol (Cel, $n = 3$) or ketamine + celastrol (Ket + Cel, $n = 5$) at PNDs 7, 9 and 11. One Way ANOVA, followed by Tukey's post hoc test F = 6.361 * $p < 0.05$; ** $p < 0.01$.

2.5. *Early Celastrol Administration Decreased NOX1 Levels in the Cerebellum of Adult Mice Per Se and Following Ketamine Exposure*

To evaluate the effects of early celastrol administration on ketamine-induced NADPH oxidase alterations in the cerebellum, we measured NOX1 and NOX2 levels in this area. NOX1 amount was significantly increased by ketamine administration in postnatal life. Celastrol, injected as single treatment at the same time point, reduced NOX1 levels compared to both saline or ketamine-treated mice. The amount of this NADPH oxidase isoform was further reduced when celastrol was administered early to ketamine-treated animals (Figure 5, One Way ANOVA, followed by Tukey's post hoc test F = 50.30, $p < 0.05$ ketamine vs. saline and ketamine + celastrol vs. celastrol; $p < 0.01$ celastrol vs. saline; $p < 0.001$ ketamine + celastrol vs. saline and vs. DMSO and ketamine vs. DMSO, celastrol and ketamine + celastrol; $p > 0.05$ saline vs. DMSO).

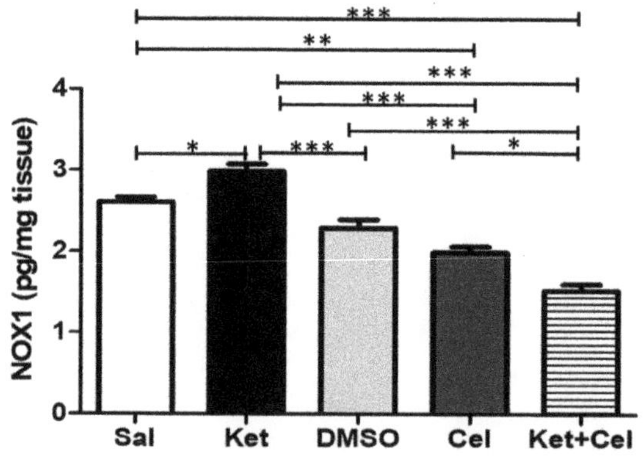

Figure 5. Celastrol administration in postnatal life decreased NOX1 levels in the cerebellum of adult mice. NOX1 levels (pg/mg tissue) in the cerebellum of adult mice receiving saline (Sal, $n = 3$) or ketamine (Ket, $n = 5$) or a 50% DMSO in PBS (DMSO, $n = 3$) or celastrol (Cel, $n = 3$) or ketamine + celastrol (Ket + Cel, $n = 5$) at PNDs 7, 9 and 11. One Way ANOVA, followed by Tukey's post hoc test F = 50.30, * $p < 0.05$; ** $p < 0.01$; *** $p < 0.001$.

Ketamine administration at PNDs 7, 9 and 11 did not significantly alter NOX2 amount in the cerebellum of adult mice, and no differences in the levels of this NADPH oxidase isoform were detected among all the other experimental groups (Figure 6, One Way ANOVA, followed by Tukey's post hoc test F = 1.158, $p > 0.05$ for all comparisons).

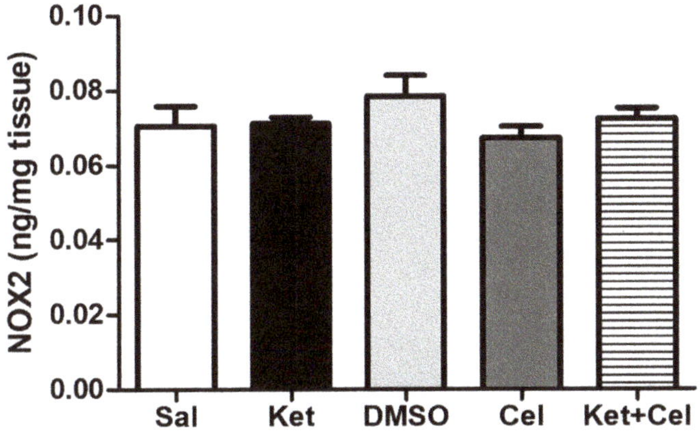

Figure 6. NOX2 levels were not altered in the cerebellum of adult mice exposed to ketamine in postnatal life. NOX2 levels (ng/mg tissue) in the cerebellum of adult mice receiving saline (Sal, $n = 3$) or ketamine (Ket, $n = 5$) or a 50% DMSO in PBS (DMSO, $n = 3$) or celastrol (Cel, $n = 3$) or ketamine + celastrol (Ket + Cel, $n = 5$) at PNDs 7, 9 and 11. One Way ANOVA, followed by Tukey's post hoc test F = 1.158 $p > 0.05$ for all comparisons.

The same was observed for cerebellar PV levels (Figure 7, One Way ANOVA, followed by Tukey's post hoc test, F = 2.632, $p > 0.05$ for all comparisons).

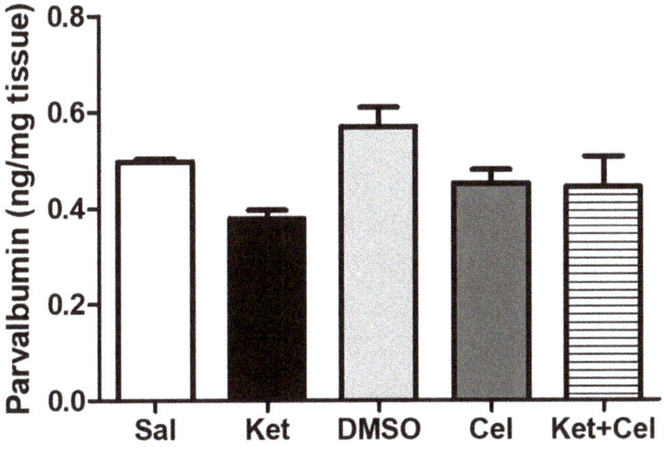

Figure 7. PV levels were not altered in the cerebellum of adult mice exposed to ketamine in postnatal life. PV levels (ng/mg tissue) in the cerebellum of adult mice receiving saline (Sal, $n = 3$) or ketamine (Ket, $n = 5$) or a 50% DMSO in PBS (DMSO, $n = 3$) or celastrol (Cel, $n = 3$) or ketamine + celastrol (Ket + Cel, $n = 5$) at PNDs 7, 9 and 11. One Way ANOVA, followed by Tukey's post hoc test F = 2.632, $p > 0.05$ for all comparisons.

2.6. Early Celastrol Administration Did not Prevent TNF-α Increase in the Cerebellum of Adult Mice Exposed to Ketamine in Postnatal Life

To investigate the effects of early celastrol administration on ketamine-induced inflammation in the cerebellum, we measured levels of TNF-α, IL-6 and IL-1β in this brain area. Ketamine administration in postnatal life determined an enhancement of cerebellar TNF-α in later adulthood compared to controls which showed comparable TNF-α amount with respect to the DMSO and celastrol-treated groups. Increased TNF-α were also detectable in adult mice receiving both ketamine and celastrol at PNDs 7, 9 and 11 (Figure 8A, One Way ANOVA, followed by Tukey's post hoc test $F = 7.382$, $p < 0.05$ ketamine vs. saline, saline vs. ketamine + celastrol and celastrol vs. ketamine + celastrol), whereas no significant alterations in the amount of IL-6 (Figure 8B, One Way ANOVA, followed by Tukey's post hoc test $F = 1.444$ $p > 0.05$ for all comparisons) and IL-1β (Figure 8C, One Way ANOVA, followed by Tukey's post hoc test $F = 2.103$ $p > 0.05$ for all comparisons) in the same brain region were found.

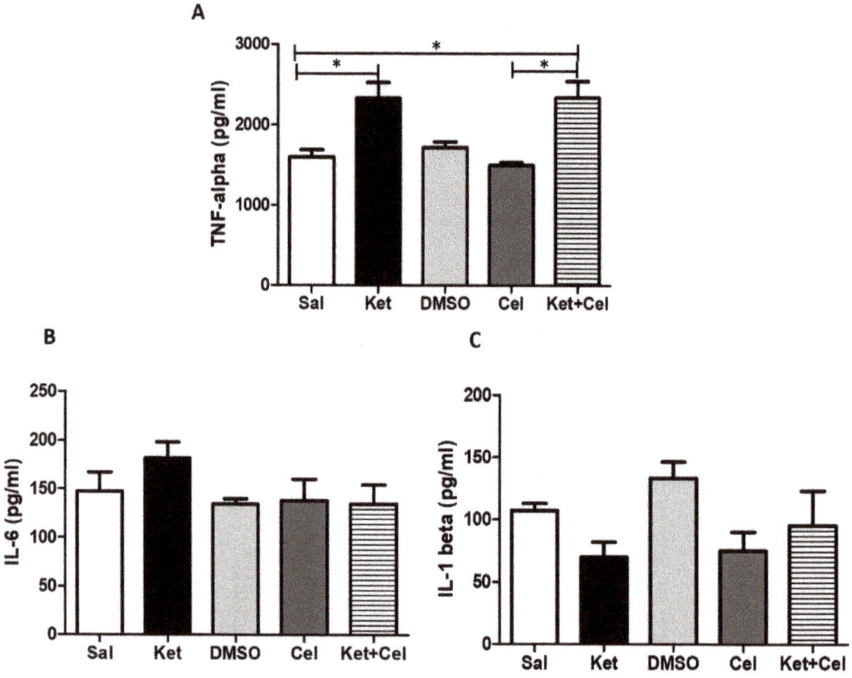

Figure 8. Celastrol administration in postnatal life did not prevent ketamine-induced TNF-α increase in the cerebellum in later adulthood. (**A**). TNF-α levels (pg/mg tissue) in the cerebellum of adult mice receiving saline (Sal, $n = 3$) or ketamine (Ket, $n = 5$) or a 50% DMSO in PBS (DMSO, $n = 3$) or celastrol (Cel, $n = 3$) or ketamine + celastrol (Ket + Cel, $n = 5$) at PNDs 7, 9 and 11. One Way ANOVA, followed by Tukey's post hoc test $F = 7.382$, * $p < 0.05$. (**B**). IL-6 levels (pg/mg tissue) in the cerebellum of adult mice receiving saline (Sal, $n = 3$) or ketamine (Ket, $n = 5$) or a 50% DMSO in PBS (DMSO, $n = 3$) or celastrol (Cel, $n = 3$) or ketamine + celastrol (Ket + Cel, $n = 5$) at PNDs 7, 9 and 11. One Way ANOVA, followed by Tukey's post hoc test $F = 1.444$, $p > 0.05$. (**C**). IL-1β levels (pg/mg tissue) in the cerebellum of adult mice receiving saline (Sal, $n = 3$) or ketamine (Ket, $n = 5$) or a 50% DMSO in PBS (DMSO, $n = 3$) or celastrol (Cel, $n = 3$) or ketamine + celastrol (Ket + Cel, $n = 5$) at PNDs 7, 9 and 11. One Way ANOVA, followed by Tukey's post hoc test $F = 2.103$ $p > 0.05$.

2.7. Early Celastrol Administration Prevented IL-10 Decrease in the Cerebellum of Adult Mice Exposed to Ketamine in Postnatal Life

To assess the effects of early celastrol administration on ketamine-induced decrease of anti-inflammatory cytokines in the cerebellum, we quantified IL-10 levels in this brain region. Mice administered with ketamine at PNDs 7, 9 and 11 showed reduced IL-10 amounts in later adulthood compared to saline-treated animals, whose levels of this cytokine were comparable to the ones detected in mice receiving DMSO or celastrol. Early celastrol administration in ketamine-treated animals was able to prevent IL-10 reduction in the cerebellum (Figure 9, One Way ANOVA, followed by Tukey's post hoc test F = 15.19, $p < 0.001$ ketamine vs. saline, ketamine vs. celastrol and ketamine vs. ketamine + celastrol; $p < 0.01$ ketamine vs. DMSO).

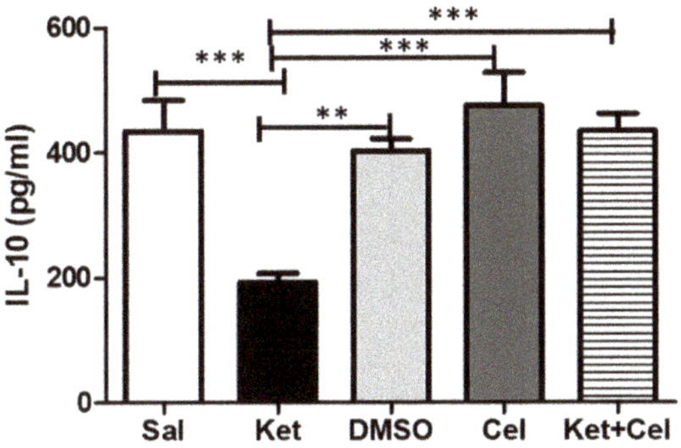

Figure 9. Celastrol administration in postnatal life prevented ketamine-induced IL-10 decrease in the cerebellum in later adulthood. IL-10 levels (pg/mL) in the cerebellum of adult mice receiving saline (Sal, $n = 3$) or ketamine (Ket, $n = 5$) or a 50% DMSO in PBS (DMSO, $n = 3$) or celastrol (Cel, $n = 3$) or ketamine + celastrol (Ket + Cel, $n = 5$) at PNDs 7, 9 and 11. One Way ANOVA, followed by Tukey's post hoc test F = 15.19, *** $p < 0.001$, ** $p < 0.01$.

3. Discussion

In this work, we demonstrated that early celastrol administration prevented discrimination ability dysfunctions, locomotor activity alterations and social behavior impairment in adult mice that had received ketamine at PNDs 7, 9 and 11. Previously published in vivo studies investigating possible beneficial effects of celastrol on CNS disorders have mainly regarded neurodegenerative disorders, including Alzheimer's disease [43–45], Parkinson's diseases [49–51], amyotrophic lateral sclerosis [42,52] and multiple sclerosis [53,54], epilepsy [55,56], cerebral ischemia and ischemic stroke [57–59] as well as traumatic brain injury [60,61]. One in vitro report indirectly investigated the impact of celastrol on the expression of specific genes, such as Fragile X Mental Retardation 1 (FMR1), linked to different psychiatric diseases, including schizophrenia [62]. Therefore, a novelty of our study with respect to the existing literature in the field is related to the evaluation of the effects of celastrol in psychotic disease by using a mouse model of the disorder. Importantly, this was obtained by negatively impacting the process of brain maturation with an early detrimental insult, represented by ketamine administration. Indeed, it has been reported that the developing brain is more vulnerable to the neurotoxicity induced by this psychoactive compound compared to the mature brain, in terms of enhanced neuronal cell death, neurogenesis alterations, disruptions of γ-aminobutyric acid (GABA)ergic interneuron development, altered NMDA-R expression, impaired synaptogenesis and increased oxidative stress production [63]. These disturbances during a critical period of brain maturation, i.e., the first 2–3 weeks of life in rodents, when brain growth spurt occurs, have been reported to trigger brain dysfunctions later in life, resulting finally in psychotic-like neuropathological and behavioral alterations [64]. Thus, our observations suggest that early administration of celastrol concomitantly to a brain insult might block the detrimental effects of ketamine with respect to the development of CNS and stop the progression of cerebral damage.

Decreased discrimination ability in rodents has been considered a behavioral feature mimicking the cognitive dysfunctions observed in psychotic patients [6]. Our findings regarding the preventive effects of early celastrol administration on ketamine-induced decrease in cognitive functions are in line with previous observations reporting a beneficial impact of this compound on learning and memory dysfunctions induced by metabolic alterations [65] or by neurodegenerative processes, induced by aggregation of specific proteins [45,66]. However, these studies were mainly focused on the behavioral effects of celastrol administration in adult life or even later, when the CNS insults leading to brain damage might have already been consolidated.

Elevations in locomotor activity in rodents are known to mimic the psychomotor agitation observed in subjects suffering from psychosis [5]. In our experimental conditions, early celastrol-treated mice, also exposed to ketamine in postnatal life, did not show an increase in locomotor activity with respect to the other experimental groups. Accordingly, the beneficial effects of celastrol on locomotor activity dysfunctions have been previously described in animal models of epilepsy, where motor function alterations were rapidly reduced by celastrol administration [67].

In this work, we also showed that ketamine administration at PNDs 7,9 and 11 induced dysfunctions in social behavior at adulthood. In particular, we reported decreased sniffing time in ketamine-treated mice with respect to controls. Together with its relation to social hierarchy in rodents, the sniffing behavior has been shown to be related to the establishment of normal social interactions [68]. Importantly, decreased social interactions in rodents have been paralleled to a negative symptom observed in psychotic patients, i.e., the social withdrawal [5]. Our findings are in line with previous work reporting a decreased sniffing time in rats treated with another NMDA-R antagonist, phencyclidine [69], together with a positive effects of antipsychotic treatment in reverting this social deficit [70]. Moreover, decreased duration of sniffing was observed in animal models of neuropsychiatric diseases also characterized by psychotic symptoms, such as autism [71]. In our experimental conditions, mice receiving ketamine in postnatal life also showed increased time spent in close-following and allogrooming. Close following is generally considered a mutual investigation behavior, while allogroming has been described as a standard behavior of altruism and reciprocal cooperation [72]. However, despite their general classification as non-aggressive behaviors, elevations in these social outcomes have been associated with subordination of the partner and abnormal dominance establishment [73], which could be seen as aggressive-like behaviors [74]. Accordingly, Becker et al. described a decrease in non-aggressive behavior in ketamine-treated rats [72]. Our findings might appear to be in contradiction with a previous work reporting that ketamine ameliorates aggressive-like behavior induced by neonatal maternal separation in mice [75]. However, in this study, lower doses of ketamine (15 mg/kg) were used and the administration time (post-natal days 35–49) was not comparable to those followed in our research procedure. In our experimental conditions, celastrol did not show beneficial effects on the ketamine-induced social withdrawal at adulthood but was able to prevent the observed increase in aggressive-like behavior. This is in line with previous findings reporting beneficial effects of antioxidant therapies in attenuating aggressive behavior induced by different stimuli [76] and describing aggressivity enhancement in mice with a genetic reduction of antioxidant functions [77]. In apparent contrast with our findings, Phensy and co-workers demonstrated that antioxidant treatment with N-acetyl cysteine was able to prevent social interaction dysfunctions induced by ketamine administration during postnatal life. However, in this work, administration of this antioxidant compound was performed throughout the entire period of brain development. Thus, we cannot exclude that prolonged administration of celastrol during brain maturation might also have an impact on social withdrawal observed at adulthood.

In our study, we found that early celastrol administration prevented elevations in cerebellar oxidative stress observed in mice treated with ketamine in postnatal life. The cerebellum has been gaining increasing importance in the pathogenic mechanisms underlying the development of psychosis [11,78–80] and of other psychiatric diseases, clinically characterized by psychotic symptoms [81]. In addition to the ketamine-induced detrimental effects on the prefrontal cortex [22,82,83], the negative impact of this NMDA-R antagonist also on the developing cerebellum has been shown in non-human primates [84]. In good agreement with our observations, previous works have reported increased direct and indirect biomarkers of oxidative stress in the cerebellum of animal models of neuropsychiatric disorders [85,86]. In particular, Filiou and co-workers described cerebellar oxidative stress-induced structural alterations in the G72/G30 transgenic schizophrenia mouse model [87]. Moreover, antipsychotic medication has been demonstrated to inhibit the activity of specific enzymes, which can also produce free radicals in rodent cerebellum [88,89]. The increased oxidative stress observed in this brain region may also be considered a possible trigger of the cerebello-thalamo-cortical network dysfunctions which have been described as predictors of disease progression in individuals at ultra-high risk for psychosis [12,90]. In support of this concept, interesting lines of evidence describe a positive effects of antioxidant treatments in preventing cerebellar dysfunctions observed in neuropsychiatric diseases also characterized by psychotic symptoms, such as autism spectrum disorder [91].

An important finding of our study consists in the observed increased cerebellar NOX1 levels in adult mice who had received ketamine in postnatal life, whereas NOX2 amount was not affected by this early detrimental insult. A physiological role of the NADPH oxidase enzymatic family in different stages of cerebellum development has been previously described [36]. Moreover, Olguín-Albuerne and Morán reported a key role of NADPH oxidase-derived ROS in controlling the development of cerebellar granule neurons during brain maturation [92]. However, in vitro and in vivo evidence highlighted a crucial role of NOX enzymes in the development of structural and functional alterations in cerebellum following different insults [93–95]. Increased NOX1 enzyme expression and activity has been implicated not only in the pathogenesis of neurodegenerative disorders [96–98], but also in neurotoxic processes mediated by sustained microglia activation [99]. Thus, the observed NOX1 increase following postnatal ketamine administration should also be considered in the context of the effects that this NMDA-R antagonist has on the inflammatory states of the brain. Supporting this perspective, it has been reported that exposure to subanesthetic doses of ketamine is able to activate neuroinflammatory pathways [83] and to induce microglia activation in rodent brains [100]. In our experimental conditions, early celastrol administration was able per se to decrease NOX1 levels in the cerebellum of adult mice which did not receive ketamine in postnatal life. Although speculative, a possible explanation for this result could be related to possible celastrol effects on other ketamine-independent events occurring in mature brain and implicating a role of the NADPH oxidase system, such as protein aggregation [101] or specific heat shock proteins expression and/or activation [102,103]. Hence, in the presence of a neurodetrimental insult, i.e., ketamine, early celastrol administration was able to further lower cerebellar NOX1 levels. With respect to these findings, additional investigations are needed to further unravel molecular mechanisms of actions of celastrol and its possible impact on NOX1 enzyme expression. Indeed, in this context, a limitation of this study is represented by the absence of the evaluation of the enzyme activation in the cerebellum. The lack of NOX2 increase following postnatal ketamine exposure observed in our experimental conditions could be explained by a region-specific effect of this NMDA-receptor antagonist in inducing an enhancement of this NADPH oxidase isoform. In line with this hypothesis, Zhang and co-workers previously described that cortical NOX2 was upregulated in adult rats treated with ketamine from PND6 to PND8 [20]. Moreover, in further support, an interesting study of Boczek et al. analyzed the effects of repeated ketamine administration on different brain areas, i.e., cortex, cerebellum, hippocampus and striatum, revealing region-specific effects of this NMDA-R antagonist [104]. However, we cannot totally exclude that the observed celastrol effects might be related to other pathways, other than the inhibition of NOX enzymes, finally resulting in decreased ROS levels, such as the enhancement of antioxidant capacity [105], the increase of antioxidant enzyme activity [106] and the targeting of mitochondria respiratory chain [107].

Decreased PV levels and loss of phenotype of PV-positive interneurons have been described in brain regions other than cerebellum, such as prefrontal cortex and hippocampus, in pharmacologic and non-pharmacologic animal models of psychosis [22,108]. With respect to this issue, a novelty of the present study is the absence, at least in our experimental conditions, of the reduction of PV amount in the cerebellum of adult mice administered with ketamine in the early stages of life, suggesting a region-specific effect of this NMDA-R antagonist. Moreover, our findings should also be considered in the light of the link existing between NADPH oxidases and PV. Indeed, NOX2 enzyme alterations have been reported to mediate cortical PV changes induced by different neurodetrimental insults, such as ketamine administration [34] or traumatic brain injury [109]. Thus, the lack of PV alterations observed in our experimental conditions might be related to the absence of NOX2 changes in the same brain region, suggesting a different mechanism of action underlying ketamine effects in the cerebellum with respect to what observed in the prefrontal cortex.

Here, we also showed that ketamine administration in early life stages caused increased levels of a specific proinflammatory cytokine, the TNF-α, in the cerebellum, without affecting cerebellar levels of IL-6 and IL-1β. Behavioral manifestations in psychiatric disorders such as schizophrenia and autism have been reported to be sustained by early neuroinflammatory processes which involve specific brain regions, including the cerebellum [110]. Moreover, patients with first psychotic episode, drug-naive schizophrenia, and subjects at ultra-high risk of psychosis have been described to share altered cerebellar-default mode network connectivity which appears to be modulate by inflammation in this brain region [111]. Moreover, in good agreement with our findings, previous evidence has reported a crucial role of TNF-α in regulating ketamine-induced neurotoxicity in the hippocampus [112,113], which is known to be functionally connected with the cerebellum [114,115]. In our experimental conditions, early celastrol administration was not able to prevent the ketamine-induced TNF-α increase in the cerebellum. This finding might appear in apparent contradiction with previous lines of evidence showing an effect of this compound in lowering TNF-α in monocytes and macrophages [45], as well as in the brain of animal models of neurodegenerative disorders, such as Alzheimer's disease [116,117], amyotrophic lateral sclerosis [42] and Parkinson's disease [50]. However, in most of the animal models on which celastrol has previously been tested for the evaluation of its effects on TNF-α, the pathological and/or neurotoxic insult leading to the neurodegenerative condition mainly occurred at adulthood. Moreover, other routes of administration (such as the oral one), as well as different doses and considered brain regions might also explain our findings. Further research is certainly needed to highlight possible different effects of celastrol on pro-inflammatory cytokines based on the time of the insult occurring in the brain. The lack of ketamine-induced cerebellar IL-6 increase that we observed might also be considered in the light of the unaltered NOX2 and PV expression we found in the same brain region. Indeed, a molecular association between IL-6, NOX2 and PV has been previously reported in the ketamine model of psychosis [35].

In this study, we also reported that early celastrol administration prevented ketamine-induced decrease of IL-10, an anti-inflammatory cytokine, in the cerebellum. Accordingly, an imbalance between pro-inflammatory and anti-inflammatory cytokines has been described in both schizophrenia [118] and other psychiatric disorders characterized by psychotic symptoms, such as bipolar disorders [119]. Intriguingly, IL-10 has been described as the most important player both in the resolution of the inflammatory cascade [120] and in the protection against possible detrimental effects following a neurotoxic insults [121,122]. Moreover, a key role of this anti-inflammatory cytokine in preventing glutamate-mediated cerebellar granule cell death has been reported [123], together with the regulation of synapses formation and functioning in the developing brain [124]. Thus, we could hypothesize that, at least in our experimental conditions, early celastrol administration might exert a protective effect against a neurotoxic insult, represented by ketamine, on the developing cerebellum, acting also on the anti-inflammatory pathways related to IL-10.

In conclusion, our study suggests that early NOX inhibition by celastrol during a crucial period of CNS maturation can prevent the development of psychotic-like behavioral dysfunctions, the increased oxidative stress and the IL-10 reduction in the cerebellum of adult mice exposed to an early neurodetrimental insult, i.e., ketamine. This might open new pharmacological insights into the possible use of this compound for neuroprotective purposes during brain development.

4. Materials and Methods

4.1. Animals

Mice were housed at constant room temperature (22 ± 1 °C) and relative humidity (55 ± 5%) under a 12 h light/dark cycle (lights on from 7:00 AM to 7:00 PM), with free access to food and water. Experimental procedures involving animals and their care were performed in conformity with the institutional guidelines of the Italian Ministry of Health (D.Lgs. n.26/2014), the Guide for the Care and Use of Laboratory Animals: Eight Edition, the Guide for the Care and Use of Mammals in Neuroscience and Behavioral Research (National Research Council, 2004), the Directive 2010/63/EU of the European Parliament and of the Council of 22 September 2010 on the protection of animals used for scientific purposes, as well as the ARRIVE guidelines. We daily monitored animal welfare during the entire period of experimental procedures. All efforts were made to minimize the number of animals used and their suffering. The experimental protocol was approved by the Italian Ministry of Health (approval number 679/2017-PR, protocol n. B2EF8.17).

4.2. Experimental Design

Five C57/Bl6 adult male mice and 10 adult females (Envigo, San Pietro al Natisone, Italy) weighing 25–30 g (8–10 weeks of age) were mated (one male and two females per cage).

Male pups were divided into the following five experimental groups:

1. pups administered with saline (10 mL/kg i.p.);
2. pups administered with ketamine (Sigma-Aldrich Corporation, Saint Louis, MO, US; 30 mg/kg i.p., dissolved in saline) [10,33];
3. pups administered with celastrol (Sigma Aldrich, Milano, Italy; 1 mg/kg i.p., dissolved in 50% DMSO/PBS) [43];
4. pups administered with a 50% DMSO/PBS solution (5 mL/kg i.p.)—we have referred to this treatment throughout the text as "DMSO";
5. pups administered with ketamine (30 mg/kg i.p., dissolved in saline, injected in the right side of the peritoneum) and celastrol (1 mg/kg i.p., dissolved in 50% DMSO/PBS, injected in the left side of the peritoneum)—we have referred to this treatment throughout the text as "ketamine + celastrol".

The above-mentioned treatments were repeated at PNDs 7, 9 and 11.

All pups were grown until adulthood, i.e., 10 weeks of age, when behavioral tests were performed. Immediately after, mice were euthanized by cervical dislocation for the collection of cerebella on which neurochemical and biomolecular analysis were conducted. The tissue was frozen in isopentane and stored at −80 °C until analysis was performed.

Body weight gain during the experimental protocol was calculated as the difference between body weight at PND 7 (the time of the first ketamine and/or celastrol injection) and body weight at 10 weeks of age (the time at which the behavioral tests were performed). No statistical differences were detected among the experimental groups (Supplementary Material A). Moreover, body weight at the time of the behavioral tests (10 weeks of age) was comparable among experimental groups (Supplementary Material B). No evident signs of hair loss and/or alopecia were observed during the experimental protocol for all the animals included in this study.

4.3. Behavioral Tests

4.3.1. NOR Test

The NOR test was performed as previously described [19,125] in a squared plastic-made arena (40 cm × 40 cm × 40 cm). For the habituation, mice were allowed to freely explore the arena for 10 min over five days. Mice were acclimatized to the testing room for one hour prior the beginning of the test. The test included two trials (training trial, T1 and testing trial, T2) of 3 min with an intertrial time of 1 min [126,127]. In T1, mice were put in the center of the arena and left free to explore two identical objects (two white light bulbs, fixed on the floor of the arena by velcro) for 3 min. In the testing trial (T2), one of the light bulbs was substituted with a novel object (a light blue plastic-made brick). At the beginning of the experimental procedure and between T1 and T2, the objects were cleaned with 20% *v*/*v* ethanol to remove any olfactory cues. Moreover, the arena was cleaned each time to remove mouse feces. Both T1 and T2 were videorecorded using a fixed camera. Then, an investigator, blind to the identity of the tested mouse, analyzed the animal behavior, including in the scoring of object sniffing and touching, as well as having moved the vibrissae while directing the nose toward the object at a distance of 1 cm. The following behaviors were not considered: sitting on, leaning against, and chewing the objects. The discrimination index was calculated using the following formula: (N − F)/(N + F) (*N* = times spent in exploration of the novel object during the T2; F = times spent in exploration of the familiar object in the T2) [19].

4.3.2. OF Test

The OF test was performed as previously described [128], in a square plastic arena (40 cm × 40 cm × 40 cm), virtually divided into nine equal squares with black horizontal and vertical lines [129]. Mice were acclimatized to the testing room for one hour prior the beginning of the test. For the habituation, mice were allowed to freely move into the arena for 10 min over five days. The day of the test, mice were initially placed in the same corner and then left to move freely in the arena for 5 min. The experimental procedures were videorecorded using a fixed camera and then analyzed by a blind investigator who manually scored as spontaneous locomotor activity the total of horizontal and vertical displacements performed during the test (squares crossed with the four paws).

4.3.3. SI Test

The SI test was performed, as previously described [130–132], in a plexiglass rectangular cage (45cm × 30cm × 25cm), located under a fixed camera. Briefly, 24 h before, as well as on the morning of the test, the cages were cleaned, the testing mouse was weighed in order to choose an appropriate intruder, which was labelled with a white, sticking tape on the tail. Mice were acclimatized to the testing room for one hour prior the beginning of the test. The testing mouse was left undisturbed in the cage for 15 min. Then, the intruder was introduced, and the social behavior was videorecorded for 10 min. Analysis of behavior was conducted by a blind researcher and the following parameters were considered for the scoring: time (seconds) spent by the testing mouse in sniffing the intruder, time (seconds) spent by the testing mouse in close following the intruder and time (seconds) spent by the testing mouse in the allogrooming to the intruder.

4.4. Enzyme-Linked Immunosorbent Assays (ELISAs)

Samples were homogenized in 10 volumes of PBS with protease inhibitors, as previously described [133,134]. Commercially available ELISA kits were used for measurement of 8-OHdG (JaICA, Shizuoka, Japan), NOX2 (MyBiosource, San Diego, CA, USA), NOX1 (MyBiosource, San Diego, CA, USA), PV (MyBiosource, San Diego, CA, USA), TNF-α (MyBiosource, San Diego, CA, USA), IL-6 (MyBiosource, San Diego, CA, USA), IL-1β (MyBiosource, San Diego, CA, USA) and IL-10 (MyBiosource, San Diego, CA, USA) in the cerebellum, according to the manufacturer's instructions. Each sample analysis was performed in duplicate to avoid intra-assay variations.

4.5. Blindness of the Study

Researchers performing data analysis were blind with respect to the treatment conditions. The blindness was maintained until the end of the analysis process.

4.6. Statistical Analysis

GraphPad 5.0 software for Windows was used to perform statistical analyses. Data were analyzed by One Way ANOVA, followed by Tukey's post hoc test. For all tests, a p value < 0.05 was considered statistically significant. Results are expressed as means ± mean standard error (SEM).

Supplementary Materials: The Supplementary Materials are available online at http://www.mdpi.com/1420-3049/24/21/3993/s1.

Author Contributions: Conceptualization, S.S., P.T., L.T. and M.G.M.; Data curation, S.S., P.T., L.T. and M.G.M.; Formal analysis, S.S. and M.G.M.; Funding acquisition, S.S., P.T. and L.T.; Investigation, S.S., P.T. and M.G.M.; Methodology, S.S., P.T. and M.G.M.; Project administration, L.T.; Resources, S.S., P.T. and L.T.; Software, S.S. and M.G.M.; Supervision, L.T.; Validation, S.S., P.T., L.T. and M.G.M.; Visualization, S.S., P.T., L.T. and M.G.M.; Writing—original draft, S.S.; Writing—review & editing, S.S., P.T., L.T. and M.G.M.

Funding: This work was supported by PRIN 2015 code 2015XSZ9A2_005 to LT, PRIN 2015 code 2015KP7T2Y to PT and "IRPF-PSE 2018 prize in the field of Central Nervous System" to SS. The APC was funded by "5 × 1000 IRPEF funds in favour of the University of Foggia, in memory of Gianluca Montel".

Acknowledgments: The authors thank Stefania Di Monte for technical support.

Conflicts of Interest: The authors declare no conflict of interests.

References

1. Curran, H.V.; Nutt, D.; de Wit, H. Psychedelics and related drugs: Therapeutic possibilities, mechanisms and regulation. *Psychopharmacology* **2018**, *235*, 373–375. [CrossRef] [PubMed]
2. Vlisides, P.E.; Bel-Bahar, T.; Nelson, A.; Chilton, K.; Smith, E.; Janke, E.; Tarnal, V.; Picton, P.; Harris, R.E.; Mashour, G.A. Subanaesthetic ketamine and altered states of consciousness in humans. *Br. J. Anaesth.* **2018**, *121*, 249–259. [CrossRef] [PubMed]
3. Pomarol-Clotet, E.; Honey, G.D.; Murray, G.K.; Corlett, P.R.; Absalom, A.R.; Lee, M.; McKenna, P.J.; Bullmore, E.T.; Fletcher, P.C. Psychological effects of ketamine in healthy volunteers. Phenomenological study. *Br. J. Psychiatry J. Ment. Sci.* **2006**, *189*, 173–179. [CrossRef]
4. Frohlich, J.; Van Horn, J.D. Reviewing the ketamine model for schizophrenia. *J. Psychopharmacol.* **2014**, *28*, 287–302. [CrossRef]
5. Powell, S.B.; Zhou, X.; Geyer, M.A. Prepulse inhibition and genetic mouse models of schizophrenia. *Behav. Brain Res.* **2009**, *204*, 282–294. [CrossRef]
6. Watson, D.J.; Marsden, C.A.; Millan, M.J.; Fone, K.C. Blockade of dopamine D(3) but not D(2) receptors reverses the novel object discrimination impairment produced by post-weaning social isolation: Implications for schizophrenia and its treatment. *Int. J. Neuropsychopharmacol. Off. Sci. J. Coll. Int. Neuropsychopharmacol.* **2012**, *15*, 471–484. [CrossRef]
7. Forrest, A.D.; Coto, C.A.; Siegel, S.J. Animal models of psychosis: Current state and future directions. *Curr. Behav. Neurosci. Rep.* **2014**, *1*, 100–116. [CrossRef]
8. Mattei, D.; Schweibold, R.; Wolf, S.A. Brain in flames—Animal models of psychosis: Utility and limitations. *Neuropsychiatr. Dis. Treat.* **2015**, *11*, 1313–1329.
9. Owen, M.J.; O'Donovan, M.C.; Thapar, A.; Craddock, N. Neurodevelopmental hypothesis of schizophrenia. *Br. J. Psychiatry J. Ment. Sci.* **2011**, *198*, 173–175. [CrossRef] [PubMed]
10. Jeevakumar, V.; Driskill, C.; Paine, A.; Sobhanian, M.; Vakil, H.; Morris, B.; Ramos, J.; Kroener, S. Ketamine administration during the second postnatal week induces enduring schizophrenia-like behavioral symptoms and reduces parvalbumin expression in the medial prefrontal cortex of adult mice. *Behav. Brain Res.* **2015**, *282*, 165–175. [CrossRef]
11. Yeganeh-Doost, P.; Gruber, O.; Falkai, P.; Schmitt, A. The role of the cerebellum in schizophrenia: From cognition to molecular pathways. *Clinics* **2011**, *66* (Suppl. S1), 71–77. [CrossRef] [PubMed]

12. Bernard, J.A.; Orr, J.M.; Mittal, V.A. Cerebello-thalamo-cortical networks predict positive symptom progression in individuals at ultra-high risk for psychosis. *Neuroimage. Clin.* **2017**, *14*, 622–628. [CrossRef] [PubMed]
13. Villanueva, R. The cerebellum and neuropsychiatric disorders. *Psychiatry Res.* **2012**, *198*, 527–532. [CrossRef] [PubMed]
14. Bernard, J.A.; Orr, J.M.; Dean, D.J.; Mittal, V.A. The cerebellum and learning of non-motor associations in individuals at clinical-high risk for psychosis. *Neuroimage Clin.* **2018**, *19*, 137–146. [CrossRef] [PubMed]
15. Schmahmann, J.D. The cerebellum and cognition. *Neurosci. Lett.* **2019**, *688*, 62–75. [CrossRef] [PubMed]
16. Andreasen, N.C.; Pierson, R. The role of the cerebellum in schizophrenia. *Biol. Psychiatry* **2008**, *64*, 81–88. [CrossRef]
17. Arasappa, R.; Rao, N.; Venkatasubramanian, G.; Jayakumar, P.; Gangadhar, B. Structural cerebellar abnormalities in antipsychotic-naive schizophrenia: Evidence for cognitive dysmetria. *Indian J. Psychol. Med.* **2008**, *30*, 83–89. [CrossRef]
18. Bielawski, M.; Bondurant, H. Psychosis following a stroke to the cerebellum and midbrain: A case report. *Cerebellum Ataxias* **2015**, *2*, 17. [CrossRef]
19. Schiavone, S.; Sorce, S.; Dubois-Dauphin, M.; Jaquet, V.; Colaianna, M.; Zotti, M.; Cuomo, V.; Trabace, L.; Krause, K.H. Involvement of NOX2 in the development of behavioral and pathologic alterations in isolated rats. *Biol. Psychiatry* **2009**, *66*, 384–392. [CrossRef]
20. Zhang, H.; Sun, X.R.; Wang, J.; Zhang, Z.Z.; Zhao, H.T.; Li, H.H.; Ji, M.H.; Li, K.Y.; Yang, J.J. Reactive oxygen species-mediated loss of phenotype of parvalbumin interneurons contributes to long-term cognitive impairments after repeated neonatal ketamine exposures. *Neurotox. Res.* **2016**, *30*, 593–605. [CrossRef]
21. Sabbagh, J.J.; Murtishaw, A.S.; Bolton, M.M.; Heaney, C.F.; Langhardt, M.; Kinney, J.W. Chronic ketamine produces altered distribution of parvalbumin-positive cells in the hippocampus of adult rats. *Neurosci. Lett.* **2013**, *550*, 69–74. [CrossRef] [PubMed]
22. Schiavone, S.; Morgese, M.G.; Bove, M.; Colia, A.L.; Maffione, A.B.; Tucci, P.; Trabace, L.; Cuomo, V. Ketamine administration induces early and persistent neurochemical imbalance and altered NADPH oxidase in mice. *Prog. Neuro-Psychopharmacol. Biol. Psychiatry* **2019**, *96*, 109750. [CrossRef] [PubMed]
23. Schwaller, B.; Meyer, M.; Schiffmann, S. 'New' functions for 'old' proteins: The role of the calcium-binding proteins calbindin D-28k, calretinin and parvalbumin, in cerebellar physiology. Studies with knockout mice. *Cerebellum* **2002**, *1*, 241–258. [CrossRef] [PubMed]
24. Bastianelli, E. Distribution of calcium-binding proteins in the cerebellum. *Cerebellum* **2003**, *2*, 242–262. [CrossRef] [PubMed]
25. Liu, F.F.; Yang, L.D.; Sun, X.R.; Zhang, H.; Pan, W.; Wang, X.M.; Yang, J.J.; Ji, M.H.; Yuan, H.M. NOX2 mediated-parvalbumin interneuron loss might contribute to anxiety-like and enhanced fear learning behavior in a rat model of post-traumatic stress disorder. *Mol. Neurobiol.* **2016**, *53*, 6680–6689. [CrossRef]
26. Schiavone, S.; Trabace, L. Pharmacological targeting of redox regulation systems as new therapeutic approach for psychiatric disorders: A literature overview. *Pharmacol. Res.* **2016**, *107*, 195–204. [CrossRef]
27. Barron, H.; Hafizi, S.; Andreazza, A.C.; Mizrahi, R. Neuroinflammation and oxidative stress in psychosis and psychosis risk. *Int. J. Mol. Sci.* **2017**, *18*, 651. [CrossRef]
28. Sorce, S.; Krause, K.H. NOX enzymes in the central nervous system: From signaling to disease. *Antioxid. Redox Signal.* **2009**, *11*, 2481–2504. [CrossRef]
29. Ibi, M.; Liu, J.; Arakawa, N.; Kitaoka, S.; Kawaji, A.; Matsuda, K.I.; Iwata, K.; Matsumoto, M.; Katsuyama, M.; Zhu, K.; et al. Depressive-like behaviors are regulated by NOX1/NADPH oxidase by redox modification of NMDA receptor 1. *J. Neurosci. Off. J. Soc. Neurosci.* **2017**, *37*, 4200–4212. [CrossRef]
30. Ma, M.W.; Wang, J.; Zhang, Q.; Wang, R.; Dhandapani, K.M.; Vadlamudi, R.K.; Brann, D.W. NADPH oxidase in brain injury and neurodegenerative disorders. *Mol. Neurodegener.* **2017**, *12*, 7. [CrossRef]
31. Schiavone, S.; Jaquet, V.; Sorce, S.; Dubois-Dauphin, M.; Hultqvist, M.; Backdahl, L.; Holmdahl, R.; Colaianna, M.; Cuomo, V.; Trabace, L.; et al. NADPH oxidase elevations in pyramidal neurons drive psychosocial stress-induced neuropathology. *Transl. Psychiatry* **2012**, *2*, e111. [CrossRef] [PubMed]
32. Schiavone, S.; Mhillaj, E.; Neri, M.; Morgese, M.G.; Tucci, P.; Bove, M.; Valentino, M.; Di Giovanni, G.; Pomara, C.; Turillazzi, E.; et al. Early loss of blood-brain barrier integrity precedes NOX2 elevation in the prefrontal cortex of an animal model of psychosis. *Mol. Neurobiol.* **2017**, *54*, 2031–2044. [CrossRef] [PubMed]

33. Sorce, S.; Schiavone, S.; Tucci, P.; Colaianna, M.; Jaquet, V.; Cuomo, V.; Dubois-Dauphin, M.; Trabace, L.; Krause, K.H. The NADPH oxidase NOX2 controls glutamate release: A novel mechanism involved in psychosis-like ketamine responses. *J. Neurosci. Off. J. Soc. Neurosci.* **2010**, *30*, 11317–11325. [CrossRef] [PubMed]
34. Behrens, M.M.; Ali, S.S.; Dao, D.N.; Lucero, J.; Shekhtman, G.; Quick, K.L.; Dugan, L.L. Ketamine-induced loss of phenotype of fast-spiking interneurons is mediated by NADPH-oxidase. *Science* **2007**, *318*, 1645–1647. [CrossRef] [PubMed]
35. Behrens, M.M.; Ali, S.S.; Dugan, L.L. Interleukin-6 mediates the increase in NADPH-oxidase in the ketamine model of schizophrenia. *J. Neurosci. Off. J. Soc. Neurosci.* **2008**, *28*, 13957–13966. [CrossRef]
36. Coyoy, A.; Olguin-Albuerne, M.; Martinez-Briseno, P.; Moran, J. Role of reactive oxygen species and NADPH-oxidase in the development of rat cerebellum. *Neurochem. Int.* **2013**, *62*, 998–1011. [CrossRef]
37. Fraguas, D.; Diaz-Caneja, C.M.; Rodriguez-Quiroga, A.; Arango, C. Oxidative stress and inflammation in early onset first episode psychosis: A systematic review and meta-Analysis. *Int. J. Neuropsychopharmacol. Off. Sci. J. Coll. Int. Neuropsychopharmacol.* **2017**, *20*, 435–444. [CrossRef]
38. Khandaker, G.M.; Cousins, L.; Deakin, J.; Lennox, B.R.; Yolken, R.; Jones, P.B. Inflammation and immunity in schizophrenia: Implications for pathophysiology and treatment. *Lancet. Psychiatry* **2015**, *2*, 258–270. [CrossRef]
39. Kirkpatrick, B.; Miller, B.J. Inflammation and schizophrenia. *Schizophr. Bull.* **2013**, *39*, 1174–1179. [CrossRef]
40. Hagberg, H.; Mallard, C. Effect of inflammation on central nervous system development and vulnerability. *Curr. Opin. Neurol.* **2005**, *18*, 117–123. [CrossRef]
41. Ng, S.W.; Chan, Y.; Chellappan, D.K.; Madheswaran, T.; Zeeshan, F.; Chan, Y.L.; Collet, T.; Gupta, G.; Oliver, B.G.; Wark, P.; et al. Molecular modulators of celastrol as the keystones for its diverse pharmacological activities. *Biomed. Pharmacother. Biomed. Pharmacother.* **2019**, *109*, 1785–1792. [CrossRef] [PubMed]
42. Kiaei, M.; Kipiani, K.; Petri, S.; Chen, J.; Calingasan, N.Y.; Beal, M.F. Celastrol blocks neuronal cell death and extends life in transgenic mouse model of amyotrophic lateral sclerosis. *Neuro-Degener. Dis.* **2005**, *2*, 246–254. [CrossRef] [PubMed]
43. Paris, D.; Ganey, N.J.; Laporte, V.; Patel, N.S.; Beaulieu-Abdelahad, D.; Bachmeier, C.; March, A.; Ait-Ghezala, G.; Mullan, M.J. Reduction of beta-amyloid pathology by celastrol in a transgenic mouse model of Alzheimer's disease. *J. Neuroinflamm.* **2010**, *7*, 17. [CrossRef] [PubMed]
44. Choi, B.S.; Kim, H.; Lee, H.J.; Sapkota, K.; Park, S.E.; Kim, S.; Kim, S.J. Celastrol from 'Thunder God Vine' protects SH-SY5Y cells through the preservation of mitochondrial function and inhibition of p38 MAPK in a rotenone model of Parkinson's disease. *Neurochem. Res.* **2014**, *39*, 84–96. [CrossRef] [PubMed]
45. Tarafdar, A.; Pula, G. The Role of NADPH Oxidases and Oxidative Stress in Neurodegenerative Disorders. *Int. J. Mol. Sci.* **2018**, *19*, E3824. [CrossRef]
46. Jaquet, V.; Marcoux, J.; Forest, E.; Leidal, K.G.; McCormick, S.; Westermaier, Y.; Perozzo, R.; Plastre, O.; Fioraso-Cartier, L.; Diebold, B.; et al. NADPH oxidase (NOX) isoforms are inhibited by celastrol with a dual mode of action. *Br. J. Pharmacol.* **2011**, *164*, 507–520. [CrossRef]
47. Schiavone, S.; Jaquet, V.; Trabace, L.; Krause, K.H. Severe life stress and oxidative stress in the brain: From animal models to human pathology. *Antioxid. Redox Signal.* **2013**, *18*, 1475–1490. [CrossRef]
48. Kawanishi, S.; Oikawa, S. Mechanism of telomere shortening by oxidative stress. *Ann. N. Y. Acad. Sci.* **2004**, *1019*, 278–284. [CrossRef]
49. Konieczny, J.; Jantas, D.; Lenda, T.; Domin, H.; Czarnecka, A.; Kuter, K.; Smialowska, M.; Lason, W.; Lorenc-Koci, E. Lack of neuroprotective effect of celastrol under conditions of proteasome inhibition by lactacystin in in vitro and in vivo studies: Implications for Parkinson's disease. *Neurotox. Res.* **2014**, *26*, 255–273. [CrossRef]
50. Cleren, C.; Calingasan, N.Y.; Chen, J.; Beal, M.F. Celastrol protects against MPTP- and 3-nitropropionic acid-induced neurotoxicity. *J. Neurochem.* **2005**, *94*, 995–1004. [CrossRef]
51. Faust, K.; Gehrke, S.; Yang, Y.; Yang, L.; Beal, M.F.; Lu, B. Neuroprotective effects of compounds with antioxidant and anti-inflammatory properties in a Drosophila model of Parkinson's disease. *BMC Neurosci.* **2009**, *10*, 109. [CrossRef] [PubMed]
52. Brown, I.R. Heat shock proteins and protection of the nervous system. *Ann. N. Y. Acad. Sci.* **2007**, *1113*, 147–158. [CrossRef] [PubMed]

53. Abdin, A.A.; Hasby, E.A. Modulatory effect of celastrol on Th1/Th2 cytokines profile, TLR2 and CD3 + T-lymphocyte expression in a relapsing-remitting model of multiple sclerosis in rats. *Eur. J. Pharmacol.* **2014**, *742*, 102–112. [CrossRef] [PubMed]
54. Wang, Y.; Cao, L.; Xu, L.M.; Cao, F.F.; Peng, B.; Zhang, X.; Shen, Y.F.; Uzan, G.; Zhang, D.H. Celastrol Ameliorates EAE Induction by Suppressing Pathogenic T Cell Responses in the Peripheral and Central Nervous Systems. *J. Neuroimmune Pharmacol. Off. J. Soc. Neuroimmune Pharmacol.* **2015**, *10*, 506–516. [CrossRef]
55. Malkov, A.; Ivanov, A.I.; Latyshkova, A.; Bregestovski, P.; Zilberter, M.; Zilberter, Y. Activation of nicotinamide adenine dinucleotide phosphate oxidase is the primary trigger of epileptic seizures in rodent models. *Ann. Neurol.* **2019**, *85*, 907–920. [CrossRef]
56. Von Ruden, E.L.; Wolf, F.; Gualtieri, F.; Keck, M.; Hunt, C.R.; Pandita, T.K.; Potschka, H. Genetic and pharmacological targeting of heat shock protein 70 in the mouse amygdala-kindling model. *ACS Chem. Neurosci.* **2019**, *10*, 1434–1444. [CrossRef]
57. Jiang, M.; Liu, X.; Zhang, D.; Wang, Y.; Hu, X.; Xu, F.; Jin, M.; Cao, F.; Xu, L. Celastrol treatment protects against acute ischemic stroke-induced brain injury by promoting an IL-33/ST2 axis-mediated microglia/macrophage M2 polarization. *J. Neuroinflamm.* **2018**, *15*, 78. [CrossRef]
58. Li, Y.; He, D.; Zhang, X.; Liu, Z.; Zhang, X.; Dong, L.; Xing, Y.; Wang, C.; Qiao, H.; Zhu, C.; et al. Protective effect of celastrol in rat cerebral ischemia model: Down-regulating p-JNK, p-c-Jun and NF-kappaB. *Brain Res.* **2012**, *1464*, 8–13. [CrossRef]
59. Zhu, F.; Li, C.; Jin, X.P.; Weng, S.X.; Fan, L.L.; Zheng, Z.; Li, W.L.; Wang, F.; Wang, W.F.; Hu, X.F.; et al. Celastrol may have an anti-atherosclerosis effect in a rabbit experimental carotid atherosclerosis model. *Int. J. Clin. Exp. Med.* **2014**, *7*, 1684–1691.
60. Kim, J.Y.; Kim, N.; Zheng, Z.; Lee, J.E.; Yenari, M.A. The 70 kDa heat shock protein protects against experimental traumatic brain injury. *Neurobiol. Dis.* **2013**, *58*, 289–295. [CrossRef]
61. Eroglu, B.; Kimbler, D.E.; Pang, J.; Choi, J.; Moskophidis, D.; Yanasak, N.; Dhandapani, K.M.; Mivechi, N.F. Therapeutic inducers of the HSP70/HSP110 protect mice against traumatic brain injury. *J. Neurochem.* **2014**, *130*, 626–641. [CrossRef] [PubMed]
62. Readhead, B.; Hartley, B.J.; Eastwood, B.J.; Collier, D.A.; Evans, D.; Farias, R.; He, C.; Hoffman, G.; Sklar, P.; Dudley, J.T.; et al. Expression-based drug screening of neural progenitor cells from individuals with schizophrenia. *Nat. Commun.* **2018**, *9*, 4412. [CrossRef] [PubMed]
63. Cheung, H.M.; Yew, D.T.W. Effects of perinatal exposure to ketamine on the developing brain. *Front. Neurosci.* **2019**, *13*, 138. [CrossRef] [PubMed]
64. Coronel-Oliveros, C.M.; Pacheco-Calderon, R. Prenatal exposure to ketamine in rats: Implications on animal models of schizophrenia. *Dev. Psychobiol.* **2018**, *60*, 30–42. [CrossRef]
65. Liao, W.T.; Xiao, X.Y.; Zhu, Y.; Zhou, S.P. The effect of celastrol on learning and memory in diabetic rats after sevoflurane inhalation. *Arch. Med Sci. AMS* **2018**, *14*, 370–380. [CrossRef]
66. Hooper, P.L.; Durham, H.D.; Torok, Z.; Hooper, P.L.; Crul, T.; Vigh, L. The central role of heat shock factor 1 in synaptic fidelity and memory consolidation. *Cell Stress Chaperones* **2016**, *21*, 745–753. [CrossRef]
67. Barker-Haliski, M.L.; Loscher, W.; White, H.S.; Galanopoulou, A.S. Neuroinflammation in epileptogenesis: Insights and translational perspectives from new models of epilepsy. *Epilepsia* **2017**, *58* (Suppl. S3), 39–47. [CrossRef]
68. Wesson, D.W. Sniffing behavior communicates social hierarchy. *Curr. Biol.* **2013**, *23*, 575–580. [CrossRef]
69. Lee, P.R.; Brady, D.L.; Shapiro, R.A.; Dorsa, D.M.; Koenig, J.I. Social interaction deficits caused by chronic phencyclidine administration are reversed by oxytocin. *Neuropsychopharmacol. Off. Publ. Am. Coll. Neuropsychopharmacol.* **2005**, *30*, 1883–1894. [CrossRef]
70. Snigdha, S.; Neill, J.C. Efficacy of antipsychotics to reverse phencyclidine-induced social interaction deficits in female rats–a preliminary investigation. *Behav. Brain Res.* **2008**, *187*, 489–494. [CrossRef]
71. Bozdagi, O.; Sakurai, T.; Papapetrou, D.; Wang, X.; Dickstein, D.L.; Takahashi, N.; Kajiwara, Y.; Yang, M.; Katz, A.M.; Scattoni, M.L.; et al. Haploinsufficiency of the autism-associated Shank3 gene leads to deficits in synaptic function, social interaction, and social communication. *Mol. Autism* **2010**, *1*, 15. [CrossRef] [PubMed]

72. Becker, A.; Peters, B.; Schroeder, H.; Mann, T.; Huether, G.; Grecksch, G. Ketamine-induced changes in rat behaviour: A possible animal model of schizophrenia. *Prog. Neuro Psychopharmacol. Biol. Psychiatry* **2003**, *27*, 687–700. [CrossRef]
73. Schweinfurth, M.K.; Stieger, B.; Taborsky, M. Experimental evidence for reciprocity in allogrooming among wild-type Norway rats. *Sci. Rep.* **2017**, *7*, 4010. [CrossRef] [PubMed]
74. Alleva, E. 7—Assessment of Aggressive Behavior in Rodents. In *Methods in Neurosciences*; Conn, P.M., Ed.; Academic Press: Cambridge, MA, USA, 1993; Volume 14, pp. 111–137.
75. Shin, S.Y.; Baek, N.J.; Han, S.H.; Min, S.S. Chronic administration of ketamine ameliorates the anxiety- and aggressive-like behavior in adolescent mice induced by neonatal maternal separation. *Korean J. Physiol. Pharmacol. Off. J. Korean Physiol. Soc. Korean Soc. Pharmacol.* **2019**, *23*, 81–87. [CrossRef] [PubMed]
76. Hira, S.; Saleem, U.; Anwar, F.; Ahmad, B. Antioxidants Attenuate Isolation- and L-DOPA-Induced Aggression in Mice. *Front. Pharmacol.* **2017**, *8*, 945. [CrossRef] [PubMed]
77. Garratt, M.; Brooks, R.C. A genetic reduction in antioxidant function causes elevated aggression in mice. *J. Exp. Biol.* **2015**, *218 Pt 2*, 223–227. [CrossRef]
78. Kim, T.; Lee, K.H.; Oh, H.; Lee, T.Y.; Cho, K.I.K.; Lee, J.; Kwon, J.S. Cerebellar structural abnormalities associated with cognitive function in patients with first-episode psychosis. *Front. Psychiatry* **2018**, *9*, 286. [CrossRef]
79. Moberget, T.; Ivry, R.B. Prediction, Psychosis, and the Cerebellum. *Biol. Psychiatry Cogn. Neurosci. Neuroimaging* **2019**, *4*, 820–831. [CrossRef]
80. Jones, C.A.; Watson, D.J.; Fone, K.C. Animal models of schizophrenia. *Br. J. Pharmacol.* **2011**, *164*, 1162–1194. [CrossRef]
81. Shinn, A.K.; Roh, Y.S.; Ravichandran, C.T.; Baker, J.T.; Ongur, D.; Cohen, B.M. Aberrant cerebellar connectivity in bipolar disorder with psychosis. *Biol. Psychiatry. Cogn. Neurosci. Neuroimaging* **2017**, *2*, 438–448. [CrossRef]
82. Yadav, M.; Parle, M.; Jindal, D.K.; Dhingra, S. Protective effects of stigmasterol against ketamine-induced psychotic symptoms: Possible behavioral, biochemical and histopathological changes in mice. *Pharmacol. Rep. Pr* **2018**, *70*, 591–599. [CrossRef] [PubMed]
83. Yadav, M.; Jindal, D.K.; Dhingra, M.S.; Kumar, A.; Parle, M.; Dhingra, S. Protective effect of gallic acid in experimental model of ketamine-induced psychosis: Possible behaviour, biochemical, neurochemical and cellular alterations. *Inflammopharmacology* **2018**, *26*, 413–424. [CrossRef] [PubMed]
84. Brambrink, A.M.; Evers, A.S.; Avidan, M.S.; Farber, N.B.; Smith, D.J.; Martin, L.D.; Dissen, G.A.; Creeley, C.E.; Olney, J.W. Ketamine-induced neuroapoptosis in the fetal and neonatal rhesus macaque brain. *Anesthesiology* **2012**, *116*, 372–384. [CrossRef] [PubMed]
85. Tobe, E.H. Mitochondrial dysfunction, oxidative stress, and major depressive disorder. *Neuropsychiatr. Dis. Treat.* **2013**, *9*, 567–573. [CrossRef] [PubMed]
86. Zhang, D.; Cheng, L.; Craig, D.W.; Redman, M.; Liu, C. Cerebellar telomere length and psychiatric disorders. *Behav. Genet.* **2010**, *40*, 250–254. [CrossRef]
87. Filiou, M.D.; Teplytska, L.; Otte, D.M.; Zimmer, A.; Turck, C.W. Myelination and oxidative stress alterations in the cerebellum of the G72/G30 transgenic schizophrenia mouse model. *J. Psychiatr. Res.* **2012**, *46*, 1359–1365. [CrossRef]
88. Streck, E.L.; Rezin, G.T.; Barbosa, L.M.; Assis, L.C.; Grandi, E.; Quevedo, J. Effect of antipsychotics on succinate dehydrogenase and cytochrome oxidase activities in rat brain. *Naunyn-Schmiedeberg's Arch. Pharmacol.* **2007**, *376*, 127–133. [CrossRef]
89. Assis, L.C.; Scaini, G.; Di-Pietro, P.B.; Castro, A.A.; Comim, C.M.; Streck, E.L.; Quevedo, J. Effect of antipsychotics on creatine kinase activity in rat brain. *Basic Clin. Pharmacol. Toxicol.* **2007**, *101*, 315–319. [CrossRef]
90. Cao, H.; Chen, O.Y.; Chung, Y.; Forsyth, J.K.; McEwen, S.C.; Gee, D.G.; Bearden, C.E.; Addington, J.; Goodyear, B.; Cadenhead, K.S.; et al. Cerebello-thalamo-cortical hyperconnectivity as a state-independent functional neural signature for psychosis prediction and characterization. *Nat. Commun.* **2018**, *9*, 3836. [CrossRef]
91. Gu, F.; Chauhan, V.; Chauhan, A. Impaired synthesis and antioxidant defense of glutathione in the cerebellum of autistic subjects: Alterations in the activities and protein expression of glutathione-related enzymes. *Free Radic. Biol. Med.* **2013**, *65*, 488–496. [CrossRef]

92. Olguin-Albuerne, M.; Moran, J. ROS produced by NOX2 control in vitro development of cerebellar granule neurons development. *ASN Neuro* **2015**, *7*. [CrossRef] [PubMed]
93. Coyoy, A.; Valencia, A.; Guemez-Gamboa, A.; Moran, J. Role of NADPH oxidase in the apoptotic death of cultured cerebellar granule neurons. *Free Radic. Biol. Med.* **2008**, *45*, 1056–1064. [CrossRef] [PubMed]
94. Sorce, S.; Nuvolone, M.; Keller, A.; Falsig, J.; Varol, A.; Schwarz, P.; Bieri, M.; Budka, H.; Aguzzi, A. The role of the NADPH oxidase NOX2 in prion pathogenesis. *PLoS Pathog.* **2014**, *10*, e1004531. [CrossRef] [PubMed]
95. Nadeem, A.; Ahmad, S.F.; Al-Harbi, N.O.; Attia, S.M.; Alshammari, M.A.; Alzahrani, K.S.; Bakheet, S.A. Increased oxidative stress in the cerebellum and peripheral immune cells leads to exaggerated autism-like repetitive behavior due to deficiency of antioxidant response in BTBR T + tf/J mice. *Prog. Neuro-Psychopharmacol. Biol. Psychiatry* **2019**, *89*, 245–253. [CrossRef] [PubMed]
96. Cristovao, A.C.; Guhathakurta, S.; Bok, E.; Je, G.; Yoo, S.D.; Choi, D.H.; Kim, Y.S. NADPH oxidase 1 mediates alpha-synucleinopathy in Parkinson's disease. *J. Neurosci. Off. J. Soc. Neurosci.* **2012**, *32*, 14465–14477. [CrossRef] [PubMed]
97. Jiang, T.; Sun, Q.; Chen, S. Oxidative stress: A major pathogenesis and potential therapeutic target of antioxidative agents in Parkinson's disease and Alzheimer's disease. *Prog. Neurobiol.* **2016**, *147*, 1–19. [CrossRef] [PubMed]
98. Belarbi, K.; Cuvelier, E.; Destée, A.; Gressier, B.; Chartier-Harlin, M.C. NADPH oxidases in Parkinson's disease: A systematic review. *Mol. Neurodegener.* **2017**, *12*, 84. [CrossRef]
99. Cheret, C.; Gervais, A.; Lelli, A.; Colin, C.; Amar, L.; Ravassard, P.; Mallet, J.; Cumano, A.; Krause, K.H.; Mallat, M. Neurotoxic activation of microglia is promoted by a nox1-dependent NADPH oxidase. *J. Neurosci. Off. J. Soc. Neurosci.* **2008**, *28*, 12039–12051. [CrossRef]
100. Nakki, R.; Nickolenko, J.; Chang, J.; Sagar, S.M.; Sharp, F.R. Haloperidol prevents ketamine- and phencyclidine-induced HSP70 protein expression but not microglial activation. *Exp. Neurol.* **1996**, *137*, 234–241. [CrossRef]
101. Vasconcellos, L.R.; Dutra, F.F.; Siqueira, M.S.; Paula-Neto, H.A.; Dahan, J.; Kiarely, E.; Carneiro, L.A.; Bozza, M.T.; Travassos, L.H. Protein aggregation as a cellular response to oxidative stress induced by heme and iron. *Proc. Natl. Acad. Sci. USA* **2016**, *113*, E7474–E7482. [CrossRef]
102. Chen, F.; Pandey, D.; Chadli, A.; Catravas, J.D.; Chen, T.; Fulton, D.J. Hsp90 regulates NADPH oxidase activity and is necessary for superoxide but not hydrogen peroxide production. *Antioxid. Redox Signal.* **2011**, *14*, 2107–2119. [CrossRef] [PubMed]
103. Troyanova, N.I.; Shevchenko, M.A.; Boyko, A.A.; Mirzoyev, R.R.; Pertseva, M.A.; Kovalenko, E.I.; Sapozhnikov, A.M. Modulating effect of extracellular HSP70 on generation of reactive oxigen species in populations of phagocytes. *Bioorganicheskaia Khimiia* **2015**, *41*, 305–315. [CrossRef] [PubMed]
104. Boczek, T.; Lisek, M.; Ferenc, B.; Wiktorska, M.; Ivchevska, I.; Zylinska, L. Region-specific effects of repeated ketamine administration on the presynaptic GABAergic neurochemistry in rat brain. *Neurochem. Int.* **2015**, *91*, 13–25. [CrossRef] [PubMed]
105. Wang, C.; Shi, C.; Yang, X.; Yang, M.; Sun, H.; Wang, C. Celastrol suppresses obesity process via increasing antioxidant capacity and improving lipid metabolism. *Eur. J. Pharmacol.* **2014**, *744*, 52–58. [CrossRef]
106. Divya, T.; Dineshbabu, V.; Soumyakrishnan, S.; Sureshkumar, A.; Sudhandiran, G. Celastrol enhances Nrf2 mediated antioxidant enzymes and exhibits anti-fibrotic effect through regulation of collagen production against bleomycin-induced pulmonary fibrosis. *Chem. Biol. Interact.* **2016**, *246*, 52–62. [CrossRef]
107. Chen, G.; Zhang, X.; Zhao, M.; Wang, Y.; Cheng, X.; Wang, D.; Xu, Y.; Du, Z.; Yu, X. Celastrol targets mitochondrial respiratory chain complex I to induce reactive oxygen species-dependent cytotoxicity in tumor cells. *BMC Cancer* **2011**, *11*, 170. [CrossRef]
108. Braun, I.; Genius, J.; Grunze, H.; Bender, A.; Möller, H.J.; Rujescu, D. Alterations of hippocampal and prefrontal GABAergic interneurons in an animal model of psychosis induced by NMDA receptor antagonism. *Schizophr. Res.* **2007**, *97*, 254–263. [CrossRef]
109. Schiavone, S.; Neri, M.; Trabace, L.; Turillazzi, E. The NADPH oxidase NOX2 mediates loss of parvalbumin interneurons in traumatic brain injury: Human autoptic immunohistochemical evidence. *Sci. Rep.* **2017**, *7*, 8752. [CrossRef]
110. Meyer, U.; Feldon, J.; Dammann, O. Schizophrenia and autism: Both shared and disorder-specific pathogenesis via perinatal inflammation? *Pediatric Res.* **2011**, *69*, 26–33. [CrossRef]

111. Wang, H.; Guo, W.; Liu, F.; Wang, G.; Lyu, H.; Wu, R.; Chen, J.; Wang, S.; Li, L.; Zhao, J. Patients with first-episode, drug-naive schizophrenia and subjects at ultra-high risk of psychosis shared increased cerebellar-default mode network connectivity at rest. *Sci. Rep.* **2016**, *6*, 26124. [CrossRef]
112. Zheng, X.; Zhou, J.; Xia, Y. The role of TNF-α in regulating ketamine-induced hippocampal neurotoxicity. *Arch. Med. Sci. AMS* **2015**, *11*, 1296–1302. [CrossRef] [PubMed]
113. Li, Y.; Shen, R.; Wen, G.; Ding, R.; Du, A.; Zhou, J.; Dong, Z.; Ren, X.; Yao, H.; Zhao, R.; et al. Effects of ketamine on levels of inflammatory cytokines IL-6, IL-1beta, and TNF-alpha in the hippocampus of mice following acute or chronic administration. *Front. Pharmacol.* **2017**, *8*, 139. [PubMed]
114. Onuki, Y.; Van Someren, E.J.W.; De Zeeuw, C.I.; Van der Werf, Y.D. Hippocampal–cerebellar interaction during spatio-temporal prediction. *Cereb. Cortex* **2013**, *25*, 313–321. [CrossRef] [PubMed]
115. Babayan, B.M.; Watilliaux, A.; Viejo, G.; Paradis, A.-L.; Girard, B.; Rondi-Reig, L. A hippocampo-cerebellar centred network for the learning and execution of sequence-based navigation. *Sci. Rep.* **2017**, *7*, 17812. [CrossRef] [PubMed]
116. Decourt, B.; Lahiri, D.K.; Sabbagh, M.N. Targeting tumor necrosis factor alpha for Alzheimer's disease. *Curr. Alzheimer Res.* **2017**, *14*, 412–425. [CrossRef]
117. Allison, A.; Cacabelos, R.; Lombardi, V.; Alvarez, X.; Vigo, C. Celastrol, a potent antioxidant and anti-inflammatory drug, as a possible treatment for Alzheimer's disease. *Prog. Neuro-Psychopharmacol. Biol. Psychiatry* **2001**, *25*, 1341–1357. [CrossRef]
118. Müller, N. Inflammation in Schizophrenia: Pathogenetic Aspects and Therapeutic Considerations. *Schizophr. Bull.* **2018**, *44*, 973–982. [CrossRef]
119. Kim, Y.-K.; Jung, H.-G.; Myint, A.-M.; Kim, H.; Park, S.-H. Imbalance between pro-inflammatory and anti-inflammatory cytokines in bipolar disorder. *J. Affect. Disord.* **2007**, *104*, 91–95. [CrossRef]
120. Garcia, J.M.; Stillings, S.A.; Leclerc, J.L.; Phillips, H.; Edwards, N.J.; Robicsek, S.A.; Hoh, B.L.; Blackburn, S.; Dore, S. Role of Interleukin-10 in Acute Brain Injuries. *Front. Neurol.* **2017**, *8*, 244. [CrossRef]
121. Stoll, G.; Jander, S.; Schroeter, M. *Cytokines in CNS Disorders: Neurotoxicity versus Neuroprotection*; Advances in Dementia Research, Vienna, 2000//; Jellinger, K., Schmidt, R., Windisch, M., Eds.; Springer Vienna: Vienna, Austria, 2000; pp. 81–89.
122. Zhu, Y.; Chen, X.; Liu, Z.; Peng, Y.P.; Qiu, Y.H. Interleukin-10 Protection against lipopolysaccharide-induced neuro-inflammation and neurotoxicity in ventral mesencephalic cultures. *Int. J. Mol. Sci.* **2015**, *17*, 25. [CrossRef]
123. Bachis, A.; Colangelo, A.M.; Vicini, S.; Doe, P.P.; De Bernardi, M.A.; Brooker, G.; Mocchetti, I. Interleukin-10 prevents glutamate-mediated cerebellar granule cell death by blocking caspase-3-like activity. *J. Neurosci.* **2001**, *21*, 3104–3112. [CrossRef] [PubMed]
124. Lim, S.H.; Park, E.; You, B.; Jung, Y.; Park, A.R.; Park, S.G.; Lee, J.R. Neuronal synapse formation induced by microglia and interleukin 10. *PLoS ONE* **2013**, *8*, e81218. [CrossRef] [PubMed]
125. Lueptow, L.M. Novel object recognition test for the investigation of learning and memory in mice. *J. Vis. Exp. Jove* **2017**, *126*, e55718. [CrossRef] [PubMed]
126. Trabace, L.; Cassano, T.; Colaianna, M.; Castrignano, S.; Giustino, A.; Amoroso, S.; Steardo, L.; Cuomo, V. Neurochemical and neurobehavioral effects of ganstigmine (CHF2819), a novel acetylcholinesterase inhibitor, in rat prefrontal cortex: An in vivo study. *Pharmacol. Res.* **2007**, *56*, 288–294. [CrossRef]
127. Carratu, M.R.; Borracci, P.; Coluccia, A.; Giustino, A.; Renna, G.; Tomasini, M.C.; Raisi, E.; Antonelli, T.; Cuomo, V.; Mazzoni, E.; et al. Acute exposure to methylmercury at two developmental windows: Focus on neurobehavioral and neurochemical effects in rat offspring. *Neuroscience* **2006**, *141*, 1619–1629. [CrossRef]
128. Nogueira Neto, J.D.; de Almeida, A.A.; da Silva Oliveira, J.; Dos Santos, P.S.; de Sousa, D.P.; de Freitas, R.M. Antioxidant effects of nerolidol in mice hippocampus after open field test. *Neurochem. Res.* **2013**, *38*, 1861–1870. [CrossRef]
129. Fortes, A.C.; Almeida, A.A.; Mendonca-Junior, F.J.; Freitas, R.M.; Soares-Sobrinho, J.L.; de La Roca Soares, M.F. Anxiolytic properties of new chemical entity, 5TIO1. *Neurochem. Res.* **2013**, *38*, 726–731. [CrossRef]
130. Crawley, J.N.; Chen, T.; Puri, A.; Washburn, R.; Sullivan, T.L.; Hill, J.M.; Young, N.B.; Nadler, J.J.; Moy, S.S.; Young, L.J.; et al. Social approach behaviors in oxytocin knockout mice: Comparison of two independent lines tested in different laboratory environments. *Neuropeptides* **2007**, *41*, 145–163. [CrossRef]
131. Silverman, J.L.; Turner, S.M.; Barkan, C.L.; Tolu, S.S.; Saxena, R.; Hung, A.Y.; Sheng, M.; Crawley, J.N. Sociability and motor functions in Shank1 mutant mice. *Brain Res.* **2011**, *1380*, 120–137. [CrossRef]

132. Kaidanovich-Beilin, O.; Lipina, T.; Vukobradovic, I.; Roder, J.; Woodgett, J.R. Assessment of social interaction behaviors. *J. Vis. Exp. Jove* **2011**, *25*, e2473. [CrossRef]
133. Schiavone, S.; Tucci, P.; Mhillaj, E.; Bove, M.; Trabace, L.; Morgese, M.G. Antidepressant drugs for beta amyloid-induced depression: A new standpoint? *Prog. Neuro-Psychopharmacol. Biol. Psychiatry* **2017**, *78*, 114–122. [CrossRef] [PubMed]
134. Morgese, M.G.; Tucci, P.; Mhillaj, E.; Bove, M.; Schiavone, S.; Trabace, L.; Cuomo, V. Lifelong nutritional omega-3 deficiency evokes depressive-like state through soluble beta amyloid. *Mol. Neurobiol.* **2017**, *54*, 2079–2089. [CrossRef] [PubMed]

Sample Availability: All the compounds used in this work are commercially available. Details about selling companies are provided in Materials and Methods.

molecules

MDPI

Article

Insights into Heterologous Biosynthesis of Arteannuin B and Artemisinin in *Physcomitrella patens*

Nur Kusaira Khairul Ikram [1,2], Arman Beyraghdar Kashkooli [3,4], Anantha Peramuna [5], Alexander R. van der Krol [3], Harro Bouwmeester [3,6] and Henrik Toft Simonsen [5,*]

1 Institute of Biological Sciences, Faculty of Science, University of Malaya, Kuala Lumpur 50603, Malaysia; nkusaira@um.edu.my
2 Centre for Research in Biotechnology for Agriculture (CEBAR), University of Malaya, Kuala Lumpur 50603, Malaysia
3 Laboratory of Plant Physiology, Wageningen University and Research, Droevendaalsesteeg 1, 6708 PB Wageningen, The Netherlands; arman.beyraghdarkashkooli@wur.nl (A.B.K.); sander.vanderkrol@wur.nl (A.R.v.d.K.); h.j.bouwmeester@uva.nl (H.B.)
4 Bioscience, Wageningen Plant Research, Wageningen University and Research, Droevendaalsesteeg 1, 6708 PB Wageningen, The Netherlands
5 Department of Biotechnology and Biomedicine, Technical University of Denmark, Søltofts Plads, 2800 Kgs. Lyngby, Denmark; aperamuna@gmail.com
6 Plant Hormone Biology group, Swammerdam Institute for Life Sciences, University of Amsterdam, 1098 XH Amsterdam, The Netherlands
* Correspondence: hets@dtu.dk

Academic Editors: Pinarosa Avato and Thomas J. Schmidt
Received: 20 June 2019; Accepted: 21 October 2019; Published: 23 October 2019

Abstract: Metabolic engineering is an integrated bioengineering approach, which has made considerable progress in producing terpenoids in plants and fermentable hosts. Here, the full biosynthetic pathway of artemisinin, originating from *Artemisia annua*, was integrated into the moss *Physcomitrella patens*. Different combinations of the five artemisinin biosynthesis genes were ectopically expressed in *P. patens* to study biosynthesis pathway activity, but also to ensure survival of successful transformants. Transformation of the first pathway gene, *ADS*, into *P. patens* resulted in the accumulation of the expected metabolite, amorpha-4,11-diene, and also accumulation of a second product, arteannuin B. This demonstrates the presence of endogenous promiscuous enzyme activity, possibly cytochrome P450s, in *P. patens*. Introduction of three pathway genes, *ADS-CYP71AV1-ADH1* or *ADS-DBR2-ALDH1* both led to the accumulation of artemisinin, hinting at the presence of one or more endogenous enzymes in *P. patens* that can complement the partial pathways to full pathway activity. Transgenic *P. patens* lines containing the different gene combinations produce artemisinin in varying amounts. The pathway gene expression in the transgenic moss lines correlates well with the chemical profile of pathway products. Moreover, expression of the pathway genes resulted in lipid body formation in all transgenic moss lines, suggesting that these may have a function in sequestration of heterologous metabolites. This work thus provides novel insights into the metabolic response of *P. patens* and its complementation potential for *A. annua* artemisinin pathway genes. Identification of the related endogenous *P. patens* genes could contribute to a further successful metabolic engineering of artemisinin biosynthesis, as well as bioengineering of other high-value terpenoids in *P. patens*.

Keywords: artemisinin; *Physcomitrella patens*; sesquiterpenoids; malaria; biotechnology

1. Introduction

Artemisinin is a potent malaria drug that is exclusively produced in the plant *Artemisia annua*. The limited production of artemisinin in glandular trichomes of leaves and flowers has led to an extensive cultivation of *Artemisia* plants to meet the needs of the patients. The complex structure of artemisinin makes the chemical synthesis difficult and expensive. Therefore, various efforts have been performed to improve the production of artemisinin in the plant. As alternative, other hosts for heterologous production have been explored, but currently artemisinin production is still mainly based on the use of cultivated plants.

All genes responsible for the biosynthesis of the direct precursor of artemisinin, dihydroartemisinic acid, have been characterized (Scheme 1) [1]. The final conversion of dihydroartemisinic acid to artemisinin is thought to be a light-induced non-enzymatic spontaneous reaction [2]. The first committed biosynthetic step is the cyclization of endogenous farnesyl diphosphate (FPP) to amorpha-4,11-diene by amorpha-4,11-diene synthase (ADS) [3–6], which is substrate for the next enzyme amorphadiene monooxygenase (CYP71AV1). CYP71AV1 is an important cytochrome P450 enzyme [7] in artemisinin biosynthesis as it catalyses three subsequent oxidations of amorpha-4,11-diene to artemisinic acid, via artemisinic alcohol and artemisinic aldehyde [8]. However, in addition the alcohol dehydrogenase 1 (ADH1, a dehydrogenase/reductase enzyme) has been identified, which specifically produces artemisinic aldehyde from artemisinic alcohol (Scheme 1). This specificity and strong expression in *A. annua* glandular trichomes likely indicates that ADH1 is mainly responsible for biosynthesis of artemisinic aldehyde [9,10]. Artemisinic aldehyde is at a branch point in the bifurcating pathway producing either dihydroartemisinic acid or artemisinic acid [9,10]. In the branch leading to artemisinin, artemisinic aldehyde is reduced to dihydroartemisinic aldehyde by artemisinic aldehyde Δ11(13)-reductase (DBR2) and subsequently is oxidized to dihydroartemisinic acid by an aldehyde dehydrogenase (ALDH1) [11–13]. Besides catalysing the oxidation of dihydroartemisinic aldehyde to dihydroartemisinic acid in one branch, in a second pathway branch ALDH1 also catalyses the oxidation of artemisinic aldehyde to artemisinic acid (a reaction also catalysed by CYP71AV1) [7,12]. Another enzyme, dihydroartemisinic aldehyde reductase (RED1) converts dihydroartemisinic aldehyde into dihydroartemisinic alcohol, a "dead end" product, which negatively affects the yield of artemisinin [11]. The final steps in the two branches of the pathway likely involves photo-oxidation of dihydroartemisinic acid and artemisinic acid to artemisinin and arteannuin B, respectively [2,7].

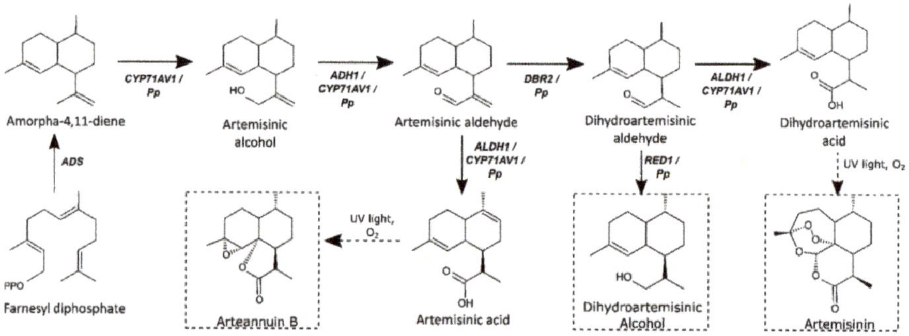

Scheme 1. The biosynthetic pathways of artemisinin and arteannuin B in *Artemisia annua*. *Pp* annotation represents possible native *P. patens* enzyme activity. *ADS*, amorphadiene synthase; *CYP71AV1*, amorphadiene oxidase; *ADH1*, alcohol dehydrogenase; *DBR2*, artemisinic aldehyde double-bond reductase; *ALDH1*, aldehyde dehydrogenase 1. The boxes indicate the products of the pathway.

Taking advantage of the elucidated artemisinin pathway, metabolic engineering has been a popular approach to improve the production of artemisinin or its precursors in heterologous hosts such as *E. coli*, yeast and tobacco. A production of amorpha-4,11-diene at 24 g/L was established through the introduction of the MVA pathway and ADS in *E. coli* along with several other modifications [14]. However, expressing plant P450s (such as CYP71AV1) in *E. coli* is not favourable. Therefore *Saccharomyces cerevisiae* (baker's yeast) was engineered to boost the MVA pathway and ADS through several modifications resulting in a yeast strain producing 153 mg/L amorpha-4,11-diene [8]. Subsequently, CYP71AV1 and a cytochrome P450 reductase (CPR) were introduced resulting in production of up to 100 mg/L of artemisinic acid [8]. The strains were further optimized by adding ADH1, ALDH1 and CYPB5, a native partner of CYP71AV1, that contributed to a significant increase of 25 g/L artemisinic acid via fermentation [9]. Although in these systems complete artemisinin biosynthesis is not accomplished, a 3-step chemical conversion from artemisinic acid to artemisinin has been developed and is currently used in commercial production of artemisinin in combination with yeast fermentation [9,15].

Introducing artemisinin pathway genes in tobacco has also been successful, using both stable and transient expression [16–21]. However, in tobacco pathway intermediates are efficiently glycosylated, resulting in low artemisinin yield [16,19]. Attempts have been made to target pathway enzymes to different compartments such as the chloroplast, and Fuentes et al. were able to produce 120 μg/g dry weight (d.w.) artemisinic acid [20], while Malhotra et al. produced 0.8 mg/g d.w. artemisinin in *Nicotiana benthamiana* [22]. All these attempts involved extensive bioengineering of precursor pathways and pathway localization, which is time consuming and with limited success in increasing final yield. Recent work has shown that *Physcomitrella patens* can be a promising heterologous host for artemisinin production, with a high yield of artemisinin after three days, prior to any production enhancements [21,23].

In the present study, various combinations of the pathway genes are assembled to study the biosynthetic route and the interplay with endogenous metabolism as well as ensuring the survival of successful transformants. We observed biosynthetic routes not previously described in the metabolic network of *P. patens* and demonstrate that some endogenous *P. patens* enzymes have promiscuous substrate recognition, which may substitute for some *A. annua* pathway enzyme activities. This provides new insight into *P. patens* metabolism and offers alternative engineering targets for production of artemisinin in this primitive plant and promising heterologous production platform.

2. Results and Discussion

2.1. Heterologous Expression of Artemisinin Biosynthesis Pathway Genes

The gene encoding the first committed enzyme in the artemisinin biosynthesis pathway (ADS) was introduced into the wild-type (WT) *P. patens*. Integration of the gene was confirmed by PCR on genomic DNA isolated from transformants (Figure S1) and metabolic profiling showed that amorpha-4,11-diene was produced in cultures up to levels up to 200 mg/L [23]. However, localization of the amorpha-4,11-diene remains unclear: is it stored in specific organelles such as lipid bodies or transported out of the cell? Several studies have shown that *P. patens* is able to ectopically produce volatile terpenoids, but the regulation of volatiles production and their potential storage within *P. patens* is yet to be explored [23–25]. Besides amorpha-4,11-diene, the transgenic lines expressing *ADS* also accumulated arteannuin B, which is thought to be derived from artemisinic acid through photo-oxidation. This suggest accumulation of artemisinic acid in the transgenic lines and reveals a promiscuous activity of an endogenous oxidative enzyme (or enzymes) such as the cytochrome P450 in *P. patens*, which can catalyse the triple oxidation of amorpha-4,11-diene via artemisinic alcohol and aldehyde to the acid. In *A. annua* these activities are catalysed by CYP71AV1 and ADH1 [8,26]. Although predominant results indicate that most plant P450s are highly specific in their substrate recognition, increasing evidence shows that some plant P450s can be promiscuous in substrate recognition, similar to mammalian P450s [27–30]. Endogenous *P. patens* oxidative enzymes fully convert amorpha-4,11-diene to artemisinic acid, since the alcohol and aldehyde intermediates were not detected in culture extracts. *P. patens* naturally produces high amounts of *ent*-kaurenoic acid from *ent*-kaurene, which is catalysed by an *ent*-kaurene oxidase (CYP701B1) through three successive oxidations [31,32]. CYP701B1 may therefore be a likely candidate for catalysing the conversion of amorpha-4,11-diene into artemisinic acid in *P. patens*. Other possible candidate enzymes are the numerous cytochrome P450s, ferrodoxin mono-oxygenases, and other oxidoreductases encoded by the *P. patens* genome.

Having established transgenic lines producing a high level of amorpha-4,11-diene, a second transformation introduced the second (*CYP71AV1*) and third (*ADH1*) artemisinin pathway genes. Likewise, the final two artemisinin pathway genes, *DBR2* and *ALDH1* were also introduced into the *ADS* background lines. Having successfully introduced two different sets of 3 artemisinin genes; *ADS-CYP71AV1-ADH1* and *ADS-DBR2-ALDH1* in *P. patens*, the remaining artemisinin pathway genes were introduced into these transgenic lines. This resulted in transgenic lines with all five artemisinin biosynthesis genes in different genomic sequential arrangements. The transgenic lines *ADS-CYP71AV1-ADH1-DBR2-ALDH1* and *ADS-DBR2-ALDH1-CYP71AV1-ADH1* were recovered and genotyping showed the presence of all five artemisinin biosynthesis genes in the genome of *P. patens* (Figure S1).

2.2. Metabolite Profiling of Transgenic P. patens Lines

In total five different transgenic lines were produced (Table 1). Metabolic profiling of these lines showed that artemisinin was produced in all lines, except for the transgenic line solely expressing *ADS*. The *ADS-CYP71AV1-ADH1* line only produced 25% of the artemisinin levels in the *ADS-DBR2-ALDH1* line. This suggests that in the *ADS-DBR2-ALDH1* line the *P. patens* oxidizing enzymes efficiently convert amorpha-4,11-diene to artemisinic aldehyde, which is then converted by DBR2 and ALDH1 to dihydroartemisinic acid (Scheme 1, Table 1). Interestingly, two other metabolites; artemisinic alcohol and dihydroartemisinic alcohol were also detected in the *ADS-DBR2-ALDH1* line. Notably, ADH1 is specific towards artemisinic alcohol [9] and absence of ADH1 in the *ADS-DBR2-ALDH1* lines may explain the accumulation of artemisinic alcohol in this line. The presence of dihydroartemisinic alcohol in the *ADS-DBR2-ALDH1* lines suggests that *P. patens* has an endogenous oxidoreductases similar to *A. annua* RED1 that catalyses the formation of dihydroartemisinic alcohol from dihydroartemisinic aldehyde in *A. annua* [11].

Table 1. Quantification of artemisinin, artemisinin intermediates and arteannuin B produced in transgenic *Physcomitrella patens* and the moss culture liquid media (from 3 weeks moss culture, average of two cultures). The content in the liquid media represents the amount of molecules that have been excreted from the moss cells.

	ADS	ADS-CYP71AV1-ADH1	ADS-CYP71AV1-ADH1-DBR2-ALDH1	ADS- DBR2-ALDH1	ADS-DBR2-ALDH1-CYP71AV1-ADH1
Content in culture liquid media (without moss)	(µg/g FW)	(µg/g FW)	(µg/g FW)	(µg/g FW)	(µg/g FW)
Artemisinic alcohol	ND	ND	ND	ND	ND
Dihydroartemisinic alcohol	ND	ND	ND	0.09	ND
Arteannuin B	1.05	0.04	0.09	1.74	ND
Content in dried moss tissue	(mg/g DW)	(mg/g DW)	(mg/g DW)	(mg/g DW)	(mg/g DW)
Artemisinin	ND	0.01	0.03	0.04	0.01
Artemisinic alcohol	ND	ND	ND	0.13	ND
Dihydroartemisinic alcohol	ND	ND	ND	0.07	ND

ND, not detected.

Arteannuin B is mostly present in the liquid media (see Figure 1, Table 1) indicating transport capacity for artemisinic acid or arteannuin B to the outside of the cells. Alternatively, this could indicate that accumulation of these compounds is toxic to the cells that then die. The artemisinic aldehyde is at the branch point of the biosynthesis pathway, leading to either dihydroartemisinic acid (precursor of artemisinin) or artemisinic acid (precursor of arteannuin B) (Scheme 1). While *DBR2* catalyses the conversion of artemisinic aldehyde toward artemisinin production, *ALDH1* and *CYP71AV1* or *P. patens* hydroxylases catalyse the formation of artemisinic acid.

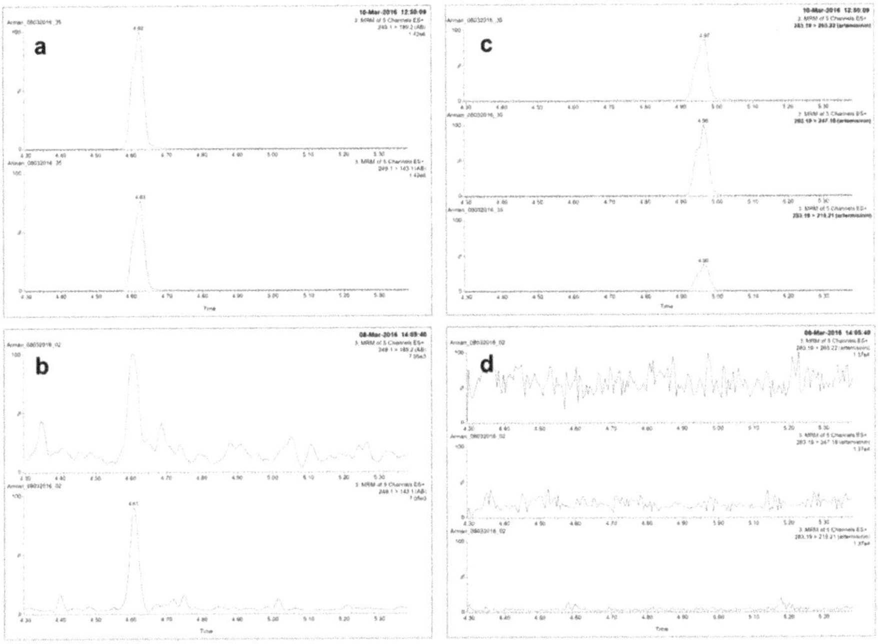

Figure 1. UPLC-MRM-MS analysis of arteannuin B. (**a**) UPLC-MRM-MS of arteannuin B standard fragmented in MRM channels of *m/z* 249.1 > 189.2; 249.1 > 143.1 (**b**) UPLC-MRM-MS analysis of arteannuin B in transformed *P. patens* with *ADS* (RT = 4.61). (**c**) UPLC-MRM-MS of artemisinin standard fragmented in MRM channels of *m/z* 283.19 > 219.21; 283.19 > 247.19 and 283.19 > 265.22 (RT = 4.96). (**d**) Demonstration of absence of artemisinin by UPLC-MRM-MS of artemisinin in fragmented in MRM channels of *m/z* 283.19 > 219.21; 283.19 > 247.19 and 283.19 > 265.22 of extracts from transformed *P. patens* with *ADS*. C+D show that artemisinin is not present in the *ADS* only lines of *P. patens*.

Our transgenic *P. patens* lines were grown under constant (24 h) high light intensity. Thus, all the produced artemisinic acid or dihydroartemisinic acid are presumably photo-chemically converted into arteannuin B and artemisinin, respectively and neither of the two acids were detected in our study.

The accumulation of arteannuin B was correlated with the amount of artemisinin. Transformants with higher levels of arteannuin B, also accumulates higher levels of artemisinin. For instance, *ADS-DBR2-ALDH1* accumulates most artemisinin as well as arteannuin B.

The accumulation of artemisinin in the *ADS-CYP71AV1-ADH1* line shows that *P. patens* has enzymes with similar activities as DBR2 and ALDH1 from *A. annua*. The lower artemisinin accumulation in the *ADS-CYP71AV1-ADH1* line suggests that the affinity of the endogenous *P. patens* enzyme for the pathway intermediates may not be as good as for *A. annua* DBR2 and ALDH1.

Although presence of endogenous enzyme activity might contribute to the accumulation of artemisinin, only arteannuin B was detected in the *ADS* expressing line (see Figure 1). One reason could be that the *P. patens* hydroxylases and oxidoreductases has lower affinity towards the heterologous substrates than the pathway enzymes, CYP71AV1, DBR2 and ALDH1. For example, higher levels of artemisinin was detected when CYP71AV1 was expressed (*ADS-CYP71AV1-ADH1*), which should accumulate artemisinic aldehyde, but this is catalysed into dihydroartemisinic acid by native hydroxylases and oxidoreductases.

Dihydroartemisinic acid spontaneously transform into artemisinin when exposed to light. Meanwhile, in the *ADS*-only line amorpha-4,11-diene accumulates and here the native hydroxylases might favour reactions resulting in a final accumulation of arteannuin B via artemisinic acid (see Scheme 1 for the pathway).

Unlike in other heterologous plants e.g., *Nicotiana benthamiana* [16], no glycosylated and/or glutathione conjugates of the artemisinin biosynthesis intermediate related products were detected in the transgenic *P. patens* lines [23]. The absence of glycosylated products could be due to the much lower number of genes encoding putative glycosyltransferases in *P. patens*, compared to that in higher (vascular) plants [33]. This could be an important feature of *P. patens* to favour full pathway activity toward the accumulation of the two products artemisinin and/or arteannuin B.

2.3. *Analysis of Artemisinin Pathway Gene Expression Profiles*

Analysis of the artemisinin biosynthetic gene expression profile was performed to investigate the correlation between gene expression and metabolite production in the transgenic lines (Figure 2). The expression of the first committed enzyme, ADS was the highest when it was introduced alone, and decreased with the increasing number of genes introduced; *ADS* > *ADS-CYP71AV1-ADH1* > *ADS-CYP71AV1-ADH1-DBR2-ALDH1*. A similar pattern was observed in the expression of the other constructs with *ADS* > *ADS-DBR2-ALDH1* > *ADS-DBR2-ALDH1-CYP71AV1-ADH1*. For *CYP71AV1*, there was no significant difference in expression between the *ADS-CYP71AV1-ADH1* and *ADS-DBR2-ALDH1-CYP71AV1-ADH1* lines. However, the expression level was 100 fold higher in the *ADS-CYP71AV1-ADH1-DBR2-ALDH1* line showing that higher amount of the enzyme could be present for the higher production of artemisinin. *ADH1* on the other hand exhibited a low expression pattern in all transgenic lines, suggesting its limited contribution to the overall artemisinin pathway in *P. patens*.

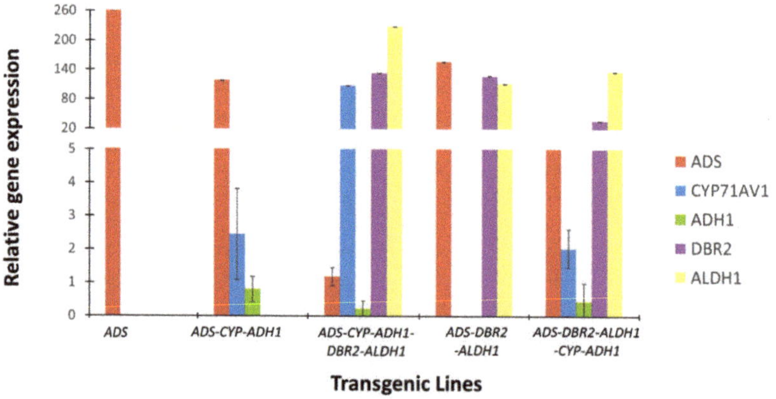

Figure 2. Relative expression of artemisinin pathway genes (*ADS, CYP71AV1, ADH1, DBR2, ALDH1*) in the five transgenic *P. patens* lines. Error bars are shown as SE (n = 3).

Overall, *ADS-DBR2-ALDH1* shows higher gene expressions for all three genes compared to the other transgenic lines and this correlates positively with the product levels. The expression level of the *ADS* gene in *ADS-DBR2-ALDH1* is the second highest, after the *ADS* only expressing line, which may lead to abundant amorpha-4,11-diene to be catalysed by *DBR2* into artemisinic aldehyde and subsequently into dihydroartemisinic acid by *ALDH1*. However, in addition, endogenous *P. patens* hydroxylases and *ALDH1* efficiently catalyse the formation of artemisinic acid, hence contributing to higher accumulation of arteannuin B than artemisinin (Table 1). The transgene expression levels in all the lines expressing *DBR2* and *ALDH1* correlate well with their end product profiles (Figure 2, Table 1). Similarly, lines *ADS-CYP71AV1-ADH1* and *ADS-DBR2-ALDH1-CYP71AV1-ADH1*, which show lower expression of *CYP71AV1*, also show lower levels of artemisinin. Results thus suggest that not only higher affinity for substrates but also abundance of the active *A. annua* enzymes has a positive impact on artemisinin levels. Improving expression and protein levels even further may therefore be targets for future research.

The expression of *DBR2* and *ALDH1* was relatively high and correlates with the amount of metabolite produced. Studies on the artemisinin pathway gene expression in different *A. annua* chemotypes: the high artemisinin producer (HAP) and low artemisinin producer (LAP) as well as the *Nicotiana benthamiana* transiently expressing the artemisinin biosynthetic pathway genes show that the expression of DBR2 is significantly higher in the HAP varieties which is similar to the gene expression pattern found in *P. patens* [16,34]. It is evident that *DBR2* and *ALDH1* appear to be of a great importance in elevating artemisinin production in *P. patens*, *A. annua* and other heterologous plant-based systems [16,20,34,35].

2.4. Lipid Body Formation in Transgenic P. patens

P. patens utilizes lipid bodies (LBs) in its life cycle [36] and because of the hydrophobic nature of artemisinin, we investigated whether ectopic expression of the artemisinin pathway in transgenic *P. patens* favours LB formation by LB staining with BODIPY. Confocal microscopy observations confirmed that abundant and large LBs are present in all transgenic lines (Figure 3). Formation of these LBs in response to production of potentially toxic compounds could indicate an alternative phytotoxic defence mechanism in *P. patens* prior to the development of alternative detoxification strategies through glycosylation as in higher plants. Glycosylation and modification by glutathione of pathway intermediates are the biggest competitor for production of artemisinin and other sesquiterpenes in heterologous plant expression systems. The absence of such detoxification mechanisms and induction of potential sequester structures like LBs in *P. patens* make this organism a potential valuable novel tool for production of artemisinin or other valuable terpenes. To address this, further research on the mechanism of lipid body formation and identification of LB composition in the transgenic *P. patens* will be valuable for an overall understanding on *P. patens* metabolic responses to heterologously produced metabolites.

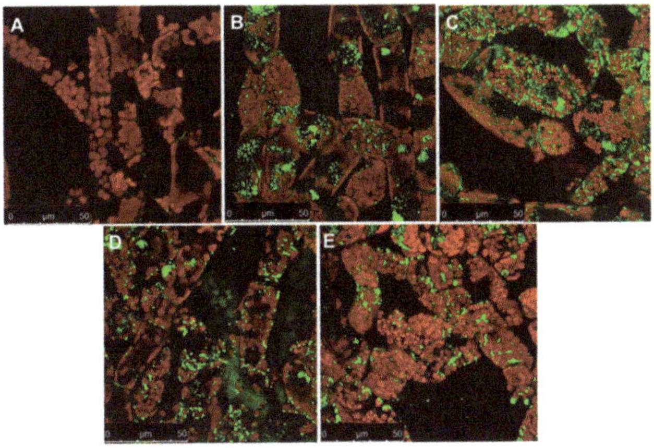

Figure 3. Projections of 8 day old moss obtained by confocal microscopy showing the accumulation of lipid bodies (green spots, stained with BODIPY) in wild type (**A**) and transgenic moss bearing (**B**) *ADS* (**C**) *ADS-CYP71AV1-ADH1* (**D**) *ADS-DBR2-ALDH1* (**E**) *ADS-CYP71AV1-ADH1-DBR2-ALDH1*. Red color represent chlorophyll autofluorescence.

3. Materials and Methods

3.1. Plant Material and Growth Conditions

P. patens (Gransden ecotype, International Moss Stock Center #40001) was grown on solid and liquid PhyB media under sterile conditions, at 25 °C with continuous 20–50 W/m^2 light intensity [37].

3.2. DNA Fragments and Genes

The Pp108 locus homologous recombination flanking regions were amplified from genomic DNA of *P. patens*. The *ADS* gene was a kind gift from Assoc. Prof. Dae Kyun Ro, University of Calgary, Calgary, AB, Canada. The synthetic genes of *CYP71AV1* (DQ268763), *ADH1* (JF910157.1), *DBR2* (EU704257.1), and *ALDH1* (FJ809784.1) were synthesized by GenScript (city, state abbrev USA) according to the *P. paten* codon usage. The synthetic genes was linked with a peptide linker LP4/2A from *Impatiens balsamina* and foot-and-mouth-disease virus (FMDV); *CYP71AV1*-LP4/2A-*ADH1*, *DBR2*-LP4/2A-*ALDH1*. The Ubiquitin promoter and Ubiquitin terminator from *Arabidopsis thaliana* (CP002686.1) synthetic genes were also synthesized by GenScript. The Maize Ubiquitin 1 promoter, *OCS* terminator and G418 selection cassettes was obtained from the pMP1355 vector, a kind gift from Professor Mark Estelle, University of California San Diego, San Diego, CA, USA.

3.3. Transformation Procedures

A detailed description of moss transformation has been previously published [37,38]. Five to seven day old *P. patens* cultures (from last blending) was harvested and digested with 0.5% DriselaseR enzyme solution in 8.5% mannitol (D9515, Sigma Aldrich) followed by incubation at room temperature for 30 to 60 min. The digested sample was then filtered through a 100 µm pored mesh-filter and the protoplast was collected by centrifugation at 150–200× *g* for 4 min with slow breaking. The pellet was washed twice with the protoplast wash solution (8.5% mannitol, 10 mM $CaCl_2$) and the protoplast density was measured using a hemocytometer before suspending in MMM solution (9.1% D-mannitol, 10% MES and 15mM $MgCl_2$) to a concentration of 1.6 × 106 protoplasts/mL. 300 µL of the protoplast suspension and 300 µL of PEG solution were added to a 15 mL tube containing 10 µg total DNA and incubated at 45 °C for 5 min and another 5 min at room temperature. 8.5% D-mannitol (300 µL) was then added five times and dilutions with 1 mL of 8.5% D-mannitol another five times. The transformed protoplasts were collected by centrifugation, resuspended in 500 µL of 8.5% D-mannitol and 2.5 mL of protoplast regeneration media (top layer; PRMT). One ml of the mixture was distributed on three plates containing protoplast regeneration media (bottom layer; PRMB) overlaid with cellophane. The plates were incubated in continuous light for 5 to 7 days at 25 °C. The cellophane and regenerating protoplasts was then transferred to PhyB media containing the appropriate selection marker for two weeks, before transferring on PhyB media without antibiotics for another 2 weeks and later transferred back to the final antibiotic selection to confirmed stable transformants.

The first committed precursor of artemisinin biosynthesis pathway, *ADS* was introduced into wildtype *P. patens* at the designated neutral locus Pp108. The transformed lines were selected on regeneration medium with geneticin (G418) for two rounds of selection. Next, we transformed the second and third: *CYP71AV1*-LP4/2A-*ADH1* as well as the fourth and fifth; *DBR2*-LP4/2A-*ALDH1* genes respectively into the *ADS*-expressing transgenic line. Both transformations are targeted to replace the previously transformed G418 selection marker with the new selection of hygromycin. Having successfully introduced three artemisinin genes; *ADS-CYP71AV1-ADH1* and *ADS-DBR2-ALDH1* in *P. patens*, we next completed the pathway with addition of the remaining artemisinin genes into both transgenic lines. For this transformation, the previously removed G418 selection marker was used again and hygromycin was targeted for recombination such that this selection marker was removed.

3.4. PCR, DNA Purification and Concentration

All DNA fragments were amplified with PhusionR High-Fidelity DNA Polymerase (New England Biolabs, County Road Ipswich, MA, USA). PCR conditions and annealing temperatures were modified depending on primers and templates used in the reaction. PCR reactions using plasmid DNA as template were digested with DpnI (NEB, County Road Ipswich, MA, USA) for 1 h at 37 °C followed by inactivation at 65 °C for 20 min to lower background after transformation. PCR products were purified using QIAquick PCR Purification Kit (Qiagen GmbH, Strasse 1, Hilden, Germany). The DNA fragments for transformations were concentrated via ethanol precipitation to a final concentration of ~1 µg/µL, determined using NanoDrop2000 (Thermo Fisher Scientific, Waltham, MA, USA). The primers used are listed in Table S1.

3.5. Metabolite Profiling

3.5.1. UPLC-MRM-MS Analysis

Fresh moss samples were harvested, snap-frozen and ground into a fine powder. Samples of 3000 mg were extracted with 3 mL citrate phosphate buffer, pH 5.4, followed by vortexing and sonication for 15 min. One mL of Viscozyme (V2010, Sigma) was added and samples were incubated at 37 °C. The whole mixture was then extracted three times with 3 mL ethyl acetate and concentrated to a volume of 1 mL and stored at −20 °C. For liquid culture extracts, 500 mL of liquid culture was harvested, passed through a filter paper and extracted with 200 mL of ethyl acetate in a separation funnel. Ethyl acetate was concentrated to a volume of 1 mL and stored at −20 °C. Ethyl acetate of both liquid culture and moss sample extracts were then dried under a flow of N_2 and resuspended into 300 µL of 75% MeOH:H_2O (*v*:*v*). Extracts were passed through a 0.45 µm membrane filter (Minisart® RC4, Sartorius, Germany) before analysis. Artemisinin and artemisinin biosynthesis pathway intermediates were measured in a targeted approach by using a Waters Xevo tandem quadrupole mass spectrometer equipped with an electrospray ionization source and coupled to an Acuity UPLC system (Waters), essentially as described [16]. For A BEH C18 column (100 × 2.1 mm × 1.7 µm; Waters) was used for chromatographic separation by applying a water:acetonitrile gradient. The gradient started from 5% (*v*/*v*) acetonitrile in water with formic acid [1:1000 (*v*/*v*)] for 1.25 min, was raised to 50% in 2.35 min and was raised to 90% at 3.65 min. This was kept for 0.75 min before returning to the 5% acetonitrile/water (*v*/*v*) with formic acid [1:1000 (*v*/*v*)] by using a 0.15 min gradient. The same solvent composition was used to equilibrate the column for 1.85 min. The flow rate was 0.5 mL/min and the column temperature was maintained at 50 °C. Injection volume was set to 10 µL. Desolvation and cone gas flow were set to 1000 and 50 L/h and the mass spectrometer was operated in positive ionization mode. Capillary voltage was set at 3.0 kV. Desolvation and source temperatures were set at 650 and 150 °C, respectively. The cone voltage was optimized for all metabolites using the Waters IntelliStart MS Console. Fragmentation by collision-induced dissociation was done in the ScanWave collision cell using argon. Multiple Reaction Monitoring (MRM) was used for detection and quantification of artemisinin and the other compounds. MRM transitions for artemisinin and pathway intermediates measurement settings were optimized for MRM channels, which are presented in Table S2. Targeted analysis of the fragmentation pattern of authenticated standard was optimized for each of the target compounds. For artemisinin three parent(/daughter) ions (expressed as channels) was obtained and for arteannuin B two channels were identified, as previously described [16,23]. The presence or absence of each compound in samples were checked by comparing the RT of compounds in standard mix with samples. As an additional quality measure the ratio between peak intensity of each compound's channels (e.g., for artemisinin the ratio of 283.19 > 219.21 to 283.19 > 247.19 in samples should be the same as the ratio in what has been measured in artemisinin standard) were checked which was the same in both standards and the identified compounds in samples. Retention time of each compound (positive ionization mode) is presented in Table S3. Artemisinin and dihydroartemisinic acid were gift from Dafra Pharma (Belgium). Other precursors were synthesized from dihydroartemisinic acid by

Chiralix (Nijmegen, the Netherlands) which was checked by NMR (>98% purity). External calibration curves were measured by using reference standards.

3.5.2. LC-QTOF-MS for Analysis of Conjugated Artemisinin Pathway Intermediates

For the artemisinin pathway intermediates glycosides and conjugations, 100 mg of fresh *P. patens* tissue was ground in liquid nitrogen and extracted with 300 µl MeOH:formic acid [1000:1 (*v*/*v*)]. Samples were briefly vortexed and sonicated for 15 min, followed by 15 min centrifugation at 13,000× *g*. Extracts were passed through a 0.45 µm membrane filter (Minisart® RC4, Sartorius) before analysis on a Water alliance 2795 HPLC connected to a QTOF Ultima V 4.00.00 mass spectrometer (Waters MS Technologies). The mass spectrometer was operated in negative ionization mode. A precolumn of 2.0 × 4 mm (Phenomenex, Denmark) was connected to the C18 analytical column (Luna 3 µm C18/2 100A; 2.0 × 150 mm; Phenomenex). Degassed eluent A and B were HPLC-grade water:formic acid [1000:1 (*v*/*v*)] and acetonitrile:formic acid [1000:1 (*v*/*v*)], respectively. The flow rate was 0.19 mL/min. The HPLC gradient started from 5% eluent B and linearly increased to 75% in 45 min. After that, the column was equilibrated for 15 min with 5% eluent B. 5 µL of each sample was used for injection.

3.6. Lipid Bodies Staining and Microscopy

Equal amount of 14 days old liquid grown cells were suspended in PBS pH 7.4 buffer and stained with a final concentration of 0.5 µg/mL of BIODIPY 505/515 (Invitrogen Molecular Probes, Thermo Fisher). Cells were incubated in the dark for 15 min and visualized with a Leica LAS AF confocal laser microscope. Lipid bodies were visualized with a 488 nm laser excitation line and a 510–530 nm emission window. Chloroplasts were visualized using the same laser line and a 650–700 nm excitation window. Z stacks were performed on each image with a line average of 4 and combined using maximum projection into a single image, and image was visualized with ImageJ [39].

3.7. Expression Profiling in P. patens

100 mg of one week old moss tissue was extracted by RNeasy Plant Mini Kit (Qiagen 74904) according to the protocol provided. The samples were treated with DNase I (Sigma AMPD1) to remove remaining genomic DNA. The RNA quality and concentration was determined by Nanodrop2000 Spectrophotometer (Thermo Fisher Scientific). cDNA synthesis was performed with 500 ng RNA samples using SuperScript III First-Strand Synthesis System for RT-PCR kit (18080-051, Life Technologies, Denmark). Real time quantitative PCR was performed using QuantiFast ® SYBR ® Green PCR (Qiagen, Denmark) according to the protocol provided and run at 95 °C for 5 min, 40 cycles at 95 °C for 10 s followed by 60 °C for 30 s on a CFX Connect Real Time PCR Detection System (BioRad, Denmark). The qPCR was performed with three biological replicates for each sample and three technical replicates for each biological sample. Primers used are listed in (Table S1). Efficiencies of all primers were estimated by generating a standard curve via cDNA serial dilutions using this formula $E = 10^{-1/slope} - 1$. E values of the primer pairs ranged between 93 to 101% (efficiency between 90 and 110% are acceptable). *P. patens* β-actin was used as the reference gene and the transcripts level was calculated as follows: $\Delta CT = CT(GOI) - CT(Actin)$, $\Delta\Delta CT$ was normalized using ΔCT and the relative change in gene expression is calculated by $2^{-\Delta\Delta CT}$ method [40].

4. Conclusions

Here we show that the anti-malaria drug, artemisinin, can be produced in *P. patens* with either complete or partial introduction and expression of the artemisinin pathway genes. The results demonstrate that *P. patens* expresses endogenous enzymes with similar activity to that of the artemisinin biosynthesis pathway in *A. annua*. This possibly affects the accumulation of artemisinin and arteannuin B. Knocking out the endogenous oxidizing enzyme(s) responsible for the conversion of amorpha-4,11-diene into artemisinic acid could possibly positively affect the yield of artemisinin as it could stimulate the flux towards dihydroartemisinic aldehyde. This work provides novel insights into the metabolic machinery of *P. patens* and shows it has enzymes with activities similar to those that catalyse the artemisinin pathway in *A. annua*. Discovery of these enzymes and the encoding genes may contribute not only to successful metabolic engineering of artemisinin biosynthesis in *P. patens*, but also to the engineering of other high-value terpenes in *P. patens*. Enzymes with promiscuous activity can be of high value for any synthetic biology adventure since they can be used for many purposes. They also shed light on general enzyme activity for the specific classes of enzymes. Work is ongoing to discover these enzymes.

Supplementary Materials: The following are available online. Figure S1 shows the Genotyping of the moss, Figures S2 and S3 show UPLC-MRM-MS analysis of artemisinin and arteannuin B, respectively from the different P. patens transgenic lines. Table S1 shows primers used in the study and Table S2 is the optimized MRM transition settings for UPLC-MRM-MS.

Author Contributions: For this paper the authors contributed as follows: Conceptualization, N.K.K.I., and H.T.S.; Methodology, N.K.K.I., A.B.K., and A.P.; Validation, N.K.K.I. and A.B.K.; Formal analysis, N.K.K.I. and A.B.K.; Investigation, N.K.K.I., A.B.K., and A.P.; Resources, N.K.K.I., A.B.K., and H.T.S.; Data curation, N.K.K.I, A.P. and A.B.K.; Writing—original draft preparation, N.K.K.I.; Writing—review and editing, N.K.K.I., A.B.K., A.P., A.R.v.d.K., H.B., and H.T.S.; Visualization, N.K.K.I., and A.B.K., Supervision, A.R.v.d.K., H.B, and H.T.S.; Project administration, H.T.S; Funding acquisition,, N.K.K.I, A.R.v.d.K., H.B., and H.T.S.

Funding: Nur Kusaira Binti Khairul Ikram was supported by a grant from the Ministry of Higher Education, Malaysia and the University of Malaya. Anantha Peramuna and Henrik Toft Simonsen was supported by The Danish Council for Independent Research (#4005-00158B).

Acknowledgments: The authors would like to thank Mark Estelle, Yuji Hiwatashi and Dae Kyun Ro for kindly providing the pMP1355, and PZAG1 vector and the ADS template.

Conflicts of Interest: All authors declare that they have no conflict of interest. HTS is co-founder of Mosspiration Biotech IVS that aim to produce fragrances in *P. patens*, but not artemisinin.

References

1. Xie, D.-Y.; Ma, D.-M.; Judd, R.; Jones, A.L. Artemisinin biosynthesis in *Artemisia annua* and metabolic engineering: Questions, challenges, and perspectives. *Phytochem. Rev.* **2016**, *15*, 1093–1114. [CrossRef]
2. Sy, L.-K.; Brown, G.D. The mechanism of the spontaneous autoxidation of dihydroartemisinic acid. *Tetrahedron* **2002**, *58*, 897–908. [CrossRef]
3. Bouwmeester, H.J.; Wallaart, T.E.; Janssen, M.H.; van Loo, B.; Jansen, B.J.; Posthumus, M.A.; Schmidt, C.O.; De Kraker, J.-W.; König, W.A.; Franssen, M.C. Amorpha-4, 11-diene synthase catalyses the first probable step in artemisinin biosynthesis. *Phytochemistry* **1999**, *52*, 843–854. [CrossRef]
4. Mercke, P.; Bengtsson, M.; Bouwmeester, H.J.; Posthumus, M.A.; Brodelius, P.E. Molecular cloning, expression, and characterization of amorpha-4, 11-diene synthase, a key enzyme of artemisinin biosynthesis in *Artemisia annua* L. *Arch. Biochem. Biophys.* **2000**, *381*, 173–180. [CrossRef] [PubMed]
5. Picaud, S.; Mercke, P.; He, X.; Sterner, O.; Brodelius, M.; Cane, D.E.; Brodelius, P.E. Amorpha-4,11-diene synthase: Mechanism and stereochemistry of the enzymatic cyclization of farnesyl diphosphate. *Arch. Biochem. Biophys.* **2006**, *448*, 150–155. [CrossRef] [PubMed]
6. Picaud, S.; Olofsson, L.; Brodelius, M.; Brodelius, P.E. Expression, purification, and characterization of recombinant amorpha-4,11-diene synthase from *Artemisia annua* L. *Arch. Biochem. Biophys.* **2005**, *436*, 215–226. [CrossRef]
7. Teoh, K.H.; Polichuk, D.R.; Reed, D.W.; Nowak, G.; Covello, P.S. *Artemisia annua* L. (Asteraceae) trichome-specific cdnas reveal CYP71AV1, a cytochrome p450 with a key role in the biosynthesis of the antimalarial sesquiterpene lactone artemisinin. *FEBS Lett.* **2006**, *580*, 1411–1416. [CrossRef]
8. Ro, D.-K.; Paradise, E.M.; Ouellet, M.; Fisher, K.J.; Newman, K.L.; Ndungu, J.M.; Ho, K.A.; Eachus, R.A.; Ham, T.S.; Kirby, J. Production of the antimalarial drug precursor artemisinic acid in engineered yeast. *Nature* **2006**, *440*, 940. [CrossRef]
9. Paddon, C.J.; Westfall, P.; Pitera, D.; Benjamin, K.; Fisher, K.; McPhee, D.; Leavell, M.; Tai, A.; Main, A.; Eng, D. High-level semi-synthetic production of the potent antimalarial artemisinin. *Nature* **2013**, *496*, 528–532. [CrossRef]
10. Olofsson, L.; Engstrom, A.; Lundgren, A.; Brodelius, P. Relative expression of genes of terpene metabolism in different tissues of *Artemisia annua* L. *BMC Plant Biol.* **2011**, *11*, 45. [CrossRef]

11. Rydén, A.-M.; Ruyter-Spira, C.; Quax, W.J.; Osada, H.; Muranaka, T.; Kayser, O.; Bouwmeester, H. The molecular cloning of dihydroartemisinic aldehyde reductase and its implication in artemisinin biosynthesis in *Artemisia annua*. *Planta Med.* **2010**, *76*, 1778. [CrossRef] [PubMed]
12. Teoh, K.H.; Polichuk, D.R.; Reed, D.W.; Covello, P.S. Molecular cloning of an aldehyde dehydrogenase implicated in artemisinin biosynthesis in *Artemisia annua* this paper is one of a selection of papers published in a special issue from the national research council of canada-plant biotechnology institute. *Botany* **2009**, *87*, 635–642. [CrossRef]
13. Zhang, Y.; Teoh, K.H.; Reed, D.W.; Maes, L.; Goossens, A.; Olson, D.J.; Ross, A.R.; Covello, P.S. The molecular cloning of artemisinic aldehyde δ11 (13) reductase and its role in glandular trichome-dependent biosynthesis of artemisinin in *Artemisia annua*. *J. Biol. Chem.* **2008**, *283*, 21501–21508. [CrossRef] [PubMed]
14. Martin, V.J.J.; Pitera, D.J.; Withers, S.T.; Newman, J.D.; Keasling, J.D. Engineering a mevalonate pathway in *Escherichia coli* for production of terpenoids. *Nat. Biotech.* **2003**, *21*, 796–802. [CrossRef]
15. Paddon, C.J.; Keasling, J.D. Semi-synthetic artemisinin: A model for the use of synthetic biology in pharmaceutical development. *Nat. Rev. Microbiol.* **2014**, *12*, 355. [CrossRef]
16. Ting, H.M.; Wang, B.; Rydén, A.M.; Woittiez, L.; Herpen, T.; Verstappen, F.W.; Ruyter-Spira, C.; Beekwilder, J.; Bouwmeester, H.J.; Krol, A. The metabolite chemotype of *Nicotiana benthamiana* transiently expressing artemisinin biosynthetic pathway genes is a function of CYP71AV1 type and relative gene dosage. *New Phytol.* **2013**, *199*, 352–366. [CrossRef]
17. Farhi, M.; Marhevka, E.; Ben-Ari, J.; Algamas-Dimantov, A.; Liang, Z.; Zeevi, V.; Edelbaum, O.; Spitzer-Rimon, B.; Abeliovich, H.; Schwartz, B. Generation of the potent anti-malarial drug artemisinin in tobacco. *Nat. Biotechnol.* **2011**, *29*, 1072–1074. [CrossRef]
18. Zhang, Y.; Nowak, G.; Reed, D.W.; Covello, P.S. The production of artemisinin precursors in tobacco. *Plant Biotechnol. J.* **2011**, *9*, 445–454. [CrossRef]
19. Wang, B.; Kashkooli, A.B.; Sallets, A.; Ting, H.-M.; de Ruijter, N.C.; Olofsson, L.; Brodelius, P.; Pottier, M.; Boutry, M.; Bouwmeester, H. Transient production of artemisinin in *Nicotiana benthamiana* is boosted by a specific lipid transfer protein from a. Annua. *Metab. Eng.* **2016**, *38*, 159–169. [CrossRef]
20. Fuentes, P.; Zhou, F.; Erban, A.; Karcher, D.; Kopka, J.; Bock, R. A new synthetic biology approach allows transfer of an entire metabolic pathway from a medicinal plant to a biomass crop. *eLife* **2016**, *5*, e13664. [CrossRef]
21. Ikram, N.K.; Simonsen, H.T. A review of biotechnological artemisinin production in plants. *Front. Plant Sci.* **2017**, *8*, 1966. [CrossRef] [PubMed]
22. Malhotra, K.; Subramaniyan, M.; Rawat, K.; Kalamuddin, M.; Qureshi, M.I.; Malhotra, P.; Mohmmed, A.; Cornish, K.; Daniell, H.; Kumar, S. Compartmentalized metabolic engineering for artemisinin biosynthesis and effective malaria treatment by oral delivery of plant cells. *Mol. Plant* **2016**, *9*, 1464–1477. [CrossRef] [PubMed]
23. Ikram, K.; Binti, N.K.; Beyraghdar Kashkooli, A.; Peramuna, A.V.; van der Krol, A.R.; Bouwmeester, H.; Simonsen, H.T. Stable production of the antimalarial drug artemisinin in the moss *Physcomitrella patens*. *Front. Bioeng. Biotechnol.* **2017**, *5*, 47. [CrossRef] [PubMed]
24. Zhan, X.; Han, L.A.; Zhang, Y.; Chen, D.; Simonsen, H.T. Metabolic engineering of the moss *Physcomitrella patens* to produce the sesquiterpenoids patchoulol and α/β-santalene. *Front. Plant Sci.* **2014**, *5*, 636. [CrossRef] [PubMed]
25. Pan, X.-W.; Han, L.; Zhang, Y.-H.; Chen, D.-F.; Simonsen, H.T. Sclareol production in the moss *Physcomitrella patens* and observations on growth and terpenoid biosynthesis. *Plant Biotechnol. Rep.* **2015**, *9*, 149–159. [CrossRef]
26. Brown, G.D.; Sy, L.-K. In vivo transformations of artemisinic acid in *Artemisia annua* plants. *Tetrahedron* **2007**, *63*, 9548–9566. [CrossRef]
27. Hamberger, B.; Bak, S. Plant P450s as versatile drivers for evolution of species-specific chemical diversity. *Philos. Trans. R. Soc. B: Biol. Sci.* **2013**, *368*, 20120426. [CrossRef]
28. Kashkooli, A.B.; van der Krol, A.; Rabe, P.; Dickschat, J.S.; Bouwmeester, H. Substrate promiscuity of enzymes from the sesquiterpene biosynthetic pathways from *Artemisia annua* and *Tanacetum parthenium* allows for novel combinatorial sesquiterpene production. *Metab. Eng.* **2019**.
29. Weitzel, C.; Simonsen, H.T. Cytochrome P450-enzymes involved in the biosynthesis of mono-and sesquiterpenes. *Phytochem. Rev.* **2015**, *14*, 7–24. [CrossRef]

30. Dueholm, B.; Krieger, C.; Drew, D.; Olry, A.; Kamo, T.; Taboureau, O.; Weitzel, C.; Bourgaud, F.; Hehn, A.; Simonsen, H.T. Evolution of substrate recognition sites (srss) in cytochromes P450 from Apiaceae exemplified by the CYP71AJ subfamily. *BMC Evol. Biol.* **2015**, *15*, 122. [CrossRef]
31. Zhan, X.; Bach, S.S.; Hansen, N.L.; Lunde, C.; Simonsen, H.T. Additional diterpenes from *Physcomitrella patens* synthesized by copalyl diphosphate/kaurene synthase (*Pp*CPS/KS). *Plant Physiol. Biochem.* **2015**, *96*, 110–114. [CrossRef] [PubMed]
32. Noguchi, C.; Miyazaki, S.; Kawaide, H.; Gotoh, O.; Yoshida, Y.; Aoyama, Y. Characterization of moss ent-kaurene oxidase (CYP701B1) using a highly purified preparation. *J. Biochem.* **2017**, *163*, 69–76. [CrossRef] [PubMed]
33. Yonekura-Sakakibara, K.; Hanada, K. An evolutionary view of functional diversity in family 1 glycosyltransferases. *Plant J.* **2011**, *66*, 182–193. [CrossRef] [PubMed]
34. Yang, K.; Monafared, R.S.; Wang, H.; Lundgren, A.; Brodelius, P.E. The activity of the artemisinic aldehyde δ11 (13) reductase promoter is important for artemisinin yield in different chemotypes of *Artemisia annua*. *Plant Mol. Biol.* **2015**, *88*, 325–340. [CrossRef] [PubMed]
35. Yuan, Y.; Liu, W.; Zhang, Q.; Xiang, L.; Liu, X.; Chen, M.; Lin, Z.; Wang, Q.; Liao, Z. Overexpression of artemisinic aldehyde δ11 (13) reductase gene–enhanced artemisinin and its relative metabolite biosynthesis in transgenic *Artemisia annua* L. *Biotechnol. Appl. Biochem.* **2015**, *62*, 17–23. [CrossRef] [PubMed]
36. Huang, C.-Y.; Chung, C.-I.; Lin, Y.-C.; Hsing, Y.-I.C.; Huang, A.H.C. Oil bodies and oleosins in *Physcomitrella* possess characteristics representative of early trends in evolution. *Plant Physiol.* **2009**, *150*, 1192–1203. [CrossRef]
37. Bach, S.S.; King, B.C.; Zhan, X.; Simonsen, H.T.; Hamberger, B. Heterologous stable expression of terpenoid biosynthetic genes using the moss *Physcomitrella patens*. In *Plant Isoprenoids. Methods in Molecular Biology (Methods and Protocols), Vol. 1153*; Humana Press: New York, NY, USA, 2014; pp. 257–271.
38. Cove, D.J.; Perroud, P.-F.; Charron, A.J.; McDaniel, S.F.; Khandelwal, A.; Quatrano, R.S. The moss *Physcomitrella patens*: A novel model system for plant development and genomic studies. *Cold Spring Harb. Protoc.* **2009**, *2009*, pdb.emo115. [CrossRef]
39. Schindelin, J.; Rueden, C.T.; Hiner, M.C.; Eliceiri, K.W. The ImageJ ecosystem: An open platform for biomedical image analysis. *Molecular Reproduction and Development* **2015**, *82*, 518–529. [CrossRef]
40. Livak, K.J.; Schmittgen, T.D. Analysis of relative gene expression data using real-time quantitative pcr and the 2− δδct method. *Methods* **2001**, *25*, 402–408. [CrossRef]

molecules

MDPI

Article

Eruca sativa Meal against Diabetic Neuropathic Pain: An H_2S-Mediated Effect of Glucoerucin

Elena Lucarini [1], Eleonora Pagnotta [2], Laura Micheli [1], Carmen Parisio [1], Lara Testai [3,4,5], Alma Martelli [3,4,5], Vincenzo Calderone [3,4,5], Roberto Matteo [2], Luca Lazzeri [2], Lorenzo Di Cesare Mannelli [1,*] and Carla Ghelardini [1]

1 Department of Neuroscience, Psychology, Drug Research and Child Health—NEUROFARBA—Pharmacology and Toxicology Section, University of Florence, 50139 Florence, Italy
2 CREA-Council for Agricultural Research and Economics, Research Centre for Cereal and Industrial Crops, 40128 Bologna, Italy
3 Department of Pharmacy, University of Pisa, 56126 Pisa, Italy
4 Interdepartmental Research Centre "Nutraceuticals and Food for Health (NUTRAFOOD)", University of Pisa, 56126 Pisa, Italy
5 Interdepartmental Research Centre of Ageing Biology and Pathology, University of Pisa, 56126 Pisa, Italy
* Correspondence: lorenzo.mannelli@unifi.it

Academic Editor: Pinarosa Avato
Received: 13 June 2019; Accepted: 7 August 2019; Published: 19 August 2019

Abstract: The management of pain in patients affected by diabetic neuropathy still represents an unmet therapeutic need. Recent data highlighted the pain-relieving efficacy of glucosinolates deriving from Brassicaceae. The purpose of this study was to evaluate the anti-hyperalgesic efficacy of *Eruca sativa* defatted seed meal, along with its main glucosinolate, glucoerucin (GER), on diabetic neuropathic pain induced in mice by streptozotocin (STZ). The mechanism of action was also investigated. Hypersensitivity was assessed by paw pressure and cold plate tests after the acute administration of the compounds. Once bio-activated by myrosinase, both *E. sativa* defatted meal (1 g kg^{-1} p.o.) and GER (100 μmol kg^{-1} p.o., equimolar to meal content) showed a dose-dependent pain-relieving effect in STZ-diabetic mice, but the meal was more effective than the glucosinolate. The co-administration with H_2S scavengers abolished the pain relief mediated by both *E. sativa* meal and GER. Their effect was also prevented by selectively blocking Kv7 potassium channels. Repeated treatments with *E. sativa* meal did not induce tolerance to the anti-hypersensitive effect. In conclusion, *E. sativa* meal can be suggested as a new nutraceutical tool for pain relief in patients with diabetic neuropathy.

Keywords: diabetic neuropathy; neuropathic pain; glucosinolates; *Eruca sativa*; glucoerucin; H_2S; Kv7 potassium channels

1. Introduction

The development of neuropathy is a common long-term complication of uncontrolled hyperglycemia and the relief of neuropathic pain still represents a therapeutic challenge in patients affected by diabetes [1]. The management of diabetic neuropathic pain consists basically in improving glycaemic control as a prophylactic therapy and using medications to alleviate pain. Unfortunately, their use is limited by side effects and by the development of tolerance [2,3]. Recent evidence highlighted the beneficial effect of synthetic and naturally occurring H_2S donors in different types of persistent pain [4,5]. Among the natural compounds able to release H_2S there are isothiocyanates, which derive from glucosinolate (GSL) hydrolysis mediated by the enzyme myrosinase (β-thioglucoside glucohydrolase, thioglucosidase, EC3.2.1.147) or by the intestinal microflora [6–8]. These phytochemicals are contained in almost all the plants belonging to the Brassicaceae family and are responsible for many of their beneficial effects in animals, as well as in humans [6,8–10]. The GSL glucoraphanin (GRA) and the derived isothiocyanate sulforaphane (SFN), are the most widely studied due to their potent anti-inflammatory, antioxidant, anti-cancer, antibiotic, as well as neuroprotective effects [6,11–16]. SFN has also been tested in humans, demonstrating an improvement of glucose levels in patients with type 2 diabetes [17]. Nevertheless, its effect on the development of diabetic neuropathy was not studied. Recent findings highlighted the anti-hyperalgesic and protective effects of SFN in an animal model of chemotherapy-induced neuropathy [18] and its capacity to potentiate the antinociceptive effects of opioids in animals with inflammatory pain or diabetic neuropathy [19,20]. As in the case of other H_2S donors, SNF properties are closely related to the release of H_2S in vivo and the consequent activation of Kv7 potassium channels [4,7,18,21–23].

SFN represents a redox couple with erucin, another isothiocyanate which is derived from the metabolism of glucoerucin (GER), the most abundant GSL in *Eruca sativa* spp. oleifera Mill seeds [24–26]. Despite the limited studies on erucin, beneficial properties similar to SFN have recently been reported [27–29], as its ability to release H_2S in vitro and to mediate vasodilatation [30,31]. This also led to assume that the effects showed by SFN in vivo could actually be due to its rapid interconversion to erucin [32]. In 2015 Franco et al. developed a system to obtain a food-safe organic material starting from *E. sativa* (*Eruca sativa* Mill. Sel. NEMAT). This pressure defatted oilseed meal enriched of GSL, suitable to produce bakery products, aimed to realize a functional food [33]. The purpose of this study was to evaluate the antihyperalgesic properties (efficacy and tolerance) of *E. sativa* defatted seed meal (DSM), along with that of its active constituent GER, in a model of diabetic neuropathic pain induced by streptozotocin (STZ) in mice. The involvement of H_2S release and Kv7 modulation in the pain-relieving activity of *E. sativa* derived products were also investigated.

2. Results

2.1. *Eruca sativa Defatted Seed Meal Characterization*

Eruca sativa DSM was characterized in its main components: Proteins, % residual oil and its fatty acid profile, GSL content and profile, total free phenolic fraction, and myrosinase activity. Proteins were the main component of *E. sativa* DSM accounting for 36% *w*/*w* of dry matter. The mild oil extraction brought to a 20% residual oil component in DSM, which was characterized for fatty acid profile and resulted in particularly rich erucic, linolenic, oleic, and linoleic acids (37%; 16%; 15%; 12%, respectively). The GSL content accounted for total 138 μmol g^{-1}, with 98.6 % GER of the total GSLs, and the remaining GRA. Total free phenolic content was 8.9 ± 0.5 mg of gallic acid equivalents (Ge) g^{-1}, according to previous studies [34]. Residual myrosinase activity was 8 ± 2 U, with one enzyme unit (U) corresponding to 1 μmol/g DSM of sinigrin transformed in 1 min. The myrosinase activity was comparable to a previous study [28] and low in comparison to the myrosinase activity of cold extracted *E. sativa* DSM, which was about 24 U [28].

2.2. *Effect of Eruca sativa Defatted Seed Meal and Glucoerucin on Diabetes-Induced Neuropathic Pain*

Figures 1 and 2s how, respectively, the effect of acute oral administration of *E. sativa* DSM (0.1–1 g kg^{-1}) and GER (30–100 μmol kg^{-1}) in STZ-treated animals with and without myrosinase bioactivation. Four weeks after the STZ injection, mice showed a significantly decreased latency to pain-related behaviours induced by a noxious mechanical stimulus (Paw pressure test, Figures 1a and 2a) as well as by a thermal non-noxious stimulus (cold plate test, Figures 1b and 2b), compared with control mice treated with vehicle (Figures 1 and 2). *Eruca sativa* DSM was able to dose-dependently relieve pain in STZ-treated mice, increasing the paw withdrawal latency to the value of controls 30 min after the administration of both doses 0.3 and 1 g kg^{-1}. Furthermore, the higher dose (1 g kg^{-1}) of *E. sativa* DSM showed a long-lasting effect, since the animal's pain threshold was significantly increased up to 90 min after the injection (Figure 1a). The pain-relieving effect of *E. sativa* DSM was also observed in the cold plate test, though it is significant only at the higher dose (Figure 1b). GER, administered in an equivalent dose to that contained in the *E. sativa* DSM (100 µmol kg^{-1}) significantly reduced mechanical hyperalgesia in STZ-treated animals, though it was less effective than the meal. By contrast, the 3-fold lower dose of GER (30 µmol kg^{-1}) was completely ineffective (Figure 2a). The same trend was observed in the cold plate test (Figure 2b). It is worth noting that both the solutions of *E. sativa*, DSM and GER, lost their effect on pain without the myrosinase-mediated bioactivation (Figures 1 and 2).

Figure 3 shows the effect of the repeated treatment with *E. sativa* DSM on STZ-induced neuropathic pain in mice. The defatted seed meal was administered once daily for 8 consecutive days to evaluate the development of tolerance in these animals. The Figure shows the animal pain threshold 60 min after the treatments. The acute pain-relieving effect of *E. sativa* DSM (1 g kg^{-1}) remained constant over time, without the onset of tolerance. On the other hand, the repeated administration of *E. sativa* DSM did not influence the animal basal threshold, which was not different from that of STZ + vehicle-treated animals before the compound administration.

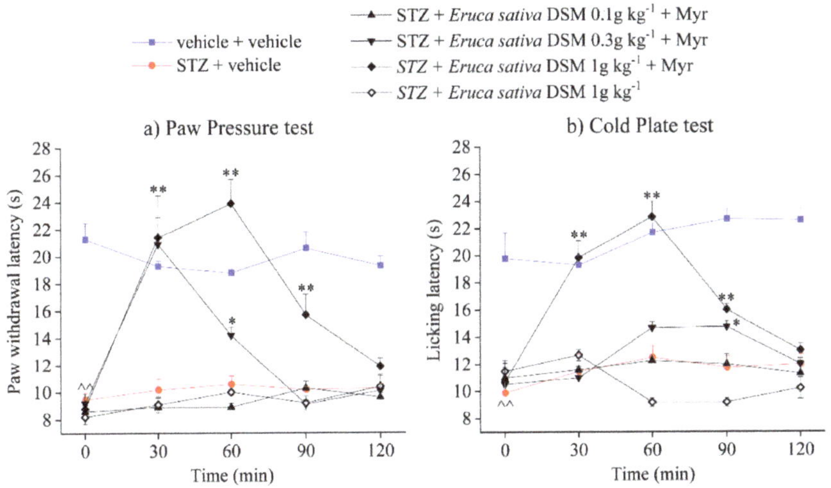

Figure 1. Effect of acute administration of bioactivated *Eruca sativa* defatted seed meal on streptozotocin (STZ)-induced neuropathic pain. The response to both a mechanical and a thermal stimulus was evaluated by measuring the latency (s) to pain-related behaviors; (**a**) withdrawal or (**b**) licking of the paw. *Eruca sativa* defatted seed meal (DSM) (0.1–1 g kg^{-1}) was bioactivated by adding 30 µL mL^{-1} of myrosinase (Myr) (32 U mL^{-1}) 15 min before the oral administration in STZ-treated animals. Tests were performed 30, 60, 90, and 120 min after the injection. ^^ $p < 0.01$ versus vehicle + vehicle-treated mice; * $p < 0.05$ and ** $p < 0.01$ versus STZ + vehicle-treated mice.

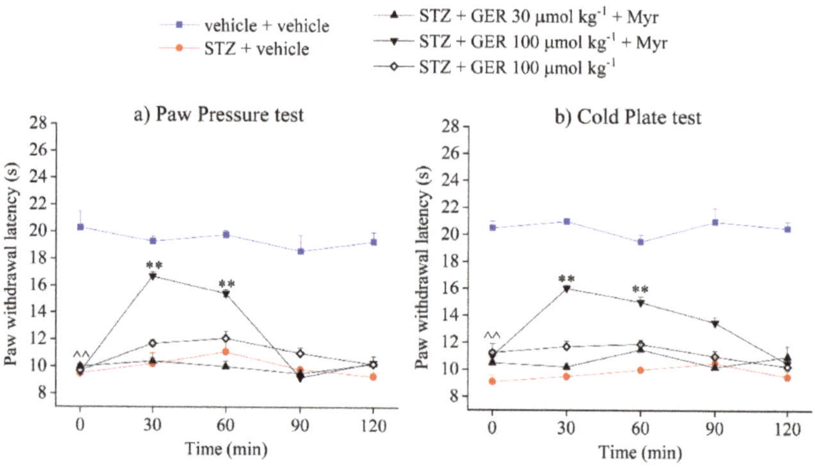

Figure 2. Effect of acute administration of bioactivated glucoerucin (GER) on streptozotocin (STZ)-induced neuropathic pain. The response to both a mechanical and a thermal stimulus was evaluated by measuring the latency (s) to pain-related behaviors; (**a**) withdrawal or (**b**) licking of the paw. GER (30–100 μkg^{-1}) was bioactivated by adding 30 $\mu L\ mL^{-1}$ of myrosinase (32 U mL^{-1}) 15 min before the oral administration in STZ-treated animals. Tests were performed 30, 60, 90, and 120 min after the injection. ^^ $p < 0.01$ versus vehicle + vehicle-treated mice; * $p < 0.05$ and ** $p < 0.01$ versus STZ + vehicle-treated mice.

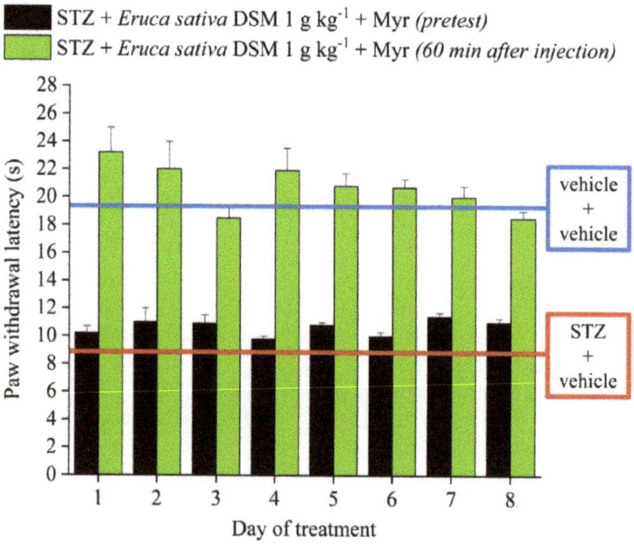

Figure 3. Effect of the repeated treatment with *Eruca sativa* defatted seed meal (DSM) on streptozotocin (STZ)-induced neuropathic pain. The response to a mechanical stimulus was evaluated by measuring the latency (s) to pain-related behaviors (paw withdrawal). The myrosinase (Myr)-bioactivated *Eruca sativa* DSM (1 g kg^{-1}) was administered once daily for 8 consecutive days in STZ-treated animals (once neuropathy was established) and pain threshold was assessed before and 60 min after the injection. ^^ $p < 0.01$ versus vehicle + vehicle-treated mice; * $p < 0.05$ and ** $p < 0.01$ versus STZ + vehicle-treated mice.

2.3. Role of Isothiocyanates and H_2S-Release in the Anti-Hyperalgesic Effect of Eruca sativa Defatted Seed Meal and Glucoerucin

To evaluate the role of H_2S in the anti-hyperalgesic effect showed from *E. sativa* DSM and GER, we administered the compounds in mixture with oxidized glutathione (GSSG), a compound able to bind the isothiocyanates, preventing the release of H_2S [35–37], and hemoglobin (Hb), a molecule able to bind H_2S [38]. The co-administration with GSSG (20 mg kg^{-1} po) was able to fully prevent the anti-hyperalgesic effect of *E. sativa* DSM (1 g kg^{-1}) as well as that of GER (100 µmol kg^{-1}): the pain threshold of animals treated with both these substances in mixture with GSSG was not significantly different from that of STZ + vehicle-treated animals (Figure 4a,b). The same result was observed by systemically administering GSSG (20 mg kg^{-1} sc) in concomitance with the oral administration of *E. sativa* DSM and GER (Figure 4a,b). Both the oral and the subcutaneous administration of GSSG (20 mg kg^{-1}) in STZ-treated animals did not elicit effects on animal pain threshold (Figure S1). The effect of the tested compounds was also abolished by co-administering Hb (300 mg kg^{-1} po) to both products (Figure 4c,d).

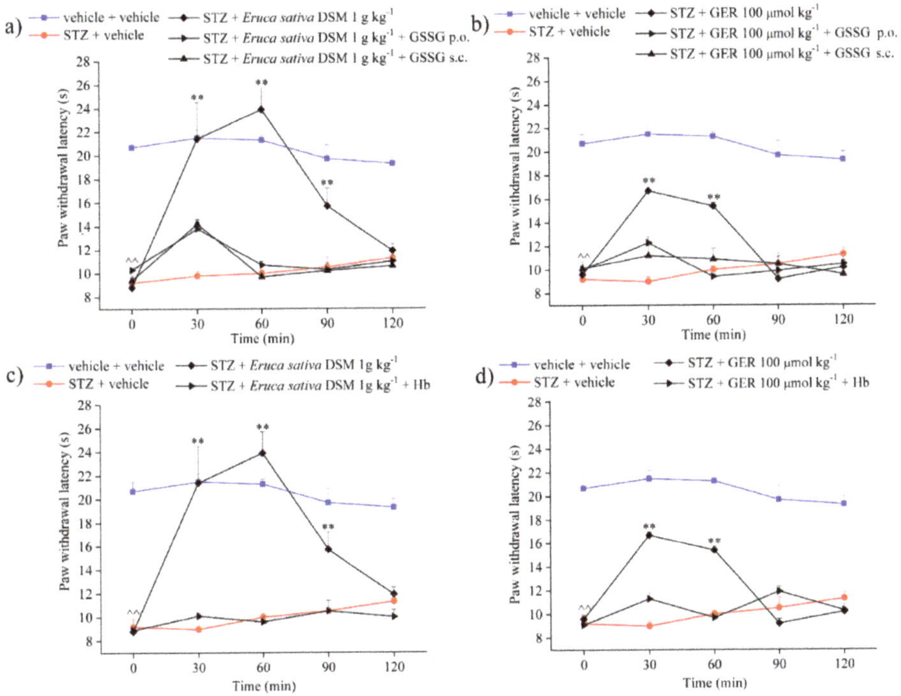

Figure 4. Role of H_2S in the pain-relieving effect of *Eruca sativa* defatted seed meal (DSM) and glucoerucin (GER). The response to a mechanical stimulus was evaluated by measuring the latency(s) to pain-related behavior (paw withdrawal). Oxidized glutathione (GSSG) (20 mg kg^{-1}) was orally and subcutaneously administered in concomitance with both (**a**) Myr-bioactivated *Eruca sativa* DSM (1 g kg^{-1}) and (**b**) GER (100 µmol kg^{-1}); tests were performed 30, 60, 90, and 120 min after injection. (**c**) Myrosinase (Myr)-bioactivated *Eruca sativa* DSM (1 g kg^{-1}) and (**d**) GER (100 µmol kg^{-1}) were orally administered alone or in mixture with human hemoglobin (Hb) (300 mg kg^{-1}); tests were performed 30, 60, 90, and 120 min after injection. ^^ $p < 0.01$ versus vehicle + vehicle-treated mice; * $p < 0.05$ and ** $p < 0.01$ versus streptozotocin (STZ) + vehicle-treated mice.

2.4. Involvement of Kv7 Potassium Channels in the Pain-Relieving Effect of Eruca sativa *Defatted Seed Meal and Glucoerucin*

To study the involvement of the Kv7 potassium channel in the anti-neuropathic effect of *E. sativa* DSM and GER, the selective Kv7 blocker, XE991, was intraperitoneally administered in concomitance with both the substances. Figure 5 shows the effect induced by *E. sativa* DSM (1g kg^{-1} po) and GER (100 μmol kg^{-1} po) on diabetes-induced neuropathic pain in comparison with that obtained by pre-treating the animals with XE991 (1 mg kg^{-1} ip). The anti-hyperalgesic effect of *E. sativa* DSM and GER was fully prevented by the intraperitoneal administration of XE991, as highlighted in Figure 5a,b, respectively.

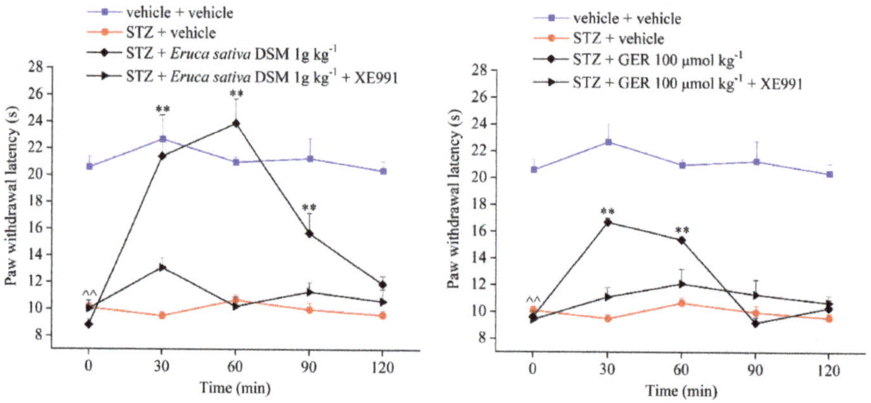

Figure 5. Involvement of Kv7 potassium channels in the pain-relieving effect of *Eruca sativa* defatted seed meal (DSM) and glucoerucin (GER). The response to a mechanical stimulus was evaluated by measuring the latency to pain-related behaviors (paw withdrawal). (**a**) Myrosinase (Myr)-bioactivated *Eruca sativa* DSM (1 g kg^{-1}) and (**b**) GER (100 μmol kg^{-1}) were orally administered in concomitance with XE991 (1 mg kg^{-1} ip); tests were performed 30, 60, 90, and 120 min after injection. ^^ $p < 0.01$ versus vehicle + vehicle-treated mice; * $p < 0.05$ and ** $p < 0.01$ versus streptozotocin (STZ) + vehicle-treated mice.

3. Discussion

This work, for the first time, highlighted the pain-relieving properties of *E. sativa*. In particular, we demonstrated that *E. sativa* DSM, along with its main GSL, GER, can counteract pain in animals affected by diabetic neuropathy induced by STZ. As in the case of other GSLs [18], the effect was mediated by H_2S release and the consequent activation of Kv7 potassium channels. However, the effect of the *E. sativa* DSM was not only attributable to the content of GER, suggesting a synergism between the GSLs and the other phytochemicals contained in this nutraceutical product.

Diabetic peripheral neuropathy is a distressing disease of the nerves in the hands and feet, it is a common complication of both type 1 and type 2 diabetes [1,39]. The symptoms most commonly experienced in these patients are burning, electric-shock type and sharp pains [39–41], while aching, itching, and cold pain are common but less prevalent manifestations [41,42]. These symptoms increase at night, predictably interfering with sleep [43]. In pre-clinical studies, the STZ model of diabetes has been shown to be associated with sensory changes including allodynia and hyperalgesia which develop starting in the few weeks following STZ administration [44,45].

The management of diabetic neuropathy involves maintaining good glycaemic control by drugs as well as by lifestyle modification, like diet and exercise [46–48]. Current therapies aiming to relieve neuropathy-related symptoms, such as pain, are helpful only in one-third of patients with 50% of efficacy [27], often achieved with troublesome side effects and low levels of satisfaction [47,49].

Evidence collected in the last few years supports a diet-based approach in the management of different types of diseases, including chronic pain syndromes [50–52]. Among the most largely studied nutraceutical products there are the GSLs, secondary metabolites that can be found in different concentrations among cruciferous vegetables [6,18]. It is thought that GSLs, together with myrosinase, are a part of a defense mechanism implemented by plants to protect themselves against biotic and abiotic stress [53]. Recently we discovered that GSLs along with their hydrolysis product, isothiocyanates, are strongly effective in relieving neuropathic pain induced by chemotherapy [18]. Interestingly, other natural and synthetic isothiocyanates-based compounds also showed broadly pain-relieving properties in animal models of persistent pain [4,5].

Eruca sativa is an edible plant indigenous of the Mediterranean area that has been traditionally used for its medicinal properties. Similar to other Brassicaceae, the characteristic pungent taste and odor of *E. sativa* leaves were attributed to GSLs. This plant has a high vitamin C content and is known for various health-promoting effects, including improvement of blood circulation, diuretic, and anti-inflammatory properties [27,54–56]. *Eruca sativa* DSM represents an enriched functional food formulated to modulate the release over time of GSLs degradation products, in order to obtain the most effective biological activity [28,57]. Accordingly, we found that the employment of *E. sativa* DSM led to a more strong and long-lasting effect in comparison with GER. The effect of both the compounds is dependent on the bioactivation mediated by myrosinase, indicating as being mainly responsible for pain relief the isothiocyanates derived from the hydrolysis of GER, erucin. The obtained result opened the way to two different hypotheses. The first is that the effect of *E. sativa* DSM is mediated not only by GSLs and the derived isothiocyanates but also by other constituents, as phenols and fatty acids. Indeed, the beneficial effects of antioxidant compounds, such as phenols, against neuropathic pain are well known [58–62]. On the other hand, the effect of *E. sativa* DSM is likely attributable to the GSL content [4,18], since its effect was completely abolished by co-administering the H_2S scavenger as well as by the oxidative cleavage of the isothiocyanate mediate by the disulfide GSSG. In particular, GSSG, systemically administered, was able to prevent the pain-relieving effect, indicating that the isothiocyanate erucin, once adsorbed in the gut, reaches the bloodstream where it probably releases H_2S. On the other hand, the administration of GSSG in a mixture with the bioactivated compounds could prevent its intestinal absorption.

The effect of *E. sativa* was also prevented blocking Kv7 potassium channels, confirming again the direct involvement of GSLs in the pain-relieving effect [4,18].

This evidence, which seems to diminish the importance of the other constituents of the meal own effect on pain modulation, actually move the attention to the second hypothesis, namely that this formulation could be able to modulate the release of the GSLs, improving their pharmacological profile. In fact, it is known that the efficacy of H_2S donors is closely linked to their pharmacokinetics—slower is the release of H_2S, higher is the efficacy [4,5]. This is mainly due to the bell-shape beneficial effect showed by H_2S in the organism [63]. In this context, the peculiar formulation of *E. sativa* DSM could determine a slow release of GSLs, allowing a sustained availability of isothiocyanates and consequently H_2S in vivo, and avoiding quick exhaustion of the pain-relieving effect.

A peculiar feature of GER is that it needs to be preventively bioactivated by myrosinase in solution before the administration in vivo. The same was observed with the *E. sativa* DSM, strengthening once again the importance of its glucosinolates content in the pain-relieving effect. This chemical property makes GER different from other GLSs, such as GRA. In fact, in our previous work, we tested the anti-hyperalgesic effect of this GLS and the derived isothiocyanate, SFN, in a model of neuropathic pain induced by chemotherapy [18]. In that case, we did not have to pre-treat the GLS with the enzyme myrosinase to get the effect. By mixing myrosinase with GER or *Eruca sativa* DSM, we are delivering the isothiocyanate erucin in vivo. It likely means that GER is ineffective. In the absence of myrosinase, GLS can be hydrolyzed to isothiocyanates by the bacteria that constitute the gut microflora. Nevertheless, it was found that the microbiome only supports poor hydrolysis, unless exposed to dietary GLSs for a period of days [64]. On the other hand, the microbiota could not have the time necessary to hydrolyze GER in the lumen if it is quickly absorbed or metabolized in different products in the gut. Anyway, the fact that these compounds need to be bioactivated does not preclude the possibility of using them but it is a point to take into account for the treatment protocol.

Another important point to consider is that the effect of *E. sativa* is eligible only after the acute administration and it does not show a therapeutic effect on the neuropathy, which also persists after the repeated treatment. By contrast, the analog, GRA, and the derived isothiocyanate, sSFN, were able to prevent the development of the neuropathy induced by chemotherapy [18]. This observation suggests that the administration of the GSLs can counteract the pathophysiological mechanisms that lead to the instauration of the neuropathies, such as the oxidative stress [5,65,66], but cannot revert it after its establishment. Anyway, in the case of diabetic neuropathy, it is difficult to apply a preventive treatment at clinical level since this type of disease is a long-term complication of uncontrolled hyperglycemia [2,39,40]. In fact, a proper treatment of hyperglycemia is the most effective and straight forward method to prevent neuropathy in diabetic patients. So, another interesting possibility could be to employ *E. sativa*-derived GLSs as a nutraceutical approach to manage pain in diabetes patients who have already developed the neuropathy, since it still represents a therapeutic problem [48,49]. Indeed, although *E. sativa* does not appear to be a resolving treatment for diabetic neuropathy, its acute anti-hyperalgesic efficacy joined to the characteristics of food supplements suggest its clinical use for treating neuropathic pain as monotherapy or in combination with drugs for sparing dosages and enhance efficacy.

In this perspective, *E. sativa* DSM proved to be a valid innovative formulation to guarantee proper delivery of GSLs in vivo and to enhance their therapeutic efficacy against pain, laying the bases for its rational use in patients affected by diabetic neuropathy.

4. Materials and Methods

4.1. *Eruca sativa Defatted Seed Meal Production and Characterization*

Eruca sativa Mill. Var. NEMAT was grown during the season 2014–2015, within a plot with a size of 1100 m^2, adopting a minimum agronomical input approach [23]. The cultivation was carried out at CREA experimental farm located at Budrio (Bologna) in the Po Valley area (Emilia Romagna region, 44°32′00″ N; 11°29′33″ E, altitude 28 m a.s.l.). The area was characterized by flat land with alluvial deep loamy soil with medium level content of total nitrogen and organic matter content. After harvesting, *E. sativa* seeds were accurately threshed with fixed small-scale threshing equipment and air-dried to reduce the high residual moisture content. *Eruca sativa* seeds were defatted using a small continuous seed crusher machine (Bracco Company model Elle.Gi type 0.90) at a temperature-controlled procedure, during which temperature was maintained at a maximum of 70 °C. *Eruca sativa* DSM was characterized by moisture, proteins, residual oil, GSL, total free phenolic content, and residual myrosinase activity according to the following methods:

(1) Moisture content was determined to evaluate the difference between its weight before and after oven-drying at 105 °C for 12 h.
(2) Proteins were determined from the total content of nitrogen determined using the elemental analyzer LECO CHN TruSpec according to the American Society for Testing Materials (ASTM D5373).
(3) Residual oil content was determined by the standard Soxhlet extraction method using hexane as a solvent and characterized for its fatty acid composition by the UNI EN ISO 5508 method (1998) [67]. Fatty acid composition of residual oil was analyzed after trans-methylation in 2N KOH methanol solution. Fatty acid methyl esters (FAMEs) were evaluated by gas chromatography and the internal normalization method [68] was used for determining the fatty acid profile.
(4) Glucosinolate content was determined following the ISO 9167-1 method with some minor modifications [69]. Briefly, 250 mg DSM were extracted in 70% ethanol at 80 °C. One milliliter of crude extract was loaded onto a DEAE Sephadex A-25 (GE Healthcare, Freiburg, Germany)

mini-column. After washing with 25 mM acetate buffer (pH 5.6), GSLs were desulfated by adding purified sulfatase (200 μL, 0.35 U/mL). The desulfo-GSLs were eluted in water (HPLC grade) and detected in HPLC-UV [69] monitoring their absorbance at 229 nm. They were identified with respect to their UV spectra and retention time, according to our library [70], and their amounts were estimated using sinigrin as an internal standard. Each extraction and analysis was performed in triplicate.

(5) Total free phenolic content was assayed with the Folin–Ciocalteu method according to [71]. Values are the mean ± SD of three independent extractions by four replicates for each measurement. *Eruca sativa* DSM extracts were obtained in acidified ethanol, ethanol/1 N HCl (85:15; *v*/*v*), after 30 min at 21 °C in 40 kHz ultrasonic bath (Sonica Sweep System, Soltec). The supernatants of a triple extraction procedure were collected and maintained at −20 °C in the dark for 48 h to facilitate macromolecule precipitation. Five serial dilutions of the filtered extracts were assayed at 765 nm, 20 °C, in an Infinite M200 NanoQuant Plate reader (Tecan, Switzerland). The slope of each calibration curve was compared to a standard gallic acid calibration curve (range 0.3–27 μg ml^{-1}, $r^2 = 0.9972$). The slope ratio of sample/standard curves was calculated, and results were expressed as mg of GAE per g of DSM.

(6) Myrosinase activity was determined by the pH-stat technique according to [28]. Briefly, 300 mg of *E. sativa* DSM were loaded in 15 mL of 1% NaCl into a reaction cell at 37 °C in a DL50 pH-Stat titrator (Mettler Toledo, Switzerland). The reaction started by adding 0.5 mL of 0.5 M sinigrin solution in distilled water, after 8–10 min of conditioning, and was monitored following NaOH additions used to maintain pH constant at 6.5, versus time in minutes. The assay was carried out in triplicate. One enzyme unit (U) corresponded to 1 μmol/g DSM of sinigrin transformed in 1 min.

4.2. Isolation of Glucoerucin

Glucoerucin was isolated starting from *E. sativa* seeds, as previously described [28]. Briefly, seeds of *E. sativa* from the Brassicaceae collection at CREA-CI, Bologna, Italy [36] were crushed in boiling 70% ethanol and the GSL was isolated as K^+ salt by two sequential steps, including ion exchange and size exclusion chromatography. Isolated GER preparation was analyzed by HPLC-UV after enzymatic desulfation according to [69] and it was identified by UV spectra and HPLC retention times according to our library [70]. The purity of GER was 97% as indicated by HPLC-UV chromatograms and 91 ± 2% on weight basis estimated using sinigrin as an internal standard. It was stored until use at −20 °C. Erucin was produced in-situ through myrosinase-catalyzed hydrolysis, as previously described [30]. Myrosinase (32 U/mL), was isolated from the seeds of *Sinapis alba* L. according to [72]. One unit of myrosinase activity is defined as the amount of enzyme capable of hydrolyzing 1 μmol sinigrin, per min, at pH 6.5 and 37 °C

4.3. Animals

Animals were male C57BL/6 mice (Envigo, Varese, Italy) weighing approximately 22–25 g at the beginning of the experimental procedure were used. Animals were housed in CeSAL (Centro Stabulazione Animali da Laboratorio, University of Florence) and used at least 1 week after their arrival. Ten mice were housed per cage (size = 26 × 41 cm); animals were fed with a standard laboratory diet and tap water ad libitum and kept at 23 ± 1 °C with a 12-hr light/dark cycle, with light at 7 a.m. All animal manipulations were carried out according to the Directive 2010/63/EU of the European Parliament and of the European Union council (September 22, 2010) on the protection of animals used for scientific purposes. The ethical policy of the University of Florence complies with the Guide for the Care and Use of Laboratory Animals of the U.S. National Institutes of Health (NIH Publication No. 85–23, revised 1996; University of Florence assurance number: A5278-01). Formal approval to conduct the described experiments was obtained from the Animal Subjects Review Board of the University of

Florence. Experiments involving animals have been reported according to ARRIVE guidelines [39]. All efforts were made to minimize animal suffering and to reduce the number of animals used.

4.4. Induction of Diabetic Neuropathy in Mice

Mice were intraperitoneally administered with STZ, (Sigma Aldrich, Milan, Italy) 100 mg kg^{-1}, followed three days after with a second dose of STZ 50 mg kg^{-1} [73]. Since streptozotocin has stability problems [74], the solution was prepared immediately before the injection. To maintain cleanliness and avoid the development of any infection due to excessive urination, animal bedding was changed frequently. Pain threshold was investigated each week after the injection of STZ and tests were performed once neuropathy was established in mice.

4.5. Assessment of Mechanical Hyperalgesia

Mechanical hyperalgesia was determined by measuring the latency in seconds to withdraw the paw away from a constant mechanical pressure exerted onto the dorsal surface [75]. A 15 g calibrated glass cylindrical rod (diameter = 10 mm) chamfered to a conical point (diameter = 3 mm) was used to exert the mechanical force. The weight was suspended vertically between two rings attached to a stand and was free to move vertically. A single measure was made per animal. A cut off time of 40 s was used.

4.6. Assessment of Thermal Allodynia

The animals were placed in a stainless-steel box (12 × 20 × 10 cm) with a cold plate as floor. The temperature of the cold plate was kept constant at 4 °C ± 1 °C. Pain-related behavior (licking of the hind paw) was observed, and the time (seconds) of the first sign was recorded. The cut-off time of the latency of paw lifting or licking was set at 30 s [76]. The results were expressed by the licking latency resulting from the compounds acute administration.

4.7. Compounds Administration

Eruca sativa DSM, GER, and myrosinase were produced according to the method described above. Compounds were acutely administered as follows. The doses of *E. sativa* DSM (0.1–1 g kg^{-1} po) were chosen based on previously published H_2S releasing and antinociceptive properties of synthetic and natural ITCs [4,5]. The doses of GER (30–100 µmol kg^{-1} po) used are equivalent to those contained in *E. sativa* DSM (0.3–1 g kg^{-1} po). Both *E. sativa* DSM and GER were bioactivated by adding 30 µL mL^{-1} of myrosinase (32 U mL^{-1}) 15 min before administering them in the animals. Behavioral tests were carried out 30, 60, 90, and 120 min after the injection. Afterward, repeated oral administrations of *E. sativa* DSM (0.3–1 g kg^{-1}) were carried out daily in the mice after the establishment of the diabetic neuropathy. Behavioral tests were performed once daily after the acute administration. In additional experiments, *E. sativa* DSM (1g kg^{-1}) and GER (100 µmol kg^{-1}) were administered in mixture with human hemoglobin 4.6 µmol kg^{-1} (300 mg kg^{-1}; Hb; Sigma-Aldrich, Italy) and with glutathione 65 µmol kg^{-1} (20 mg kg^{-1}; GSSG; Sigma-Aldrich, Milan, Italy). The effect of the subcutaneous administration of GSSG 15 min before *E. sativa* DSM (1g kg^{-1} po) and GER (100 µmol kg^{-1} po) was also evaluated. The Kv7 potassium channel blocker XE991 (Tocris Bioscience, Italy; 2.66 µmol kg^{-1}; 1 mg kg^{-1}; [77]) was dissolved in saline solution and intraperitoneally administered in concomitance with the tested compounds injection.

4.8. Statistical Analysis

Behavioral measurements were performed on 10 mice for each treatment carried out in two different experimental sets. Investigators were blind to all experimental procedures. Results were expressed as mean ± S.E.M. The analysis of variance of data was performed by one-way analysis of variance, and a Bonferroni's significant difference procedure was used as post hoc comparison.

p values of less than 0.05 or 0.01 were considered significant. Data were analyzed using the "Origin 9" software (OriginLab, Northampton, MA, USA).

Supplementary Materials: Figure S1: Effect of acute administration of GSSG on STZ-induced neuropathic pain.

Author Contributions: L.L. and L.D.C.M. designed the experimental protocol. E.L. and C.P. performed the experiments. E.P. and R.M. provided the compounds used in the work and their characterization. L.T., A.M., and L.M. collaborated in the data analysis and in the conceptualization of the project. The main manuscript was written by E.L., L.D.C.M., and extended by E.P., C.G. and V.C. performed the statistical analysis and revised the manuscript.

Funding: This research was funded by the Italian Ministry of Instruction, University and Research (MIUR), PON "Ricerca e Innovazione" 2014-2020-Azione II, by the COMETA research project "Colture autoctone mediterranee e loro valorizzazione con tecnologie avanzate di chimica verde" (Native Mediterranean crops and their enhancement with advanced green chemistry technologies) (ARS01_00606). Grant decree COMETA prot. n. 1741 of 05/07/2018, CUP B26G18000200004—COR 545910.

Conflicts of Interest: The authors declare no conflict of interest.

References

1. Abbott, C.A.; Malik, R.A.; Van Ross, E.R.; Kulkarni, J.; Boulton, A.J. Prevalence and characteristics of painful diabetic neuropathy in a large community based diabetic population in the U.K. *Diabetes Care* **2011**, *34*, 2220–2224. [CrossRef] [PubMed]
2. Tesfaye, S.; Boulton, A.J.; Dickenson, A.H. Mechanisms and management of diabetic painful distal symmetrical polyneuropathy. *Diabetes Care* **2013**, *36*, 2456–2465. [CrossRef] [PubMed]
3. Boyle, J.; Eriksson, M.E.; Gribble, L.; Gouni, R.; Johnsen, S.; Coppini, D.V.; Kerr, D. Randomized, placebo-controlled comparison of amitriptyline, duloxetine, and pregabalin in patients with chronic diabetic peripheral neuropathic pain: Impact on pain, polysomnographic sleep, daytime functioning, and quality of life. *Diabetes Care* **2012**, *35*, 2451–2458. [CrossRef]
4. Di Cesare Mannelli, L.; Lucarini, E.; Micheli, L.; Mosca, I.; Ambrosino, P.; Soldovieri, M.V.; Martelli, A.; Testai, L.; Taglialatela, M.; Calderone, V.; et al. Effects of natural and synthetic isothiocyanate-based H_2S-releasers against chemotherapy-induced neuropathic pain: Role of Kv7 potassium channels. *Neuropharmacology* **2017**, *121*, 49–59. [CrossRef] [PubMed]
5. Lucarini, E.; Micheli, L.; Martelli, A.; Testai, L.; Calderone, V.; Ghelardini, C.; Di Cesare Mannelli, L. Efficacy of isothiocyanate-based compounds on different forms of persistent pain. *J. Pain Res.* **2018**, *11*, 2905–2913. [CrossRef] [PubMed]
6. Dinkova-Kostova, A.T.; Kostov, R.V. Glucosinolates and isothiocyanates in health and disease. *Trends Mol. Med.* **2012**, *18*, 337–347. [CrossRef] [PubMed]
7. Citi, V.; Martelli, A.; Testai, L.; Marino, A.; Breschi, M.C.; Calderone, V. Hydrogen sulfide releasing capacity of natural isothiocyanates: Is it a reliable explanation for the multiple biological effects of Brassicaceae? *Planta Medica* **2014**, *80*, 610–613. [CrossRef] [PubMed]
8. Mithen, R.; Ho, E. Isothiocyanates for Human Health. *Mol. Nutr. Food Res.* **2018**, *62*, 1870079. [CrossRef] [PubMed]
9. Ishida, M.; Hara, M.; Fukino, N.; Kakizaki, T.; Morimitsu, Y. Glucosinolate metabolism, functionality and breeding for the improvement of Brassicaceae vegetables. *Breed. Sci.* **2014**, *64*, 48–59. [CrossRef]
10. Fahey, J.W.; Wade, K.L.; Wehage, S.L.; Holtzclaw, W.D.; Liu, H.; Talalay, P.; Fuchs, E.; Stephenson, K.K. Stabilized sulforaphane for clinical use: Phytochemical delivery efficiency. *Mol. Nutr. Food Res* **2017**, *61*, 1600766. [CrossRef] [PubMed]
11. Guerrero-Beltran, C.E.; Calderon-Oliver, M.; Pedraza-Chaverri, J.; Chirino, Y.I. Protective effect of sulforaphane against oxidative stress: Recent advances. *Exp. Toxicol. Pathol.* **2012**, *64*, 503–508. [CrossRef] [PubMed]
12. Zhang, Y.; Kensler, T.W.; Cho, C.G.; Posner, G.H.; Talalay, P. Anticarcinogenicactivities of sulforaphane and structurally related synthetic norbornylisothiocyanates. *Proc. Natl. Acad. Sci. USA* **1994**, *91*, 3147–3150. [CrossRef]

13. Pu, D.; Zhao, Y.; Chen, J.; Sun, Y.; Lv, A.; Zhu, S.; Luo, C.; Zhao, K.; Xiao, Q. Protective effects of sulforaphane on cognitive impairments and ad-like lesions in diabetic mice are associated with the upregulation of Nrf2 transcription activity. *Neuroscience* **2018**, *381*, 35–45. [CrossRef] [PubMed]
14. Silva Rodrigues, J.F.; Silva, E.; Silva, C.; França Muniz, T.; De Aquino, A.F.; Neuza da Silva Nina, L.; Fialho Sousa, N.C.; Nascimento da Silva, L.C.; De Souza, B.G.G.F.; Da Penha, T.A.; et al. Sulforaphane Modulates Joint Inflammation in a Murine Model of Complete Freund's Adjuvant-Induced Mono-Arthritis. *Molecules* **2018**, *23*, 988. [CrossRef] [PubMed]
15. Tarozzi, A.; Angeloni, C.; Malaguti, M.; Morroni, F.; Hrelia, S.; Hrelia, P. Sulforaphane as a Potential Protective Phytochemical against Neurodegenerative Diseases. *Oxidative Med. Cell Longev.* **2013**, *2013*, 415078. [CrossRef] [PubMed]
16. Yanaka, A. Daily intake of broccoli sprouts normalizes bowel habits in human healthy subjects. *J. Clin. Biochem. Nutr.* **2018**, *62*, 75–82. [CrossRef] [PubMed]
17. Axelsson, A.S.; Tubbs, E.; Mecham, B.; Chacko, S.; Nenonen, H.A.; Tang, Y.; Fahey, J.W.; Derry, J.M.J.; Wollheim, C.B.; Wierup, N.; et al. Sulforaphane reduces hepatic glucose production and improves glucose control in patients with type 2 diabetes. *Sci. Transl. Med.* **2017**, *9*, 394. [CrossRef] [PubMed]
18. Lucarini, E.; Micheli, L.; Trallori, E.; Citi, V.; Martelli, A.; Testai, L.; De Nicola, G.R.; Iori, R.; Calderone, V.; Ghelardini, C.; et al. Effect of glucoraphanin and sulforaphane against chemotherapy-induced neuropathic pain: Kv7 potassium channels modulation by H_2S release in vivo. *Phytother. Res.* **2018**, *32*, 2226–2234. [CrossRef]
19. McDonnell, C.; Leánez, S.; Pol, O. The induction of the transcription factor Nrf2 enhances the antinociceptive effects of delta-opioid receptors in diabetic mice. *PLoS ONE* **2017**, *12*, e0180998. [CrossRef]
20. Redondo, A.; Chamorro, P.A.F.; Riego, G.; Leánez, S.; Pol, O. Treatment with sulforaphane produces antinociception and improves morphine effects during inflammatory pain in mice. *J. Pharmacol. Exp. Ther.* **2017**, *363*, 293–302. [CrossRef]
21. Martelli, A.; Testai, L.; Breschi, M.C.; Lawson, K.; McKay, N.G.; Miceli, F.; Taglialatela, M.; Calderone, V. Vasorelaxation by hydrogen sulphide involves activation of Kv7 potassium channels. *Pharmacol. Res.* **2013**, *70*, 27–34. [CrossRef] [PubMed]
22. Hedegaard, E.R.; Gouliaev, A.; Winther, A.K.; Arcanjo, D.D.; Aalling, M.; Renaltan, N.S.; Wood, M.E.; Whiteman, M.; Skovgaard, N.; Simonsen, U. Involvement of Potassium Channels and Calcium-Independent Mechanisms in Hydrogen Sulfide-Induced Relaxation of Rat Mesenteric Small Arteries. *J. Pharmacol. Exp. Ther.* **2016**, *356*, 53–63. [CrossRef] [PubMed]
23. Martelli, A.; Testai, L.; Citi, V.; Marino, A.; Bellagambi, F.G.; Ghimenti, S.; Breschi, M.C.; Calderone, V. Pharmacological characterization of the vascular effects of aryl isothiocyanates: Is hydrogen sulfide the real player? *Vasc. Pharmacol.* **2014**, *60*, 32–41. [CrossRef] [PubMed]
24. Platz, S.; Piberger, A.L.; Budnowski, J.; Herz, C.; Schreiner, M.; Blaut, M.; Hartwig, A.; Lamy, E.; Hanske, L.; Rohn, S. Bioavailability and biotransformation of sulforaphane and erucin metabolites in different biological matrices determined by LC-MS-MS. *Anal. Bioanal. Chem.* **2015**, *407*, 1819–1829. [CrossRef] [PubMed]
25. Valgimigli, L.; Iori, R. Antioxidant and pro-oxidant capacities of ITCs. *Environ. Mol. Mutagen.* **2009**, *50*, 222–237. [CrossRef] [PubMed]
26. Lazzeri, L.; Errani, O.; Leoni, M.; Venturi, G. *Eruca sativa* spp. oleifera: A new non-food crop. *Ind. Crops Prod.* **2004**, *20*, 67–73. [CrossRef]
27. Fuentes, E.; Alarcón, M.; Fuentes, M.; Carrasco, G.; Palomo, I. A novel role of *Eruca sativa* Mill. (Rocket) extract: Antiplatelet (NF-kB inhibition) and antithrombotic activities. *Nutrients* **2014**, *6*, 5839–5852. [CrossRef] [PubMed]
28. Sadiq, A.; Hayat, M.Q.; Mall, S.M. Qualitative and quantitative determination of secondary metabolites and antioxidant potential of *Eruca sativa*. *Nat. Prod. Chem. Res.* **2014**, *2*, 1000137. [CrossRef]
29. Sarwar Alam, M.; Kaur, G.; Jabbar, Z.; Javed, K.; Athar, M. *Eruca sativa* seeds possess antioxidant activity and exert a protective effect on mercuric chloride induced renal toxicity. *Food Chem. Toxicol.* **2007**, *45*, 910–920. [CrossRef]
30. Martelli, A.; Piragine, E.; Citi, V.; Testai, L.; Pagnotta, E.; Ugolini, L.; Lazzeri, L.; Di Cesare Mannelli, L.; Manzo, O.L.; Bucci, M.; et al. Erucin exhibits vasorelaxing effects and antihypertensive activity by H2 S-releasing properties. *Br. J. Pharmacol.* **2019**. [CrossRef]

31. Citi, V.; Piragine, E.; Pagnotta, E.; Ugolini, L.; Di Cesare Mannelli, L.; Testai, L.; Ghelardini, C.; Lazzeri, L.; Calderone, V.; Martelli, A. Anticancer properties of erucin, an H2 S-releasing isothiocyanate, on human pancreatic adenocarcinoma cells (AsPC-1). *Phytother. Res.* **2019**, *33*, 845–855. [CrossRef] [PubMed]
32. Clarke, J.D.; Hsu, A.; Riedl, K.; Bella, D.; Schwartz, S.J.; Stevens, J.F.; Ho, E. Bioavailability and inter-conversion of sulforaphane and erucin in human subjects consuming broccoli sprouts or broccoli supplement in a cross-over study design. *Pharmacol. Res.* **2011**, *64*, 456–463. [CrossRef] [PubMed]
33. Franco, P.; Spinozzi, S.; Pagnotta, E.; Lazzeri, L.; Ugolini, L.; Camborata, C.; Roda, A. Development of a liquid chromatography-electrospray ionization-tandem mass spectrometry method for the simultaneous analysis of intact glucosinolates and isothiocyanates in Brassicaceae seeds and functional foods. *J. Chromatogr. A* **2016**, *1428*, 154–161. [CrossRef] [PubMed]
34. Zaka, M.; Abbasi, B.H. Effects of bimetallic nanoparticles on seed germination frequency and biochemical characterisation of *Eruca sativa*. *IET Nanobiotechnol.* **2017**, *11*, 255–260. [CrossRef] [PubMed]
35. Oliviero, T.; Verkerk, R.; Dekker, M. Isothiocyanates from Brassica Vegetables—Effects of Processing, Cooking, Mastication, and Digestion. *Mol. Nutr. Food Res.* **2018**, *62*, 1701069. [CrossRef] [PubMed]
36. Dinkova-Kostova, A.T.; Fahey, J.W.; Kostov, R.V.; Kensler, T.W. KEAP1 and done? Targeting the NRF2 pathway with sulforaphane. *Trends Food Sci. Technol.* **2017**, *69*, 257–269. [CrossRef] [PubMed]
37. Rohwerder, T.; Sand, W. The sulfane sulfur of persulfides is the actual substrate of the sulfur-oxidizing enzymes from *Acidithiobacillus* and *Acidiphilium* spp. *Microbiology* **2003**, *149*, 1699–1710. [CrossRef]
38. Mishanina, T.V.; Libiad, M.; Banerjee, R. Biogenesis of reactive sulfur species for signaling by hydrogen sulfide oxidation pathways. *Nat. Chem. Biol.* **2015**, *11*, 457–464. [CrossRef]
39. Schreiber, A.K.; Nones, C.F.; Reis, R.C.; Chichorro, J.G.; Joice, M.; Cunha, J.M. Diabetic neuropathic pain: Physiopathology and treatment. *World J. Diabetes* **2015**, *6*, 432–444. [CrossRef]
40. Callaghan, B.C.; Cheng, H.T.; Stables, C.L.; Smith, A.L.; Feldman, E.L. Diabetic neuropathy: Clinical manifestations and current treatments. *Lancet Neurol.* **2012**, *11*, 521–534. [CrossRef]
41. Galer, B.S.; Gianas, A.; Jensen, M.P. Painful diabetic polyneuropathy: Epidemiology, pain description, and quality of life. *Diabetes Res. Clin. Pract.* **2000**, *47*, 123–128. [CrossRef]
42. Themistocleous, A.C.; Ramirez, J.D.; Shillo, P.R.; Lees, J.G.; Selvarajah, D.; Orengo, C.; Tesfaye, S.; Rice, A.S.; Bennett, D.L. The Pain in Neuropathy Study (PiNS): A cross-sectional observational study determining the somatosensory phenotype of painful and painless diabetic neuropathy. *Pain* **2016**, *157*, 1132–1145. [CrossRef] [PubMed]
43. Gore, M.; Brandenburg, N.A.; Dukes, E.; Hoffman, D.L.; Tai, K.S.; Stacey, B. Pain severity in diabetic peripheral neuropathy is associated with patient functioning, symptom levels of anxiety and depression, and sleep. *J. Pain Symptom Manag.* **2005**, *30*, 374–385. [CrossRef] [PubMed]
44. Malcangio, M.; Tomlinson, D.R. A pharmacologic analysis of mechanical hyperalgesia in streptozotocin/diabetic rats. *Pain* **1998**, *76*, 151–157. [CrossRef]
45. Murakami, T.; Iwanaga, T.; Ogawa, Y.; Fujita, Y.; Sato, E.; Yoshitomi, H.; Sunada, Y.; Nakamura, A. Development of sensory neuropathy in streptozotocin-induced diabetic mice. *Brain Behav.* **2013**, *3*, 35–41. [CrossRef] [PubMed]
46. Tesfaye, S. Recent advances in the management of diabetic distal symmetrical polyneuropathy. *J. Diabetes Investig.* **2011**, *2*, 33–42. [CrossRef]
47. Pop-Busui, R.; Boulton, A.J.; Feldman, E.L.; Bril, V.; Freeman, R.; Malik, R.A.; Sosenko, J.M.; Ziegler, D. Diabetic Neuropathy: A Position Statement by the American Diabetes Association. *Diabetes Care* **2017**, *40*, 136–154. [CrossRef]
48. Tesfaye, S.; Vileikyte, L.; Rayman, G.; Sindrup, S.H.; Perkins, B.A.; Baconja, M.; Vinik, A.I.; Boulton, A.J. The Toronto expert Panel on Diabetic Neuropathy. Painful diabetic peripheral neuropathy: Consensus recommendations on diagnosis, assessment and management. *Diabetes Metab. Res. Rev.* **2011**, *27*, 629–638. [CrossRef]
49. Tölle, T.; Xu, X.; Sadosky, A.B. Painful diabetic neuropathy: A cross-sectional survey of health state impairment and treatment patterns. *J. Diabetes Complicat.* **2006**, *20*, 26–33. [CrossRef]
50. Wang, A.; Leong, D.J.; Cardoso, L.; Sun, H.B. Nutraceuticals and osteoarthritis pain. *Pharmacol. Ther.* **2018**, *187*, 167–179. [CrossRef]

51. Crawford, C.; Boyd, C.; Berry, K.; Deuster, P. HERB Working Group. Dietary Ingredients Requiring Further Research Before Evidence-Based Recommendations Can Be Made for Their Use as an Approach to Mitigating Pain. *Pain Med.* **2019**. [CrossRef]
52. Brain, K.; Burrows, T.L.; Rollo, M.E.; Chai, L.K.; Clarke, E.D.; Hayes, C.; Hodson, F.J.; Collins, C.E. A systematic review and meta-analysis of nutrition interventions for chronic noncancer pain. *J. Hum. Nutr. Diet.* **2019**, *32*, 198–225. [CrossRef] [PubMed]
53. Martínez-Ballesta, M.C.; Moreno, D.A.; Carvajal, M. The Physiological Importance of Glucosinolates on Plant Response to Abiotic Stress in Brassica. *Int. J. Mol. Sci.* **2013**, *14*, 11607–11625. [CrossRef] [PubMed]
54. Hetta, M.H.; Owis, A.I.; Haddad, P.S.; Eid, H.M. The fatty acid-rich fraction of *Eruca sativa* (rocket salad) leaf extract exerts antidiabetic effects in cultured skeletal muscle, adipocytes and liver cells. *Pharm. Biol.* **2017**, *55*, 810–818. [CrossRef] [PubMed]
55. Khoobchandani, M.; Ojeswi, B.K.; Ganesh, N.; Srivastava, M.M.; Gabbanini, S.; Matera, R.; Iori, R.; Valgimigli, L. Antimicrobial properties and analytical profile of 850 traditional *Eruca sativa* seed oil: Comparison with various aerial and root plant extracts. *Food Chem.* **2010**, *120*, 217–224. [CrossRef]
56. Bennett, R.N.; Rosa, E.A.; Mellon, F.A.; Kroon, P.A. Ontogenic profiling of glucosinolates, flavonoids, and other secondary metabolites in *Eruca sativa* (salad rocket), *Diplotaxis erucoides* (wall rocket), *Diplotaxis tenuifolia* (wild rocket), and *Bunias orientalis* (Turkish rocket). *J. Agric. Food Chem.* **2006**, *54*, 4005–4015. [CrossRef] [PubMed]
57. Lazzeri, L.; Leoni, O.; Manici, L.M.; Palmieri, S.; Patalano, G. Use of Seed Flour as Soil Pesticide. U.S. Patent No. 7749549, 6 July 2010.
58. Rajanandh, M.G.; Kosey, S.; Prathiksha, G. Assessment of antioxidant supplementation on the neuropathic pain score and quality of life in diabetic neuropathy patients—A randomized controlled study. *Pharmacol. Rep.* **2014**, *66*, 44–48. [CrossRef] [PubMed]
59. Stepanović-Petrović, R.; Micov, A.; Tomić, M.; Pecikoza, U. Levetiracetam synergizes with gabapentin, pregabalin, duloxetine and selected antioxidants in a mouse diabetic painful neuropathy model. *Psychopharmacology (Berl.)* **2017**, *234*, 1781–1794. [CrossRef] [PubMed]
60. Aswar, M.; Patil, V. Ferulic acid ameliorates chronic constriction injury induced painful neuropathy in rats. *Inflammopharmacology* **2016**, *24*, 181–188. [CrossRef] [PubMed]
61. Hasanein, P.; Mohammad Zaheri, L. Effects of rosmarinic acid on an experimental model of painful diabetic neuropathy in rats. *Pharm. Biol.* **2014**, *52*, 1398–1402. [CrossRef] [PubMed]
62. Sun, J.; Chen, F.; Braun, C.; Zhou, Y.Q.; Rittner, H.; Tian, Y.K.; Cai, X.Y.; Ye, D.W. Role of curcumin in the management of pathological pain. *Phytomedicine* **2018**, *48*, 129–140. [CrossRef] [PubMed]
63. Wallace, J.L.; Wang, R. Hydrogen sulfide-based therapeutics: Exploiting a unique but ubiquitous gasotransmitter. *Nat. Rev. Drug Discov.* **2015**, *14*, 329–345. [PubMed]
64. Angelino, D.; Dosz, E.B.; Sun, J.; Hoeflinger, J.L.; van Tassell, M.L.; Chen, P.; Harnly, J.M.; Miller, M.J.; Jeffery, E.H. Myrosinase-dependent and–independent formation and control of isothiocyanate products of glucosinolate hydrolysis. *Front. Plant Sci.* **2015**, *6*, 1345. [CrossRef] [PubMed]
65. Vincent, A.M.; Russell, J.W.; Low, P.; Feldman, E.L. Oxidative stress in the pathogenesis of diabetic neuropathy. *Endocr. Rev.* **2004**, *25*, 612–628. [PubMed]
66. Di Cesare Mannelli, L.; Zanardelli, M.; Failli, P.; Ghelardini, C. Oxaliplatin-induced neuropathy: Oxidative stress as pathological mechanism. Protective effect of silibinin. *J. Pain.* **2012**, *13*, 276–284. [CrossRef] [PubMed]
67. UNI EN ISO. *Animal and Vegetable Fats 536 and Oils—Analysis by Gaschromatography of Methyl Esters of Fatty Acids, Oli E Grassi Animali E Vegetali—Analisi Gascromatografica Degli Esteri Metilici Degli Acidi Grassi;* Ente Nazionale Italiano di Unificazione: Milan, Italy, 1998.
68. ISO. *Animal and Vegetable Fats and Oils—Gas Chromatography of Fatty acid Methyl Esters—Part 4: Determination by Capillary Gas Chromatography;* International Organization for Standardization: Geneva, Switzerland, 2015.
69. Pagnotta, E.; Agerbirk, N.; Olsen, C.E.; Ugolini, L.; Cinti, S.; Lazzeri, L. Hydroxyl and Methoxyl Derivatives of Benzylglucosinolate in Lepidium densiflorum with Hydrolysis to Isothiocyanates and non-Isothiocyanate Products: Substitution Governs Product Type and Mass Spectral Fragmentation. *J. Agric. Food Chem.* **2017**, *65*, 3167–3178. [CrossRef] [PubMed]

70. Abdull Razis, A.F.; Bagatta, M.; De Nicola, G.R.; Iori, R.; Plant, N.; Ioannides, C. Characterization of the temporal induction of hepatic xenobiotic- metabolizing enzymes by glucosinolates and isothiocyanates: Requirement for at least a 6 h exposure to elicit complete induction profile. *J. Agric. Food Chem.* **2012**, *60*, 5556–5564. [CrossRef]
71. Singleton, V.L.; Orthofer, R.; Lamuela-Raventos, R.M. Analysis of total phenols and other oxidant substrates and antioxidants by mean of Folin-Ciocalteu reagent. *Methods Enzymol.* **1999**, *299*, 152–178.
72. Pessina, A.; Thomas, R.M.; Palmieri, S.; Luisi, P.L. An improved method for the purification of myrosinase and its physicochemical characterization. *Arch. Biochem Biophys.* **1990**, *280*, 383–389. [CrossRef]
73. Obrosov, A.; Shevalye, H.; Coppey, L.J.; Yorek, M.A. Effect of tempol on peripheral neuropathy in diet-induced obese and high-fat fed/low-dose streptozotocin-treated C57Bl6/J mice. *Free Radic Res.* **2017**, *51*, 360–367. [CrossRef]
74. Rakieten, N.; Rakieten, M.L.; Nadkarni, M.V. Studies on the diabetogenic action of streptozotocin. *Cancer Chemother. Rep.* **1963**, *29*, 91–98. [PubMed]
75. Russo, R.; D'Agostino, G.; Mattace Raso, G.; Avagliano, C.; Cristiano, C.; Meli, R.; Calignano, A. Central administration of oxytocin reduces hyperalgesia in mice: Implication for cannabinoid and opioid systems. *Peptides* **2012**, *38*, 81–88. [CrossRef] [PubMed]
76. Di Cesare Mannelli, L.; Maresca, M.; Farina, C.; Scherz, M.W.; Ghelardini, C. A model of neuropathic pain induced by sorafenib in the rat: Effect of dimiracetam. *Neurotoxicology* **2015**, *50*, 101–107. [CrossRef] [PubMed]
77. Blackburn-Munro, G.; Jensen, B.S. The anticonvulsant retigabine attenuates nociceptive behaviours in rat models of persistent and neuropathic pain. *Eur. J. Pharmacol.* **2003**, *460*, 109–116. [CrossRef]

Sample Availability: Samples of the compounds are available from the authors.

molecules

MDPI

Article

Discovery of Lipid Peroxidation Inhibitors from *Bacopa* Species Prioritized through Multivariate Data Analysis and Multi-Informative Molecular Networking

Tongchai Saesong [1], Pierre-Marie Allard [2], Emerson Ferreira Queiroz [2], Laurence Marcourt [2], Nitra Nuengchamnong [3], Prapapan Temkitthawon [1], Nantaka Khorana [4], Jean-Luc Wolfender [2,*] and Kornkanok Ingkaninan [1,*]

[1] Department of Pharmaceutical Chemistry and Pharmacognosy, Faculty of Pharmaceutical Sciences and Center of Excellence for Innovation in Chemistry, Naresuan University, Phitsanulok 65000, Thailand
[2] School of Pharmaceutical Sciences, EPGL, University of Geneva, University of Lausanne, CMU Rue Michel Servet 1, 1211 Geneva 4, Switzerland
[3] Science Lab Center, Faculty of Science, Naresuan University, Phitsanulok 65000, Thailand
[4] Division of Pharmaceutical Sciences, School of Pharmaceutical Sciences, University of Phayao, Phayao 56000, Thailand
* Correspondence: jean-luc.wolfender@unige.ch (J.-L.W.); k_ingkaninan@yahoo.com (K.I.)

Academic Editor: Pinarosa Avato
Received: 29 June 2019; Accepted: 15 August 2019; Published: 17 August 2019

Abstract: A major goal in the discovery of bioactive natural products is to rapidly identify active compound(s) and dereplicate known molecules from complex biological extracts. The conventional bioassay-guided fractionation process can be time consuming and often requires multi-step procedures. Herein, we apply a metabolomic strategy merging multivariate data analysis and multi-informative molecular maps to rapidly prioritize bioactive molecules directly from crude plant extracts. The strategy was applied to 59 extracts of three *Bacopa* species (*B. monnieri*, *B. caroliniana* and *B. floribunda*), which were profiled by UHPLC-HRMS^2 and screened for anti-lipid peroxidation activity. Using this approach, six lipid peroxidation inhibitors **1–6** of three *Bacopa* spp. were discovered, three of them being new compounds: monnieraside IV (**4**), monnieraside V (**5**) and monnieraside VI (**6**). The results demonstrate that this combined approach could efficiently guide the discovery of new bioactive natural products. Furthermore, the approach allowed to evidence that main semi-quantitative changes in composition linked to the anti-lipid peroxidation activity were also correlated to seasonal effects notably for *B. monnieri*.

Keywords: metabolomics; multivariate data analysis; molecular network; *Bacopa monnieri*; LC-MS

1. Introduction

Natural products (NPs) play an important role as a source of various pharmaceuticals and biologically active substances. However, the discovery of new bioactive NPs is challenging because of the inherent complex composition of crude natural extracts. Such extracts contain hundreds, if not thousands, of chemical constituents and the purification and identification of bioactive NPs by conventional methods is a time consuming multi-step procedure. Moreover, bioactive substances can be lost during purification and effort can be wasted in the unnecessary re-isolation of known NPs. Therefore, it is important to pinpoint bioactive candidates and recognize known metabolites (dereplication) early in the purification process in order to avoid the redundant isolation of known molecules [1,2].

Recently, metabolomics combined with multivariate data analysis (MVA) has proven to be an efficient tool to predict bioactive constituents in NP research [3–7]. Metabolomics aims at providing comprehensive qualitative and quantitative analysis of the whole set of metabolites (metabolome) present in a complex biological sample [8,9]. The most used analytical techniques in metabolomics are nuclear magnetic resonance (NMR) and mass spectrometry (MS) [10]. Generally metabolite profiling of natural extracts is achieved via high resolution ultra-high performance liquid chromatography (UHPLC), coupled to high resolution tandem mass spectrometry ($HRMS^2$), which provides molecular formula and fragmentation information on most NPs in extracts in an untargeted manner [11]. Unsupervised or supervised multivariate data analysis such as principal components analysis (PCA) or orthogonal partial least squares (OPLS) are then needed to mine such data and highlight biomarkers. Alternative strategies have been developed to explore LC-$HRMS^2$ metabolite profiling datasets with the aim of highlighting structural similarities between analytes and efficiently identify new compounds with potential therapeutic interest. Molecular network analysis (MN) [12,13] is a computer-based approach allowing the organization of fragmentation spectra from MS-based metabolomics experiments in order to dereplicate and eventually prioritize natural products of interest [14–16]. MN is generated based on the similarities of fragmentation patterns and, thus, indirectly allows the grouping of analytes with closely related structures. Networks can be built using the Global Natural Product Social Molecular Networking (GNPS) platform [17] or software such as Metgem or MS-Dial [18,19].

Bacopa is a genus of aquatic plants belonging to the Plantaginaceae family. Three species occur in Thailand: *B. monnieri*, *B. caroliniana* and *B. floribunda* [20]. Among them, only *B. monnieri* (Brahmi) has been reported as a herbal medicine in Ayurvedic medicine for learning and memory improvement [21]. The safety and efficacy of Brahmi extracts in animal models [22,23] and in clinical trials [24–28] have been proven and support its traditional uses. Intake of Brahmi has been reported to exert undesirable effects on the gastrointestinal tract, such as nausea, increased stool frequency and abdominal cramps [25,29], which might be explained by a cholinergic effect [30]. In addition, severe liver toxicity has been detected in women taking Brahmi products for vitiligo disease. Nevertheless, their liver function returned to normal after discontinuation of products' usage [31]. Other reports however indicated that Brahmi possessed hepatoprotective activity [32,33]. Notwithstanding such adverse effects and considering the positive effects of the plant in relation with cognition improvements, further investigations are still worth to identify bioactive principles.

The compounds responsible for the memory enhancing effects of Brahmi have been reported to be triterpenoid saponins i.e., bacoside A_3, bacopaside I, bacopaside II, bacopasaponin C and bacopaside X [34,35]. They are considered as markers of Brahmi [36–41], and their level is assessed for quality control purposes. Usually, the level of plant specialized metabolites is highly variable according to environmental factors. In Brahmi, the levels of such markers were found to vary significantly depending on the part of used (leaves, stems, shoots etc.), collection area and season [42–45].

Moreover, this plant also contains other classes of NPs such as sterols [46], flavonoids [47] and phenylethanoids [48,49] that may play roles in the pharmacological activities of the plant. It has also been reported that part of the neuroprotective effects of Brahmi appeared to result from its antioxidant activities that suppress neuronal oxidative stress. Brahmi has been found to inhibit the lipid peroxidation reaction of brain homogenate in a dose-dependent manner [50].

In this study, we aimed at searching for compounds that could be involved in the memory improvement activity of Brahmi through lipid peroxidation inhibitory activity. In addition, the anti-lipid peroxidation activity of two other *Bacopa* species has been investigated. To achieve these goals, a metabolomic strategy combining multivariate data analysis (MVA) and bioactivity informed molecular maps [14] was used as a guide to highlight bioactive constituents early in the phytochemical study process and directly target their isolation.

2. Results and Discussion

Fifty-nine extracts of three *Bacopa* species from different regions of Thailand and harvested at various seasons [summer (March to June), rainy season (July to October) and winter (November to February)] were collected for this study. All extracts were profiled by UHPLC-HRMS^2 to generate data that could be used to monitor metabolite profile variations across the whole dataset and provide high quality data dependent MS^2 spectra for annotation. In parallel, all of the extracts were screened for their anti-lipid peroxidation activity. Variations in the profiles were then linked to bioactivity modulation through MVA in order to highlight possible bioactive metabolites. In addition, the MS^2 dataset was organized using the GNPS platform to generate a MN, which was visualized using Cytoscape software. The bioactivity and taxonomy of plant extracts were mapped on the MN in order to pinpoint cluster(s) of potentially bioactive metabolite(s). The lists of prioritized candidates from MVA and MN were finally compared and the common metabolites were then selected as bioactive candidates. They were annotated based on their MS^2 spectra compared with experimental or in silico MS/MS database (GNPS libraries and DNP–ISDB). Both known and possibly novel compounds were isolated to establish their bioactivities and their structures were unambiguously determined by NMR. A summary of the prioritization workflow is presented in Figure 1.

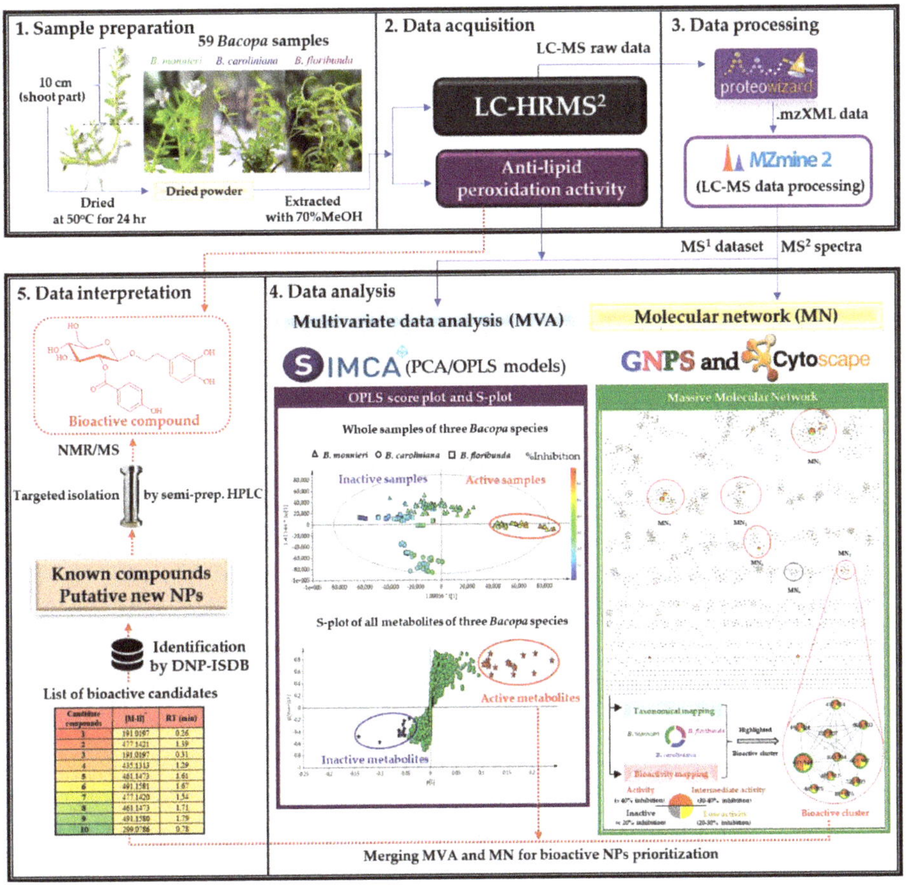

Figure 1. Schematic diagram of lipid peroxidation inhibitor discovery from LC-HRMS^2 analyses of 59 *Bacopa* extracts combining metabolomics MVA and multi-informative MN.

2.1. *Lipid Peroxidation Inhibitory Activity Evaluation of the Extracts*

The fifty-nine extracts of three *Bacopa* species collected from different regions of Thailand in rainy season, winter and summer were submitted to a thiobarbituric acid reactive substances (TBAR) assay. A significant variation of lipid peroxidation inhibitory activities between groups of related samples was observed (Figure 2A–C). In particular, *B. monnieri* harvested in summer (Figure 2C) exhibited stronger inhibitory effects (around 2-fold) than *B. monnieri* collected in other seasons or than other *Bacopa* species.

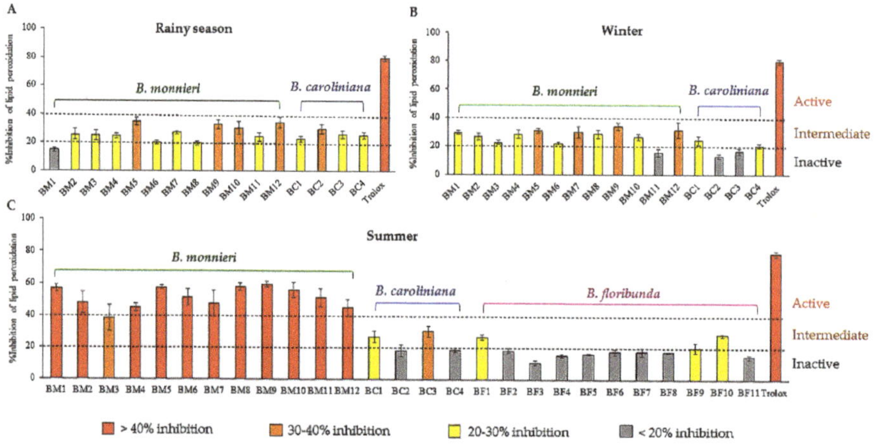

Figure 2. Anti-lipid peroxidation activities of three *Bacopa* species i.e., *B. monnieri* (BM), *B. caroliniana* (BC), and *B. floribunda* plant (BF) collected from different regions in the (**A**) rainy, (**B**) winter and (**C**) summer seasons. Samples giving >40% inhibition were considered active, 30-40% inhibition was intermediate activity, 20-30% inhibition was low activity, and those exhibiting <20% inhibition were considered inactive. Trolox (100 µg/mL) was used as a positive control.

2.2. *Potential Bioactive Metabolites Prioritized through Multivariate Statistical Analysis and Molecular Networking*

2.2.1. Organization and Pre–Treatment of the Metabolite Profiling Data

All extracts that were screened for bioactivity were profiled by UHPLC-HRMS^2 using a generic gradient in negative ionization (NI) mode to provide MS^1 and MS^2 data of all metabolites in the *Bacopa* samples. The NI mode was used because it provided far more molecular ion features than the positive ionization (PI) mode for the samples considered. This was in good agreement with the rich polyphenolic content of *Bacopa* species.

After profiling, the LC–HRMS^2 data was treated by MZmine [51] for mass detection, chromatogram building, deconvolution, isotopic peak grouping, alignment and gap filling. This resulted in a peaklist of 6082 features which was further filtered to a peaklist of 4191 features having associated MS^2 spectra. This peaklist of 4191 features was exported as input for the MVA (MS^1 data only) and for MN generation (MS^1 and MS^2 data). These data were correlated to the extract's bioactivity results in order to highlight bioactive compounds responsible for anti–lipid peroxidation in *Bacopa* species.

2.2.2. Multivariate Data Analysis

As a preliminary step, the whole MS^1 dataset (consisting of *m/z* values, retention times (RT), and intensities) was analyzed by principal component analysis (PCA) to investigate the differences of metabolite profiles of three *Bacopa* species and the effects on quality of regional cultivation and seasonal harvesting of BM and BC samples. The PCA scatter plot (normalized by Pareto-scaling) is presented in Figure 3A. It showed obvious discrimination among *B. monnieri* (BM), *B. caroliniana* (BC) and *B. floribunda* (BF), exhibiting 65.50% of the total variance in the dataset (46.10% of the variance for PC1 and 19.40% for PC2). This plot exhibited obvious inter–species variations, while intra–species variation of BM and BC samples could only be observed in the PCA plots generated from the individual datasets of BM and BC (Figure 3B,C). Interestingly, the PCA plot of the BM dataset showed a clear separation between BM samples collected in summer versus those harvested in the rainy season and winter (Figure 3B). For BC, the samples were clustered into three groups, according to the harvesting season (Figure 3C). These results demonstrated that the metabolite profiles of BM and BC in different seasons were different and could thus impact the bioactivity of these samples. Therefore, notably for BM, which is used as a food supplement, the harvesting season clearly needs to be taken in consideration to favor the sought-after bioactivity. On the other hand, the PCA plots indicated that the sample composition did not seem to be affected by the region of provenance.

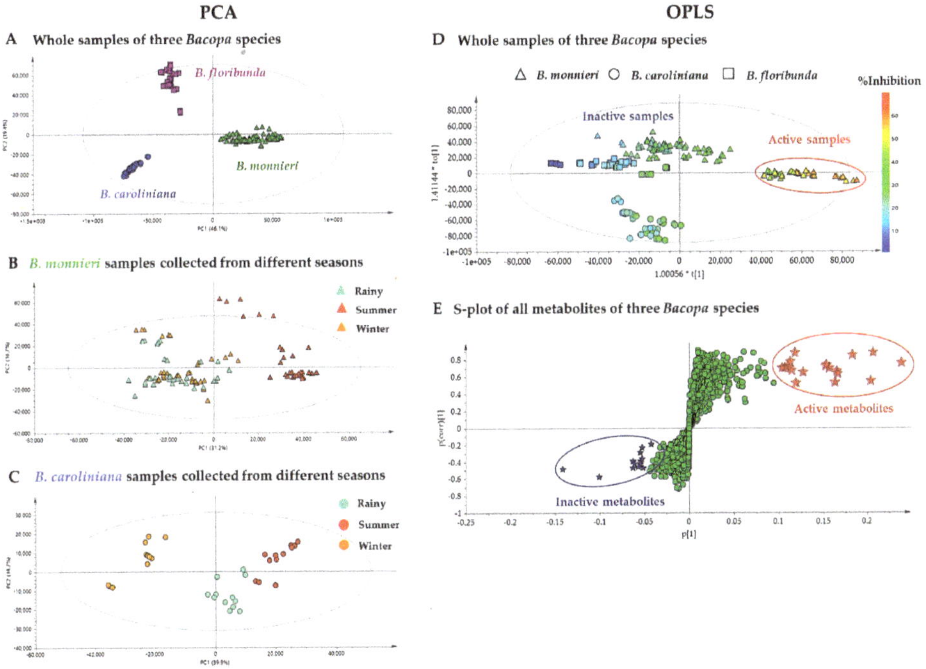

Figure 3. (**A**) PCA score plot based on chemical profiles of 59 extracts of three *Bacopa* species. (**B**,**C**) PCA score plots based on chemical profiles of 36 extracts of *B. monnieri* and 12 extracts of *B. caroliniana*, respectively from different sources in three seasonal collections. (**D**) OPLS score plot based on the chemical profiles and anti-lipid peroxidation activity of all *Bacopa* extracts. (**E**). S-plot presenting nineteen candidate active features with high p[1] values (red filled star) and inactive features with low p[1] value (blue filled star).

In order to correlate the variations observed in bioactivities with the metabolite profiles of all extracts, the data was analyzed by a supervised method (OPLS), which is a regression extension of PCA allowing maximization of the separation between groups of observations and pinpointing of variables contributing to the separation. The peaklist consisting of *m/z* values, RT, and intensities was used as X variables (similarly to what had been done for PCA) and the %inhibitions of lipid peroxidation were used as the Y variables. A significant separation between the active and the inactive groups was observed, as shown in the OPLS score plot (Figure 3D), where a reddish color represents a high %lipid peroxidation inhibition. As expected from the initial screening results (see Figure 2), all samples exhibiting an activity higher than 40% were grouped (BM samples collected in summer). From the S-plot of all metabolites in the *Bacopa* samples (Figure 3E), 19 features at the upper right corner (highlighted with red stars) were identified as the most discriminating features between the active and non-active samples, and were thus potentially responsible for the observed anti-lipid peroxidation effects. In contrast, the features at the lower left corner corresponded to metabolites that were likely non-actives. These nineteen features with high p[1] values were thus ranked as putative bioactive features (Table 1). Using the *m/z* and RT of each feature (labeled **F–n°** in the Table 1), we found that seventeen features corresponded to unique compounds and that two other features, **F2** and **F8** were adduct and dimer forms of **F18** and **F3**, respectively. Therefore, seventeen bioactive candidates were prioritized from the S-plot. In parallel to this MVA treatment, the same dataset was explored using the multi-informative MN strategy.

2.2.3. Multi-Informational Molecular Map

Multi-informative MN is a strategy that has previously been demonstrated to effectively prioritize bioactive compounds in natural extract collections [14]. For this, the MS^1–MS^2 peaklist was analyzed using such approach in order to visually highlight the clusters of compounds possibly responsible for the observed anti-lipid peroxidation activity. Here, the 4191 features presenting MS^2 were organized using the GNPS platform to generate a single MN. In this MN, the nodes representing each feature were grouped into 602 clusters by similarity of fragmentation patterns. A multi-informational molecular map was created by merging this MN with biological results and taxonomical information (Figure 4A). All nodes in the MN were color-labeled according to the corresponding lipid peroxidation inhibition level of the extracts (bioactive mapping). This allowed a rapid highlighting of potential bioactive molecular families. Additionally, a taxonomical mapping was applied. The species were differentiated by colored tags on the border of each node (Figure 4A). This additional layout was used to indicate the distribution of plant species for each node. If a given node was most abundantly found in bioactive species, it could be hypothesized that this node was potentially related to an NP responsible for the observed bioactivity of the extract of the corresponding species. Using such mapping, twenty putative bioactive clusters with a minimum of five nodes, corresponding to more than a hundred features were selected by visual inspection based on their dominant red color tags indicating presence in bioactive extracts (Figure S1). The colors of the border (taxonomical origin mapping) suggested that the active nodes were mainly found in *B. monnieri*, while only a few were related to other species. The size of the nodes was based on the MS intensity, which was obtained from an average of the corresponding signal across all samples. In a MN, molecular families tend to cluster together, thus leading to similar ionization behaviours within clusters. Consequently, we hypothesized that the MS intensity of these molecules within a cluster was indicative of their relative abundance. According to this logic, five bioactive clusters (MN_1–MN_5, Figure 4B), were further prioritized based on the five largest nodes, leading to a selection of 25 potential bioactive features (Table 1). Among these, seventeen features corresponded to unique molecules, whereas the other neighboring nodes connected to these features were dimeric or adduct forms. Thus, seventeen compounds from MN_1-MN_5 were considered as bioactive candidates from MN (Table 1). An example of unprioritized cluster (MN_6), potentially linked to non-active metabolites, with dominant grey color tags is also shown in Figure 4C for comparison purposes.

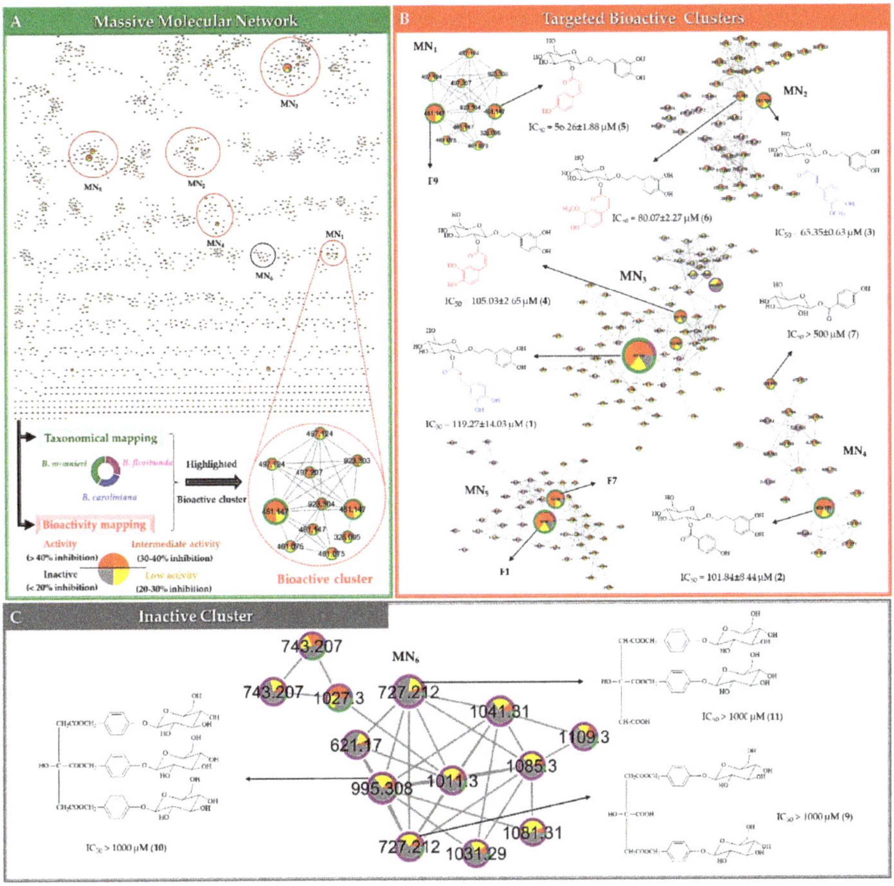

Figure 4. Multi-informational molecular map obtained from the analyses of 59 extracts of three *Bacopa* species mapping with taxonomy and anti-lipid peroxidation activity. Taxonomies of the samples are shown in different colors on the border of each node. Green, blue and purple represent BM, BC and BF, respectively. Bioactivities of the samples are shown in different colors inside each node. The active extracts with an inhibition higher than 40% are represented in red and inactive extracts with less than 40% inhibition are represented in gray. The size of each node is based on the peak height intensity. (**A**) A multi-informative massive molecular network created from MS^2 datasets. (**B**) Five selected bioactive clusters, MN_1-MN_5 with two potential candidates in each cluster, (**C**) an inactive cluster, MN_6. Chemical structures of the active compounds in Figure 4B,C are expressed with IC_{50} values of anti-lipid peroxidation activity.

Table 1. The nineteen bioactive candidate features (**F1–F19**) ranked by p[1] value from S-plot of MVA and twenty-five bioactive candidates selected from prioritized clusters of MN (MN_1–MN_5). Ten potential bioactive compounds prioritized from the merging of MVA and MN approach are highlighted (one color per cluster). IC_{50} values of the compounds on anti-lipid peroxidation activity are expressed in μM and as an average from triplicate experiments ± standard deviation.

ID	*m/z*	RT (min)	p[1] Value*	Selected Bioactive Cluster	Chemical Formula	Δ ppm	Dereplicated Compounds (MSMS Based Identification)**	Isolated Compounds (NMR Identification)	Anti-Lipid Peroxidation Activity (IC_{50} (μM))
F1	191.0197[M − H]⁻	0.25	0.239	MN_5	$C_6H_8O_7$	0.14	Idaric acid-1,4-lactone		
F2	217.0487[M + Cl]⁻	0.23	0.207	NS	$C_6H_{14}O_6$	−1.20	Adduct of **F18**		
F3	477.1420[M − H]⁻	1.38	0.204	MN_3	$C_{23}H_{26}O_{11}$	−3.91	Plantainoside B[b]	Plantainoside B (**1**)	119.27 ± 14.03
F4	377.0873[M − H]⁻	0.24	0.183	NS	$C_{18}H_{18}O_9$	1.08	4,8-Dihydroxy-1,2,3,6,7-pentamethoxy-9H-xanthen-9-one		
F5	315.1099[M − H]⁻	0.60	0.166	NS	$C_{14}H_{20}O_8$	−4.31	2-(3,5-Dihydroxyphenyl)ethanol-3′-*O*-*β*-D-glucopyranoside	3,4-dihydroxyphenethyl glucoside (**8**)	>500
F6	435.1313[M − H]⁻	1.28	0.165	MN_4	$C_{21}H_{24}O_{10}$	−3.74	Monnieraside III[a]	Monnieraside III (**2**)	101.84 ± 8.44
F7	191.0197[M − H]⁻	0.31	0.163	MN_5	$C_6H_8O_7$	0.14	Idaric acid-1,4-lactone isomer		
F8	955.2917[2M − H]⁻	1.38	0.156	MN_3	$C_{23}H_{26}O_{11}$	−4.91	Dimer of **F3**		
F9	461.1473[M − H]⁻	1.60	0.154	MN_1	$C_{23}H_{26}O_{10}$	−4.29	8-*O*-(6′-*O*-*trans*-Coumaroyl-*β*-D-glucopyranosyl)-3,4-dihydroxyphenylethanol		
F10	491.1580[M − H]⁻	1.67	0.152	MN_2	$C_{24}H_{28}O_{11}$	−4.51	Monnieraside II[a]	Monnieraside II (**3**)	65.35 ± 0.63
F11	1063.4467[M − H]⁻	3.07	0.128	NS	$C_{49}H_{76}O_{23}S$	−3.92	Unidentified[c]		
F12	477.1420[M − H]⁻	1.53	0.119	MN_3	$C_{23}H_{26}O_{11}$	−3.91	Plantainoside B[b]	Monnieraside IV[e] (**4**)	105.03 ± 2.65
F13	219.0458[M − H]⁻	0.23	0.118	NS	$C_{15}H_8O_2$	−3.41	Unidentified[c]		
F14	461.1473[M − H]⁻	1.71	0.115	MN_1	$C_{23}H_{26}O_{10}$	−4.29	8-*O*-(6′-*O*-*trans*-Coumaroyl-*β*-D-glucopyranosyl)-3,4-dihydroxyphenylethanol	Monnieraside V[e] (**5**)	56.26 ± 1.88
F15	491.1579[M − H]⁻	1.78	0.113	MN_2	$C_{24}H_{28}O_{11}$	−4.31	Monnieraside II[a]	Monnieraside VI[e] (**6**)	80.07 ± 2.27
F16	977.4458[M − H]⁻	3.00	0.112	NS	$C_{46}H_{74}O_{20}S$	−3.75	Bacopaside I[a]		>1000[f]
F17	299.0786[M − H]⁻	0.78	0.110	MN_4	$C_{13}H_{16}O_8$	−4.54	4-Hydroxybenzoyl glucose[b]	4-hydroxybenzoyl glucose (**7**)	>500
F18	181.0717[M − H]⁻	0.23	0.107	NS	$C_6H_{14}O_6$	−0.21	Mannitol[d]		
F19	631.2274[M − H]⁻	0.60	0.104	NS	$C_{46}H_{32}O_3$	0.74	Unidentified[c]		
F20	497.1243[M + Cl]⁻	1.58	0.033	MN_1	$C_{23}H_{26}O_{10}$	−4.63	Adduct of **F9**		
F21	461.0749[M − H]⁻	1.56	0.003	MN_1	$C_{21}H_{18}O_{12}$	−5.09	3′,4′,5,7-Tetrahydroxyflavone5-*O*-*β*-D-glucurono-pyranoside		
F22	497.1243[M + Cl]⁻	1.71	0.029	MN_1	$C_{23}H_{26}O_{10}$	−4.63	Adduct of **F14**		
F23	521.1685[M − H]⁻	1.66	0.053	MN_2	$C_{25}H_{30}O_{12}$	−3.93	Aucubigenin-10-*O*-(4-hydroxy-3- methoxy-cinnamoyl), 1-*O*-*β*-D-glucopyranoside[b]		
F24	983.3235[2M − H]⁻	1.67	0.084	MN_2	$C_{24}H_{28}O_{11}$	−4.53	Dimer of **F10**		
F25	527.1347[M + Cl]⁻	1.67	0.030	MN_2	$C_{24}H_{28}O_{11}$	−4.05	Adduct of **F10**		
F26	341.0893[M − H]⁻	0.66	0.064	MN_3	$C_{15}H_{18}O_9$	−4.37	Chaenorrhinoside[b]		
F27	477.1421[M − H]⁻	1.62	0.043	MN_3	$C_{23}H_{26}O_{11}$	−3.90	Plantainoside B[b]		
F28	871.2706[2M − H]⁻	1.29	0.077	MN_4	$C_{21}H_{24}O_{10}$	−4.57	Dimer of **F6**		
F29	471.1084[M + Cl]⁻	1.29	0.033	MN_4	$C_{21}H_{24}O_{10}$	−4.36	Adduct of **F6**		
F30	599.1642[2M − H]⁻	0.79	0.068	MN_4	$C_{13}H_{16}O_8$	−4.07	Dimer of **F17**		
F31	421.0046[M − H]⁻	0.31	0.008	MN_5	$C_{17}H_{10}O_{13}$	0.63	Unidentified[c]		
F32	405.0308[M − H]⁻	0.31	0.057	MN_5	$C_{14}H_{14}O_{14}$	0.69	Unidentified[c]		
F33	191.0198[M − H]⁻	0.38	0.027	MN_5	$C_6H_8O_7$	−0.38	Idaric acid-1,4-lactone		
Three isolated inactive compounds selected from inactive cluster (MN_6) of the MN and in S-plot of MVA									
F34	727.2125[M − H]⁻	1.20	−0.026	MN_6	$C_{32}H_{40}O_{19}$	−4.67	Unidentified[c]	Parishin C (**9**)	>1000
F35	995.3078[M − H]⁻	1.40	−0.037	MN_6	$C_{45}H_{56}O_{25}$	−4.03	Parishin A[d]	Parishin A (**10**)	>1000
F36	727.2123[M − H]⁻	1.12	−0.060	MN_6	$C_{32}H_{40}O_{19}$	−4.40	Unidentified[c]	Parishin B (**11**)	>1000

* The values obtained from S-plot of OPLS and ** DNP-ISDB in silico fragmented results unless specified (Top 1 result only are reported). [a,b] The compound has been previously reported in *B. monnieri* and Plantaginaceae family, respectively, [c] No matching with DNP-ISDB or GNPS libraries, [d] Annotated compound from GNPS spectral libraries, [e] New compound and [f] Standard compound. NS: not selected from bioactive clusters (MN_1–MN_5) but from other clusters in MN.

2.2.4. Merging MVA and MN for Bioactive Candidate Prioritization

The S-plot of MVA brings statistical correlation between features and bioactivity but can however be biased by scaling and normalization processes. On the other side, the bioactivity-informed MN approach allows to highlight structural relations between putative bioactive compounds and thus, despite the lack of statistics, allows to indirectly discriminate possible MS artefacts from specialized metabolites features. In order to prioritize unique bioactive molecules from the merging of MVA and MN, common features found in both approaches were highlighted with color tags (see in Table 1) and prioritized as potential bioactive candidates. The two largest nodes found in each five selected clusters (MN_1-MN_5, Figure 4B) represented features also found in the list of putative bioactive candidates in MVA. Therefore, these ten features (**F1, F3, F6, F7, F9, F10, F12, F14, F15** and **F17**) were prioritized as potential bioactive compounds for this study (Table 1).

2.3. DNP-ISDB Dereplication and Purification of Bioactive Candidates

In the MN, the acquired MS^2 spectra of each node from the whole MN were matched automatically against GNPS spectral libraries and then annotated against an in silico spectral database build from the Dictionary of Natural Products (DNP-ISDB) as previously described [1] thus providing an identification of level 2 [52]. These spectra were subsequently matched against with a subset of the DNP-ISDB restricted to Plantaginaceae specialized metabolites in order to refine the dereplication results. The top five candidate structures with highest spectral similarity scores were retrieved and the chemical structures for each node was directly visualized within the network using Cytoscape and the ChemViz plugin. The candidate structures for each node were ranked according to their spectral similarity score and the structure with the highest score was reported (Table 1).

Compounds **F1** and **F7** (*m/z* 191.0197 $[M - H]^-$) were isomers, which were both annotated as idaric acid-1,4-lactone. The other three pairs of isomers i.e., **F3** and **F12** (*m/z* 477.1421 $[M - H]^-$), **F9** and **F14** (*m/z* 461.1473 $[M - H]^-$) and **F10** and **F15** (*m/z* 491.1581 $[M - H]^-$), were proposed to be plantainoside B, 8-*O*-(6′-*O*-trans-coumaroyl-*β*-D-glucopyranosyl)-3,4-dihydroxyphenylethanol and monnieraside II, respectively. The **F6** was predicted to be monnieraside III. The unprioritized features, **F34–36**, did not match with MS^2 spectra libraries from DNP–ISDB, however **F35** was matched against the GNPS spectral library entry parishin A. From these dereplication results, the four pairs of isomers could not be differentiated and two inactive features were given no annotation. Therefore, they may have been new compounds. To establish their structures and evaluate their bioactivity potential, targeted purification of these potential bioactive and inactive compounds was carried out. In order to isolate these compounds, the active extract of *B. monnieri* was fractionated by medium pressure liquid chromatography coupled to an ultraviolet detector (MPLC-UV). The conditions of this separation were first developed by HPLC–UV using a column with identic stationary phase. After this, the analytical HPLC conditions were geometrically transferred to semi–preparative MPLC-UV [53]. All of the MPLC fractions obtained were systematically analyzed by LC-MS. Using the retention time and molecular weight, it was possible to localize the ten potential bioactive candidates (**F1, F3, F6, F7, F9, F10, F12, F14, F15** and **F17**) and three unprioritized features (**F34–36**). MPLC fractions were further purified by semi–preparative HPLC. As for the separation using MPLC, the conditions of the semi–preparative HPLC were first developed in an analytical method using a column with a similar stationary phase chemistry. After this step, the condition was successfully transferred to the semi–preparative HPLC [54] (Figure S2). In order to avoid loss of resolution, the sample was introduced into the semi–preparative HPLC column by dry load according to a recently developed protocol [55]. Thanks to this approach, it was possible to obtain a high–resolution separation of the majority of the polar compounds, allowing them to be obtained in a high degree of purity. Using this system, seven bioactive candidates prioritized by MVA and MN (compounds **1–7**, corresponding to features **F3, F6, F10, F12, F14, F15** and **F17**, respectively) and one compound highlighted MVA only (compound **8**, corresponding to feature **F5**) were isolated. In addition, compounds **9–11** (features **F34–36**), which were all found in a non–prioritized cluster (MN_6, Figure 4C) and in an area of the S-plot indicative of potential inactive compounds (lower left corner, Figure 3E), were also isolated.

2.4. *Identification and Structure Elucidation of Compounds* **1–11**

After purification, all isolated compounds were fully characterized by extensive 2D NMR experiments, which complemented the $HRMS^2$ results. Compounds **1–3** and **7–11**, were identified as plantainoside B (**1**), monnieraside III (**2**), monnieraside II (**3**) [48], 4-hydroxybenzoyl glucose (**7**) [56], 3,4-dihydroxyphenethyl glucoside (**8**) [57], parishin C (**9**), parishin A (**10**) and parishin B (**11**) [58], respectively, by comparing their spectral data with literature. Compounds **4–6** were isolated for the first time and identified as new phenylethanoid glycosides: monnieraside IV (**4**), monnieraside V (**5**), and monnieraside VI (**6**). The ^1H and ^{13}C-NMR of **4–6** are provided in Table 2 and their COSY, HMBC and ROESY correlations are shown in Figure 5.

Table 2. ^1H- and ^{13}C-NMR (600/151 MHz, in CD_3OD) of **4–6**.

Position	Monnieraside IV (4)		Monnieraside V (5)		Monnieraside VI (6)	
	δ_C	δ_H (J in Hz)	δ_C	δ_H (J in Hz)	δ_C	δ_H (J in Hz)
1	131.5		131.3		131.2	
2	117.0	6.61, d (2.1)	116.8	6.62, d (2.1)	116.6	6.61, d (2.1)
3	146.0		145.8		145.8	
4	144.6		144.4		144.3	
5	116.3	6.61, d (8.1)	116.1	6.61, d (8.1)	116.2	6.60, d (8.1)
6	121.4	6.49, dd (8.1, 2.1)	121.1	6.50, dd (8.1, 2.1)	121.1	6.48, dd (8.1, 2.1)
7	36.5	2.68, t (7.2)	36.3	2.68, m	36.3	2.67, t (7.1)
8	71.9	3.64, dt (9.8, 7.2) 4.00, dt (9.8, 7.2)	71.5	3.63, dt (9.4, 7.3) 4.01, dt (9.4, 6.9)	71.6	3.63, dt (9.8, 7.1) 4.00, dt (9.8, 7.1)
1'	102.3	4.45, d (8.1)	102.0	4.44, d (8.1)	102.1	4.46, d (8.0)
2'	74.9	4.79, dd (9.3, 8.1)	74.6	4.79, dd (9.3, 8.1)	74.7	4.79, dd (9.3, 8.0)
3'	76.2	3.51, t (9.3)	75.9	3.50, t (9.3)	76.0	3.52, t (9.3)
4'	71.8	3.38, t (9.3)	71.5	3.38, t (9.3)	71.5	3.38, t (9.3)
5'	78.1	3.29 (overlapped)	77.9	3.28 (overlapped)	77.9	3.30 (overlapped)
6'	62.6	3.69, dd (12.0, 5.7) 3.88, dd (12.0, 2.3)	62.4	3.69, dd (11.9, 5.8) 3.88, dd (11.9, 1.8)	62.4	3.69, dd (12.0, 5.8) 3.88, dd (12.0, 2.3)
1"	128.2		127.6		127.9	
2"	118.7	7.38, d (2.1)	133.4	7.60, d (8.7)	114.8	7.72, d (2.0)
3"	145.7		115.5	6.74, d (8.7)	148.0	
4"	148.3		159.8		149.1	
5"	115.7	6.72, d (8.2)	115.5	6.74, d (8.7)	115.4	6.76, d (8.2)
6"	125.1	7.08, dd (8.2, 2.1)	133.4	7.60, d (8.7)	126.4	7.12, dd (8.2, 2.0)
7"	145.1	6.81, d (12.8)	144.6	6.88 d (12.7)	145.1	6.87, d (12.8)
8"	116.7	5.73, d (12.8)	116.6	5.76, d (12.7)	116.5	5.77, d (12.8)
9"	167.4		167.3		167.1	
OCH_3					56.2	3.85, s

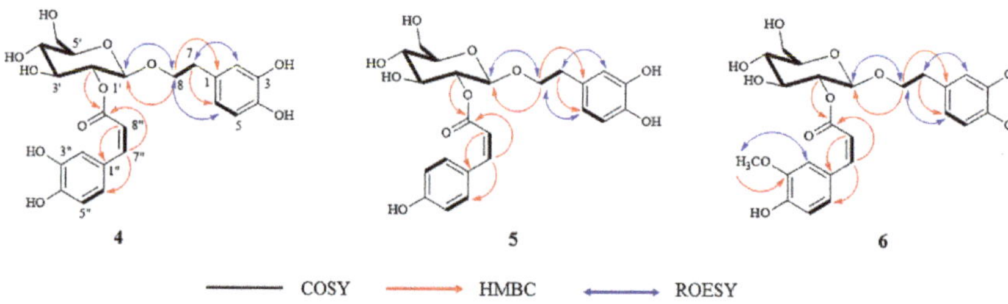

Figure 5. The COSY, HMBC and ROESY correlations of new compounds **4–6**.

The 2D NMR spectra and HRMS spectra are provided as supplementary data (Figures S3–S21). The structures of seven isolated bioactive candidates are displayed on the prioritized clusters in Figure 4B and structure of the three unprioritized compounds are provided in Figure 4C.

Compound **4** was obtained as a white amorphous powder. The HRESIMS of this compound exhibited a deprotonated molecular ion at *m/z* 477.1420 $[M - H]^-$ corresponding to the molecular formula $C_{23}H_{26}O_{11}$ (calcd. 477.1402), indicating an isomer of plantainoside B (**1**). The NMR data of **4** showed close similarities to those of plantainoside B except that the value of the coupling constant between the two ethylenic protons at δ_H 5.73 (H-8") and 6.81 (H-7") of 12.8 Hz indicated a *cis*-form for the caffeoyl group in **4**. The structure of **4** was therefore established as 8-*O*-(2′-*O*-*cis*-caffeoyl-*β*-D-glucopyranosyl)-3,4-dihydroxyphenylethanol (monnieraside IV).

Compound **5** was obtained as a white amorphous powder and it showed a deprotonated molecular ion at *m/z* 461.1473 $[M - H]^-$, which was consistent with the molecular formula $C_{23}H_{26}O_{10}$ (calcd. 461.1453). The NMR data of **5** exhibited a *para*-disubstituted moiety at δ_H 6.74 (2H, d, J = 8.7 Hz, H-3", H-5") and 7.60 (2H, d, J = 8.7 Hz, H-2", H-6") instead of the tri-substituted group of the *cis*-caffeoyl of **4**. The 16 Da mass difference between these two compounds was consistent with this NMR observation. The structure of **5** was established as 8-*O*-(2′-*O*-*cis*-coumaroyl-*β*-D-gluco-pyranosyl)-3,4-dihydroxyphenylethanol (monnieraside V).

The molecular formula of compound **6** (white amorphous powder) was calculated as $C_{24}H_{28}O_{11}$ by analysis of its HRESIMS (*m/z* 491.1580 $[M - H]^-$, calcd. 491.1559). The NMR data of **6** showed similarities with those of compound **3** (monnieraside II) both of them being isomers. A *cis*-feruoyl group was present in **6**, as confirmed by the coupling constant value of 12.8 Hz between H-7" and H-8" protons. The structure of **6** was thus established as 8-*O*-(2′-*O*-*cis*-feruloyl-*β*-D-glucopyranosyl)-3,4-dihydroxyphenylethanol (monnieraside VI).

According to DNP-ISDB dereplication results for the eleven isolated compounds (**1-11**), four compounds; plantainoside B (**1**), monnieraside III (**2**), monnieraside II (**3**) and 4-hydroxybenzoyl glucose (**7**) were correctly annotated as confirmed by NMR results (Table 1). Compound **8** was attributed an incorrect structure (2-(3,5-dihydroxyphenyl)ethanol-3'-*O*-*β*-D-glucopyranoside) by MS^2 dereplication, however this annotation was related to the structure later established by NMR (3,4-dihydroxyphenethyl glucoside). In addition, DNP-ISDB dereplication proposed the structure of **F9** and **5** (*m/z* 461.1473 $[M - H]^-$) as 8-*O*-(6′-*O*-*trans*-coumaroyl-*β*-D-glucopyranosyl)-3,4-dihydroxy-phenylethanol. However, NMR data of **5** suggested it as 8-*O*-(2′-*O*-*cis*-coumaroyl-*β*-D-glucopyranosyl)-3,4-dihydroxyphenylethanol. This indicated that the structure of **F9** could indeed be the dereplicated *trans*–isomer. Furthermore, previous observation showed that the *trans*-isomers of phenylpropanoid derivatives (compounds **1** and **3**) had shorter retention time than their *cis*-isomers counterpart (compounds **4** and **6**). The same phenomenon was also observed for **F9** and **5**. Consequently, **F9** could therefore correspond to as 8-*O*-(2′-*O*-*trans*-coumaroyl-*β*-D-glucopyranosyl)-3,4-dihydroxy-phenylethanol. In addition, we found that the annotation against GNPS spectral libraries of compound **10** (parishin A) was correct, as confirmed by NMR structural elucidation. In MN_6, the annotation of node *m/z* 995.3078 $[M - H]^-$ with parishin A and the mass difference of 268.0950 with two neighboring nodes at *m/z* 727.2121 $[M - H]^-$, RT 1.19 min and 727.2124 $[M - H]^-$, RT 1.10 min indicated a possible loss of the 4-(*β*-D-glucopyranosyloxy)benzyl alcohol moiety ($-C_{13}H_{16}O_6$, calcd. 268.0946) present on parishin A. After isolation and NMR identification structural elucidation, **9** and **11** were indeed found to be parishin C and parishin B, respectively, illustrating the interest of MN for dereplication purposes.

2.5. Evaluation of the Anti-Lipid Peroxidation Activity of the Isolated Compounds

In order to verify the bioactivity potential of the compound prioritized by the combination of MVA and multi-informative MN, the seven isolated compounds were tested for their anti-lipid peroxidation activity with the TBAR assay. Six compounds, **1–6**, showed inhibitory activity with IC_{50} values < 120 μM and one compound, **7**, had lower activity (IC_{50} > 500 μM) (Table 1). The positive control (Trolox) showed an IC_{50} value of 13.92 ± 0.32 μM. For this study, we defined compounds presenting IC_{50} values not higher than 10-fold of the control's IC_{50} value as active compounds.

Some prioritized features (**F1**, **F7** and **F9**) could not be isolated, their bioactivity potential is however discussed according to the following evidences. Features **F1** and **F7** were proposed to be idaric acid-1,4-lactone and its isomer by MS^2. TheD enantiomer,D-glucaric-1,4-lactone, has been reported to exert anti-lipid peroxidation and anti-oxidant activities [59]. Compound **F9** was also likely to exhibit anti-lipid peroxidation activity similar to its isomer (**5**), in the same fashion as isomeric compounds **1/4** and **3/6** also shared the same range of anti-lipid peroxidation activity. Given the structure similarity of **1–6**, their inhibitory activities were compared. The activity of the compounds tends to decrease when C3'' was substituted with methoxy (**3**, **6**) and hydroxy groups (**1**, **4**), respectively (Figure 4B). Such substitutions might reduce the ability of the compounds to protect the oxidation of Fe^{2+} to Fe^{3+} in the lipid peroxidation process.

To verify that the proposed merging of MVA and MN decreased the numbers of false positive candidate compounds, two features **F5** and **F16** (identified to bacopaside I using standard comparison) highlighted by MVA only were assayed. Both showed low levels of activity with IC_{50} values > 500 µM and > 1000 µM, respectively. This indicated that the combination of both prioritization approaches could help to further refine the prioritization process and lower the rate of false positives isolation.

Additionally, three unprioritized compounds **9–11** were isolated and their anti-lipid peroxidation activity assayed. We found that these three compounds displayed very low inhibition of lipid peroxidation with the IC_{50} values > 1000 µM, indicating that the employed strategy was effective to highlight bioactive compounds from complex mixtures of NPs prior to isolation.

Further investigations of ten prioritized bioactive features **F1**, **F7**, **F9** and compounds **1–7** revealed that they were differently distributed (% of MS intensities) in the three *Bacopa* species (Figure 6). The highest mean distribution of these compounds was observed in *B. monnieri* (77%), followed by *B. floribunda* (21%). This result agreed with the finding that *B. monnieri* had higher anti-lipid peroxidation activity than *B. floribunda* (Figure 2), suggesting that these compounds are the bioactives responsible for the anti–lipid peroxidation effects observed in *B. monnieri* and *B. floribunda*. Even though *B. caroliniana* presented the lowest level of these active compounds (~2%), it still showed some inhibition of lipid peroxidation, which could indicate the presence of other bioactive compounds in the plant.

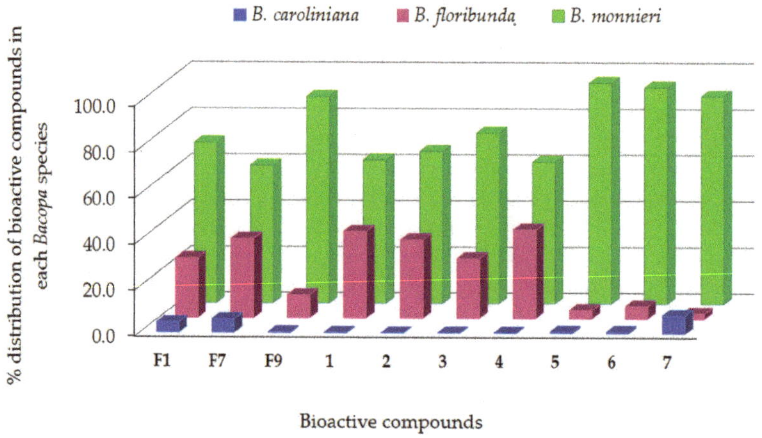

Figure 6. Percentage distribution of ten bioactive compounds in each *Bacopa* species, calculated by division of the average MS signal intensity of the compound in each species by a sum of signal intensities of the compound in three *Bacopa* species ×100.

The biological evaluation of the compounds prioritized by merging MVA and MN, indicated the validity of the approach. However, some bioactive compounds could be missed since the selection in MN was partly based on MS signal intensity, which is non–quantitative and highly dependent on the chemical structure of the analytes. The hyphenation of MS analytical platforms with universal detectors such as evaporative light scattering detector (ELSD) should offer a more accurate view of the precise quantitative repartition of metabolites within complex matrices, hence enhancing the power of MS–based prioritization approaches.

3. Materials and Methods

3.1. Chemicals and Plant Materials

All chemicals used were of analytical grade and obtained from Sigma-Aldrich (St. Louis, MO, USA). All solvents were HPLC and LC-MS grades. Acetonitrile (ACN), methanol (MeOH) and formic acid were purchased from Merck (Darmstadt, Germany). Water was purified by a Milli–Q purification system from Millipore (Bedford, MA, USA).

Three *Bacopa* species i.e., 36 samples of *B. monnieri* (BM1-12), 12 samples of *B. caroliniana* (BC1-4), and 11 samples of *B. floribunda* (BF1 from nature and BF2-11 from tissue culture) were collected from different regions and seasons. Only collected BM and BC samples were planted under the same growing conditions in the Faculty of Pharmaceutical Sciences, Naresuan University and subsequently harvested during different seasons in 2017: January (represented winter), April (summer), and July (rainy season) to enable an evaluation of the effect of these seasonal conditions. These plants species were identified by Dr. Pranee Nangngam and their voucher specimens (Saesong001-17) have been deposited at Department of Biology, Faculty of Science, Naresuan University. The codes and information regarding the samples are presented in Table 3.

Table 3. The geographical details of the *Bacopa* samples collected in this study. Samples 1–16 were collected in 3 seasons i.e., winter, summer, and rainy season (48 samples). Only sample 17 was collected in summer (1 sample). Plant tissue cultures of *B. floribunda* (samples 18–27) were collected in April, 2017 (10 samples).

No.	Code	*Bacopa* spp.	Sources
1	BM1	*B. monnieri*	Perth, Australia
2	BM2	*B. monnieri*	Wat Phra Sri Mahathat, Bangkok, Thailand
3	BM3	*B. monnieri*	Samphan garden, Nakhon Pathom, Thailnd
4	BM4	*B. monnieri*	Naresuan University, Phitsanulok, Thailand
5	BM5	*B. monnieri*	Kasetsart University, Bangkok, Thailand
6	BM6	*B. monnieri*	Nakhon Nayok, Thailand
7	BM7	*B. monnieri*	Chatuchak Market, Bangkok, Thailand
8	BM8	*B. monnieri*	Ayutthaya, Thailand
9	BM9	*B. monnieri*	Fukuoka, Japan (originated in India)
10	BM10	*B. monnieri*	Siriraj hospital, Bangkok, Thailand
11	BM11	*B. monnieri*	Chatuchak Market, Bangkok, Thailand
12	BM12	*B. monnieri*	Phetchabun, Thailand (originated in India)
13	BC1	*B. caroliniana*	Naresuan University, Phitsanulok, Thailand
14	BC2	*B. caroliniana*	Nakhon Nayok, Thailand
15	BC3	*B. caroliniana*	Chiang Mai, Thailand
16	BC4	*B. caroliniana*	Bangkok, Thailand
17	BF1	*B. floribunda*	Sakolnakorn, Thailand
18–27	BF2 to BF11	*B. floribunda*	Plant tissue cultures obtained from Department of Biology, Faculty of Science, Naresuan University

The shoot part (10 cm) of each *Bacopa* sample was collected based on a previous method [45]. Then it was cleaned and dried at 50 °C in a hot air oven for 24 h. The dried plants were crushed and passed through a 60 mesh sieve and stored in plastic containers under refrigeration at −20 °C until used.

3.2. *Sample Preparation*

Metabolites of *Bacopa* were extracted by adding 1 mL of 70%MeOH to a powdered sample (20 mg). The solution was then sonicated at room temperature for 15 min and filtered through a 0.45 µm nylon filter. Each extract solution was analyzed by UPHLC-HRMS^2 and tested for anti-lipid peroxidation activity in parallel.

3.3. *TBAR Assay*

Lipid peroxidation inhibitory activity was tested by TBARs assay, with minor modification to a previous study [50]. In this process, 20 µL of sample and 140 µL of homogenate rat brain (contained 5.72 mg/mL total protein) were mixed and incubated at 37 °C for 30 min. Then, 20 µL of 4 mM Fe_2SO_4 and 2 mM ascorbic acid were added to the mixture solution and incubated at 37 °C for 1 h. After incubation, 200 µL of TBARs reagent (40% trichloroacetic acid, 1.4% thiobarbituric acid, and 8% HCl) was added and incubated at 90 °C for 60 min. The mixture was then allowed to cool to room temperature and centrifuged at 10,000 rpm at 4 °C for 5 min to pelletize the precipitated protein. The absorbance of the supernatant was read at 530 nm by a microplate reader (BioTek Instruments, Winooski, Vermont, USA). The inhibition was calculated by comparison with the negative control. The homogenized rat brain in this assay was prepared in 1x PBS buffer (pH 7.4). The protein content in the homogenized rat brain was measured using a bicinchoninic acid (BCA) assay [60].

3.4. *UHPLC-ESI-HRMS^2 Analysis*

The UHPLC–HRMS^2 was carried out on a Waters Acquity UPLC IClass system system interfaced to a Q-Exactive Focus mass spectrometer (Thermo Scientific, Bremen, Germany), using a heated electrospray ionization (HESI-II) source. Chromatographic separation was performed on a Waters BEH C18 column (50 × 2.1 mm, 1.7 µm), the mobile phase consisted of 0.1% formic acid in water (A) and 0.1% formic acid in acetonitrile (B), the flow rate was 600 µL/min, the injection volume was 1 µL, and the linear gradient elution initially increased from 5–100% B for 7 min, followed by isocratic conditions at 100% B for 1 min, and then decreased to 5% B for the final step for 2 min. The negative ionization mode was applied in this study because the molecular ion peak of the most important metabolites could not be observed in positive ion mode. The optimized HESI-II parameters were set as follows: source voltage, 3.5 kV; sheath gas flow rate (N_2), 48 units; auxiliary gas flow rate, 11 units; spare gas flow rate, 2.0 units; capillary temperature, 300 °C, S-Lens RF Level, 55. The mass analyzer was calibrated using a mixture of caffeine, methionine-arginine-phenylalanine-alanine-acetate (MRFA), sodium dodecyl sulfate, sodium taurocholate, and Ultramark 1621 in an acetonitrile/methanol/water solution containing 1% formic acid by direct injection. The data-dependent MS/MS events were performed on the three most intense ions detected in full scan MS (Top3 experiment). The MS/MS isolation window width was 2 Da, and the normalized collision energy (NCE) was set to 35 units. In data-dependent MS/MS experiments, full scans were acquired at a resolution of 35,000 fwhm (at *m/z* 200) and MS/MS scans at 17,500 fwhm, both with a maximum injection time of 50 ms. After being acquired in a MS/MS scan, parent ions were placed in a dynamic exclusion list for 3.0 s. All samples were performed by UHPLC-HRMS^2 in one batch and a single pool of all samples was used as a quality control (QC). The QC sample was processed to monitor the reproducibility and stability of the system, which was injected at the beginning, then once every ten tested samples, and at the end of the batch analysis.

3.5. *MZmine data preprocessing*

The UHPLC–HRMS^2 raw data were converted to .mzXML format using MSConvert software, part of the ProteoWizard package and processed with MZmine version 2.32. Six main steps, consisting in mass detection, chromatogram building, deconvolution, isotopic peak grouping, alignment and gap filling, were carried. The mass detection was set in centroid mode and the noise level was kept at 1×10^6 for MS^1 and 0 for MS^2. The ADAP chromatogram builder was selected and run using a minimum group size in number of scans of 5, minimum height of 1×10^6, and *m/z* tolerance of 0.001 Da (or 5 ppm). The chromatogram deconvolution was set as follows: wavelets (ADAP) was used as the algorithm for peak recognition, *m/z* and RT range for MS^2 scan pairing were 0.3 Da and 0.1 min, S/N threshold was 20, minimum feature height was 1×10^6, coefficient/area threshold was 110, peak duration range was 0.01–1.0 min, and the RT wavelets range was 0.001–0.04. Chromatograms were then deisotoped by isotopic peaks a grouper algorithm with a *m/z* tolerance of 0.001 Da and an RT tolerance of 0.05 min. Peak alignment was carried out using a join aligner, with *m/z* tolerance set at 0.001 Da, absolute RT tolerance at 0.05 min, and weight for *m/z* and RT at 30. The missing peaklist after alignment was filled by gap filling of same RT and *m/z* range gap filler module with a *m/z* tolerance of 0.001 Da. After gap filling, all peaklists were done with identification of adduct search, complex search, and molecular formula prediction. This resulted in a peaklist of 6082 features which was further filtered to a peaklist of 4191 features having an associated data dependent MS^2 spectra. This resulting peaklist of 4191 features was exported as input for the MVA (MS^1 data only) and for MN generation (MS^1 and MS^2 data).

3.6. Multivariate Analysis

After data treatment with MZmine, a three-dimensional data matrix comprising of retention time, *m/z* value and peak height were analyzed by SIMCA-P software (version 13.0, Umerics, Umea, Sweden). Pareto-scaling was applied to normalize data for PCA and OPLS analysis. In addition, R^2 and Q^2 (cum) were used for model evaluation. Values of both parameters close to 1.0 indicated a good fitness for the created model. OPLS, a supervised multivariate statistical method, was completed with percent inhibition of lipid peroxidation activity as the Y input. The features with potential bioactivity from S-plot in OPLS model were selected based on their p[1] values.

3.7. Molecular Networking Analyses

The MN of MS^2 spectra of the *Bacopa* species was generated using the online workflow of the Global Natural Products Social Molecular Networking (GNPS). The MS^2 spectra were then clustered with MS-Cluster with a parent mass tolerance at 0.02 Da and a fragment ion mass tolerance at 0.02 Da to create consensus spectra, and consensus spectra containing less than two spectra were discarded. A network was then created, where edges were filtered to have a cosine score above 0.7 and more than 6 matching peaks. Furthermore, the edges between two nodes were kept in the network if each of the nodes appeared in each other's respective top 10 most similar nodes. The spectra in the network were automatically searched against GNPS spectral libraries and then against DNP-ISDB according to a previously described methodology [1]. ChemViz 1.3 plugin (freely available at [61]) was used to display the structure of the dereplication hits directly within Cytoscape 3.6.1. The generated MN in this study can be seen in [62] and the MASSIVE datasets contained all raw data was provided in the link of [63].

3.8. Purification of Candidate Bioactive Compounds

3.8.1. Extraction Procedure

The dried powder of BM4 (100 g) was macerated three times with MeOH and shaken for 24 h to give 24.2 g of MeOH extract. The polar substances (sugar) of the extract were removed using solid phase extraction prior to purification using the following protocol. The 200 g of C18 (ZEOprep® 60 C18, 40–63 µm) was packed in a column and activated by MeOH (1 L), followed by conditioning with water (1 L). Then, 2 g of Brahmi extract in 10 mL water was loaded and the column was washed with water (1 L) to remove polar substances. Remaining compounds were finally eluted with MeOH (1 L).

3.8.2. Purification Methods

The isolation steps of candidate compounds were performed by MPLC and followed by semi–preparative HPLC. A system of MPLC was carried out on an LC instrument conducted with a 681-pump module C-615, UV-Vis module C-640, and a fraction collector module C-660 (Buchi, Flawil, Switzerland). Fractionation was performed with an ZEOprep® C18 column (70 × 460 mm, 15–25 μm) with elution of 0.1% formic acid in water (A) and 0.1% formic acid in acetonitrile (B). The gradient elution started from 0-20 min of 35% B and then increased to 100% B for 284 min. The flow rate was 20 mL/min. This condition was first optimized on an analytical HPLC column (250 × 4.6 mm i.d., 15–25 μm, Zeochem, Uetikon am See, Switzerland) packed with the same stationary phase and then geometrically transferred to the preparative scale [53]. The extract was introduced into the MPLC column by dry injection by mixing 5.62 g of the extract with 18.30 g of the Zeoprep C18 stationary phase (40–63 μm, Zeochem). The mixture was conditioned in a dry-load cell (11.5 × 2.7 cm i.d.) and it was connected subsequently between the pumps and the MPLC column. Twenty-five fractions were collected by peak-based detection under UV at 205, 254 and 366 nm. When there were no peaks, 250 mL of each of the fractions was collected. The candidate compounds in the fractions were tracked down by LC-MS using the same conditions as mentioned in session 3.4.

The candidate bioactive compounds (**1–8**) and inactive compounds (**9–11**) were isolated from fraction 3 of MPLC using semi–preparative HPLC, which was performed on a HPLC-UV instrument with SPD-20A UV-Vis, a LC-20AP Pump, a FRC-10A fraction collector and a sample injector (Shimadzu, USA). The separation was carried out on an XBridge C18 OBD prep column (19 × 250 mm, 5 μm, Waters, Milford, MA, USA) with a guard column (4 × 20 mm, 5 μm), using an isocratic system of 0.1% formic acid in water and in acetonitrile at ratios of 86 and 14 as mobile phase. The separation time was 65 min with a post run of 10 min and the flow rate set at 17 mL/min. This semi–preparative HPLC condition was optimized on an analytical HPLC using a column with a similar stationary phase (XBridge C18, 4.6 × 250 mm, 5 μm) and then the optimum condition was geometrically transferred to the semi-preparative scale [54]. In order to avoid loss of resolution, the sample was loaded into the column by dry loading according to a recently developed protocol [55], which made it possible to obtain a high–resolution separation of the majority of the polar compounds to ensure a high degree of purity. Using this preparative system, eighty-four fractions were collected by peak-based detection under UV absorption of 205, 254 and scan 200–600 nm and volume based collection (8 mL of each fraction). All collected fractions were dried by speed vacuum (Genevac HT-4X, Genevac Ltd., North Carolina, USA). Isolation was achieved and afforded candidate bioactive compounds of **1** (8.5 mg), **2** (2.2 mg), **3** (0.9 mg), **4** (1.4 mg) **5** (0.1 mg) **6** (0.6 mg) and **7** (0.8 mg) and **8** (3.0 mg) and three inactive compounds of **9** (0.4 mg), **10** (3.0 mg) and **11** (1.2 mg). The purity and structure elucidation of each isolated compound was checked with HPLC, MS and NMR.

3.8.3. Identification Procedures

The NMR spectra of each isolated compound was recorded on a Bruker Avance Neo 600 MHz spectrometer equipped with a QCI 5mmCryoprobe and a SampleJet automated sample changer (Bruker BioSpin, Rheinstetten, Germany) (600). Chemical shifts (δ) were recorded in parts per million in methanol-d_4 using the residual solvent signal (δ_H 3.31; δ_C 49.0) as internal standards for ^{1}H and ^{13}C-NMR, respectively. Mass spectrometric data were obtained on a Waters Acquity UPLC IClass system system interfaced to a Q-Exactive Focus mass spectrometer (Thermo Scientific).

4. Conclusions

In this work, the integration of MVA and multi-informative MN based on LC–HRMS^2 metabolite profiling with bioactivity data was proven to be an efficient way to identify bioactive constituents in closely related plant extracts. The data generated allowed a rapid prioritization of bioactive compounds on a specific target from crude *Bacopa* extracts. Thanks to this approach the potential bioactivity for individual compounds could be anticipated prior to any physical separation process. This allowed the targeted isolation of six phenylethanoid glycosides **1–6** of *Bacopa* species with lipid-peroxidation inhibitory activity three of them being novel compounds i.e., monnieraside IV (**4**), monnieraside V (**5**) and monnieraside VI (**6**).

Additionally, the results in MVA and MN showed significant difference between Brahmi samples harvested in summer and other seasons in term of overall biological activity and amount of bioactive compounds. To our knowledge, Brahmi is collected throughout the year in Thailand and, based on our study, seasonal effects are important to consider and might affect the medicinal properties claimed for Brahmi. The described bioactive compounds could be used as biomarkers for quality control of this plant.

Supplementary Materials: The following are available online. Figure S1: Twenty candidate bioactive clusters observed by visual inspection based on dominant red color tag and five selected bioactive clusters in red square box (MN_1-MN_5) were nominated based on node size; Figure S2: Representative HPLC chromatograms from method transfer between HPLC (A) and semi-preparative HPLC (B) for separation of compounds **1–11** in fraction 3 (from MPLC) of *B. monnieri* extract; Figure S3: HRESIMS spectrum of compound **4** (negative ionization); Figure S4: ^{1}H-NMR spectrum of compound **4** in CD_3OD at 600 MHz; Figure S5: COSY NMR spectrum of compound **4** in CD_3OD; Figure S6. ^{13}C-DEPTQ NMR spectrum of compound **4** in CD_3OD at 151 MHz; Figure S7: Edited-HSQC-NMR spectrum of compound **4** in CD_3OD; Figure S8: HMBC-NMR spectrum of compound **4** in CD_3OD; Figure S9: ROESY NMR spectrum of compound **4** in CD_3OD; Figure S10: HRESIMS spectrum of compound **5** (negative ionization); Figure S11: 1H-NMR spectrum of compound **5** in CD_3OD at 600 MHz; Figure S12: COSY NMR spectrum of compound **5** in CD_3OD; Figure S13: Edited-HSQC-NMR spectrum of compound **5** in CD_3OD; Figure S14: HMBC-NMR spectrum of compound **5** in CD_3OD; Figure S15: ROESY NMR spectrum of compound **5** in CD_3OD; Figure S16: HRESIMS spectrum of compound **6** (negative ionization); Figure S17: ^{1}H-NMR spectrum of compound **6** in CD_3OD at 600 MHz; Figure S18: COSY NMR spectrum of compound **6** in CD_3OD; Figure S19: Edited-HSQC-NMR spectrum of compound **6** in CD_3OD; Figure S20: HMBC-NMR spectrum of compound **6** in CD_3OD; Figure S21: ROESY NMR spectrum of compound **6** in CD_3OD.

Author Contributions: T.S. performed whole experiments, data analysis, and prepared manuscript, P.-M.A. acquired UHPLC-HRMS^2 data and supervised data analysis, E.F.Q. helped for isolation, L.M. analyzed the NMR and structure elucidations, N.N. helped for data analysis, P.T. helped for data analysis, N.K. helped for data analysis, T.S., P.-M.A., J.-L.W. and K.I. conceived and designed the study. All authors reviewed the results and approved the final version of the manuscript.

Funding: This work was supported by the Royal Golden Jubilee PhD Program [PHD/0039/2557 to Tongchai Saesong and Kornkanok Ingkaninan], the Thailand Research Fund [DBG6080005, IRN61W0005], Naresuan University, the Center of Excellence for Innovation in Chemistry (PERCH-CIC), Ministry of Higher Education, Science, Research and Innovation. The School of Pharmaceutical Sciences of the University of Geneva (Jean-Luc Wolfender) is thankful to the Swiss National Science Foundation for the support in the acquisition of the NMR 600 MHz (SNF R'Equip grant 316030_164095).

Acknowledgments: We are gratefully to Pranee Nangngam for providing *Bacopa* samples and her help in plant identification. Additionally, we would like to thank the Bioactive Natural Products Unit, University of Geneva, Switzerland, who provided laboratory facilities.

Conflicts of Interest: The authors declare no conflict of interest.

References

1. Allard, P.-M.; Péresse, T.; Bisson, J.; Gindro, K.; Marcourt, L.; Pham, V.C.; Roussi, F.; Litaudon, M.; Wolfender, J.-L. Integration of molecular networking and In-Silico MS/MS fragmentation for natural products dereplication. *Anal. Chem.* **2016**, *88*, 3317–3323. [CrossRef] [PubMed]
2. Hubert, J.; Nuzillard, J.-M.; Renault, J.-H. Dereplication strategies in natural product research: How many tools and methodologies behind the same concept? *Phytochem. Rev.* **2017**, *16*, 55–95. [CrossRef]
3. Yuliana, N.D.; Khatib, A.; Choi, Y.H.; Verpoorte, R. Metabolomics for bioactivity assessment of natural products. *Phytother. Res.* **2011**, *25*, 157–169. [CrossRef] [PubMed]
4. Li, P.; AnandhiSenthilkumar, H.; Wu, S.-b.; Liu, B.; Guo, Z.-y.; Fata, J.E.; Kennelly, E.J.; Long, C.-l. Comparative UPLC-QTOF-MS-based metabolomics and bioactivities analyses of *Garcinia oblongifolia*. *J. Chromatogr. B* **2016**, *1011*, 179–195. [CrossRef] [PubMed]

5. D'Urso, G.; Pizza, C.; Piacente, S.; Montoro, P. Combination of LC–MS based metabolomics and antioxidant activity for evaluation of bioactive compounds in *Fragaria vesca* leaves from Italy. *J. Pharm. Biomed. Anal.* **2018**, *150*, 233–240. [CrossRef]
6. Ayouni, K.; Berboucha-Rahmani, M.; Kim, H.K.; Atmani, D.; Verpoorte, R.; Choi, Y.H. Metabolomic tool to identify antioxidant compounds of *Fraxinus angustifolia* leaf and stem bark extracts. *Ind. Crops. Prod.* **2016**, *88*, 65–77. [CrossRef]
7. Caesar, L.K.; Kellogg, J.J.; Kvalheim, O.M.; Cech, N.B. Opportunities and Limitations for Untargeted Mass Spectrometry Metabolomics to Identify Biologically Active Constituents in Complex Natural Product Mixtures. *J. Nat. Prod.* **2019**, *82*, 469–484. [CrossRef]
8. Patti, G.J.; Yanes, O.; Siuzdak, G. Innovation: Metabolomics: The apogee of the omics trilogy. *Nat. Rev. Mol. Cell Biol.* **2012**, *13*, 263–269. [CrossRef]
9. Kim, H.K.; Choi, Y.H.; Verpoorte, R. NMR-based plant metabolomics: Where do we stand, where do we go? *Trends Biotechnol.* **2011**, *29*, 267–275. [CrossRef]
10. Wolfender, J.-L.; Rudaz, S.; Hae Choi, Y.; Kyong Kim, H. Plant Metabolomics: From Holistic Data to Relevant Biomarkers. *Curr. Med. Chem.* **2013**, *20*, 1056–1090.
11. Wolfender, J.-L.; Nuzillard, J.-M.; van der Hooft, J.J.J.; Renault, J.-H.; Bertrand, S. Accelerating Metabolite Identification in Natural Product Research: Toward an Ideal Combination of Liquid Chromatography–High-Resolution Tandem Mass Spectrometry and NMR Profiling, in Silico Databases, and Chemometrics. *Anal. Chem.* **2019**, *91*, 704–742. [CrossRef]
12. Yang, J.Y.; Sanchez, L.M.; Rath, C.M.; Liu, X.; Boudreau, P.D.; Bruns, N.; Glukhov, E.; Wodtke, A.; de Felicio, R.; Fenner, A.; et al. Molecular networking as a dereplication strategy. *J. Nat. Prod.* **2013**, *76*, 1686–1699. [CrossRef]
13. Wang, M.; Carver, J.J.; Phelan, V.V.; Sanchez, L.M.; Garg, N.; Peng, Y.; Nguyen, D.D.; Watrous, J.; Kapono, C.A.; Luzzatto-Knaan, T.; et al. Sharing and community curation of mass spectrometry data with Global Natural Products Social Molecular Networking. *Nat. Biotechnol.* **2016**, *34*, 828. [CrossRef]
14. Olivon, F.; Allard, P.-M.; Koval, A.; Righi, D.; Genta-Jouve, G.; Neyts, J.; Apel, C.; Pannecouque, C.; Nothias, L.-F.; Cachet, X.; et al. Bioactive natural products prioritization using massive multi-informational molecular networks. *Acs Chem. Biol.* **2017**, *12*, 2644–2651. [CrossRef]
15. Naman, C.B.; Rattan, R.; Nikoulina, S.E.; Lee, J.; Miller, B.W.; Moss, N.A.; Armstrong, L.; Boudreau, P.D.; Debonsi, H.M.; Valeriote, F.A.; et al. Integrating molecular networking and biological assays to target the isolation of a cytotoxic cyclic octapeptide, samoamide A, from an American Samoan Marine Cyanobacterium. *J. Nat. Prod.* **2017**, *80*, 625–633. [CrossRef]
16. Nothias, L.-F.; Nothias-Esposito, M.; da Silva, R.; Wang, M.; Protsyuk, I.; Zhang, Z.; Sarvepalli, A.; Leyssen, P.; Touboul, D.; Costa, J.; et al. Bioactivity-based molecular networking for the discovery of drug leads in natural product bioassay-guided fractionation. *J. Nat. Prod.* **2018**, *81*, 758–767. [CrossRef]
17. Global Natural Product Social Molecular Networking. Available online: http://gnps.ucsd.edu (accessed on 10 Aprile 2018).
18. Olivon, F.; Elie, N.; Grelier, G.; Roussi, F.; Litaudon, M.; Touboul, D. MetGem Software for the Generation of Molecular Networks Based on the t-SNE Algorithm. *Anal. Chem.* **2018**, *90*, 13900–13908. [CrossRef]
19. Kind, T.; Tsugawa, H.; Cajka, T.; Ma, Y.; Lai, Z.; Mehta, S.S.; Wohlgemuth, G.; Barupal, D.K.; Showalter, M.R.; Arita, M.; et al. Identification of small molecules using accurate mass MS/MS search. *Mass Spectrom. Rev.* **2018**, *37*, 513–532. [CrossRef]
20. Tem, S. *Thai Plant Names*, 2014 ed.; The Forest Herbarium, Royal Forest Department: Bangkok, Thailand, 2014.
21. Mukherjee, G.D.; Dey, C.D. Clinical trial on Brahmi. I. *J. Exp. Med. Sci.* **1966**, *10*, 5–11.
22. Vollala, V.R.; Upadhya, S.; Nayak, S. Effect of *Bacopa monniera* Linn. (brahmi) extract on learning and memory in rats: A behavioral study. *J. Vet. Behav.* **2010**, *5*, 69–74. [CrossRef]
23. Saraf, M.K.; Prabhakar, S.; Khanduja, K.L.; Anand, A. *Bacopa monniera* attenuates scopolamine-induced impairment of spatial memory in mice. *Evid. Based Complement. Alternat. Med.* **2011**, *2011*, 10. [CrossRef]
24. Nathan, P.J.; Clarke, J.; Lloyd, J.; Hutchison, C.W.; Downey, L.; Stough, C. The acute effects of an extract of *Bacopa monniera* (Brahmi) on cognitive function in healthy normal subjects. *Hum. Psychopharmacol. Clin. Exp.* **2001**, *16*, 345–351. [CrossRef]

25. Stough, C.; Lloyd, J.; Clarke, J.; Downey, L.A.; Hutchison, C.W.; Rodgers, T.; Nathan, P.J. The chronic effects of an extract of *Bacopa monniera* (Brahmi) on cognitive function in healthy human subjects. *Psychopharmacology* **2001**, *156*, 481–484. [CrossRef]
26. Peth-Nui, T.; Wattanathorn, J.; Muchimapura, S.; Tong-Un, T.; Piyavhatkul, N.; Rangseekajee, P.; Ingkaninan, K.; Vittaya-areekul, S. Effects of 12-week *Bacopa monnieri* consumption on attention, cognitive processing, working memory, and functions of both cholinergic and monoaminergic systems in healthy elderly volunteers. *Evid. Based Complement. Alternat. Med.* **2012**, *2012*, 606424. [CrossRef]
27. Kongkeaw, C.; Dilokthornsakul, P.; Thanarangsarit, P.; Limpeanchob, N.; Norman Scholfield, C. Meta-analysis of randomized controlled trials on cognitive effects of *Bacopa monnieri* extract. *J. Ethnopharmacol.* **2014**, *151*, 528–535. [CrossRef]
28. Roodenrys, S.; Booth, D.; Bulzomi, S.; Phipps, A.; Micallef, C.; Smoker, J. Chronic effects of Brahmi (*Bacopa monnieri*) on human memory. *Neuropsychopharmacology* **2002**, *27*, 279–281. [CrossRef]
29. Morgan, A.; Stevens, J. Does Bacopa monnieri Improve Memory Performance in Older Persons? Results of a Randomized, Placebo-Controlled, Double-Blind Trial. *J. Altern. Complementary Med.* **2010**, *16*, 753–759. [CrossRef]
30. Gour, S.; Tembhre, M. Cholinergic inhibitory effects of bacopa monnieri and acephate in the kidney of rat. *Int. J. Curr. Adv. Res.* **2018**, *7*, 14136–14141.
31. Teschke, R.; Bahre, R. Severe hepatotoxicity by Indian Ayurvedic herbal products: A structured causality assessment. *Ann. Hepatol.* **2009**, *8*, 258–266. [CrossRef]
32. Sumathi, T.; Nongbri, A. Hepatoprotective effect of Bacoside-A, a major constituent of Bacopa monniera Linn. *Phytomedicine* **2008**, *15*, 901–905. [CrossRef]
33. Menon, B.R.; Rathi, M.A.; Thirumoorthi, L.; Gopalakrishnan, V.K. Potential Effect of Bacopa monnieri on Nitrobenzene Induced Liver Damage in Rats. *Indian J. Clin. Biochem.* **2010**, *25*, 401–404. [CrossRef]
34. Singh, H.; Dhawan, B.N. Neuropsychopharmacological effects of the ayurvedic nootropic *Bacopa monnieri* Linn. *Indian J. Pharmacol.* **1997**, *29*, 359–365.
35. Russo, A.; Borrelli, F. *Bacopa monniera*, a reputed nootropic plant: An overview. *Phytomedicine* **2005**, *12*, 305–317. [CrossRef]
36. Deepak, M.; Sangli, G.K.; Arun, P.C.; Amit, A. Quantitative determination of the major saponin mixture bacoside A in *Bacopa monnieri* by HPLC. *Phytochem. Anal.* **2005**, *16*, 24–29. [CrossRef]
37. Ganzera, M.; Gampenrieder, J.; Pawar, R.S.; Khan, I.A.; Stuppner, H. Separation of the major triterpenoid saponins in *Bacopa monnieri* by high-performance liquid chromatography. *Anal. Chim. Acta* **2004**, *516*, 149–154. [CrossRef]
38. Murthy, P.B.; Raju, V.R.; Ramakrisana, T.; Chakravarthy, M.S.; Kumar, K.V.; Kannababu, S.; Subbaraju, G.V. Estimation of twelve bacopa saponins in *Bacopa monnieri* extracts and formulations by high-performance liquid chromatography. *Chem. Pharm. Bull. (Tokyo)* **2006**, *54*, 907–911. [CrossRef]
39. Phrompittayarat, W.; Wittaya-Areekul, S.; Jetiyanon, K.; Putalun, W.; Tanaka, H.; Ingkaninan, K. Determination of saponin glycosides in *Bacopa monnieri* by reversed phase high performance liquid chromatography. *Thai Pharm. Health Sci. J.* **2007**, *2*, 26–32.
40. Bhandari, P.; Kumar, N.; Singh, B.; Singh, V.; Kaur, I. Silica-based monolithic column with evaporative light scattering detector for HPLC analysis of bacosides and apigenin in *Bacopa monnieri*. *J. Sep. Sci.* **2009**, *32*, 2812–2818. [CrossRef]
41. British Pharmacopoeia Commission. *The British Pharmacopoeia 2016*; The Stationery Office: London, UK, 2016; Volume 1.
42. Mathur, S.; Sharma, S.; Gupta, P.M.; Kumar, S. Evaluation of an Indian germplasm collection of the medicinal plant Bacopa monnieri (L.) Pennell by use of multivariate approaches. *Euphytica* **2003**, *133*, 255–265. [CrossRef]
43. Bansal, M. Diversity among wild accessions of Bacopa monnieri (L.) Wettst. and their morphogenetic potential. *Acta Physiol. Plant.* **2014**, *36*, 1177–1186. [CrossRef]
44. Bansal, M.; Reddy, M.S.; Kumar, A. Seasonal variations in harvest index and bacoside A contents amongst accessions of Bacopa monnieri (L.) Wettst. collected from wild populations. *Physiol. Mol. Biol. Plants* **2016**, *22*, 407–413. [CrossRef]

45. Phrompittayarat, W.; Jetiyanon, K.; Wittaya-Areekul, S.; Putalun, W.; Tanaka, H.; Khan, I.; Ingkaninan, K. Influence of seasons, different plant parts, and plant growth stages on saponin quantity and distribution in *Bacopa monnieri*. *SJST* **2011**, *33*, 193–199.
46. Bhandari, P.; Kumar, N.; Singh, B.; Kaul, V.K. Bacosterol Glycoside, a New 13,14-Seco-steroid Glycoside from *Bacopa monnieri*. *Chem. Pharm. Bull. (Tokyo)* **2006**, *54*, 240–241. [CrossRef]
47. Bhandari, P.; Kumar, N.; Gupta, A.P.; Singh, B.; Kaul, V.K. A rapid RP-HPTLC densitometry method for simultaneous determination of major flavonoids in important medicinal plants. *J. Sep. Sci.* **2007**, *30*, 2092–2096. [CrossRef]
48. Chakravarty, A.K.; Sarkar, T.; Nakane, T.; Kawahara, N.; Masuda, K. New Phenylethanoid Glycosides from *Bacopa monniera*. *Chem. Pharm. Bull. (Tokyo)* **2002**, *50*, 1616–1618. [CrossRef]
49. Ohta, T.; Nakamura, S.; Nakashima, S.; Oda, Y.; Matsumoto, T.; Fukaya, M.; Yano, M.; Yoshikawa, M.; Matsuda, H. Chemical structures of constituents from the whole plant of Bacopa monniera. *J. Nat. Med.* **2016**, *70*, 404–411. [CrossRef]
50. Limpeanchob, N.; Jaipan, S.; Rattanakaruna, S.; Phrompittayarat, W.; Ingkaninan, K. Neuroprotective effect of *Bacopa monnieri* on beta-amyloid-induced cell death in primary cortical culture. *J. Ethnopharmacol.* **2008**, *120*, 112–117. [CrossRef]
51. Katajamaa, M.; Miettinen, J.; Orešič, M. MZmine: Toolbox for processing and visualization of mass spectrometry based molecular profile data. *Bioinformatics* **2006**, *22*, 634–636. [CrossRef]
52. Schymanski, E.L.; Jeon, J.; Gulde, R.; Fenner, K.; Ruff, M.; Singer, H.P.; Hollender, J. Identifying Small Molecules via High Resolution Mass Spectrometry: Communicating Confidence. *Environ. Sci. Technol.* **2014**, *48*, 2097–2098. [CrossRef]
53. Challal, S.; Queiroz, E.F.; Debrus, B.; Kloeti, W.; Guillarme, D.; Gupta, M.P.; Wolfender, J.L. Rational and Efficient Preparative Isolation of Natural Products by MPLC-UV-ELSD based on HPLC to MPLC Gradient Transfer. *Planta Med.* **2015**, *81*, 1636–1643. [CrossRef]
54. Guillarme, D.; Nguyen, D.T.T.; Rudaz, S.; Veuthey, J.-L. Method transfer for fast liquid chromatography in pharmaceutical analysis: Application to short columns packed with small particle. Part I: Isocratic separation. *Eur. J. Pharm. Biopharm.* **2007**, *66*, 475–482. [CrossRef]
55. Queiroz, E.F.; Alfattani, A.; Afzan, A.; Marcourt, L.; Guillarme, D.; Wolfender, J.-L. Utility of dry load injection for an efficient natural products isolation at the semi-preparative chromatographic scale. *J. Chromatogr. A* **2019**, *1598*, 85–91. [CrossRef]
56. Tabata, M.; Umetani, Y.; Ooya, M.; Tanaka, S. Glucosylation of phenolic compounds by plant cell cultures. *Phytochemistry* **1988**, *27*, 809–813. [CrossRef]
57. Bianco, A.; Mazzei, R.A.; Melchioni, C.; Romeo, G.; Scarpati, M.L.; Soriero, A.; Uccella, N. Microcomponents of olive oil—III. Glucosides of 2(3,4-dihydroxy-phenyl)ethanol. *Food Chem.* **1998**, *63*, 461–464. [CrossRef]
58. Jer-Huei, L.; Yi-Chu, L.; Jiing-Ping, H.; Kuo-Ching, W. Parishins B and C from rhizomes of Gastrodia elata. *Phytochemistry* **1996**, *42*, 549–551. [CrossRef]
59. Saluk-Juszczak, J.; Olas, B.; Nowak, P.; Staroń, A.; Wachowicz, B. Protective effects of D-glucaro-1,4-lactone against oxidative modifications in blood platelets. *Nutr. Metab. Cardiovasc. Dis.* **2008**, *18*, 422–428. [CrossRef]
60. Smith, P.K.; Krohn, R.I.; Hermanson, G.T.; Mallia, A.K.; Gartner, F.H.; Provenzano, M.D.; Fujimoto, E.K.; Goeke, N.M.; Olson, B.J.; Klenk, D.C. Measurement of protein using bicinchoninic acid. *Anal. Biochem.* **1985**, *150*, 76–85. [CrossRef]
61. ChemViz: Cheminformatics Plugin for Cytoscape. Available online: http://www.cgl.ucsf.edu/cytoscape/chemViz/ (accessed on 10 July 2018).
62. Global Natural Product Social Molecular Networking. Available online: https://gnps.ucsd.edu/ProteoSAFe/status.jsp? (accessed on 19 June 2018).
63. MASSIVE datasets. Available online: ftp://massive.ucsd.edu/MSV000083989 (accessed on 18 June 2019).

Sample Availability: Samples of the compounds **1–11** are available upon request from the authors.

molecules

MDPI

Article

Insights into the Phytochemistry of the Cuban Endemic Medicinal Plant *Phyllanthus orbicularis*: Fideloside, a Novel Bioactive 8-*C*-glycosyl 2,3-Dihydroflavonol

Antonio Francioso [1,2,3,*], Katrin Franke [1], Claudio Villani [4], Luciana Mosca [2], Maria D'Erme [2], Stefan Frischbutter [5,6], Wolfgang Brandt [1], Angel Sanchez-Lamar [3] and Ludger Wessjohann [1,*]

1 Department of Bioorganic Chemistry, Leibniz Institute of Plant Biochemistry, 06120 Halle (Saale), Germany
2 Department of Biochemical Sciences "A. Rossi Fanelli", Sapienza University of Rome, 00185 Roma, Italy
3 Department of Plant Biology, Faculty of Biology, University of Havana, 10 200 La Habana, Cuba
4 Department of Chemistry and Technology of Drugs, Sapienza University of Rome, 00185 Roma, Italy
5 Department of Dermatology and Allergy, Charité, Universitätsmedizin Berlin, 10117 Berlin, Germany
6 German Rheumatism Research Centre, a Leibniz Institute, 10117 Berlin, Germany
* Correspondence: Antonio.francioso@uniroma1.it (A.F.); Ludger.Wessjohann@ipb-halle.de (L.W.)

Academic Editor: Pinarosa Avato
Received: 5 July 2019; Accepted: 3 August 2019; Published: 6 August 2019

Abstract: *Phyllanthus orbicularis* (Phyllanthaceae) is an endemic evergreen tropical plant of Cuba that grows in the western part of the island and is used in traditional medicine as an infusion. The aqueous extract of this plant presents a wide range of pharmacological activitiessuch as antimutagenic, antioxidant and antiviral effects. Given the many beneficial effects and the great interest in the development of new pharmacological products from natural sources, the aim of this work was to investigate the phytochemistry of this species and to elucidate the structure of the main bioactive principles. Besides the presence of several known polyphenols, the major constituent was hitherto not described. The chemical structure of this compound, here named Fideloside, was elucidated by means of HR-ESIMS/MS^n, 1D/2D NMR, FT-IR, and ECD as (2*R*,3*R*)-(−)-3′,4′,5,7-tetrahydroxydihydroflavonol-8-*C*-β-D-glucopyranoside. The compound, as well as the plant aqueous preparations, showed promising bioactive properties, i.e., anti-inflammatory capacity in human explanted monocytes, corroborating future pharmacological use for this new natural C-glycosyl flavanonol.

Keywords: *Phyllanthus orbicularis*; C-glycoside; flavonoid; natural products; traditional medicine; Cuba; *Phyllanthus chamacristoides*; chromatography; mass spectrometry; NMR; circular dichroism; stereochemistry; Fideloside; cytokines; anti-inflammatory activity

1. Introduction

Natural products represent a very important traditionalsource of novel drugs. They are also a relevant inspiration for the synthesis of novel molecules of pharmaceutical interest. Among the plethora of potential pharmaceutical and nutritional plant-derived molecules, phenolics represent a dominant group of compounds with crucialnatural antioxidantsand flavors [1–4].

With 7500 species of flowering plants, of which 50% are endemic, Cuba hosts more than half of all Caribbean flora [5], that is also the reason why the use of "green" medicine to prevent or treat different illnesses is deeply rooted in Cuban popular traditions. About 1250 species in180 families from Cuba are used as medicinal plants, in which the Euphorbiaceae family is one of the most broadly represented [6,7]. Euphorbiaceae and the segregated Phyllanthraceae are commonly very rich in bioactive metabolites. The genus *Phyllanthus* of this family includes Cuban endemic species which are widely used by traditional medical practitioners for the treatment of different types of diseases [8]. Indeed, other *Phyllanthus* species have worldwide applications including reports from China, the Philippines, Nigeria, East and West Africa, and Latin America comprising further Caribbean countries [9]. Several therapeutic properties have been attributed to this genus, such as antipyretic, antibacterial, antiparasitic, anticontraceptive, and antiviral activities [10,11]. Crude extracts of species such as *Phyllanthus amarus* and *Phyllanthus emblica* have been reported to provide antioxidant and anti-genotoxic activities [12].

Phyllanthus orbicularis Kunth is an endemic evergreen plant of Cuba that grows in the western side of the island in Pinar del Rio district. This plant, commonly known as "Alegrìa", is used in traditional medicine as an infusion for its anti-pyretic and antiviral properties [13–15]. In vitro tests showed that the aqueous extract from this species has a marked antiviral activity [16]. In sight of this, several preclinical studies have been carried out with the aim to use this extract as a pharmacological alternative in hepatitis B and human herpes virus type-2 therapy [15,17]. In addition, *P. orbicularis* aqueous extract has anti-mutagenic properties against hydrogen peroxide-induced clastogenicity and mutagenicity exhibiting protective effects against pro-mutagenic aromatics [18–20]. Moreover, the extract exhibits a photo-protective activity against γ-radiation, both in pre- and post-irradiation treatments [21,22]. Recent data demonstrated the protective effect of aqueous extracts from Cuban endemic *P. orbicularis* against UV-light induced DNA damage and genotoxicity [23–25].

To gain insight into the chemical principles responsible for the biological effects, a complete characterization of the phytochemical profile of Cuban endemic *Phyllanthus* species is required. To date only limited data are available, obtained by GC/MS and HPLC analyses of organic or aqueous extracts, which demonstrate the presence of known bioactive terpenoids and flavonoids [15,26]. *P. orbicularis* aqueous extract is the most interesting preparation from a pharmacological point of view, being the most effective and most studied in biological models, and the most relevant in application. However, despite its beneficial biological activities, the phytochemical composition of this plant is still not completely known. Of all previous works describing *P. orbicularis* aqueous extract chemistry, none offer a complete profile and a detailed chemical characterization. Given its common use in Cuba and the many beneficial effects of the plant, and the still increasing interest in the development of new pharmacological products from natural sources, the aim of this work is to investigate the phytochemistry of the Cuban endemic *P. orbicularis* compared to the endemic *P.chamacristoides*, which is not used in traditional medicine. The focus will be laid on the elucidation of the structures of the still unknown main bioactive principles.

2. Results

2.1. Phytochemical Characterization of Cuban Phyllanthus Species

UPLC-DAD profiles (280 nm) of aqueous extracts from two endemic Cuban *Phyllanthus* species (*P. orbicularis* and *P. chamacristoides*) analyzed at the same concentration and in the same chromatographic conditionsare shown in Figure 1. We compared the metabolite profile of the medicinal plant *Phyllanthus orbicularis* with that from *Phyllanthus chamacristoides* not used in traditional medicine. The chromatograms can be divided virtually in three regions, representing three different classes of molecules. From the beginning of the chromatographic run to 3.5 min there is the elution of hydrophilic phenolic acids, the central part of the chromatogram (from 3.5 to 4.8 min) is characterized by the presence of catechins and procyanidins (monomers and polymers), and from 4.8 min to the end of the gradient the last eluting molecules of these extracts are represented by more complex flavonoids. Analyzed compounds were numbered from **1** to **9** (Suppl., Figure S1) in order of their retention times and correspond to the major compounds detected (Table 1). In accordance with previously reported data, our results reveal the presence of catechin (peak **4**, Rt 3.85 min), procyanidin B2 (peak **5**, Rt 4.07 min), epicatechin (peak **6**, Rt 4.23 min) and rutoside (peak **8**, Rt 4.51 min) in *P. orbicularis*. The identity of these compounds was confirmed by the analysis of authentic analytical standards. As Figure 1 shows, peak **3** is the major compound in *P. orbicularis* and is present only in this species. Negative mode HRESIMS analyses of the other eluting peaks evidenced deprotonated ions [M−H]$^-$(UVλ$_{max}$) at *m*/*z* 315.0717 (255,sh290 nm), *m*/*z* 355.0668 (326 nm), *m*/*z* 465.1039(290 nm), *m*/*z* 865.1984 (280 nm), and *m*/*z* 593.1514 (255 and 354 nm) corresponding, respectively, to compounds **1**, **2**, **3**, **7** and **9**. Collected samples were first submitted to direct infusion ESI-MS/MS fragmentation and then the whole extracts were analyzed by LC-HRESI-MS^n for further structural elucidations. Molecular fragments obtained by both methods were in accordance with standards and literature data for all compounds investigated. The UV-Vis absorption features of compound **1** ($C_{13}H_{16}O_9$, Rt 3.49 min) fit with the presence of a protocatechuic moiety (255 nm; sh 290 nm). The MS^2 fragmentation pattern of the parent ion (*m*/*z* 315.0717) is consistent with protocatechuic acid glucoside, showing the presence of the major fragment at *m*/*z* 153.0196 derived from the loss of the sugar moiety. MS^3 of this fragment gives rise to an ion at *m*/*z* 109 in accordance with the structure of this molecule [27,28]. Compound **2** ($C_{15}H_{16}O_{10}$, Rt 3.52 min) shows an UV-Vis spectrum with λ$_{max}$ at 326 nm typical of hydroxycinnamate conjugated systems. ESI-MS^2 fragmentation of the pseudomolecular ion at *m*/*z* 355.0668 generates fragments at *m*/*z* 147.0301 and *m*/*z* 163.0405, resulting from two different cleavages of the ester bond, and two complementary fragments at *m*/*z* 209.0304 ($C_6H_9O_8^-$) and *m*/*z* 191.0198, referring to glucaric acid and its dehydration product, respectively [29–31]. MS^3 of the fragment at *m*/*z* 191 gives rise to subsequent glucaric acid decarboxylation products at *m*/*z* 147.1865 and *m*/*z* 85.0297. Peak **2** was consequently identified as *p*-cumaroyl-glucaric acid. Compounds **7** (Rt 4.35 min) and **9** (Rt 4.6 min) were already detected in *Phyllanthus orbicularis* extracts and were re-identified by means of their chromatographic behavior, spectroscopic features and ESI-HRMS/MS^n fragmentation patterns [15]. Compound **7** shows a molecular ion at *m*/*z* 865.1986 and a UV-vis λ$_{max}$ at 281 nm. This molecule was previously identified in this extract as the epicatechin trimer procyanidin C1. The MS/MS fragmentation of the precursor ion generates the dimer at *m*/*z* 577.1353 with the same subsequent MS/MS fragmentation pattern as procyanidin B1/B2 type molecules, confirming the nature of this compound [32]. Peak **9** was identified as the flavonol glycoside nicotiflorin in accordance to the literature data for this plant constituent. MS/MS fragmentation of the pseudomolecular ion (*m*/*z* 593.1514 [M-H]$^-$) gives rise to the aglycone part at *m*/*z* 285.0403, corresponding to a kaempferol moiety. Further MS/MS of the fragment at *m*/*z* 285 generates fragments at *m*/*z* 255, 227 and 151 [33].

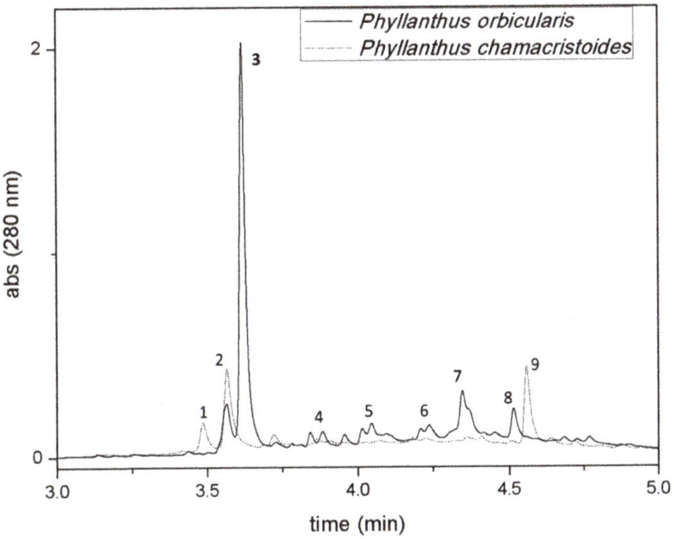

Figure 1. UPLC-DAD (280 nm) chromatograms of *Phyllanthus orbicularis* and *Phyllanthus chamacristoides* aqueous extracts and assignments of eluting peaks.

Table 1. Spectroscopic and spectrometric data of identified compounds.

Peak	Retention Time (min)	Compound	Molecular Formula	λ_{max}abs(nm)	MS[1] [M − H]⁻(*m/z*)	MS[2] [M − H]⁻(*m/z*)	MS[3][M − H]⁻(*m/z*)
1	3.49	Protocatechuic acid glucoside	$C_{13}H_{16}O_9$	290	315.0717	153.0196	109
2	3.52	*p*-Cumaroyl-glucaric acid	$C_{15}H_{16}O_{10}$	326	355.0668	191.0198	147; 85
3	**3.65**	**Fideloside**	$\mathbf{C_{21}H_{22}O_{12}}$	**290**	**465.1039**	**345.0620**	**277; 179; 167**
4 *	3.85	Catechin	$C_{15}H_{14}O_6$	278	289.0720	271.0620; 245.0825	
5 *	4.07	Procyanidin B2	$C_{30}H_{26}O_{12}$	280	577.1352	451.1036; 425.088; 289.0720	
6 *	4.23	Epicatechin	$C_{15}H_{14}O_6$	278	289.0720	271.0620; 245.0825	
7	4.35	Procyanidin C1	$C_{45}H_{38}O_{18}$	281	865.1986	847.1882; 739.1667; 695.1407; 577.1353	[865 → 577] 289
8 *	4.51	Rutoside	$C_{27}H_{30}O_{16}$	355	609.1460		
9	4.60	Nicotiflorin	$C_{27}H_{30}O_{15}$	343	593.1514	285.0403	255; 227; 151

* confirmed by analytical standard injection.

2.2. *Structure Elucidation of Compound 3 (Fideloside)*

Although compound **3** is the major metabolite of *P. orbicularis* (*m/z* 465.1039 [M-H]⁻, Rt 3.65 min), no previous chemical identification was reported [17]. The UV-Vis absorption features of this molecule (λ_{max} at 290 nm) suggested a not completely conjugated flavonoid system and the HRESI-MS derived molecular formula of $C_{21}H_{22}O_{12}$ indicates the presence of one hexose moiety. MS/MS fragmentation of the precursor ion at *m/z* 465.1039 [M-H]⁻ gives rise to a *m/z* 345.0620 [(M − H) − 120]⁻ fragment, generated by the cleavage in the glycoside portion on position 2″. These data are consistent with a C-type glycosidic structure [34,35]. Further MS/MSof *m/z* 345 generates ions at *m/z* 179and 167 resulting from the retro-Diels–Alder fragmentation of flavonoid ring C, indicating the position of the glycoside moiety to be on ring A. Another ion generated by MS^3 fragmentation of *m/z* 345 is the *m/z* 277 ion generated by a cleavage in the B ring (Figure 2).

For completechemical characterization, compound **3** was isolated and the structure was elucidated by means of $^1H/^{13}C$ 1D and 2D NMR and IR spectroscopy. Table 2 reports NMR data for compound **3**. ^1H/NMR and ^{13}C/NMR spectra in DMSO-d6 display an array of signals in agreement with the hypothesized structure and consistent with literature data of similar flavonoid *C*-glycosides (Suppl., Figures S2–S7) [35–37]. HMBC correlations from the anomeric sugar proton (H-1″) to C-8, C-7 and C-9 established the presence of the glycosidic moiety at C-8. The diaxial coupling of H-2 and H-3 in the ^1H NMR spectrum indicates a *trans*-type dihydro-saturation at positions C-2 and C-3. Furthermore, NOESY experiments suggest the positions of phenolic OH groups at C-3′ and C-4′ (Figure 3). The infrared spectrum of compound **3** (Suppl., Figure S8) is in agreement with the structure, showing representative IR vibrational bands at 3233 cm^{-1} (O–H stretching), 1633 cm^{-1} (C=O stretching), 1362 cm^{-1} (phenolic C–O and O–H vibrational modes), 1277 cm^{-1} (C–O–C stretching in =C–O–C– groups) [38].

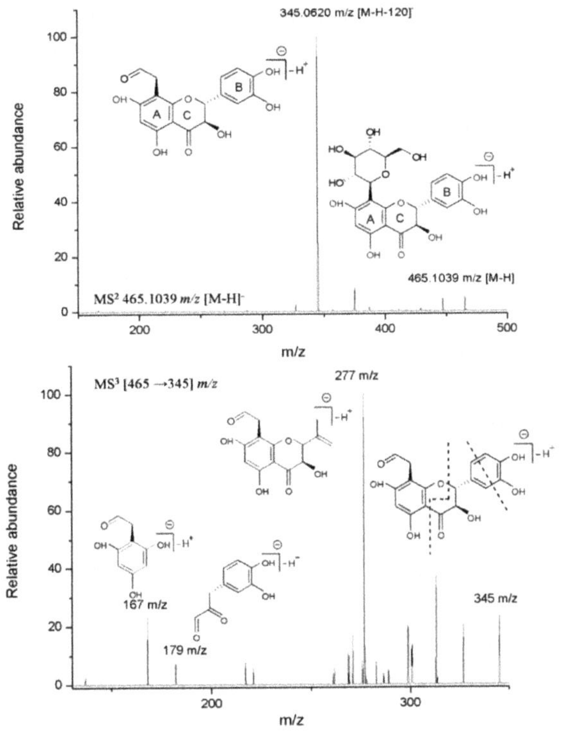

Figure 2. Fideloside (**3**) MS/MS^n fragmentation.

Table 2. 1D and 2D $^1H/^{13}C$ NMR data of Fideloside (**3**) in DMSO-d6 as solvent.

Nr.	δ c	DEPT	δ H (J in Hz)	^1H-^1H COSY	NOESY	HMBC
2	82.1	CH	5.02 (d, 11.02)	H-3	H-3-; H-6′; H-2′	H-2′;H-6′; OH-3
3	72.1	CH	4.25 (m)	H-2; OH-3	H-2′, H-6′; OH-3	OH-3; H-2
4	197.9	C				H-2; H-6;OH-3
5	162.1	C				H-6; OH-5
6	95.6	CH	6.04 (s)			OH-5
7	165.7	C				H-6; H-1″
8	105.5	C				H-6; H-1″-H; H-2″
9	161.4	C				H-2; H-1″
10	100.5	C				H-6; OH-5
1′	128.4	C				H-2; H-5′; H-2′
2′	115.0	CH	6.94 (brs)	H-6′	H-3; H-2	H-2; H-5′
3′	144.6	C				H-5′
4′	145.1	C				H-2′; H-6′
5′	115.0	CH	6.73 (d, 8.09)	H-6′	H-6′	H-2′; H-6′
6′	118.3	CH	6.84 (brd, 8.09)	H-2′; H-5′	H-2; H-5′; H-3	H-2′; H-2
1″	73.0	CH	4.45 (d, 9.63)	H-2″	H-3″	H-2″; H-6
2″	70.2	CH	3.82 (brt, 9.53)	H-1″; H-3″, OH-2″	H-4″; H-3″; H-1″	H-1″
3″	78.6	CH	3.11 (m)	H-2″; H-4″; OH-3″	H-1″; H-2″	H-1″; H-2″
4″	70.4	CH	2.95 (br)	H-3″; H-5″; OH-4″	H-2″; OH-4; H_2-6″	H-5″; H-3″; H-1″
5″	81.3	CH	3.09 (m)	H-6″	H-2″; Hb-6″	H-1″
6″	61.7	CH_2	Ha: 3.70 (m) Hb: 3.43 (m)	H-5″; H-6″; OH-6″	H-6″; H-4″	
3-OH			5.82(d, 6.13)	H-3	H-3	
5-OH			12.01(s)		H-6	
7-OH			-			
3′-OH			8.87 (brs)		H-2′	
4″-OH			9.00 (brs)		H-5′	
2″-OH			4.62 (brs)	H-2″		
3″-OH			4.83 (brs)	H-3″	H-2″, H-4″	
4″-OH			4.84 (brs)	H-4″		
6″-OH			4.57 (brs)	H_2-6″		

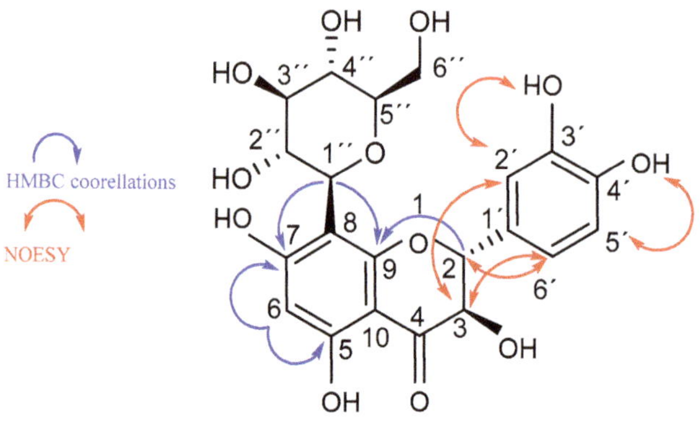

Figure 3. Fideloside (**3**) chemical structure with selected key NMR correlations.

The absolute configuration was elucidated by comparison of experimental and calculated circular dichroism spectra. The measured spectrum shows the presence of a negative Cotton effect at 295 nm and positive Cotton effect at 331 nm, which correspond to the (2*R*,3*R*) isomer (Figure 4), as previously reported for flavanonols [37,39,40].

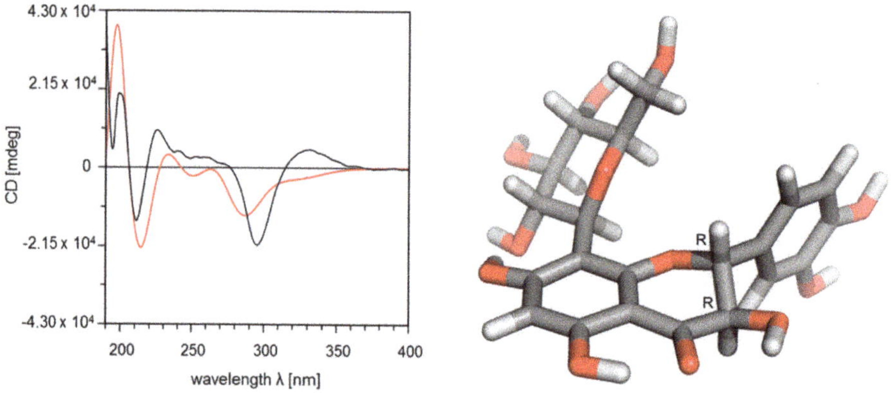

Figure 4. Left: comparison of experimental CD spectrum (black line) with Boltzmann weighted calculated CD spectrum for the (2*R*,3*R*)-enantiomer of compound **3** with a similarity factor S = 0.7099 for sigma = 0.3 eV and 18 nm shift. Right: calculated most stable conformation of the (2*R*,3*R*)-enantiomer.

The calculated relative conformational energies of the DFT optimized structures are listed in Table 3. The comparison of the Boltzmann weighted calculated CD spectra with the experimental ones clearly indicate that compound **3** adopts a (2*R*,3*R*)-configuration, since the fit with the experimental spectrum for this configuration is much better (Figure 4) than for the (2*S*,3*S*)-configuration (Suppl., Figure S9, Table S1).

Table 3. Results of DFT calculations for the (2*R*,3*R*) enantiomer of compound **3**.

Conformation	O-C2-C1′-C2′ (in°)	C2′-C3′-O-H (in°)	Energy (kcal/mol)	Boltzmann Weight	CD-Fit
1	−61.8	−179.5	0	59.4	0.6757
2	122.8	2.4	0.66	19.5	0.5712
3	−54.7	1.0	0.97	11.5	0.7065
4	121.9	−179.0	1.08	9.6	0.5974
Boltzmann					**0.7099**

On the basis of all experimental and calculated data, the chemical structure of this molecule is elucidated as (2*R*,3*R*)-(−)-3′,4′,5,7-tetrahydroxydihydroflavonol-8-C-β-D-glucopyranoside, a structure never reported previously for the genus *Phyllanthus* or in any other plant. We suggest to name this new natural compound '*Fideloside*' as the start of our work on this Cuban natural product coincided with the death of the long term Cuban leader Fidel Castro Ruz (Birán, 1927–La Habana, 2016).

2.3. Modulation of Cytokine Production

Since flavonoids can act in multiple way on inflammatory processes and Fideloside comprises the bioactive aglycon taxifolin, we investigated whether it is able to modulate interleukin production in human monocytes. Figure 5 shows a first biological assessment of pro-inflammatory (IL-1beta, IL-6) and anti-inflammatory (IL-10) cytokine production in human monocytes treated with poly-IC as a pro-inflammatory stimulus.

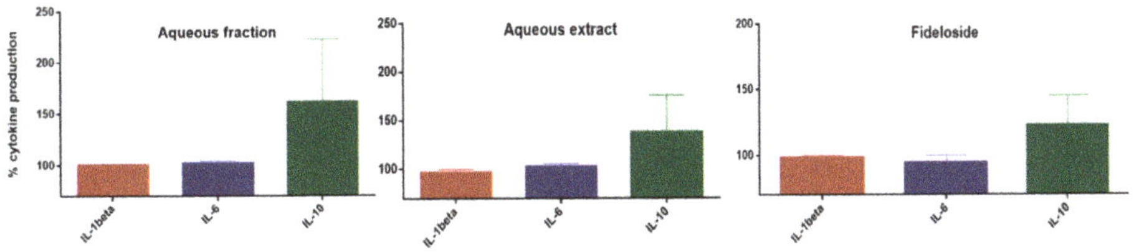

Figure 5. Anti-inflammatory capacity of extracts (3 μg/mL) and isolated Fideloside (1 μM) from *Phyllanthus orbicularis*. Levels of pro- and anti-inflammatory cytokines after poly-IC stimuli (CTRL+, 100%) of human monocytes.

These initial results show that the profile of interleukins secretion, in particular IL-10, seems to be modulated by Fideloside similarly to the aqueous extract and aqueous fraction suggesting a crucial role for this compound in the aqueous preparation used in Cuban traditional medicine.

3. Discussion

As expected, different polyphenols are the main secondary metabolites in both Cuban *Phyllanthus* species, i.e., *P. orbicularis* and *P. chamacristoides*. *P. orbicularis* presents a more diverse profile of polyphenolic compounds compared to *P. chamacristoides*, and especially a before unidentified dominating compound. Alvarez and co-workers investigated *P. orbicularis* extracts by bioactivity-guided fractionation and determined some phenolic compounds, like catechins and procyanidins, as anti HSV-2 compounds [15]. However, these authors did not characterize the main compound, which together with the identification of several minor constituents, was still lacking [15,17]. Our results demonstrate the presence of phenolic compounds unidentified in previous investigations in the two plant species and, most importantly, of a new C-glycoside flavonoid from *P. orbicularis* which represents the main component (circa 70%) of the aqueous infusion. This compound, and C-glycoside flavonoids in general, were not described for the genus *Phyllanthus* until now. C-glycoside flavonoids are a rare and very interesting class of organic natural compounds, considering that many of them have demonstrated their effectiveness as therapeutic agents such as anti-inflammatory, antioxidant, anticancer and antidiabetic drugs [41]. Compared to common glycosides (*O*- and *N*-), *C*-glycosides present minimal conformational differences with the advantage of being resistant to enzymatic or acidic hydrolysis, since the anomeric center of the acetal group is converted to an ether moiety.

Our finding is highly relevant from both a pharmacological and an analytical point of view, because of its potential as a chemotaxonomic and drug quality analysis tool for the recognition and distinction of effective *P. orbicularis* extracts versus, e.g., closely related species. The other consideration rises up from the evidence that *P. orbicularis* is used in traditional medicine as an aqueous extract whereas *P. chamacristoides* is not. Other than *O*-glycosides, *C*-glycosides are much more stable to hydrolysis during extraction and especially stomach passage (acidic cleavage), as well as in the further absorption and metabolism in humans, i.e., in terms of an increased bioavailability and half-life time in vivo [41]. *C*-linked glycosides, as well as the enzymes involved in their metabolism (*C*-glycosyltranferases and *C*-glycosidases), are extremely rare in nature and absent in human metabolism. These features can confer to the molecule a very unique pharmacokinetic profile and distribution.

Fideloside (**3**) as major flavonoid was tested for its anti-inflammatory capacity on human monocytes and demonstrated an increasing effect on the production of IL-10 anti-inflammatory cytokine with respect to pro-inflammatory mediators. The aqueous extract and the aqueous fraction of *P. orbicularis* show a closely related activity profile, suggesting that the newly discovered natural product could act as the major compound responsible for the pharmacological properties of this medicinal plant. In addition to the biochemical features, its physico-chemical properties are very interesting and promising from a pharmacological point of view. The C-glycosidic moiety strongly increases the water solubility and the bioavailability of the molecule, and, as pointed out above, suggests that its amphiphilic behavior could be longer retained if applied orally. For the same reason, its "green"water extraction is possible not only for direct consumption as in traditional applications, but also should allow for easier processing into standardized formulations. Fideloside is the *C*-8-glycosylated form of taxifolin, a well-known flavanonol found in a wide range of vegetables with strong antioxidant capacity and recently published interesting bioactive properties, including anti-inflammatory activity [42–45]. To date, the only known natural *C*-glycosylated taxifolin is the *C*-6 glycoside with (2*S*,3*S*) stereochemistry (Ulmoside), which biological activity is still under investigation [37,46].

As mentioned before, *C*-linked glycosidic phenols are a very unique class of compounds with future potential in different fields. These modifications of plant secondary metabolites are biochemically and evolutionally not well studied and characterized. Enzymes involved in C-glycosyl bond formation are very little known, or minor amounts of C-glycosides are formed as minor byproduct of O-glycosylation [47]. The latter case is highly unlikely here, thus the elucidation of this new peculiar product from the Cuban endemic *Phyllanthus orbicularis* can represent a starting point for the study and characterization of novel enzymes involved in *C*-glycosyl phenolics biosynthesis.

4. Materials and Methods

4.1. Chemicals, Reagents and General Procedures

TLC was carried out on silica gel 60 F_{254} plates (Merck, Germany). Spots were visualized under UV light (254 and 365 nm) or by heating after spraying with 2% vanillin solution (in 96%H_2SO_4). Low resolution ESI-MS analyses were performed on a SCIEX API-3200 instrument (Applied Biosystems, Concord, Ontario, Canada) combined with a HTC-XT autosampler (CTC Analytics, Zwingen, Switzerland). The samples were introduced via autosampler and 2 μL loop injection. ^{1}H, ^{13}C NMR and 2D (COSY, HSQC, HMBC and NOESY) spectra were recorded on an Agilent DD2 400 NMR spectrometer and the chemical shifts were referenced to TMS or the solvent residual peak. UV spectra were measured with a Jasco V-560 UV/Vis spectrophotometer. CD spectra were acquired on a Jasco J-815 CD spectrophotometer and the specific rotation was measured with a Jasco P-2000 polarimeter. Infrared spectra (ATR) were recorded using a Thermo Nicolet 5700 FT-IR spectrometer. Rutoside, (+)-catechin and (−)-epicatechin analytical standards were obtained from Sigma Aldrich (Germany). Procyanidin B2 was used from the IPB-NWC in-house reference compound library (isolated from *Bumelia sartorum* Mart.) [48]. All the reagents and solvents used were of analytical and LC-MS grade.

4.2. Plant Material

Phyllanthus orbicularis Kunth was collected in February 2007 from Cajálbana, Pinar del Río, Cuba. The specimens were authenticated and stored at the Cuban Botanical Garden (No.7/220 HAJB). *Phyllanthus chamaecristoides* was collected in spring 2011 from Guantánamo region, Cuba (20° 28″ 32.7″″

N, 74° 43″ 45.4″″ W). The specimens were authenticated by specialists of Cuban Botanical Garden, and stored in this scientific institution as: *Phyllanthus chamaecristoides* Urbano subsp. *baracoensis* (TB4452).

4.3. Extraction and Compound Isolation

The plant material aerial parts were extracted with two different methods according to literature data affording an aqueous extract (AE) and a crude methanolic extract (CE).

The aqueous extracts (AEs) were obtained from dried aerial parts (ground leaves and stems) following previously described methods [16,25]. Briefly, dry plant material was extracted in bi-distilled water under continuous shaking (1 g: 7.5 mL) for 4 h at 37 °C, or 2 h at 70 °C. After filtration and lyophilization, the material was stored in a dry, cool place until subsequent analyses.

Crude extracts (CEs) were obtained by extracting grounddry plant aerial parts with 10 volumes (*w*/*v*) of aqueous methanol (80% MeOH). After an initial 15 min of ultrasonication (bath), the plant material was extracted other two times for 2h with 10 volumes each of 80%MeOH at room temperature without sonication and one last time overnight at room temperature with the same procedure. The combined extracts were filtered and the solvents were evaporated to dryness under reduced pressure using a rotary evaporator. The isolation and purification of compound **3** was performed as follows: 25 g of *Phyllanthus orbilucularis* dry material were extracted with 80% MeOH as described above to obtain CE. The dry extract was resuspended in H_2O and partitioned by liquid–liquid extraction, first with *n*-hexane and then with ethyl acetate, to give the respective H_2O fraction (AF, 2.2 gr), *n*-hexane fraction (HF, 129 mg) and EtOAc fraction (EF 159 mg). Before purification, every fraction was dissolved to the same concentration and checked by TLC and UHPLC-DAD-MS. Then, 550 mg of AF were chromatographed on a Sephadex LH-20 (Pharmacia) column using pure MeOH as eluent to obtain 20 mg of **3** (Rf 0.43; silica gel;EtOAc:MeOH:H_2O/6:1:1) (*2R,3R*)-(−)-3′,4′,5,7-tetrahydroxydihydroflavonol-8-C-β-D-glucopyranoside (Fideloside):

Yellow amorphous. $[\alpha]^{25}_D$−10.46 (c 0.5; MeOH). CD (c 0.005; MeOH) $[\theta]_{295}$−21,139, $[\theta]_{331}$ +5001. UV λ_{max};MeOH: 290 nm. IR data: 3233 cm^{-1}, 1633 cm^{-1}, 1362 cm^{-1}, 1277 cm^{-1}.^1H NMR: (DMSO-d6, 400 MHz) and δ: ^{13}C NMR: (DMSO-d6, 101 MHz) see Table 2 HRESIMS $[M-H]^-$ calculated for $C_{21}H_{21}O_{12}^-$: 465.1038, found 465.1039.

4.4. UPLC-DAD-MS and ESI-MS/MS

UPLC-DAD-MS was performed on a Waters Acquity H-Class UPLC system (Waters, Milford, MA, USA), including a quaternary solvent manager (QSM),a sample manager with a flow through needle system (FTN), a photodiode array detector (PDA) anda single-quadruple mass detector with electrospray ionization source (ACQUITY QDa). Chromatography was performed on a Waters C18 HSST3 column (100 mm × 2.1 mm i.d., 1.7 μm particle size). Solvent A was 0.1% aqueous HCOOH and solvent B was 0.1% HCOOH in CH_3CN. Flow rate was 0.5 mL/min and column temperature was set at 25 °C. Elution was performed isocratically for the first minute with 2% B; from minute 1 to minute 6 solvent B was linearly increased to 55%; from 6 to 10 min 20%A and 80%B; then, in 0.5 min solvent B was set at 100% and maintained for 2 min. The column was re-equilibrated with 98% A and 2%B before the next injection. Samples were dissolved in the mobile phase and 10 μL injected through the needle. The PDA detector was set up in the range 200 to 600nm. Mass spectrometric detection was performed in the negative electrospray ionization mode using nitrogen as nebulizer gas. Analyses were performed in the Total Ion Current (TIC) mode in a mass range 50–1000 *m*/*z*. Capillary voltage was 0.8 kV, cone voltage 30 V, ion source temperature 120°C and probe temperature 600 °C. Direct infusion ESI-MS/MS analyses were performed on UHPLC-DAD collected pure peaks.

4.5. LC-High Resolution-MS^n

Separations were performed with the same chromatographic method described above ona Waters C18 HSST3 column (100 mm × 1 mm i.d., 1.7 μm particle size) using a Dionex Ultimate 3000 UHPLC System, equipped with a quaternary pump, autosampler (100 μL sample loop, partial injection mode,

2 µL injection volume, sample temperature 8 °C), and DAD Detector (Thermo Fisher Scientific, Bremen, Germany). The effluent from the PDA detector was connected on-line to an LTQ-Orbitrap Elite mass spectrometer equipped with a high-temperature electrospray ionization (HESI) ion source, controlled by the Excalibur 2.7 software (Thermo Fisher Scientific, Bremen, Germany) and operated in the negative ion mode. The ion spray voltage was set to 4.0 kV, sheath and auxiliary gases on 20 and 5 psi, respectively. The Orbitrap-MS spectra were acquired within the *m*/*z* range of 50–2000 and resolution of 30,000. The tandem mass spectra were acquired by collision induced dissociation (CID) in linear ion trap (LIT) at 35% normalized collision energy and isolation width of 2.0 *m*/*z*. The fragments were detected at anFT-resolution of 30,000.

4.6. Molecular Modeling and DFT Calculations

NMR-measurements of compound **3** clearly indicate a *trans* conformation for C2-C3 hydrogen atoms, which are possible only for a (2*S*,3*S*) or (2*R*,3*R*) configuration even when an axial orientation of the dihydroxybenzyl moiety is taken into consideration. Therefore, CD-spectra where calculated for the two enantiomers and compared with the experimental one. The models were constructed using the Molecular Operating Environment (MOE) software and energy optimized using the MMFF94 molecular mechanics force field [49,50]. Conformational analysis was performed with the low mode conformational search module implemented in MOE. As first result, four conformations for each enantiomer with almost identical energies appeared for the dihydroxybenzyl moiety. The resulting most stable conformation for the sugar moiety was incorporated in an identical fashion for all further calculations. For validation of the obtained results for the entire compounds, corresponding calculations were performed with removed sugar moiety. All four low energy conformations of each enantiomer were optimized by using density functional theory (DFT) with BP86 functional and the def2-TZVPP basis set implemented in the ab initio ORCA 3.0.3 program package [51–56]. The influence of the solvent MeOH was included in the DFT calculations using the COSMO model [56]. For the simulation of the CD spectra, the first 50 excited states of each enantiomer were calculated by applying the long-range corrected hybrid functional TD CAM-B3LYP with the def2-TZVP(-f) and def2-TZVP/J basis sets. The CD curves were visualized and compared with the experimental ones with the help of the software SpecDis 1.64 [57].

4.7. Human Monocyte Isolation andAssessment of Cytokine Release

PBMCs (peripheral blood mononuclear cells) were isolated from the fresh blood of healthy donors (DRK Berlin, in accordance with the recommendations of the local ethics committee on human studies, Charité, Berlin, Germany) by density gradient centrifugation. Briefly, blood was added to Leucosep tubes (Greiner Bio-one GmbH, Frickenhausen, Germany) containing 15 mL of Leukocyte separation medium (Ficoll-Paque Plus, GE Healthcare Biosciences AB, Uppsala, Sweden) and centrifuged at 840× *g* for 20 min without breaks at room temperature. The interphase (PBMCs) was harvested and washed two times with PBS/BSA/EDTA (PBS + 0.2% BSA + 2 mM EDTA) and centrifuged (20 °C, 15 min, 200× *g*) to remove platelets. Monocytes were isolated using the monocyte isolation Kit II (Miltenyi Biotech GmbH Bergisch Gladbach, Germany) following the manufacturer's instructions. The purity of monocytes as assessed by flow cytometry was between 90% and 95% (±2%). Cells were seeded at 1 × 105 cells/well in serum free medium (X-Vivo 15, Lonza, Verviers, Belgium) in a round-bottom 96 well plate (Sarstedt AG & Co. KG, Nümbrecht, Germany) in the presence of the extracts or compounds or 0.1% DMSO (as control) and activated with 3 µg/mL poly-IC (Sigma Aldrich, Taufkirchen, Germany). Extracts or compound concentrations used for anti-inflammatory activity assay were previously assessed non-toxic for the cells by flow cytometry analyses. After 24 h of incubation at 37 °C supernatants were harvested and cytokine release was measured using a bead-based multiplex cytokine assay (Cytokine 25-Plex human Procarta Plex Panel 1B, Thermo Fisher Scientific, Darmstadt, Germany) and the Bioplex 200 system (Bio-Rad Laboratories GmbH, München, Germany).

5. Conclusions

Our results demonstrate the presence of a new bioactive natural product, (2*R*,3*R*)-(−)-3′,4′,5,7-tetrahydroxydihydroflavonol-8-*C*-*β*-D-glucopyranoside (Fideloside, **3**), here reported for the first time, belonging to the rare but highly-valued class of *C*-glycosylated phenols. The compound was isolated and purified from the endemic Cuban medicinal plant *Phyllanthus orbicularis*, and the chemical structure was unequivocally assessed as C8-glucoside of (2*R*,3*R*)-taxifolin by means of spectrometric, experimental and molecular modeling techniques. While is already taxifolin endowed with antioxidant and anti-inflammatory activities, the *C*-glycosylation could give to this derivative even better pharmacological and pharmaceutical properties. Preliminary experimental results on human monocytes demonstrated a promising bioactivity profile, with a positive modulation of anti-inflammatory mediators with respect to pro-inflammatory ones after cellular pro-inflammatory stimulus. In view of the above, Fideloside and *P. orbicularis* represent an important starting point for further bioactivity studies and of both the development of a standardized phytopharmaceutical product and the biochemistry of *C*-glycosylation.

Supplementary Materials: The following are available online, Figure S1: chemical structures; Figures S2–S7: NMR spectra; Figure S8: infrared spectrum; Figure S9: (2S,3S) enantiomer CD spectrum and conformation; Table S1: DFT calculations for (2S,3S) enantiomer.

Author Contributions: Conceptualization, A.F., L.W., A.S.-L. and L.M.; methodology, A.F., A.S.-L., K.F., S.F., C.V. and W.B.; software, A.F., L.W. and W.B.; validation, L.M., K.F. and M.D.; formal analysis, K.F. and A.F.; investigation, A.F.; resources, L.W. and A.S.-L.; data curation, A.F., W.B. and S.F.; writing—original draft preparation, A.F.; writing—review and editing, K.F., L.M., A.F., M.D., L.W. and A.S.-L.; visualization, A.F.; supervision, A.F., L.M., K.F., A.S.-L. and L.W.; project administration, A.F. and L.W.; funding acquisition, A.F. and L.W.", please turn to the CRediT taxonomy for the term explanation. Authorship is limited to those who have contributed substantially to the work reported.

Funding: This research was supported by Leibniz-DAAD grant to A.F and Leibniz SAS (Leibniz Research Alliance BCB interaction fund).

Acknowledgments: The authorsthankAndrea Porzel for NMR spectral analyses, and Aldrin Vasco-Vidal, Manuel Garcia-Ricardo, Alfredo Rodriguez-Puentesand TuvshinjargalBudragchaafortheir technical support.

Conflicts of Interest: The authors declare no conflict of interest.

References

1. Shahidi, F.; Ambigaipalan, P. Phenolics and polyphenolics in foods, beverages and spices: Antioxidant activity and health effects—A review. *J. Funct. Foods* **2015**, *18*, 820–897. [CrossRef]
2. Mastromarino, P.; Capobianco, D.; Cannata, F.; Nardis, C.; Mattia, E.; De Leo, A.; Restignoli, R.; Francioso, A.; Mosca, L. Resveratrol inhibits rhinovirus replication and expression of inflammatory mediators in nasal epithelia. *Antiviral Res.* **2015**, *123*, 15–21. [CrossRef] [PubMed]
3. Lim, C.-G.; Koffas, M.A.G. Bioavailability and Recent Advances in the Bioactivity of Flavonoid and Stilbene Compounds. *Curr. Org. Chem.* **2010**, *14*, 1727–1751. [CrossRef]
4. Mattioli, R.; Francioso, A.; d'Erme, M.; Trovato, M.; Mancini, P.; Piacentini, L.; Casale, A.; Wessjohann, L.; Gazzino, R.; Costantino, P.; et al. Anti-Inflammatory Activity of A Polyphenolic Extract from Arabidopsis thaliana in In Vitro and In Vivo Models of Alzheimer's Disease. *Int. J. Mol. Sci.* **2019**, *20*, 708. [CrossRef] [PubMed]
5. Menes, M.D.O. Dos nuevasvariedades de *Portulaca brevifolia* Urb. (Portulacaceae) para la Flora de Cuba. *FeddesRepert* **2007**. [CrossRef]
6. Hammer, K.; Esquivel, M.; Fuentes, V.; Lima, H.; Knüpffer, H. Additional notes to the cheklist of cuban cultivated plants (1). *Die Kult.* **1990**, *38*, 325–343. [CrossRef]
7. Riverón-Giró, F.B.; Sánchez, C. Two new species of Tectaria (Tectariaceae) from Cuba. *Willdenowia* **2015**, *45*, 189–196. [CrossRef]
8. Ihantola-Vormisto, A.; Summanen, J.; Kankaanranta, H.; Vuorela, H.; Asmawi, Z.M.; Moilanen, E. Anti-inflammatory activity of extracts from leaves of *Phyllanthus emblica*. *Planta Med.* **1997**, *63*, 518–524. [CrossRef]

9. Thyagarajan, S.P.; Thirunalasundari, T.; Subramanian, S.; Venkateswaran, P.S.; Blumberg, B.S. Effect of phyllanthusamarus on chronic carriers of hepatitis b virus. *Lancet* **1988**, *332*, 764–766. [CrossRef]
10. Kuttan, R.; Harikumar, K.B. *Phyllanthus Species: Scientific Evaluation and Medicinal Applications*; CRC Press: Boca Raton, FL, USA, 2011; ISBN 1439821445.
11. Joy, K.L.; Kuttan, R. Inhibition by *Phyllanthus amarus* of Hepatocarcinogenesis Induced by N-Nitrosodiethylamine. *J. Clin. Biochem. Nutr.* **2011**, *24*, 133–139. [CrossRef]
12. Gowrishanker, B.; Vivekanandan, O.S. In vivo studies of a crude extract of *Phyllanthus amarus* L. in modifying the genotoxicity induced in *Viciafaba* L. by tannery effluents. *Mutat. Res. Toxicol.* **1994**, *322*, 185–192. [CrossRef]
13. Gaitén, Y.I.G.; Martínez, M.M.; Alarcón, A.B.; Vãzquez, M.M.; Hernãndez, J.L.F.; Roche, L.D.; Rastrelli, L. Anti-inflammatory and antioxidant activity of a methanolic extract of phyllanthus orbicularis and its derived flavonols). *J. Essent. Oil Res.* **2011**, *23*, 50–53. [CrossRef]
14. Quintero, A.R.; Gutiérrez, I.S.; Díaz, L.M.; del Barrio Alonso, G. Effect of Phyllanthus orbicularis on the cell viability and the hepatitis B surface antigen in PLC/PRF/5 cells. *Rev. Cuba. Farm.* **2011**, *45*, 536–544.
15. Álvarez, Á.L.; Dalton, K.P.; Nicieza, I.; Diñeiro, Y.; Picinelli, A.; Melón, S.; Roque, A.; Suárez, B.; Parra, F. Bioactivity-guided fractionation of phyllanthus orbicularis and identification of the principal anti HSV-2 compounds. *Phyther. Res.* **2012**, *26*, 1513–1520. [CrossRef] [PubMed]
16. Del Barrio, G.; Parra, F. Evaluation of the antiviral activity of an aqueous extract from Phyllanthus orbicularis. *J. Ethnopharmacol.* **2000**, *72*, 317–322. [CrossRef]
17. Álvarez, Á.L.; del Barrio, G.; Kourí, V.; Martínez, P.A.; Suárez, B.; Parra, F. In vitro anti-herpetic activity of an aqueous extract from the plant *Phyllanthus orbicularis*. *Phytomedicine* **2009**, *16*, 960–966. [CrossRef] [PubMed]
18. Sànchez-Lamar, A.; Fiore, M.; Cundari, E.; Ricordy, R.; Cozzi, R.; De Salvia, R. Phyllanthus orbicularis aqueous extract: Cytotoxic, genotoxic, and antimutagenic effects in the CHO cell line. *Toxicol. Appl. Pharmacol.* **1999**, *161*, 231–239. [CrossRef] [PubMed]
19. Ferrer, M.; Sánchez-Lamar, A.; Fuentes, J.L.; Barbé, J.; Llagostera, M. Studies on the antimutagenesis of *Phyllanthus orbicularis*: Mechanisms involved against aromatic amines. *Mutat. Res. Genet. Toxicol. Environ. Mutagen.* **2001**, *498*, 99–105. [CrossRef]
20. Ferrer, M.; Cristófol, C.; Sánchez-Lamar, A.; Fuentes, J.L.; Barbé, J.; Llagostera, M. Modulation of rat and human cytochromes P450 involved in PhIP and 4-ABP activation by an aqueous extract of *Phyllanthus orbicularis*. *J. Ethnopharmacol.* **2004**, *90*, 273–277. [CrossRef]
21. Vernhes, M.; González-Pumariega, M.; Alonso, A.; Baly, L.; Menck, C.F.M.; Sánchez-Lamar, A. Photoprotective effect phyllanthus orbicularis HBK in *E. coli* cells. *Vaccimonitor* **2010**, *19*, 233.
22. Alonso, A.; Fuentes, J.L.; Sánchez-Lamar, A.; Llagostera, M. Antimutagenic Effect of Phyllanthus orbicularis against γ-radiation. *Lat. Am. J. Pharm.* **2010**, *29*, 148–152.
23. Vernhes, M.; González-Pumariega, M.; Passaglia, A.; Martins, F.C.; Sánchez-Lamar, A. Aqueous extract of *Phyllanthus orbicularis* K protects the plasmid DNA from the damage induced by ultraviolet radiation. *Ars Pharm.* **2013**, *54*, 1.
24. Tamayo, M.V.; Schuch, A.P.; Yagura, T.; Gil, L.B.; Menck, C.F.M.; Sánchez-Lamar, A. Genoprotective Effect of *Phyllanthus orbicularis* Extract Against UVA, UVB, and Solar Radiation. *Photochem. Photobiol.* **2018**, *94*, 1026–1031. [CrossRef] [PubMed]
25. Menéndez-Perdomo, I.M.; Wong-Guerra, M.; Fuentes-León, F.; Carrazana, E.; Casadelvalle, I.; Vidal, A.; Sánchez-Lamar, A. Antioxidant, photoprotective and antimutagenic properties of *Phyllanthus* spp. from Cuban flora. *J. Pharm. Pharmacogn. Res.* **2017**, *5*, 251–261.
26. Gutiérrez, Y.; Miranda, M.; Henriques, A.; del Barrio, G. Flavonoids analysis of a butanol fraction obtained from *Phyllanthus orbicularis* HBK. *Univ. Revista Cubana de Farmacia* **2010**, *44*, 367–373.
27. Catarino, M.D.; Silva, A.M.S.; Saraiva, S.C.; Sobral, A.J.F.N.; Cardoso, S.M. Characterization of phenolic constituents and evaluation of antioxidant properties of leaves and stems of *Eriocephalus africanus*. *Arab. J. Chem.* **2018**, *11*, 62–69. [CrossRef]
28. Jaiswal, R.; Halabi, E.A.; Karar, M.G.E.; Kuhnert, N. Identification and characterisation of the phenolics of *Ilex glabra* L. Gray (Aquifoliaceae) leaves by liquid chromatography tandem mass spectrometry. *Phytochemistry* **2014**, *106*, 141–155. [CrossRef] [PubMed]

29. Elliger, C.A.; Lundin, R.E.; Haddon, W.F. Caffeyl esters of glucaric acid in *Lycopersiconesculentum* leaves. *Phytochemistry* **1981**, *20*, 1133–1134. [CrossRef]
30. Coutinho, I.D.; Baker, J.M.; Ward, J.L.; Beale, M.H.; Creste, S.; Cavalheiro, A.J. Metabolite profiling of sugarcane genotypes and identification of flavonoid glycosides and phenolic acids. *J. Agric. Food Chem.* **2016**, *64*, 4198–4206. [CrossRef]
31. Risch, B.; Herrmann, K.; Wray, V. (E)-O-p-Coumaroyl-, (E)-O-Feruloyl-derivatives of glucaric acid in citrus. *Phytochemistry* **1988**, *27*, 3327–3329. [CrossRef]
32. Lin, L.Z.; Sun, J.; Chen, P.; Monagas, M.J.; Harnly, J.M. UHPLC-PDA-ESI/HRMSnprofiling method to identify and quantify oligomeric proanthocyanidins in plant products. *J. Agric. Food Chem.* **2014**, *62*, 9387–9400. [CrossRef] [PubMed]
33. Chen, Y.; Yu, H.; Wu, H.; Pan, Y.; Wang, K.; Jin, Y.; Zhang, C. Characterization and quantification by LC-MS/MS of the chemical components of the heating products of the flavonoids extract in *Pollen typhae* for transformation rule exploration. *Molecules* **2015**, *20*, 18352–18366. [CrossRef] [PubMed]
34. Geng, P.; Sun, J.; Zhang, M.; Li, X.; Harnly, J.M.; Chen, P. Comprehensive characterization of C-glycosyl flavones in wheat (*Triticum aestivum* L.) germ using UPLC-PDA-ESI/HRMSn and mass defect filtering. *J. Mass Spectrom.* **2016**, *51*, 914–930. [CrossRef] [PubMed]
35. Dokkedal, A.L.; Lavarda, F.; Dos Santos, L.C.; Vilegas, W. Xeractinol—A new flavanonol C-glucoside from *Paepalanthus argenteus* var. argenteus (Bongard) Hensold (Eriocaulaceae). *J. Braz. Chem. Soc.* **2007**, *18*, 437–439. [CrossRef]
36. Mbafor, J.T.; Fomum, Z.T.; Promsattha, R.; Sanson, D.R.; Tempesta, M.S. Isolation and characterization of taxifolin 6-c-glucoside from garcinia epunctata. *J. Nat. Prod.* **1989**, *52*, 417–419. [CrossRef] [PubMed]
37. Rawat, P.; Kumar, M.; Sharan, K.; Chattopadhyay, N.; Maurya, R. Ulmosides A and B: Flavonoid 6-C-glycosides from *Ulmuswallichiana*, stimulating osteoblast differentiation assessed by alkaline phosphatase. *Bioorg. Med. Chem. Lett.* **2009**, *19*, 4684–4687. [CrossRef] [PubMed]
38. Sokolová, R.; Nycz, J.E.; Ramešová, Š.; Fiedler, J.; Degano, I.; Szala, M.; Kolivoška, V.; Gál, M. Electrochemistry and spectroelectrochemistry of bioactive hydroxyquinolines: A mechanistic study. *J. Phys. Chem. B* **2015**, *119*, 6074–6080. [CrossRef]
39. Nonaka, G.-I.; Goto, Y.; Kinjo, J.-E.; Nohara, T.; Nishioka, I. Tannins and related compounds. LII Studies on the constituents of the leaves of *Thujopsisdolabrata* SIEB. et ZUCC. *Chem. Pharm. Bull.* **2011**, *35*, 1105–1108. [CrossRef]
40. Tofazzal Islam, M.; Tahara, S. Dihydroflavonols from *Lanneacoromandelica*. *Phytochemistry* **2000**, *54*, 901–907. [CrossRef]
41. Xiao, J.; Capanoglu, E.; Jassbi, A.R.; Miron, A. Advance on the Flavonoid *C-gly* cosides and Health Benefits. *Crit. Rev. Food Sci. Nutr.* **2016**, *56*, S29–S45. [CrossRef]
42. Gocer, H.; Topal, F.; Topal, M.; Küçük, M.; Teke, D.; Gülçin, I.; Alwasel, S.H.; Supuran, C.T. Acetylcholinesterase and carbonic anhydrase isoenzymes i and II inhibition profiles of taxifolin. *J. Enzyme Inhib. Med. Chem.* **2016**, *31*, 441–447. [CrossRef] [PubMed]
43. Kuang, H.; Tang, Z.; Zhang, C.; Wang, Z.; Li, W.; Yang, C.; Wang, Q.; Yang, B.; Kong, A.N. Taxifolin activates the Nrf2 anti-oxidative stress pathway in mouse skin epidermal JB6 P+ cells through epigenetic modifications. *Int. J. Mol. Sci.* **2017**, *18*, 1546. [CrossRef] [PubMed]
44. Saito, S.; Yamamoto, Y.; Maki, T.; Hattori, Y.; Ito, H.; Mizuno, K.; Harada-Shiba, M.; Kalaria, R.N.; Fukushima, M.; Takahashi, R.; et al. Taxifolin inhibits amyloid-β oligomer formation and fully restores vascular integrity and memory in cerebral amyloid angiopathy. *Acta Neuropathol. Commun.* **2017**, *5*, 26. [CrossRef] [PubMed]
45. Sun, X.; Chen, R.C.; Yang, Z.H.; Sun, G.B.; Wang, M.; Ma, X.J.; Yang, L.J.; Sun, X.B. Taxifolin prevents diabetic cardiomyopathy in vivo and in vitro by inhibition of oxidative stress and cell apoptosis. *Food Chem. Toxicol.* **2014**, *63*, 221–232. [CrossRef] [PubMed]
46. Gupta, P.; Singh, A.; Tiwari, S.; Mishra, A.; Maurya, R.; Singh, S. Ulmosides A: Flavonoid 6-C-glycosides from Ulmuswallichiana attenuates lipopolysacchride induced oxidative stress, apoptosis and neuronal death. *Neurotoxicology* **2019**, *73*, 100–111. [CrossRef] [PubMed]
47. Enzymatic C-Alkylation of Aromatic Compounds. In *Biocatalysis in Organic Synthesis*; hieme E-Books & E-Journals Partner: Stuttgart, Germany, 2016.

48. Ruela, H.S.; Leal, I.C.R.; de Almeida, M.R.A.; dos Santos, K.R.N.; Wessjohann, L.A.; Kuster, R.M. Antibacterial and antioxidant activities and acute toxicity of *Bumeliasartorum* Mart., Sapotaceae, a Brazilian medicinal plant. *Rev. Bras. Farmacogn.* **2011**, *21*, 86–91. [CrossRef]
49. Chemical Computing Group ULC. Molecular Operating Environment (MOE). Available online: https://www.chemcomp.com/ (accessed on 5 August 2019).
50. Halgren, T.A. MMFF VI. MMFF94s option for energy minimization studies. *J. Comput. Chem.* **1999**, *20*, 720–729. [CrossRef]
51. Becke, A.D. Density-functional exchange-energy approximation with correct asymptotic behavior. *Phys. Rev. A* **1988**, *38*, 3098. [CrossRef]
52. Perdew, J.P. Density-functional approximation for the correlation energy of the inhomogeneous electron gas. *Phys. Rev. B* **1986**, *33*, 8822. [CrossRef]
53. Karton, A.; Tarnopolsky, A.; Lamère, J.F.; Schatz, G.C.; Martin, J.M.L. Highly accurate first-principles benchmark data sets for the parametrization and validation of density functional and other approximate methods. Derivation of a robust, generally applicable, double-hybrid functional for thermochemistry and thermochemical. *J. Phys. Chem. A* **2008**, *112*, 12868–12886. [CrossRef]
54. Schäfer, A.; Horn, H.; Ahlrichs, R. Fully optimized contracted Gaussian basis sets for atoms Li to Kr. *J. Chem. Phys.* **1992**, *97*, 2571–2577. [CrossRef]
55. Weigend, F.; Ahlrichs, R. Balanced basis sets of split valence, triple zeta valence and quadruple zeta valence quality for H to Rn: Design and assessment of accuracy. *Phys. Chem. Chem. Phys.* **2005**, *7*, 3297–3305. [CrossRef] [PubMed]
56. Sinnecker, S.; Rajendran, A.; Klamt, A.; Diedenhofen, M.; Neese, F. Calculation of solvent shifts on electronic g-tensors with the conductor-like screening model (COSMO) and its self-consistent generalization to real solvents (direct COSMO-RS). *J. Phys. Chem. A* **2006**, *110*, 2235–2245. [CrossRef] [PubMed]
57. Bruhn, T.; Schaumlöffel, A.; Hemberger, Y.; Bringmann, G. SpecDis: Quantifying the comparison of calculated and experimental electronic circular dichroism spectra. *Chirality* **2013**, *25*, 243–249. [CrossRef] [PubMed]

molecules

MDPI

Article

The Effects of 2′,4′-Dihydroxy-6′-methoxy-3′,5′-dimethylchalcone from *Cleistocalyx operculatus* Buds on Human Pancreatic Cancer Cell Lines

Huynh Nhu Tuan [1,†], Bui Hoang Minh [2,†], Phuong Thao Tran [3], Jeong Hyung Lee [3], Ha Van Oanh [1], Quynh Mai Thi Ngo [4], Yen Nhi Nguyen [5], Pham Thi Kim Lien [6] and Manh Hung Tran [6,*]

1 Hanoi University of Pharmacy, 13 Le Thanh Tong Street, Hoan Kiem District, Hanoi 100100, Vietnam
2 Faculty of Pharmacy, Nguyen Tat Thanh University, 300C Nguyen Tat Thanh Street, District 4, Hochiminh City 72820, Vietnam
3 Department of Biochemistry, College of Natural Sciences, Kangwon National University, Chuncheon, Gangwon-Do 24414, Korea
4 College of Pharmacy, Hai Phong University of Medicine and Pharmacy, 72A Nguyen Binh Khiem, Hai Phong 180000, Vietnam
5 Faculty of Biology and Biotechnology, University of Science, Vietnam National University Hochiminh City, 227 Nguyen Van Cu, District 5, Hochiminh City 748000, Vietnam
6 Biomedical Sciences Department, Institute for Research & Executive Education (VNUK), The University of Danang, 158A Le Loi, Hai Chau District, Danang City 551000, Vietnam
* Correspondence: tmhung801018@gmail.com
† These authors contributed equally to this research.

Academic Editor: Pinarosa Avato
Received: 3 May 2019; Accepted: 8 July 2019; Published: 11 July 2019

Abstract: 2′,4′-Dihydroxy-6′-methoxy-3′,5′-dimethylchalcone (DMC), a principal natural chalcone of *Cleistocalyx operculatus* buds, suppresses the growth of many types of cancer cells. However, the effects of this compound on pancreatic cancer cells have not been evaluated. In our experiments, we explored the effects of this chalcone on two human pancreatic cancer cell lines. A cell proliferation assay revealed that DMC exhibited concentration-dependent cytotoxicity against PANC-1 and MIA PACA2 cells, with IC_{50} values of 10.5 ± 0.8 and 12.2 ± 0.9 μM, respectively. Treatment of DMC led to the apoptosis of PANC-1 by caspase-3 activation as revealed by annexin-V/propidium iodide double-staining. Western blotting indicated that DMC induced proteolytic activation of caspase-3 and -9, degradation of caspase-3 substrate proteins (including poly[ADP-ribose] polymerase [PARP]), augmented bak protein level, while attenuating the expression of bcl-2 in PANC-1 cells. Taken together, our results provide experimental evidence to support that DMC may serve as a useful chemotherapeutic agent for control of human pancreatic cancer cells.

Keywords: *Cleistocalyx operculatus*; 2′,4′-dihydroxy-6′-methoxy-3′,5′-dimethylchalcone (DMC); pPancreatic cancer; PANC-1

1. Introduction

Pancreatic cancer (PC) causes significant mortality in the USA and other countries [1]. The GLOBOCAN 2012 summit reported that PC is responsible for over 331,000 deaths annually, and is the seventh leading cause of cancer deaths in both males and females [2,3]. PC includes adenocarcinomas, accounting for approximately 85% of cases, with an overall 5-year survival rate of 5–10%, and endocrine tumors constituting less than 5% of all cases [2,3]. The causes remain insufficiently known; however, previous studies have established that the risk factors include obesity, a genetic predisposition, diabetes, a poor diet, and physical inactivity. In addition, smoking was recognized to be a risk factor of PC. [4,5]. Over the past 10 years, PC mortality has increased in both genders in the USA, Europe, Japan, and China [4,5]. Currently, there are no effective screening recommendations for PC; therefore a better understanding of the cause and identification of risk factors is essential to prevent this disease [6]. Several therapies for PC such as radiotherapy, chemotherapy, and immunotherapy have been developed; however, drug development for this cancer remains challenging. In the search for new anti-PC drugs, natural products have been identified as potential sources for the development of new drugs [7,8].

Cleistocalyx operculatus, a member of Myrtaceae family, had been used as a beverage since ancient times in Vietnam for the treatment of cold, fever, inflammation, and gastrointestinal disorders [9]. A bud water extract increased contractility and decreased the frequency of contraction in an isolated rat heart perfusion system. Moreover, data from several studies also suggested that this extract protected lipid peroxidation in rat liver microsomes and the trauma of PC12 cells; and inhibited α-glucosidase, rat-intestinal maltase, and sucrase activities [10–13]. The plant contains chalcones, flavanones, flavones, and triterpenoids exhibiting many pharmaceutical activities, including anti-tumor effects; inhibition of cancer cell growth; and anti-cholinesterase, anti-oxidation, anti-hyperglycemia, anti-influenza, and anti-inflammation activities [14–18]. Of the active compounds, the chalcone 2′,4′-dihydroxy-6′-methoxy-3′,5′-dimethylchalcone (DMC) exhibited both cytotoxic and anti-tumor effects in vivo and was cytotoxic to several cancer cell lines in vitro. DMC could reverse multi-drug resistance in HCC cell lines. Moreover, this compound displayed hepatoprotection and neuroprotection, promoted glucose uptake, affected the differentiation of 3T3-L1 cells into adipocytes; and reduced drug efflux by suppressing Nrf2/ARE signaling in human HCC BEL-7402/5-FU cells [19–22]. DMC triggers SMMC-7721 cell apoptosis via the mitochondrion-dependent pathway, inhibiting Bcl-2 expression and thus causing outer mitochondrial membrane disintegration [23]. DMC is the most cytotoxic agent isolated from the plant to date. Here, we isolated DMC (Figure 1A) from buds of C. operculatus using several chromatographic steps, and explored the effects thereof on some human cancer cell lines. We also provide the first evidence that DMC induces apoptosis of the human pancreatic cancer cell lines PANC-1.

2. Results

2.1. Cell Proliferation Activity

To investigate the effects of DMC on the human pancreatic cancer cell lines PANC-1 and MIA PACA2 growth, cells were treated with DMC (3–30 μM) for 48 h, and after that, cell numbers and viability were measured using a Dojindo kit. DMC significantly inhibited PANC-1 (Figure 1B) and MIA PACA2 cell proliferation (Figure 1C) in concentration-dependent manners, with IC_{50} values of 10.5 ± 0.8 and 12.2 ± 0.9 μM, respectively. Inverted microscopy revealed that exposure to DMC for 24 h greatly affected the number of cell death of PANC-1 cells (Figure 1D). Considering that DMC showed stronger toxicity against PANC-1 than MIA PACA2 our subsequent studies focused on the mechanism of action of DMC in PANC-1.

2.2. Caspase-3 activity

Caspase-3 is a member of the cysteine-aspartic acid protease family and usually exists as an inactive precursor of 32 kDa in size. When it is in activation mode, this causes the death of cell by an apoptosis pathway via cleavage of proteins into heterozygous substances. DMC (3–30 μM) was added to PANC-1 cells (1×10^6/well) followed by incubation for 12, 24, and 48 h; this enhanced caspase-3 activation was measured by assaying the levels of Ac-Asp-Glu-Val-Asp-8- amino-4-trifluoromethylcoumarin (Av-DEVD-AFC).

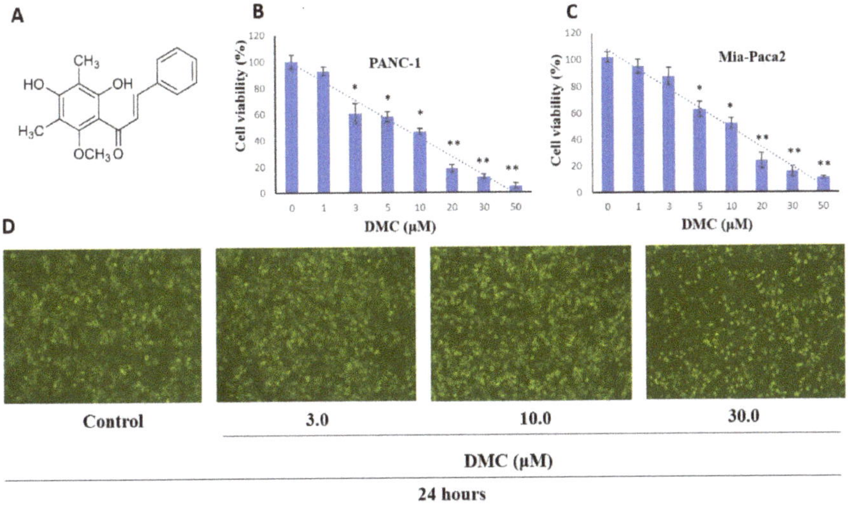

Figure 1. (**A**) Chemical structure of DMC; Effect of DMC on PANC-1 (**B**), and MIA-PACA2 (**C**) cell viability; and (**D**) PANC-1 cell morphology visualized by light microscopy (scale bar 500 μm), cells were seeded into 6-well plates at 1 × 10^5 cells/well and treated with the indicated concentration of DMC for 24 h. Data are presented as the mean ± standard deviation of three independent experiments performed in duplicate (*$p < 0.01$; **$p < 0.05$).

Figure 2 shows that caspase-3 activity increased 3–9-fold in a dose-dependent manner, when DMC-induced activities were compared to those of the vehicle.

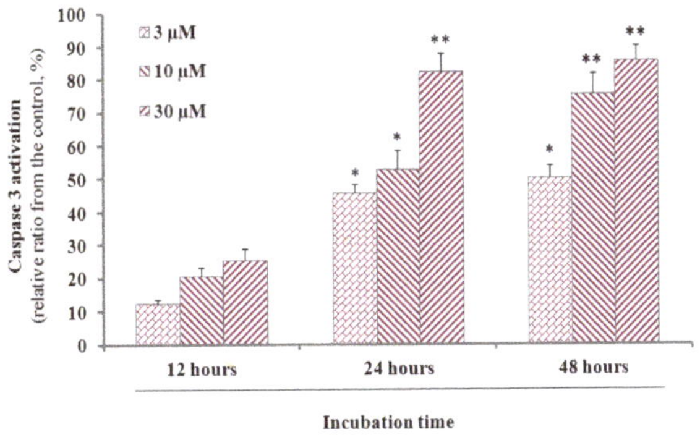

Figure 2. The increment of caspase-3 activity in PANC-1 cells treated by DMC in vitro. After 12 h, 24 h and 48 h incubation with DMC (3–30 μM), the cell lysates were incubated at 37 °C with caspase-3 substrate (Ac-DEVD-AFC) for 1 h. The fluorescence intensity of the cell lysates was measured to determine the caspase-3 activity. The blank group was used as 0.1% DMSO-treated cells. Data are presented as the mean ± SD of results from three independent experiments (* $p < 0.01$; ** $p < 0.05$).

2.3. Induction of Apoptosis by DMC

Next, PANC-1 cells (5 × 10^5) were treated with DMC (3–30 μM) for 48 h, stained with annexin V/PI, and subjected to flow cytometry using a BD Biosciences platform. Early and late apoptotic cells, and necrotic cells, were counted; and total and early apoptosis quantified (Figure 3). Apoptotic cell numbers increased in a DMC dose-dependent manner.

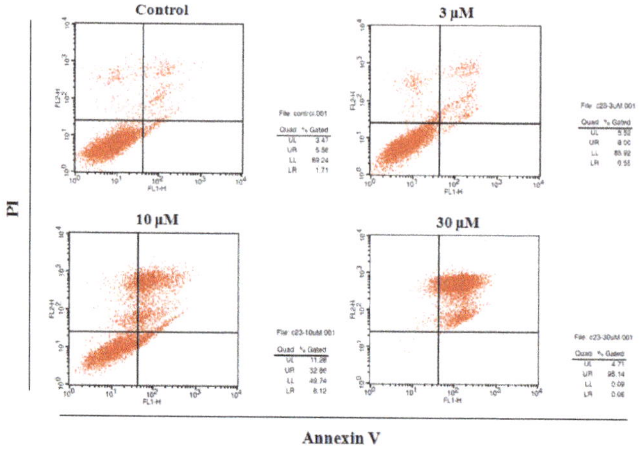

	LL (Annexin V−/PI−)	LR (Annexin V+/PI−)	UL (Annexin V−/PI+)	UR (Annexin V+/PI+)
Control	92.4 ± 3.7	2.8 ± 1.0	3.50 ± 0.8	6.1 ± 0.9
DMC (3 µM)	85.4 ± 2.3	0.5 ± 0.2	5.5 ± 1.0	8.2 ± 1.4
DMC (10 µM)	50.7 ± 4.4	6.2 ± 1.5	12.0 ± 2.5	32.8 ± 2.8
DMC (30 µM)	1.0 ± 0.3	0.1 ± 0.1	5.2 ± 0.5	95.1 ± 1.6

Figure 3. Effect of DMC on apoptosis of PANC-1 cells. Apoptosis quantification using annexin V/PI double staining assay after treatment with DMC (3–30 µM) for 48 h. PANC-1 cells were harvested and stained with PI and annexin V-FITC in darkness for 15 min. Data are presented as the mean ± SD of results from three independent experiments.

2.4. *Effect of DMC on the Expression of Apoptosis-Related Protein*

As the apoptotic cell population thus increased dramatically, we next measured the levels of apoptotic proteins. We used western blotting to detect death receptors and pro-apoptotic ligands that might be involved in DMC (3–30 µM)-induced PANC-1 apoptosis. As shown in Figure 4, DMC significantly inhibited expression of the anti-apoptotic Bcl-2 protein in a dose-dependent manner. Notably, the levels of the pro-apoptotic Bax protein were also changed by DMC. Recent evidences have suggested that the mitochondrial mutilation expedited cytochrome c (Cyt-c) which was discharged from mitochondria into the cytoplasm, triggering apoptotic progression. This process caused the stimulation of the caspase signaling and mitochondria-facilitated apoptosis so we assessed whether DMC triggers apoptosis via this mechanism in PANC-1 cells. We used western blotting to measure Cyt-c protein levels. DMC upregulated cytosolic Cyt-c expression and downregulated Bcl-2 synthesis compared to untreated cells (Figure 5). One of the other substrates for caspase during apoptosis is PARP, an enzyme that appears to be involved in DNA repair and genome surveillance and integrity in response to environmental stress. The beginning of caspase signaling activation might cause PARP cleavage which was considered as the main pathway in triggering apoptosis. As shown in Figure 4, exposure to DMC (3–30 µM) for 48 h triggered progressive PARP proteolytic cleavage and/or downregulation. We used western blotting to quantitate the levels of cleaved caspase-3 and -9; DMC upregulated cleavage of both proteins (Figure 4), explaining the Bcl-2 downregulation evident in Figure 5.

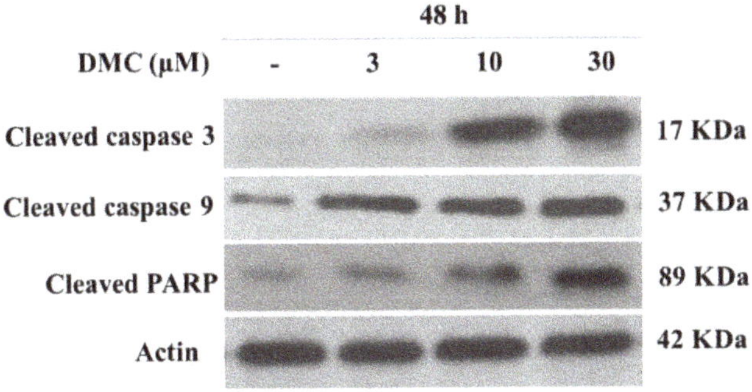

Figure 4. Effect of DMC on caspase activation and PARP degradation protein expression in PANC-1 cells. Cells were treated with DMC (3–30 μM) for 48 h. Protein 50 μg/lane from cells lysates were electrophoresed on SDS-PAGE gels, then transferred to total blot PVDF membranes. β-Actin was used as a control, (–), 0.1% DMSO-treated cells. The experiments were carried out in three replicates.

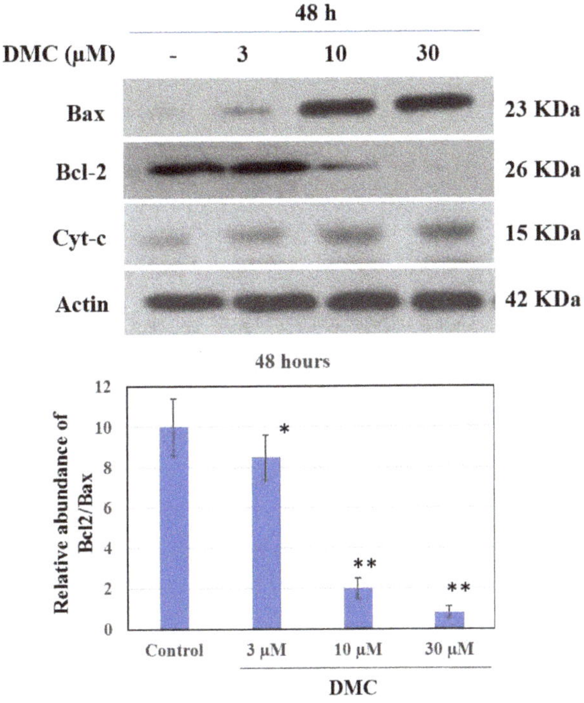

Figure 5. Effect of DMC on Bcl-2, Bax and Cyt-c protein expression in PANC-1 cells. Cells were treated with DMC (3–30 μM) for 48 h. Protein 50 μg/lane from cells lysates were electrophoresed on SDS-PAGE gels, then transferred to total blot PVDF membranes. β-Actin was used as a control, (–) 0.1% DMSO-treated cells. The experiments were carried out in three replicates. * $P < 0.05$ and $P < 0.01$ compared with control group.

3. Discussion

The pear-shaped pancreas—an abdominal organ located horizontally behind the lower part of the stomach—is an important component of the digestive system, secreting hormones, including insulin, that regulate sugar metabolism and digestive enzymes. Pancreatic cancer begins in the tissues of the pancreas. This cancer usually has a poor prognosis, even when the patient is diagnosed at the early stage because its signs and symptoms are hard to identify. The symptoms of pancreatic cancer generally mostly appear at the advanced stages of the disease. Some of the signs and symptoms of pancreatic cancer patients that might be identified include upper abdominal pain that spreads to the back, jaundice, yellow eyes, loss of appetite, weight loss, and depression. At present, the causes of the cancer remain unclear. There are two types of pancreatic cancer, including cancer formed in the pancreas (adenocarcinoma) and cancer formed in hormone-producing cells which is called endocrine. Pancreatic cancer is one of the most prevalent malignant tumors in the world and the treatment regimens for pancreatic cancer primarily depend on the cancer stages [7,8]. Nowadays, about 15–20% of patients undergo surgery and only 5% of them survive to 5 years [8]. The recent increase in cancer incidence, the absence of a cure, and severe side effects of existing drugs render it essential to find new effective therapeutics. In Vietnam, both Western and Oriental (natural plant) medicines are used to treat pancreatic cancer. Oriental medicines have fewer side effects and are less expensive than Western drugs. The herbal remedies used also target cancer-related impacts on the spleen, and sputum production. The recommended medicines include Radix Astragali membranacei, *Scutellaria barbata*, *Plumbago zeylanica*, *Poria cocos*, *Angelica sinensis*, and Rhizoma atrclylodis macrocephalae [9]. However, one of the limitations in the treatment of this disease by traditional oriental medicine method is due to the lack of scientific research perspectives in using of medicinal herbs with different ingredients and amounts.

In the last 10 years, many natural medicinal products have been used to treat pancreatic cancer. Fucoidan from a seaweed collected in Okinawa destroyed pancreatic tumor cells, and tumors regressed after 4–5 years of treatment [24]. α-Bisabolol (a sesquiterpene essential oil ingredient) reduced proliferation and survival of the pancreatic cancer cell lines KLM1, KP4, Panc1, and MIA Paca2; but not a pancreatic epithelial cell line (ACBRI515) [25]. Daily intake of plants rich in flavonoids and proanthocyanidins reduces the risk of pancreatic cancer by 25% [26–28]. Ethyl acetate extracts of *Coreopsis tinctoria* rich in flavonoids such as marein and flavanomarein kill pancreatic tumor cells by inducing apoptosis [29]. *Scutellaria baicalensis* extracts containing baicalein, wogonin, oroxylin A, and a glucuronide effectively countered pancreatic cancer in a mouse xenograft model [30,31]. The natural flavonoids and chalcons have many pharmaceutical applications, including antioxidant and anticancer ones. 2′,4′-Dihydroxy-6′-methoxy-3′,5′-dimethylchalcone (DMC) is also an important natural chalcone that has been shown to exhibit tremendous pharmacological activities which include anticancer activity against the wide range of cancer types. However, the anti-pancreatic cancer activity of DMC has not been previously investigated. In this study, DMC was selected to investigate the capability against PANC-1 cell lines. To clarify mechanism responsible for its anticancer activity, DMC at the concentration of 3–30 μM enhanced annexin-V uptake in PANC-1 cells signifying traslocation of the cell membrane phospholpids, phosphatidylsenin, from inner face to the outer surface of plasma membrane of PANC-1 cells then led to the cell apoptosis (Figure 3). Apoptosis, however, is known to be triggered by different routes, and the mitochondrials enhancement is a popularly crucial signalling pathway in the induction of apoptosis progress. Among these mitochindrials, the Bcl-2 family proteins are frequently main factors in apoptotic pathway due to their natural functional property. Bcl-2 family proteins play major roles in apoptosis and it has been suggested that such proteins exert either pro- or anti-apoptotic effects. The proteins either activate or inactivate transport through inner mitochondrial membrane pores, thus regulating the matrix Ca^{2+} level, the pH, and the cell membrane potential. Some pro-apoptotic Bcl-2 proteins may induce cytochrome c (Cyt-c) release to the cytosol; anti-apoptotic Bcl-2 proteins may inhibit such release. Cytosolic Bcl-2 proteins activated caspase-9 and -3, triggering apoptosis, meanwhile Bax was once termed Bcl-2-like protein 4, and is a pro-apoptotic protein; Bcl-2 is a major anti-apoptotic protein. Bax in the outer mitochondrial membrane enables the release of Cyt-c and activates caspase-9, a cysteine-aspartic protease involved in apoptosis and cytokine signaling. Caspase-3 is activated by proteolytic cleavage of caspase 9 to play a key role in apoptosis, further stimulating Cyt-c release by mitochondria and activating apaf-1 (the apoptosome), which then cleaves the caspase-9 pro-enzyme to the active dimer. In human cancer cells, this enzyme is regulated via phosphorylation mediated by an allosteric inhibitor, inhibiting dimerization and inducing a conformational change. Stimulation of caspase signaling and the accompanying cleavage of PARP are the principal features of the apoptotic cascade. We found that DMC activated enzymes and the PARP pathway to induce PANC-1 cell death, augmented by changes in Bcl-2 and Bax expression levels. DMC triggered the dose-dependent release of Cyt-c from mitochondria into the cytoplasm of PANC-1 cells.

DMC induces apoptosis in several human cancer cell lines including SMMC-7721 (human hepatocarcinoma cancer cells), 8898 (pancreas cancer cells), HeLa (cervical cancer cells), SPC-A-1 (lung cancer cells), 95-D (metastatic lung carcinoma cells), and GBC-SD (gall bladder carcinoma cells). When SMMC-7721 cells were treated with DMC for 48 h, the DNA became fragmented and the chromatin condensed. Also, the proportion of hypodiploid SMMC-7721 cells increased after DMC treatment [32]. At a low concentration, DMC inhibited proliferation of the human leukemia cell line K562. Notably, DMC downregulated Bcl-2 protein expression but did not affect Bax protein expression, thus reducing the Bcl-2:Bax ratio [33]. DMC was not toxic to normal human liver L-02 or normal human fetal lung fibroblast HFL-1 cell lines. In SMMC-7721 cells, DMC induced apoptosis by increasing intracellular ROS generation via inhibition of N-acetylcysteine activity [23]. Our data partly explained why DMC triggers PANC-1 cell apoptosis. We conclude that DMC exhibits significant anti-PANC-1 cancer cell activity; however, further in vivo evaluation in a mouse model of pancreatic cancer is essential.

4. Material and Methods

4.1. General Experimental Procedures

NMR experiments were conducted on a Unity INOVA 400 spectrometer (Varian, IL, USA). ^{1}H- and ^{13}C-NMR spectra were recorded at 400 and 100 MHz, respectively, and tetramethylsilane was used as the internal standard. ESI MS analyses were performed on a Micromass QTQF2 mass spectrometer (Water, Milford, MA, USA). The untraviloet (UV) was measured with a Shimadzu UV-1800 UV-Vis spectrophotometer (Shimadzu, Japan). IR spectrum was measured with a Shimadzu IR-408 spectrophotometer in $CHCl_3$ solution (Shimadzu, Japan). TLC was carried out on silica gel F_{254}-precoated glass plates and RP-18 F_{254S} plates (Merck, Germany). Dulbecco's modified Eagle medium (DMEM), fetal bovine serum (FBS), trypsin-EDTA 0.25%, streptomycin and penicillin were obtained from Hyclone (Logan, UT, USA). Dimethyl sulfoxide (DMSO), and a Dojindo Kit was purchased from Dojindo Molecular Technology INC (Maryland, USA). Annexin V-FITC/PI double staining detection kit, mitochondrial membrane potential assay kit with caspase-3 activity assay kit, propidium iodide (PI) were purchased from Beyotime (Beyotime Institute of Biotechnology, Shanghai, China). All used chemicals and reagents were of analytical grade.

4.2. Plant Material

The buds of *Cleistocalyx operculatus* were collected at Quang Nam province, Vietnam, in July 2017 and identified by Dr Pham Cong Tuan, Danang Traditional Medicine Hospital (Danang city, Vietnam). A voucher specimen (TMH-22-2017) was deposited in the Pharmaceutical Biology Laboratory of the University of Danang (Danang city, Vietnam).

4.3. Isolation of DCM

The air-dried buds (2.0 kg) were extracted with 70% ethanol (2 liters × 3 times). The 70% EtOH extract was combined and concentrated in vacuo to yield a residue which was suspended in water and then successively partitioned with *n*-hexane, EtOAc, and *n*-BuOH. After removal of solvent *in vacuo*, the *n*-hexane fraction was obtained (16.8 g). The *n*-hexane soluble fraction (HEX) was separated by silica gel column chromatography using a gradient of *n*-hexane–EtOAc (from 40:1 to 1:1) to yield 20 fractions (HEX.1 ~ HEX.20) according to their TLC profiles. Fraction HEX-5 (5.62 g) was further fractionated on a Sephadex LH-20 column eluting with MeOH to divide to six sub-fractions

(HEX.5.1-HEX.5.6). 2′,4′-Dihydroxy-6′-methoxy-3′,5′-dimethylchalcone (DMC, 1.6 g) was obtained from HEX.5.2 by crystallization from MeOH.

2′,4′-Dihydroxy-6′-methoxy-3′,5′-dimethylchalcone (DMC): Orange yellow needles (MeOH), mp 124–125 °C, UV λ_{max} (MeOH) nm (log ε): 284 (4.15), 320 (4.13); IR (KBr) cm^{-1}: 3460, 2875, 2750, 1630, 1550, 1450; ESI-MS *m/z* 312.1 $[M]^+$ (calcd for $C_{18}H_{16}O_5$), for ^1H and ^{13}C-NMR spectral data please see Supplementary Materials and in the comparison with previous reference [10].

4.4. Cell Lines and Culture

The human pancreatic cancer cell lines PANC-1 (human pancreas) and MIA-PACA2 (human pancreatic carcinoma) were obtained from the American Type Culture Collection (ATCC, Manassas, VA, USA). The cells were maintained in DMEM (GibcoBRL, NY, USA) with 10% fetal bovine serum (FBS) supplemented with 2% penicillin and 100 μg/mL of streptomycin at 37 °C in a 95% humidified atmosphere containing 5% CO_2.

4.5. Cell Proliferation Activity Assay

Cell proliferation activity of DMC was determined against PANC-1 and MIA-PACA2 cancer cell lines using a Dojindo kit with a slight modification. Viable cells were seeded in the growth medium into 96-well microtiter plates (95 μL, concentration 1×10^4 cells/well) and incubated at 37 °C in a 5% CO_2 incubator. The test sample DCM was dissolved in DMSO and adjusted to final sample concentrations ranging from 3 to 30 μM by diluting with the growth medium. Each sample was prepared in triplicate. The final DMSO concentration was adjusted to <0.1%. After standing for 4 h, the test sample was added to each well. The same volume of medium with 0.1% DMSO was added to the control wells. After 48 h incubation, Dojindo reagent was added to the each well (10 μL). 4 h later, the plate was removed from incubator and the optical density (O.D) was measured at 450 nm using a Molecular Devices microplate reader (Molecular Devices, Sunnyvale, CA, USA). The IC_{50} value was defined as the concentration of sample which reduced absorbance by 50% relative to the vehicle-treated control.

4.6. Caspase-3 Actyivation Assay

Caspase-3 enzyme activity was measured by proteolytic cleavage of the fluorogenic substrate Ac-DEVD-AFC by counting on a fluorescence plate reader (Twinkle LB970 microplate fluorometer, Berthold Technologies, Bad Wildbad, Germany). PANC-1 cells (1×10^5 cell/well) were treated with DCM (3–30 μM). After incubation for 24 h, cells were harvested and washed with cold PBS. The pellets were lyzed using 15 μL of lysis buffer [10 mM Tris-HCL (pH 8.0), 10 mM EDTA, 0.5% Triton X-100] at room temperature for 10 min, and then placed on ice; 100 μL of assay buffer [100 mM Hepes (pH 7.5), 10 mM dithiothreitol, 10% (*w*/*v*) sucrose, 0.1% (*v*/*v*) Chaps, 0.1% (*v*/*v*) BSA] and 10 μL of substrate solutin (200 μm substrate in assay buffer) were added. After incubation at 37 °C for 1 h, fluorescence was measured with excitation at 370 nm and emission at 505 nm.

4.7. Detection of Apoptosis by Double Stanning

The Annexin V-FITC/PI staining kit was used to detect the phosphatidylserine translocation, an important characteristic at an early stage of cell apoptosis. Briefly, PANC-1 cells were seeded in 6 well plates at a density of 2×10^5 cells/mL and incubated for 24 h. After that, cells were treated with different concentrations of DMC for 48 h. The cells were collected and washed in PBS, then were resuspended in 195 μL binding buffer, and incubated with 10 μL Annexin V-FITC and 5 μL PI in the dark for 20 min. Thereafter, the solutions were immediately measured by FCM (Beckman, Fullerton, CA, USA).

4.8. Preparation of Total Cell Extract and Immuno Blot Analysis

Immunoblot analysis, and immunoreactive proteins were visualized by an enhanced chemiluminescence (ECL) procedure according to the manufacturer's protocol. PANC-1 cells

(5×10^5 cells/mL) were treated with DMC (3-30 μM) for 24 h at 37 °C. Cell lysates were prepared in 100 μL of lysis buffer (Sigma, Ronkonkoma, NY, USA) containing a protease inhibitor cocktail (Roche, Mannheim, Germany). Insoluble material was removed by centrifugation at 14,000 rpm for 10 min. And then the protein contents in the supernatant were measured using a Bio-Rad DC protein assay kit. The protein extract (50 μg/well) was separated by SDS-PAGE and then transferred onto PVDF membranes (Bio-Rad, Hercules, CA, USA). The membranes were bloked with 5% (*w*/*v*) non-fat dry milk in TBS-T [Tris-buffered saline containing 0.1% (*v*/*v*) Tween-20] at 4 °C overnight and incubated with primary antibodies at room temperature for 1.5 h. The membranes were washed three times with TBS-T, and blotted with secondary antibodies conjugated with horse-radish peroxidase at room temperature for 1.5 h, followed by washing three times in TBST-T. Immunoreactive proteins were visualized by an enhanced chemiluminescence (ECL) procedure according to the manufacturer's protocol (Santa Cruz Biotechnology, Santa Cruz, CA, USA) and exposed to X ray films. Protein contents were normalized by reprobing the same membrane with anti-β-actin detection; previously used membranes were soaked in stripping buffer (Gene Bio-Application Ltd., Yavne, Israel) at room temperature for 20 min.

4.9. Statistical Analysis

All treatments were conducted in triplicate and the results are presented as the mean ± standard deviation (S.D). The statistical significance of all treatment effects was evaluated by Student's *t*-test with a probability limit for significance of $p < 0.05$, $p < 0.001$.

Supplementary Materials: The following are available online, Figure 1: ^{1}H NMR spectra of DMC (600 MHz, MeOD). Figure 2: ^{13}C NMR of DCM (125 MHz, MeOD).

Author Contributions: M.H.T., P.T.K.L. carried out the conception and designed the experiments. H.N.T., B.H.M., P.T.T., Q.M.T.N. and Y.N.N. performed sampling, extractions, and bioassay activities. H.V.O. performed identification and description of the plant. J.H.L. and M.H.T. performed N.M.R. experiments. J.H.L., P.T.K.L. and M.H.T. contributed to the preparation of the manuscript.

Funding: This research is funded by Vietnam Ministry of Education and Training under grant number YD-01 (2016-2018, TMH, The University of Danang).

Conflicts of Interest: We declare that we have no conflict of interest.

References

1. Howlader, N.; Noone, A.M.; Krapcho, M.; Miller, D.; Bishop, K.; Altekruse, S.F.; Kosary, C.L.; Yu, M.; Ruhl, J.; Tatalovich, Z.; et al. *SEER Cancer Statistics Review, 1975–2013*; National Cancer Institute: Bethesda, MD, USA, 2016.
2. Ferlay, J.; Soerjomataram, I.; Dikshit, R.; Eser, S.; Mathers, C.; Rebelo, M.; Parkin, D.M.; Forman, D.; Bray, F. *GLOBOCAN 2012 v1.0, Cancer Incidence and Mortality Worldwide: IARC CancerBase No. 11*; International Agency for Research on Cancer: Lyon, France, 2013.
3. Ferlay, J.; Soerjomataram, I.; Dikshit, R.; Eser, S.; Mathers, C.; Rebelo, M. Cancer incidence and mortality worldwide: Sources, methods and major patterns in GLOBOCAN 2012. *Int. J. Cancer* **2015**, *136*, E359–E386. [CrossRef] [PubMed]
4. Hidalgo, M.; Cascinu, S.; Kleeff, J.; Labianca, R.; Löhr, J.M.; Neoptolemos, J.; Real, F.X.; Van Laethem, J.L.; Heinemann, V. Addressing the challenges of pancreatic cancer: Future directions for improving outcomes. *Pancreatology* **2013**, *15*, 8–18. [CrossRef] [PubMed]
5. Vincent, A.; Herman, J.; Schulick, R.; Hruban, R.H.; Goggins, M. Pancreatic cancer. *Lancet* **2011**, *378*, 607–620. [CrossRef]
6. Ilic, M.; Ilic, I. Epidemiology of pancreatic cancer. *World J. Gastroenterol.* **2016**, *22*, 9694–9705. [CrossRef] [PubMed]
7. Chhoda, A.; Lu, L.; Clerkin, B.M.; Risch, H.; Farrell, J.J. Current approaches to pancreatic cancer screening. *Am. J. Pathol.* **2019**, *189*, 22–35. [CrossRef] [PubMed]

8. Cheng, X.; Zhao, G.; Zhao, Y. Combination Immunotherapy Approaches for Pancreatic Cancer Treatment. *Can. J. Gastroenterol. Hepatol.* **2018**, *2018*, 6240467. [CrossRef] [PubMed]
9. Loi, D.T. *Vietnamese Medicinal Plants and Ingredients*; Medical Publishing House: Hanoi, Vietnam, 2001; pp. 423–424.
10. Ye, C.L.; Lu, Y.H.; Wei, D.Z. Flavonoids from Cleistocalyx operculatus. *Phytochemistry* **2004**, *65*, 445–447. [CrossRef]
11. Woo, A.Y.; Waye, M.M.; Kwan, H.S.; Chan, M.C.; Chau, C.F.; Cheng, C.H. Inhibition of ATPases by Cleistocalyx operculatus. A possible mechanism for the cardiotonic actions of the herb. *Vasc. Pharmacol.* **2002**, *38*, 163–168. [CrossRef]
12. Mai, T.T.; Chuyen, N.V. Anti-hyperglycemic activity of an aqueous extract from flower buds of Cleistocalyx operculatus (Roxb.) Merr and Perry. *Biosci. Biotechnol. Biochem.* **2007**, *71*, 69–76. [CrossRef]
13. Mai, T.T.; Thu, N.N.; Tien, P.G.; Van Chuyen, N. Alpha-glucosidase inhibitory and antioxidant activities of Vietnamese edible plants and their relationships with polyphenol contents. *J. Nutr. Sci. Vitaminol.* **2007**, *53*, 267–276. [CrossRef]
14. Wang, C.; Wu, P.; Tian, S.; Xue, J.; Xu, L.; Li, H.; Wei, X. Bioactive pentacyclic triterpenoids from the leaves of Cleistocalyx operculatus. *J. Nat. Prod.* **2016**, *79*, 2912–2923. [CrossRef] [PubMed]
15. Su, J.C.; Wang, S.; Cheng, W.; Huang, X.J.; Li, M.M.; Jiang, R.W.; Li, Y.L.; Wang, L.; Ye, W.C.; Wang, Y. Phloroglucinol derivatives with unusual skeletons from Cleistocalyx operculatus and their in vitro antiviral activity. *J. Org. Chem.* **2018**, *83*, 8522–8532. [CrossRef] [PubMed]
16. Ha, T.K.; Dao, T.T.; Nguyen, N.H.; Kim, J.; Kim, E.; Cho, T.O.; Oh, W.K. Antiviral phenolics from the leaves of Cleistocalyx operculatus. *Fitoterapia* **2016**, *110*, 135–141. [CrossRef] [PubMed]
17. Min, B.S.; Cuong, T.D.; Lee, J.S.; Shin, B.S.; Woo, M.H.; Hung, T.M. Cholinesterase inhibitors from Cleistocalyx operculatus buds. *Arch. Pharm. Res.* **2010**, *33*, 1665–1670. [CrossRef] [PubMed]
18. Dung, N.T.; Bajpai, V.K.; Yoon, J.I.; Kang, S.C. Anti-inflammatory effects of essential oil isolated from the buds of Cleistocalyx operculatus (Roxb.) Merr and Perry. *Food Chem. Toxicol.* **2009**, *47*, 449–453. [CrossRef] [PubMed]
19. Huang, H.Y.; Niu, J.L.; Zhao, L.M.; Lu, Y.H. Reversal effect of 2′,4′-dihydroxy-6′-methoxy-3′,5′-dimethylchalcone on multi-drug resistance in resistant human hepatocellular carcinoma cell line BEL-7402/5-FU. *Phytomedicine* **2011**, *18*, 1086–1092. [CrossRef] [PubMed]
20. Huang, H.Y.; Niu, J.L.; Lu, Y.H. Multidrug resistance reversal effect of DMC derived from buds of Cleistocalyx operculatus in human hepatocellular tumor xenograft model. *J. Sci. Food Agric.* **2012**, *92*, 135–140. [CrossRef]
21. Yu, W.G.; Qian, J.; Lu, Y.H. Hepatoprotective effects of 2′, 4′-dihydroxy-6′-methoxy-3′, 5′-dimethylchalcone on CCl4-induced acute liver injury in mice. *J. Agric. Food Chem.* **2011**, *59*, 12821–12829. [CrossRef]
22. Su, M.Y.; Huang, H.Y.; Li, L.; Lu, Y.H. Protective effects of 2′, 4′-dihydroxy-6′-methoxy-3′, 5′-dimethylchalcone to PC12 cells against cytotoxicity induced by hydrogen peroxide. *J. Agric. Food Chem.* **2011**, *59*, 521–527. [CrossRef]
23. Ye, C.L.; Lai, Y.F. 2′,4′-Dihydroxy-6′-methoxy-3′,5′-dimethylchalcone, from buds of *Cleistocalyxoperculatus*, induces apoptosis in human hepatoma SMMC-7721 cells through a reactive oxygen species-dependent mechanism. *Cytotechnology* **2016**, *68*, 331–341. [CrossRef]
24. Fitton, J.H.; Stringer, D.N.; Karpiniec, S.S. Therapies from Fucoidan: An Update. *Mar. Drugs* **2015**, *13*, 5920–5946. [CrossRef] [PubMed]
25. Seki, T.; Kokuryo, T.; Yokoyama, Y.; Suzuki, H.; Itatsu, K.; Nakagawa, A.; Mizutani, T.; Miyake, T.; Uno, M.; Yamauchi, K.; et al. Antitumor effects of α-bisabolol against pancreatic cancer. *Cancer Sci.* **2011**, *102*, 2199–2205. [CrossRef] [PubMed]
26. Paluszkiewicz, P.; Smolińska, K.; Dębińska, I.; Turski, W.A. Main dietary compounds and pancreatic cancer risk. The quantitative analysis of case-control and cohort studies. *Cancer Epidemiol.* **2012**, *36*, 60–67. [CrossRef] [PubMed]
27. Jansen, R.J.; Robinson, D.P.; Stolzenberg-Solomon, R.Z.; Bamlet, W.R.; de Andrade, M.; Oberg, A.L.; Hammer, T.J.; Rabe, K.G.; Anderson, K.E.; Olson, J.E.; et al. Fruit and vegetable consumption is inversely associated with having pancreatic cancer. *Cancer Causes Control* **2011**, *22*, 1613–1625. [CrossRef] [PubMed]
28. Rossi, M.; Lugo, A.; Lagiou, P.; Zucchetto, A.; Polesel, J.; Serraino, D.; Negri, E.; Trichopoulos, D.; La Vecchia, C. Proanthocyanidins and other flavonoids in relation to pancreatic cancer: A case-control study in Italy. *Ann. Oncol.* **2012**, *23*, 1488–1493. [CrossRef] [PubMed]

29. Dias, T.; Liu, B.; Jones, P.; Houghton, P.J.; Mota-Filipe, H.; Paulo, A. Cytoprotective effect of Coreopsis tinctoria extracts and flavonoids on tBHP and cytokine-induced cell injury in pancreatic MIN6 cells. *J. Ethnopharmacol.* **2012**, *139*, 485–492. [CrossRef] [PubMed]
30. Lu, Q.Y.; Zhang, L.; Moro, A.; Chen, M.C.; Harris, D.M.; Eibl, G.; Go, V.L. Detection of baicalin metabolites baicalein and oroxylin-a in mouse pancreas and pancreatic xenografts. *Pancreas* **2012**, *41*, 571–576. [CrossRef] [PubMed]
31. Wu, X.; Zhang, H.; Salmani, J.M.; Fu, R.; Chen, B. Advances of wogonin, an extract from Scutellaria baicalensis for the treatment of multiple tumors. *Onco Targets Ther.* **2016**, *9*, 2935–2943. [PubMed]
32. Ye, C.L.; Liu, J.W.; Wei, D.Z.; Lu, Y.H.; Qian, F. In vitro anti-tumor activity of 2′, 4′-dihydroxy-6′-methoxy-3′, 5′-dimethylchalcone against six established human cancer cell lines. *Pharmacol. Res.* **2004**, *50*, 505–510. [CrossRef]
33. Ye, C.L.; Qian, F.; Wei, D.Z.; Lu, Y.H.; Liu, J.W. Induction of apoptosis in K562 human leukemia cells by 2′, 4′-dihydroxy-6′-methoxy-3′, 5′-dimethylchalcone. *Leuk. Res.* **2005**, *29*, 887–892. [CrossRef]

Sample Availability: Samples of the compounds are not available from the authors.

molecules

MDPI

Article

Quality Assessment of Commercial Spagyric Tinctures of *Harpagophytum procumbens* and Their Antioxidant Properties

Pinarosa Avato * and Maria Pia Argentieri

Dipartimento di Farmacia-Scienze del Farmaco, Università degli Studi di Bari Aldo Moro, via Orabona 4, 70125 Bari, Italy; mariapia.argentieri@uniba.it

* Correspondence: pinarosa.avato@uniba.it; Tel.: +39-080-5442785

Received: 26 March 2019; Accepted: 14 June 2019; Published: 17 June 2019

Abstract: Preparations from the dried tubers of *Harpagophytum procumbens* (Burch.) DC ex Meisn, commonly known as devil's claw, are mainly used in modern medicine to relieve joint pain and inflammation in patients suffering from rheumatic and arthritic disorders. This paper describes for the first time the chemical profile of a commercial spagyric tincture (named 019) prepared from the roots of the plant. For comparison purposes, a commercial not-spagyric devil's claw tincture (NST) was also analyzed. Chemical investigation of the content of specialized metabolites in the three samples indicated that harpagoside was the main compound, followed by the two isomers acteoside and isoacteoside. Compositional consistence over time was obtained by the chemical fingerprinting of another spagyric tincture (named 014) from the same producer that was already expired according to the recommendation on the label of the product. The two spagyric preparations did not show significant compositional differences as revealed by HPLC and MS analyses, except for a decrease in harpagide content in the expired 014 tincture. Moreover, their antioxidant capacities as assessed by 2,2′-di-phenyl-1-picrylhydrazyl (DPPH) and 2.2′-azin-bis (3-ethylbenzothiazoline-6-sulfonic acid) (ABTS) methods resulted in very similar IC50 values. The expired 014 tincture showed instead a lower IC50 value compared to the 019 and NST tinctures with the ferric reducing antioxidant potential (FRAP) assay, indicating a higher ferric-reducing antioxidant ability. Overall, these results indicated that the two preparations could generally maintain good stability and biological activity at least for the four years from the production to the expiration date.

Keywords: *Harpagophytum procumbens*; devil's claw; harpagoside; spagyric tincture; antioxidant activity

1. Introduction

Harpagophytum procumbens (Burch.) DC ex Meisn, commonly known as devil's claw, is a plant native to southern Africa, where it is traditionally used as a bitter tonic and a stomachic and also for the treatment of fever, gout, myalgia, and arthritis [1,2]. Accordingly, preparations from the dried tubers of the plant are mainly used in modern medicine and as health products to relieve joint pain and inflammation in patients suffering from rheumatic and arthritic disorders. Clinical studies have in fact shown that extracts from the roots of this plant are good therapeutic remedies for degenerative diseases of the musculoskeletal and locomotor systems [1,3]. In addition, the use of devil's claw secondary tubers is also approved in preparations for the relief of mild digestive disorders and for the temporary loss of appetite [4,5].

The European Medicines Agency (EMA) recommends preparations obtained by comminuting or powdering the roots of the plant. Liquid, soft, or dry extracts for oral use made in ethanol or water are also included in the recommendation [4,5]. Spagyric tinctures based on *H. procumbens* are also available on the market for articular and rheumatic complaints.

The manufacturing of a spagyric tincture is based on two main stages, namely maceration and fermentation of the drug in alcohol. Processing of the plant material is accomplished in dark thick-walled glass flasks hermetically closed and maintained in greenhouses under a controlled temperature of about 37 °C for 28 days. After this period, the tincture is decanted, and the drug residue is removed from the solution, completely dried, and burnt to ashes to recover the inorganic elements of the plant material. Ashes from the calcined drug are then dissolved in the alcoholic solution from maceration, and the final spagyric preparation is left to stand for 12 days before use.

The practice of "spagyria" dates back to Paracelsus (1493–1541), who first coined the term to mean "separate" (*spao*) and "combine" (*ageiro*), indicating that spagyric preparations are based on "separation", "extraction", and "recombination" of the active extractives, including mineral components [6].

The quality control of herbal products aims to assure their consistency, efficacy, and safety. The overall quality of botanicals depends on several factors, including the selection of raw plant materials, harvest time, seasonal changes, and post-harvest processing, and it also relies on extraction procedures and product preparations. All of these factors can primarily affect the plant/drug content of bioactive constituents and impair the efficacy of the final formulation.

The determination of chemical fingerprinting can be a powerful tool to verify the quality of botanicals [7–10]. Thus, the selection of specific chemical markers of a drug sample/preparation is considered to be crucial for the analysis of its quality. According to the EMA, chemical markers are of interest for quality control regardless of whether they possess any therapeutic or physiological activity, although ideal chemical markers should be unique metabolites that contribute to the biological efficacy of the drug or its preparation [11,12].

The use of fingerprinting in the analytical control of herbal preparation is now a widely accepted official method [7–10] to assess quality and stability over time and eventually disclose some variation in the chemical content that could reflect a decline in biological activity.

Bitter iridoid glucosides such as harpagoside and harpagide are widely regarded as the active constituents responsible for the pharmacological anti-inflammatory properties of *H. procumbens* [13–16]. Other components reported as present in the drug are the iridoid procumbide, 8-*O*-*p*-coumaroyl-harpagide, 6′-*O*-*p*-coumaroyl-procumbide, phenylethyl glycosides (such as acteoside and isoacteoside), polyphenolic acids, and flavonoids. All of these phytochemicals are considered to have antioxidant properties and to provide protection against lipid peroxidation [17]. According to the *European Pharmacopoeia* [18], roots from *H. procumbens* must contain ≥1.2% harpagoside. Therefore, a chromatographic profile based on the content of the above main components, taken as the reference chemical markers, should be used in the analytical control of preparations from the roots of *H. procumbens*.

The present manuscript aims to assess quality in terms of the quantitative and qualitative fingerprinting of selected chemical markers of a commercial spagyric preparation based on *H. procumbens*. Compositional data of specialized metabolites were compared to those from a commercial not-spagyric devil's claw tincture (NST) with June 2020 as the declared expiration date. In addition, an evaluation of possible deterioration of the chemical profile was carried out through chemical fingerprinting of an *H. procumbens* spagyric food supplement from the same manufacturer that was already expired according to the recommendation published on the label of the product. Finally, the antioxidant activity of the two spagyric preparations was determined and compared to possibly reveal any variation in activity due to the aging of the products and degradation of the bioactive phytochemicals.

2. Results

2.1. Chemical Analysis

As shown in Figure 1, the two spagyric tinctures 014 and 019 did not show significant compositional differences as revealed by thin layer chromatography-TLC. No substantial compositional differences were also observed when compared to the NST. As indicated, harpagoside, acteoside, and harpagide could be detected in all of the samples as the main specialized metabolites.

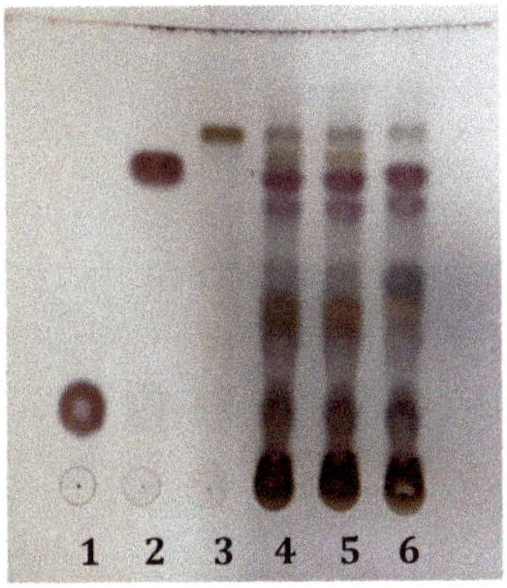

Figure 1. TLC analysis of the two spagyric tinctures, 014 and 019. Mobile phase: EtOAc/HCOOH/ CH_3CO_2H/H_2O (100:11:11:26 *v*/*v*); visualization with AS (see Section 4.4). Harpagide, 1; harpagoside, 2; acteoside, 3; 014, 4; 019, 5; not-spagyric tincture (NST), 6.

In agreement with TLC analyses, a comparison of the HPLC-DAD (diode-array detector) chromatograms indicated that the three samples 019, 014, and NST did not differ in their general composition (Figure 2). Typical UV absorptions (Table 1) detecting around 217, 246–248, 290, and 325–330 nm for compounds **1** and **2** indicated the presence of phenylethanoid glycosides [19], while the detection of UV maxima at 217 and 280 nm were consistent with an iridoid enol ether system, including a cinnamoyl chromophore in compounds **5** and **6** [20]. In addition, UV absorptions at around 224 and 311 nm suggested the presence of *p*-coumaric acid moieties in compounds **3** and **4**.

Consistent with the above observations, the chemical profile investigated by combining HPLC-DAD and LC–MS/MS and through spiking it with available reference compounds confirmed that the main peak (t_R = 39.58 min) in both samples was represented by harpagoside (Figure 2, peak 5).

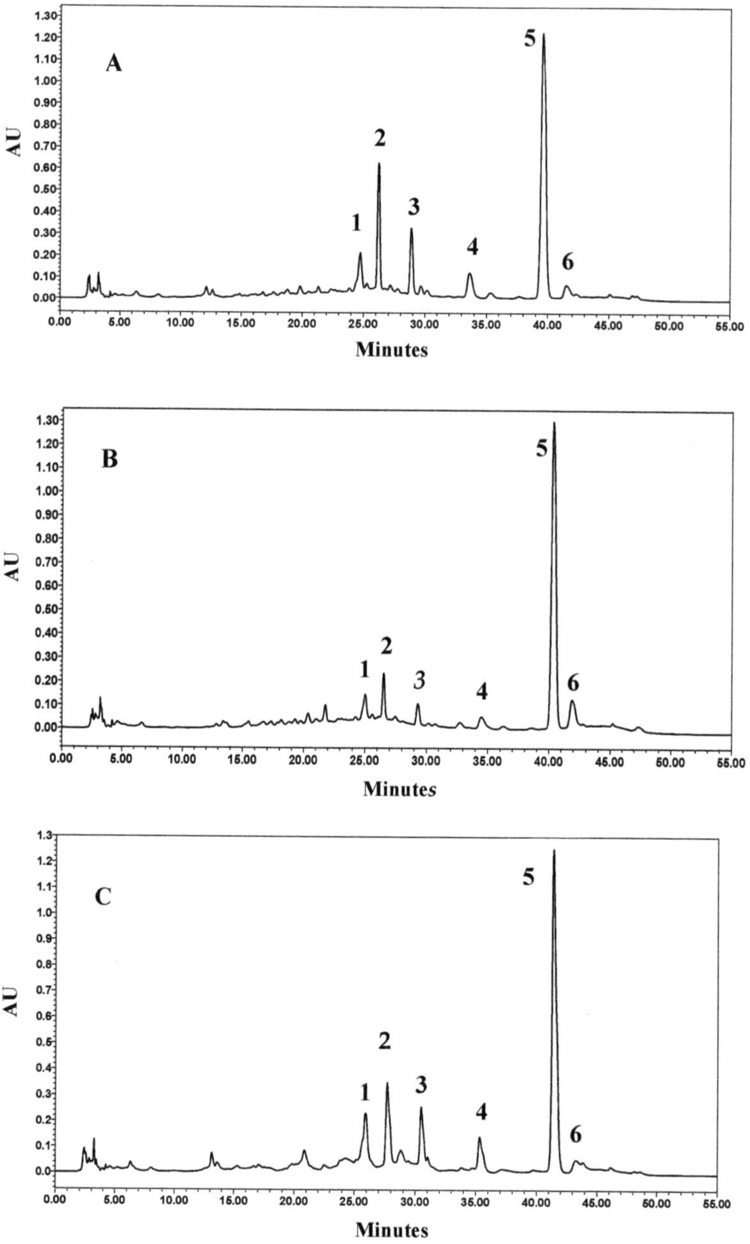

Figure 2. HPLC-DAD (270 nm) chromatograms of the tinctures 019 (**A**), 014 (**B**), and the NST (**C**). For peak naming, see Table 1.

Table 1. MS fragmentation and UV-VIS absorption data of compounds detected in the tinctures of Harpagophytum procumbens by HPLC-DAD (270 nm).

Number *	R_t (min)	Name	UV (λ max, nm)	ms1	ms2
				m/z (%)	
1	24.70	Acteoside	216.6, 246.5 sh, 290.5 sh, 325.7	623.0 (100) $[M-H]^-$	461.0 (100) $[(M-H)\text{-}162]^-$; 315.0 (4) $[(M-H)\text{-}162\text{-}146]^-$; 179.0 (2), [caffeoyl moiety]$^-$
2	26.20	Isoacteoside	217.7, 248.5 sh, 292.3 sh, 326.9	623.0 (100) $[M-H]^-$	461.0 (100) $[(M\text{-}H)\text{-}162]^-$; 315.0 (4) $[(M-H)\text{-}162\text{-}146]^-$; 179.0 (2), [caffeoyl moiety]$^-$
3	28.87	8-*O*-*p*-Coumaroyl-harpagide	224.8, 311.4	533.1 (100) $[M+Na]^+$	369.2 (100) $[(M+Na)\text{-}164]^+$; 351.0 (44) $[(M+Na)\text{-}164\text{-}18]^+$; 203.0 (6) [harpagide-162]$^+$
4	33.60	Pagoside	224.8, 311.4	491.0 (100) $[M-H]^-$	311.2 (100) $[(M-H)\text{-}162\text{-}18]^-$; 163.0 (31) [coumaric acid]$^-$
5	39.58	Harpagoside	217.7, 280.4	1011.5 (5) $[2M+Na]^+$ /517.2 (100) $[M+Na]^+$	369.2 (100) $[(M+Na)\text{-}148]^+$; 351.0 (44) $[(M+Na)\text{-}148\text{-}18]^+$; 203.0 (6) $[(M+Na)\text{-}148\text{-}166]^+$
6	41.64	8-Cinnamoylmyoporoside	217.7, 278.1	501.0 (100) $[M+Na]^+$	353.1 (100) $[(M+Na)\text{-}148]^+$; 335.2 (69) $[(M+Na)\text{-}148\text{-}18]^+$; 339.0 (41) $[(M+Na)\text{-}162]^+$; 203.0 (6) harpagide-162]$^+$

* For peak numbers, see text and Figure 2.

The UV spectrum showing two absorption bands at 217.7 and 280.4 (max) nm and the LC–MS/MS fragmentation pattern ([*m/z* 1011.5 (5) 2M + Na]$^+$, [*m/z* 517.2 (100) M + Na]$^+$, [*m/z* 369.2 (100) (M + Na)-148, cinnamic acid]$^+$, [*m/z* 351.0 (44) (M + Na)-148-18]$^+$, [*m/z* 203.0 (6) (M + Na)-148-166, harpagide]$^+$) were in fact unequivocally consistent with the identification of harpagoside [12,17]. The identity of harpagoside was also acquired by its isolation as a pure constituent through a fast and reliable solid-phase extraction (SPE) optimization method (see Section 4.4). The other major peaks (Figure 2) were respectively identified as peak 1, acteoside (verbascoside), (t_R = 24.70 min), UV 216.6, 246.5 (sh), 290.5 (sh), and 325.7 (max) nm, fragmentation pattern ([*m/z* 623.0 (100) M − H]$^-$, [*m/z* 461 (100) (M − H)-162, glucose]$^-$, [*m/z* 315.0 (4) (M − H)-162-146, rhamnose]$^-$, [*m/z* 179.0 (2), caffeoyl moiety]$^-$); peak 2, isoacteoside, (t_R = 26.20 min), UV 217.7, 248.5 (sh), 292.3 (sh), and 326.9 (max) nm, fragmentation pattern ([*m/z* 623.0 (100) M − H]$^-$, [*m/z* 461 (100) (M − H)-162, glucose]$^-$, [*m/z* 315.0 (4) (M − H)-162-146, rhamnose]$^-$, [*m/z* 179.0 (2), caffeoyl moiety]$^-$); peak 3, 8-p-coumaroyl-harpagide, (t_R = 28.87 min), UV 224.8, 311.4 (max) nm, fragmentation pattern ([*m/z* 533.1 (100) M + Na]$^+$, [*m/z* 369.2 (100) (M + Na)-164, coumaric acid]$^+$, [*m/z* 351.0 (44) (M + Na)-164-18]$^+$, [*m/z* 203.0 (6) harpagide-162, glucose]$^+$); peak 4, pagoside, (t_R = 33.60 min), UV 224.8 and 311.4 (max) nm, fragmentation pattern ([*m/z* 491.0 (100) M − H]$^-$, [*m/z* 311.2 (100) (M − H)-18-162, glucose]$^-$, [*m/z* 163.0 (31), coumaric acid]$^-$); peak 6, 8-cinnamoylmyoporoside (t_R = 41.64 min), UV 217.7 (max) and 278.1 nm, fragmentation pattern ([*m/z* 501.0 (100) M + Na]$^+$, [*m/z* 353.1 (100) (M + Na)-148, cinnamic acid]$^+$, [*m/z* 335.2 (69) (M + Na)-148-18]$^+$, [*m/z* 339.0 (41) (M + Na)-162, glucose]$^+$, [*m/z* 203.0 (6) harpagide-162, glucose]$^+$). The presence of harpagide (lacking absorbance at 270 nm), already detected by TLC, was confirmed by HPLC-ELSD (evaporative light scattering detector) analysis (Figures 1 and 3) and by coelution with an authentic compound, and it was in addition identified through its mass spectrum: ([*m/z* 365.0 (100) M + H]$^+$, [*m/z* 347.1 (36) (M + H)-18]$^+$, [*m/z* 305.1 (75) (M + H)-42-18]$^+$, [*m/z* 275.1 (41) (M + H)-90]$^+$, [*m/z* 203.0 (100) (M + H)-162]$^+$, [*m/z* 185.0 (68) (M + H)-162-18]$^+$). The identification of constituents of the two spagyric tinctures was also supported by the available literature [13,21–24].

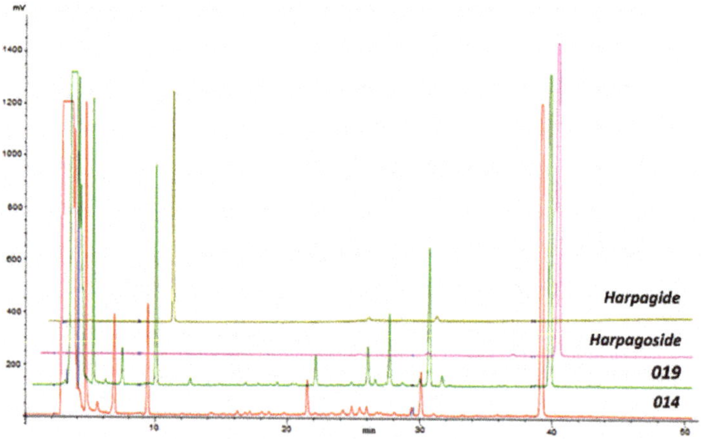

Figure 3. HPLC-ELSD chromatograms of the two spagyric tinctures, 014 and 019: Harpagoside and harpagide.

In addition to a similar chemical profile, the two spagyric tinctures also showed to a large extent a comparable quantitative composition (Table 2). A quantification of harpagoside as determined by HPLC-DAD against the calibration curve indicated that the compound was equally abundant in the two extracts, amounting respectively to 14.97 ± 0.09 µg/mg ext (59.47%) in the 019 sample and to 13.68 ± 0.19 µg/mg ext (69.68%) in the 014 sample. Other major metabolites were represented by acteoside (019: 1.99 ± 0.23 µg/mg ext, 7.90%; 014: 1.49 ± 0.02 µg/mg ext, 7.59%) and isoacteside (019:

3.94 ± 0.006 µg/mg ext, 15.65%; 014: 1.87 ± 0.14 µg/mg ext, 9.52%). A relatively higher amount of 8-*O*-*p*-coumaroyl-harpagide (019: 2.21 ± 0.0003 µg /mg ext, 8.78%; 014: 0.68 ± 0.006 µg/mg ext, 3.46%) and pagoside (019: 1.37 ± 0.01 µg/mg ext 5.44%; 014: 0.53 ± 0.009 µg/mg ext, 2.70%) was detected in the 019 sample, while 8-cinnamoylmyoporoside was more abundant in 014, 1.38 ± 0.009 µg/mg, 7.03%, versus 0.69 ± 0.008 µg/mg ext, 2.74%, in 019. The same specialized metabolites in the NST sample amounted, respectively, to acteoside, 1.35 ± 0.15 µg/mg ext, 7.39%; isoacteoside, 1.55 ± 0.04 µg/mg ext, 8.48%; 8-*O*-*p*-coumaroyl-harpagide, 0.95 ± 0.04 µg/mg ext, 5.20%; pagoside, 0.72 ± 0.02 µg/mg ext, 3.94%; harpagoside, 13.25 ± 0.07 µg/mg ext, 75.52%; 8-cinnamoylmyoporoside, 0.45 ± 0.005 µg/mg ext, 2.46% (Table 2).

Table 2. Specialized metabolites identified in 019, 014, and the NST.

Compound	014		019		NST	
	µg/mg ext	%	µg/mg ext	%	µg/mg ext	%
1	1.49 ± 0.02	7.59	1.99 ± 0.23	7.90	1.35 ± 0.15	7.39
2	1.87 ± 0.14	9.52	3.94 ± 0.006	15.65	1.55 ± 0.04	8.48
3	0.68 ± 0.006	3.46	2.21 ± 0.0003	8.78	0.95 ± 0.04	5.2
4	0.53 ± 0.009	2.70	1.37 ± 0.01	5.44	0.72 ± 0.02	3.94
5	13.68 ± 0.19	69.68	14.97 ± 0.09	59.47	13.25 ± 0.07	72.52
6	1.38 ± 0.009	7.03	0.69 ± 0.008	2.74	0.45 ± 0.005	2.46

For peak naming, see Table 1.

Due to the lack of a chromophore in the molecule, harpagide quantitation was achieved by HPLC-ELSD, which indicated that the content of this phytochemical was slightly higher in the 019 preparation (15.98 ± 0.23 µg/mg ext) compared to the 014 sample (8.50 ± 0.32 µg/mg ext). Similarly to the 019 tincture, harpagide extract accounted for 19.53 ± 0.17 µg/mg ext in the NST.

2.2. Antioxidant Activity

The antioxidant capacity of the two spagyric tinctures of *H. procumbens* was evaluated by in vitro DPPH, ABTS, and FRAP assays (see Sections 4.9–4.11) and compared to quercetin and acteoside. As shown in Figure 4, the free radical scavenging activity determined by the DPPH and ABTS methods and the ferric-reducing power calculated by the FRAP assay gave almost superimposable behaviors for the two samples, 019 and 014. They displayed a good dose-dependent inhibition of DPPH activity in the range of tested concentrations (up to 89–90% inhibition for 019 and 014, respectively) at 330 µg/mL and up to 98% inhibition of ABTS activity at 260 µg/mL. The ferric-reducing antioxidant power results were instead already high at lower concentrations (52–69% inhibition at 26 µg/mL and up to 76–83% at 60 µg/mL for 019 and 014, respectively).

With regard to the NST sample, its free radical scavenging activity and its ferric-reducing activity (determined by DPPH, ABTS, and FRAP assays) gave results almost superimposable on those obtained for the two spagyric tinctures, with a good dose versus % inhibition correlation.

However, compared to quercetin and acteoside, all three tinctures (019, 014, and the NST) displayed lower antioxidant activity (Figure 4). Both of these two compounds showed antiradical activity reaching 96–100% of DPPH inhibition at concentrations between 26 and 50 µg/mL for quercetin and acteoside. Similarly, quercetin and acteoside were very effective in scavenging the $ABTS^+$ radical cation, displaying 100% inhibition between 7 and 13 µg/mL. In addition, they showed discrete FRAP values amounting to 330 (quercetin) and 67 (acteoside) µg/mL to obtain 95% inhibition.

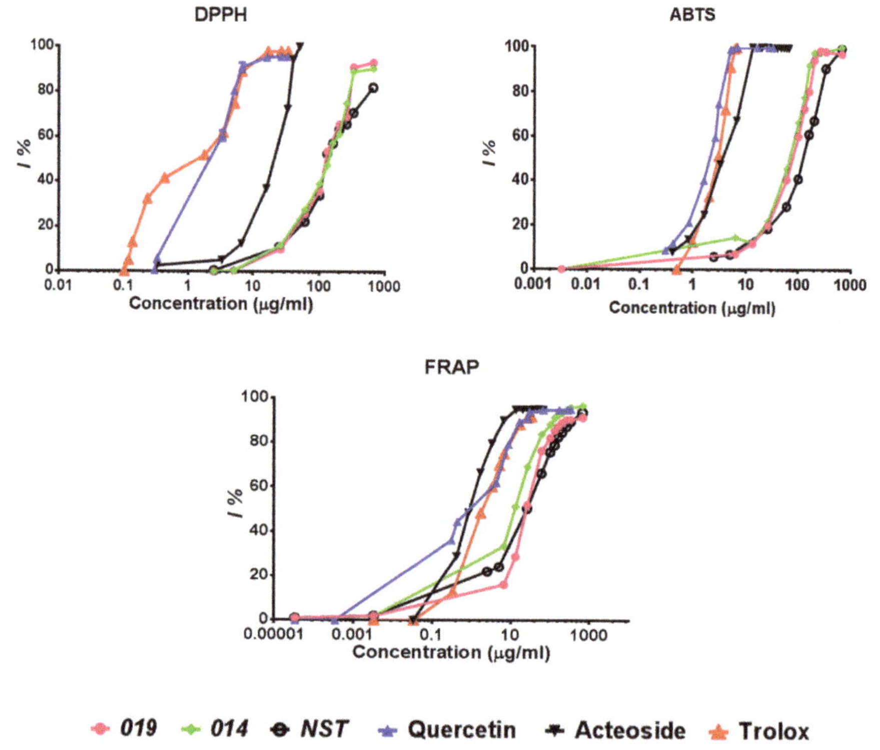

Figure 4. Antioxidant activity of spagyric tinctures 019 and 014, the NST, quercetin, acteoside, and Trolox as a positive control, as determined by DPPH, ABTS, and FRAP methods.

Values of their IC50 (concentration that gives half-maximal response), expressed as mEq of Trolox, are reported in Table 3. Both the 019 and 014 samples showed similar IC50 values of free radical scavenging activity in DPPH and ABTS, amounting to 92.53 ± 0.31 (019) and 93.33 ± 0.25 (014) mEq Trolox and 22.89 ± 0.19 (019) and 19.49 ± 0.13 (014) mEq Trolox, respectively. In contrast to the above, the expired 014 tincture showed a lower IC50 value compared to the 019 tincture in the FRAP method, indicating a higher ferric-reducing antioxidant ability. IC50 values obtained for the NST (Table 3) in the three assays (DPPH, ABTS, and FRAP) were very close to those detected for 019 and even slightly lower, indicating slightly higher antioxidant activity.

Table 3. Antioxidant activity (IC50) of the spagyric tinctures 019 and 014 and the NST of *H. procumbens*.

Sample	IC50 (mEq Trolox) ± SD		
	DPPH	ABTS	FRAP
019	92.53 ± 0.31	22.89 ± 0.19	14.11 ± 0.08
014	93.33 ± 0.25	19.49 ± 0.13	6.69 ± 0.07
NST	83.02 ± 0.28	17.78 ± 0.12	11.32 ± 0.08
Acteoside	13.83 ± 0.09	0.96 ± 0.05	0.44 ± 0.04
Quercetin	1.38 ± 0.01	0.60 ± 0.07	0.38 ± 0.02

The IC50 values of quercetin and acteoside were much lower than those of 019 and 014, indicating the better antioxidant capacity of these two pure reference compounds. Moreover, the IC50 values of quercetin and acteoside, as assessed by the ABTS and FRAP methods, were very similar, while quercetin displayed a more powerful capacity for DPPH reduction than acteoside did (Table 3).

The DPPH assay was also applied to harpagoside, the major iridoid present in the two samples: The IC50 result was higher than 330 ± 0.05 μg/mL, and therefore its antioxidant potency was not tested with the other methods, ABTS and FRAP.

3. Discussion

To the best of our knowledge, this is the first report on the phytochemical and biological characterization of spagyric preparations. In this study, we compared the compositional profile of two commercial food supplements (declared to be spagyric tinctures (019 and 014) and provided by the same producer company) with the aim of assessing the quality of the preparations in terms of chemical fingerprinting and biological activity. One of the two spagyric tinctures (014) was already expired according to the recommendation published on the label of the product, and therefore evaluation of the antioxidant activity (using three different methods) was important to display a correlation with the chemical profile and eventually with the aging of the preparation.

The major phytochemicals that have been detected in root extracts from *H. procumbens* include iridoids and phenolic glycosides [13,14,25]. Harpagoside, harpagide, and procumbide are regarded as the most representative iridoid glycosides isolated from the drug, along with the two phenylpropanoid glycosides acteoside and isoacteoside. Several other compounds have been isolated over time in different investigations [13,14,26], such as conjugated esters of iridoid glycosides (8-*O*-*p*-coumaroyl-harpagide, 6′-*O*-*p*-coumaroyl-procumbide, 8-*O*-feruloyl-harpagide, 8-cinnamoylmyoporoside).

As shown in Figure 2, the adopted HPLC analytical method provided a good separation of the phytochemical constituents of the commercial spagyric tinctures. In addition, the method fulfilled all of the validation criteria, showing good linearity of the calibration curve and good limit of detection (LoD) and limit of quantification (LoQ) values, including precision parameters, therefore showing validated repeatability and reproducibility. Compositional requirements in terms of specific chemical markers were also fulfilled in that the two spagyric tinctures, analyzed through TLC, HPLC, UV, and MS methods, displayed the expected phytochemical profile, with harpagoside as the main component along with harpagide, acteoside, and isoacteoside (Table 1).

In addition, the validation of the compositional requirements of both spagyric samples was also confirmed by the analysis of the NST sample, which showed a similar chemical profile, with harpagoside as the most abundant component, followed by acteoside and isoacteoside. Interestingly, the content of harpagide in the NST tincture was comparable (19.53 ± 0.17 μg/mg ext vs 15.98 ± 0.23 μg/mg ext) to that of 019, the tincture that was still not expired.

Spagyric preparations are not conventional herb preparations, but they are based on old alchemic procedures dating back to Paracelsus, who first developed this methodology and described it in his medical treatise *Opus Paramirum*. Our results indicated that the spagyric method allowed us to obtain preparations of good quality based on the presence of marker compounds.

In addition, considering that the two products differed by at least five years in their expiration date and presumably in their production date, fingerprinting analysis and the quantitative determination of the representative constituents in the expired spagyric preparation 014 allowed us to prove a general significant long-term stability of *H. procumbens* active metabolites. A significant decrease of harpagide content was, however, observed in the expired 014 tincture compared to 019 (Table 2).

Preparations based on devil's claw are mainly used to relieve pain and inflammation due to arthritis and other painful disorders, although the mechanism of action has not yet been fully elucidated. It is known that the generation of oxygen-free radicals is involved in the development of inflammation. Radicals freed from phagocytes are implicated in the activation of nuclear factors, which in turn induces the synthesis of cytokines. Then, a synergic action of oxygen-free radicals and cytokines promotes the synthesis of inflammatory mediators. Maintenance of an adequate antioxidant status may thus help to attenuate the symptoms of inflammation.

There are some indications that the antioxidant properties of some of the specialized metabolites also contribute to the anti-inflammatory effects of pharmaceutical preparations based on *H. procumbens* [14,15,25,27]. However, the antioxidant activity of devil's claw has not been extensively investigated, and there have been no previous investigations on the antioxidant bioactivity of spagyric preparations. Previous studies have only reported moderate antioxidant activity in methanolic root extracts of *H. procumbens*, while an aqueous extract containing 2.6% harpagoside was shown to have a good capacity to scavenge DPPH. In addition, intraperitoneal administration of a 53% ethanolic extract of devil's claw to male Wistar rats indicated antioxidant effects similar to those induced by selegiline [4,14,28].

Based on this, we evaluated the antioxidant potency of the two spagyric tinctures to eventually detect any variation in their bioactivity due to the aging of the product and possible degradation of the bioactive phytochemicals. A comparison of the chemicals in and the bioactivity of these two tinctures was also made with a commercial NST.

As for the chemical analysis, significant stability in bioactivity over the long term was also demonstrated by the almost identical antioxidant activity (as determined by the DPPH and ABTS methods (Figure 4)) and the relative IC50 values (Table 3) calculated for the two spagyric preparations, 019 and 014.

An unexpected exception was represented by the lower IC50 value (Table 3) calculated for the expired 014 tincture compared to the 019 tincture in the FRAP method, indicating a higher ferric-reducing antioxidant ability. Reasonably, this might have been due to some species (likely formed upon the aging of the product and not detectable in the used analytical conditions) that were present in the 014 sample and able to efficiently react with the ferric tripyridyltriazine complex.

For instance, it has been reported that the deglycosylation of harpagide gives a degradation product called H-harpagide (2-(formylmethyl)-2,3,5-trihydroxy-5-methylcyclopentane carbaldehyde) that is able to induce the inhibition of the COX-2 enzyme in vitro, in contrast to the parent molecule, which is instead completely inactive [29]. Due to its structure, this molecular species might also undergo oxidation and possibly be more powerful as a ferric-reducing agent. We can suggest that if such a reaction happened upon the aging of the 014 product, it could account for the lower IC50 observed with the FRAP method and the lower amount of harpagide detected in this sample.

Further support for this hypothesis might come from the observation that in the NST tincture, harpagide was present almost in the same amount as in 019 (19.53 ± 0.17 µg/mg ext vs 15.98 ± 0.23 µg/mg ext), and the IC50 values for the antioxidant activity of this sample were very similar to those obtained for the 019 tincture in the three bioassays, including the FRAP test. A deeper investigation should, however, be carried out to clarify this point.

As already reported [13,14,16,30], we also found that acteoside was a powerful antioxidant, while harpagoside did not display antioxidant capacity. Thus, acteoside might reasonably have a role in the antioxidant activity displayed by the two spagyric extracts.

In this study, an evaluation of the antioxidant activity (using three different methods) of the two spagyric tinctures aimed to show a correlation between the chemical profile and eventually the aging of the products. Thus, based on the obtained results, the two analyzed preparations should both be considered to have good biological activity, even when compared to an NST.

4. Materials and Methods

4.1. *Solvents and Reagents*

All solvents (HPLC grade and analytical grade) were obtained from Sigma/Aldrich, Italy. Phosphomolybdic acid spray reagent and anisaldehyde for TLC visualization were purchased from Sigma/Aldrich, Italy. Reagents used for the antioxidant bioassays, including DPPH (2,2′-di-phenyl-1-picrylhydrazyl), TPTZ (2,4,6-tripyridyl-s-triazine), Trolox (6-hydroxy-2,5,7,8-tetramethylchroman-2-ca rboxylic acid), and ABTS (2,2′-azino-bis (3-ethylbenzothiazoline-6-sulfonic acid) were all purchased from Sigma/Aldrich, Italy.

4.2. Samples

Two commercial samples of food supplements (kindly provided by Erbenobili, Italy) consisting of spagyric tinctures (40% ethanol) of *H. procumbens* roots were used in this study. The two samples differed in their shelf-life date: 2014 and 2019, respectively. That is, one of the two samples, conventionally named 014, was already expired when analyzed, while the other one, named 019, was still valid. For comparison purposes, a commercial NST (40% ethanol) was also analyzed.

4.3. Thin Layer Chromatography (TLC)

The composition of devil's claw extracts 019 and 014 was first investigated by TLC (precoated silica gel 60 F254 aluminum plates, Merck, Milan, Italy) eluted with EtOAc/HCOOH/CH_3CO_2H/H_2O (100:11:11:26 *v*/*v*) or with $CHCl_3$/MeOH (90:10 *v*/*v*). Visualization of the components was obtained with phosphomolybdic acid reagent (10% EtOH) or alternatively with anisaldehyde-sulphuric acid reagent (0.5 mL anisaldehyde in 10 mL glacial acetic acid, 85 mL of MeOH in 5 mL of H_2SO_4) (AS). After spraying, TLC plates were heated at 110 °C for 5–10 min and observed under visible 254-nm or UV 366-nm light. For TLC and further analyses, the two spagyric tinctures 019 and 014 and the reference NST were died under vacuum and redissolved in 80% MeOH to obtain a 60-mg/mL solution.

4.4. Harpagoside Isolation

Harpagoside purification from the two tinctures 019 and 014 was achieved by solid-phase extraction (SPE) on Waters Sep-Pak Vac 1 cc C18 cartridges by using an SPE Extraction Manifold-20 position (Waters, Italy). Cartridges were first conditioned with 5 mL of MeOH and with 10 mL of H_2O in that order. Then, 1 mL from each of the two samples 019 and 014 was dried under vacuum, redissolved in 80% MeOH, and loaded onto the SPE cartridge. Harpagoside elution was obtained by flushing the cartridge with H_2O (5 × 1 mL), followed by subsequent elutions with MeOHaq 10% (5 × 1 mL), MeOHaq 50% (5 × 1 mL), and finally MeOHaq 70% (5 × 1 mL). All of the fractions were analyzed by TLC and HPLC. Pure harpagoside was obtained in fractions eluted with MeOHaq 70%.

4.5. HPLC-DAD-ELSD

HPLC-DAD-ELSD analyses were performed with a Waters HPLC 600 Liquid Chromatograph equipped with a diode array detector, DAD 2998 Waters, and an evaporative light scattering detector, ELSD 2424 Waters. Data were processed with EmpowerTM 2 Waters Software (Waters S.p:A, Sesto San Giovanni, Milan, Italy). Nitrogen was used as the driving gas for nebulization at 60 psi. Helium was used as the degassing solvent. Extracts were separated with a Gemini C18 (Phenomenex) column (250 × 4.60 mm, 5-μm particle size) equipped with a Security Guard C18 Cartridge (4 × 3 mm, Phenomenex). The following elution system was used with DAD detection: Solvent A, H_2O; solvent B, CH_3CN. The elution gradient was 5% B in A increasing to reach 25% B at 20 min and 40% B at 40 min. UV spectra of each extract were conventionally recorded at 210, 270, 310, and 350 nm. The presence of harpagide in the two samples was monitored by acquiring the HPLC-DAD trace at 210 nm. Alternatively, the presence of harpagide was detected by ELSD at the following parameters: Drift tube temperature, 55 °C; gain, 1000. Nitrogen was used as the driving gas for nebulization at 60 psi. Helium was used as the degassing solvent. Reference harpagoside and harpagide were analyzed in the same analytical conditions. All of the HPLC analyses were run in triplicate.

4.6. Validation

The quantification of iridoid components in the tinctures under investigation was made by HPLC-DAD against a calibration curve obtained with harpagoside (Phytolab) at six different concentrations in the linear range of 1000–31 μg/mL in MeOHaq 80%. The correlation coefficient (r^2) of the standard curve in the linear plot was r^2 = 0.9999 ($y = 4E + 07x + 391{,}135$), indicating good linearity between peak areas and concentrations within the used concentration range. The quantitation of harpagide was made by HPLC-ELSD against a calibration curve obtained with harpagide at six different concentrations in the linear range of 2000–62.5 μg/mL. The correlation coefficient (r^2) of the standard curve in the linear plot of log-transformed data was r^2 = 0.9992 ($y = 1.7569x - 1.7101$), indicating good linearity between the log-transformed areas and log-transformed concentrations within the tested concentration range.

The limit of detection (LoD) and limit of quantification (LoQ) were calculated according to conventional guidelines [31,32] on the basis of signal-to-noise ratios (S/Ns) of 3:1 and 10:1, respectively, by injecting a series of dilute solutions of known concentrations of harpagoside in the range of 31–0.061 μg/mL. The LoD for harpagoside in the adopted analytical conditions was 0.061 μg/mL, while the LoQ was 0.210 μg/mL.

The precision of the analytical HPLC method was assessed by calculating intraday repeatability and interday intermediate precision [33]. Multiple injections of harpagoside solutions (0.03125 μg/mL) were performed within the same day for intraday precision, while for interday precision, analyses were run in triplicate over three consecutive days. Precision was expressed as the percent relative standard deviation (RSD%) of retention times and peak areas resulting from the analysis of the spagyric tinctures. The intraday and interday variabilities of harpagoside in the two spagyric tinctures 019 and 014 were also calculated with the same procedure. Intraday precision of the chromatographic method for harpagoside was observed in the range of 0.25–0.59% for retention times and between 0.87% and 0.90% for peak areas. Interday RSD values were 0.28% and 0.95% for retention times and peak areas, respectively. The intraday RSD values of retention times and peak areas for the 6 major analytes in the spagyric tinctures were in the range of 0.10–1.10% and 0.50–3.00%, respectively. Percent RSD values of retention times and peak areas for interday evaluation were in the range of 0.21–3.47% and 0.17–3.55%, respectively. Overall, the results obtained indicated that the method applied for the compositional analysis was precise and accurate.

4.7. LC-ESI-MS/MS

Flow injection LC-ESI-MS/MS analyses were performed on a 1100 Series Agilent LC/MSD Trap-System VL (Agilent Technologies Italia SpA, Cernusco sul Naviglio, Milan, Italy). The chromatographic conditions were as described above for the HPLC-DAD analyses. An Agilent Chemstation (LC/MSD TrapSoftware 4.1, (Agilent Technologies Italia SpA, Cernusco sul Naviglio, Milan, Italy) was used for the acquisition and processing of the data. The mass spectrometer operated in the positive and negative ion mode under the following settings: Capillary voltage, 47 V; nebulizer gas (N_2), 5 psi; drying gas (N_2), heated at 220 °C and introduced at a flow rate of 10 μL/mL. Data were acquired in the MS scanning mode over the range of 150–1500 *m/z* with a scan time of 13000 *m/z*/s. Automated MS/MS was performed by isolating the base peaks (pseudomolecular ions) using an isolation width of 4.0 *m/z*, a fragmentation amplitude of 1.0 V, the threshold set at 100, and the ion charge control on, with the maximum acquire time set at 300 ms. Samples were dissolved in MeOHaq 80% and injected at a flow rate of 0.2 mL/min.

4.8. Antioxidant Activity

Antioxidant activity of the three tinctures of *H. procumbens* (019, 014, and NST) was determined by different methods: DPPH, ferric-reducing antioxidant power (FRAP) assay, and Trolox/ABTS equivalent antioxidant capacity [34–36]. For comparative purposes, the antioxidant activity of quercetin (Sigma/Aldrich, Italy), harpagoside (Phytolab, Germany), and acteoside (Sigma-Aldrich S.r.l., Milan, Italy) were also determined with the same procedures. Determinations were carried out in triplicate.

4.9. DPPH

The scavenging activity for DPPH (Sigma, Milan, Italy) free radicals was measured according to Brand–Williams (1995), with some modifications. To 2.9 mL of a 10×10^{-5}-M solution of DPPH in MeOH, 0.1 mL of a properly diluted MeOH sample test solution was added and vortexed, that is, different dilutions of each test sample (019, 014) were prepared to determine the actual IC50 values. After 30 min of incubation in the dark at room temperature, the UV absorbance (Perkin-Elmer Lambda Bio 20 Spectrophotometer) of each sample was recorded at 515 nm against the blank (reagent solution without the test sample). All determinations were carried out in triplicate. The inhibition percentage (I%) of DPPH radicals in the test samples was calculated with the following equation: $I\% = [(A_{\text{blank}} - A_{\text{sample}})/A_{\text{blank}}] \times 100$, where A_{blank} is the absorbance of the blank solution at $t = 0$, and A_{sample} is the absorbance of the test sample at $t = 30$ min. The IC50 concentration is the amount of drug necessary to give 50% inhibition of the DPPH radicals. Acteoside, quercetin, and harpagoside were used as reference compounds.

4.10. FRAP

The following stock solutions were prepared for the bioassay according to Benzie and Strain (1996): a) a 300-mM acetate buffer solution, pH 3.6; b) a 10-mM TPTZ (2,4,6-tripyridyl-*s*-triazine) solution in MeOH; and c) a 20-mM $FeCl_3 \cdot 6\ H_2O$ solution. The FRAP working solution was prepared by mixing TPTZ and $FeCl_3 \cdot 6\ H_2O$ and acetate buffer in a ratio of 1:1:10. Test samples and reference compounds (100 µL) were added to 2.6 mL of FRAP reagent, along with 300 µL of H_2O, and allowed to react for 30 min at 37 °C in dark conditions. Absorbance readings (ferrous tripyridyltriazine complex) were taken at 595 nm. A blank solution consisted of FRAP solutions above and in water. The standard curve was ($r^2 = 0.9992$; $y = 0.0005x + 0.0005$) using a concentration range of $FeSO_4$ between 0.42 µg/mL and 20 µg/mL.

4.11. Trolox/ABTS

Radical scavenging capacity was also studied based on the reduction of ABTS+· radicals by the test samples. An ABTS+· radical cation was obtained by mixing an ABTS stock solution (7 mM in H_2O) with 2.5 mM of potassium persulfate, $K_2S_2O_8$. This solution was allowed to stand at room temperature in the dark for 12–16 h before use. For the analyses, the ABTS+· solution was diluted with water to an absorbance of 0.7 (±0.02) at 734 nm. For the UV determinations, 2.9 mL of the ABTS+· solution and 100 µL of each of the test samples were mixed, and an absorbance reading was taken at 734 nm, 2–6 min after mixing. Appropriate ABTS blanks were run in each assay. All solutions were freshly prepared for the daily experiments. The scavenging activity of each test sample was compared to that of Trolox (6-hydroxy-2,5,7,8-tetramethylchroman-2-carboxylic acid) as the positive control. A linear calibration curve ($r^2 = 0.9970$; $y = 0.0005x + 0.0005$) was constructed using Trolox in a range from 4 µM to 26 µM.

4.12. Statistical Analysis

The quantitative results for each analysis and bioassay were expressed as the mean ± standard deviation (SD) of at least three replicates for each experiment. Microsoft Office Excel 2017 was used for processing the data.

Author Contributions: P.A. conceived of and designed the experiments; M.P.A. performed the experiments; P.A. and M.P.A. analyzed the data; P.A. wrote the paper.

Funding: This research received no external funding.

Acknowledgments: The authors thank Erbenobili s.r.l. for supplying the spagyric tinctures.

Conflicts of Interest: The authors declare no conflicts of interest.

References

1. Stewart, K.M.; Cole, D. The commercial harvest of devil's claw (*Harpagophytum* spp.) in southern Africa: The devil's in the details. *J. Ethnopharmacol.* **2005**, *100*, 225–236. [CrossRef] [PubMed]
2. van Wyk, B.-E. A broad review of commercially important southern African medicinal plants. *J. Ethnopharmacol.* **2008**, *119*, 342–355. [CrossRef] [PubMed]
3. Wegener, T.; Lüpke, N.-P. Treatment of patients with artrosis of hip and knee with an aqueous extract of devil's claw (*Harpagophytum procumbens* D.C.). *Phytother. Res.* **2003**, *17*, 1165–1172. [CrossRef] [PubMed]
4. *European Union Herbal Monograph on Harpagophytum Procumbens DC. and/or Harpagophytum zeyheri Decne., Radix*; EMA/HMPC/627057/2015; European Medicines Agency: Amsterdam, The Netherlands, 2016; pp. 2–8.
5. *Devil's Claw Root-Harpagophytum Procumbens DC. and/or Harpagophytum zeyheri Decne., radix*; EMA/571858/2016; European Medicines Agency: Amsterdam, The Netherlands, 2016; pp. 1–2.
6. Moritz, S. Alchemy and contemporary spagyric medicine: A historical and socio-scientific approach. *Interdiscip. Sci. Rev.* **2016**, *41*, 13–27. [CrossRef]
7. Li, S.; Han, Q.; Qiao, C.; Song, J.; Cheng, C.L.; Xu, H. Chemical markers for the quality control of herbal medicines: An overview. *Chinese Med.* **2008**, 1–16. [CrossRef]
8. Zhang, Y.; Sun, S.; Dai, J.; Wang, W.; Cao, H.; Wu, J.; Gou, X. Quality control method for herbal medicine–Chemical fingerprinting analysis. In *Quality Control of Herbal Medicines and Related Areas*; Shoyama, Y., Ed.; InTech: Rijeka, Croatia, 2011; pp. 171–194. [CrossRef]
9. Donno, D.; Boggia, R.; Zunin, P.; Cerutti, A.K.; Guido, M.; Mellano, M.G.; Prgomet, Z.; Beccaro, G.L. Phytochemical fingerprinting and chemometrics for natural food preparation pattern recognition: An innovative technique in food supplement quality control. *J. Food Sci. Technol.* **2016**, *53*, 1071–1083. [CrossRef]
10. Xie, P.; Chen, S.; Liang, Y.; Wang, X.; Tian, R.; Upton, R. Chromatographic fingerprint analysis—A rational approach for quality assessment of traditional Chinese herbal medicine. *J. Chromatog. A* **2006**, *1112*, 171–180. [CrossRef]
11. *Reflection Paper on Markers Used for Quantitative and Qualitative Analysis of Herbal Medicinal Products and Traditional Herbal Medicinal Products*; EMEA/HMPC/253629/2007; European Medicines Agency: Amsterdam, The Netherlands, 2008; pp. 1–6.
12. *Guideline on Quality of Herbal Medicinal Products/Traditional Herbal Medicinal Products. Final*; European Medicines Agency: Amsterdam, The Netherlands, 2011; pp. 1–13.
13. Boje, K.; Lechtenberg, M.; Nahrstedt, A. New and known iridoid- and phenylethanoid glycosides from *Harpagophytum procumbens* and their in vitro inhibition of human leukocyte elastase. *Planta Med.* **2003**, *69*, 820–825.
14. Mncwangi, N.; Chen, W.; Vermaak, I.; Viljoen, A.M.; Gericke, N. Devil's claw–A review of the ethnobotany, phytochemistry and biological activity of *Harpagophytum procumbens*. *J. Ethnopharmacol.* **2012**, *143*, 755–771. [CrossRef]
15. Viljioen, A.; Mncwangi, N.; Vermaak, I. Anti-inflammatory iridoids of botanical origin. *Curr. Med. Chem.* **2012**, *19*, 2104–2127. [CrossRef]
16. Ahmed, B.; Al-Rehaily, A.J.; Al-Howiriny, T.A.; El-Sayed, K.A.; Ahmad, M.S. Scropoloside D_2 and harpagoside–B: Two new iridoid glycosides from *Scrophularia deserti* and their antidiabetic and anti-inflammatory activity. *Biol. Pharm. Bull.* **2003**, *26*, 462–467. [CrossRef] [PubMed]
17. Schaffer, L.F.; Peroza, L.R.; Boligon, A.A.; Althayde, M.L.; Alves, S.H.; Faschinetto, R.; Wagner, C. *Harpagophytum procumbens* prevents oxidative stress and loss of cell viability in vitro. *Neurochem. Res.* **2013**, *38*, 2256–2267. [CrossRef] [PubMed]
18. European Pharmacopoeia (Ph. Eur.) 9th Edition. Available online: https://www.edqm.eu/en/european-pharmacopoeia-ph-eur-9th-edition (accessed on 26 February 2019).
19. Li, L.; Tsao, R.; Liu, Z.; Liu, S.; Yang, R.; Young, J.C.; Zhu, H.; Deng, Z.; Xie, M.; Fu, Z. Isolation and purification of acteoside and isoacteoside from *Plantago psyllium* L. by high-speed counter-current chromatography. *J. Chromatogr. A* **2005**, *1063*, 161–169. [CrossRef] [PubMed]
20. Nguyen, A.-T.; Fontaine, J.; Malonne, H.; Clayes, M.; Luhmer, M.; Duez, P. A sugar ester and an iridoid glycoside from *Scrophularia ningpoensis*. *Phytochemistry* **2005**, *66*, 1186–1191. [CrossRef] [PubMed]

21. Clarkson, C.; Staerk, D.; Hansen, S.H.; Smith, P.J.; Jaroszewski, J.W. Identification of major and minor constituents of *Harpagophytum procumbens* (Devil's claw) using HPLC-SPE-NMR and HPLC-ESIMS/APCIMS. *J. Nat. Prod.* **2006**, *69*, 1280–1288. [CrossRef] [PubMed]
22. Wu, Q.; Yuan, Q.; Liu, E.-H.; Qi, L.-W.; Bi, Z.-M.; Li, P. Fragmentation study of iridoid glycosides and phenylpropanoid glycosides in *Radix scrophulariae* by rapid-resolution liquid chromatography with diode-array detection and electrospray ionization time-of-flight mass spectrometry. *Biomed. Chromatogr.* **2010**, *24*, 808–819. [CrossRef] [PubMed]
23. Karioti, A.; Fani, E.; Vincieri, F.F.; Bilia, A.R. Analysis and stability of the constituents of *Curcuma longa* and *Harpagophytum procumbens* tinctures by HPLC-DAD and HPLC-ESI.MS. *J. Pharm. Biomed. Anal.* **2011**, *55*, 479–486. [CrossRef] [PubMed]
24. Qi, J.; Chen, J.-J.; Cheng, Z.-H.; Zhou, J.-H.; Yu, B.-Y.; Qiu, S.X. Iridoid glycosides from *Harpagophytum procumbens* DC. (devil's claw). *Phytochemistry* **2006**, *67*, 1372–1377. [CrossRef] [PubMed]
25. Georgiev, M.I.; Ivanovska, N.; Alipieva, K.; Dimitrova, P.; Veerporte, R. Harpagoside: From Kalahari desert to pharmacy shelf. *Phytochemistry* **2013**, *92*, 8–15. [CrossRef]
26. Kikuchi, T.; Matsuda, S.; Kubo, Y.; Namba, T. New iridoids glucoisdes from *Harpagophytum procumbens* DC. *Chem. Pharm. Bull.* **1983**, *31*, 2296–2301. [CrossRef]
27. Schopohl, P.; Grüneberg, P.; Melzig, M.F. The influence of harpagoside and harpagide on TNFα-secretion and cell adhesion molecule mRNA-expression in IFNγ/LPS-stimulated THP-1 cells. *Fitoterapia* **2016**, *110*, 157–165. [CrossRef] [PubMed]
28. Barnes, J.; Anderson, L.A.; Phillipson, J.D. *Herbal Medicines*, 3rd ed.; Pharmaceutical Press: London, UK, 2007; pp. 207–214.
29. Zhang, L.; Fenbg, L.-F.; Jia, Q.; Xu, J.; Wang, R.; Wang, Z.; Wu, Y.; Li, Y. Effects of ß-glucisidase hydrolyzed products of harpagide and harpagoside on cyclooxygenase-2 (COX-2) in vitro. *Biorg. Med. Chem.* **2011**, *19*, 4882–4886. [CrossRef] [PubMed]
30. Arthur, H.; Joubert, E.; De Beer, D.; Malherbe, C.J.; Witthuhn, R.C. Phenylethanoid glycosides as major antioxidants in *Lippia multiflora* herbal infusion and their stability during steam pasteurization of plant material. *Food Chem.* **2011**, *127*, 581–588. [CrossRef] [PubMed]
31. Jenke, D.R. Chromatographic method validation: A review of current practices and procedures. II. Guidelines for primary validation parameters. *J. Liq. Chromatogr. Relat. Technol.* **1996**, *19*, 737–757. [CrossRef]
32. Vial, J.; Jardy, A. Experimental comparison of the different approaches to estimate LOD and LOQ for an HPLC method. *Anal. Chem.* **1999**, *71*, 2672–2677. [CrossRef]
33. Carbonara, T.; Pascale, R.; Argentieri, M.P.; Papadia, P.; Fanizzi, F.P.; Villanova, L.; Avato, P. Phytochemical analysis of a herbal tea from *Artemisia annua* L. *J. Pharm. Biomed. Anal.* **2012**, *62*, 79–86. [CrossRef] [PubMed]
34. Thaipong, K.; Boonprakob, U.; Crosby, K.; Cisneros-Zevallos, L.; Byrne, D.H. Comparison of ABTS, DPPH, FRAP and ORAC assays for estimating antioxidant activity from guava fruit extracts. *J. Food Compo. Anal.* **2006**, *19*, 669–6775. [CrossRef]
35. Brand-Williams, W.; Cuvelier, M.E.; Berset, C. Use of a free radical method to evaluate antioxidant activity. *Lebensm. Wiss. Technol.* **1995**, *28*, 25–30. [CrossRef]
36. Benzie, I.F.F.; Strain, J.J. The ferric reducing ability of plasma (FRAP) as a measure of "antioxidant power": The FRAP assay. *Anal. Biochem.* **1996**, *239*, 70–76. [CrossRef]

Sample Availability: Samples of the tinctures 019, 014 and NST are available from the authors.

molecules

MDPI

Article

Spectroscopic Characterization and Cytotoxicity Assessment towards Human Colon Cancer Cell Lines of Acylated Cycloartane Glycosides from *Astragalus boeticus* L.

Vittoria Graziani [1], Assunta Esposito [1], Monica Scognamiglio [2,*], Angela Chambery [1], Rosita Russo [1], Fortunato Ciardiello [3], Teresa Troiani [3], Nicoletta Potenza [1], Antonio Fiorentino [1,4,*] and Brigida D'Abrosca [1,4]

1 Dipartimento di Scienze e Tecnologie Ambientali Biologiche e Farmaceutiche (DiSTABiF), Università degli Studi della Campania "Luigi Vanvitelli", via Vivaldi 43, I-81100 Caserta, Italy; vittoria.graziani@unicampania.it (V.G.); assunta.esposito@unicampania.it (A.E.); angela.chambery@unicampania.it (A.C.); rosita.russo@unicampania.it (R.R.); nicoletta.potenza@unicampania.it (N.P.); brigida.dabrosca@unicampania.it (B.D.A.)

2 Department of Biochemistry, Max Planck Institute for Chemical Ecology-Beutenberg Campus, Hans-Knöll-Straße, 8 D-07745 Jena, Germany

3 Dipartimento di Medicina di Precisione, Università degli Studi della Campania "Luigi Vanvitelli" - Via Pansini, 5, 80131 Napoli, Italy; fortunato.ciardiello@unicampania.it (F.C.); teresa.troiani@unicampania.it (T.T.)

4 Dipartimento di Biotecnologia Marina, Stazione Zoologica Anton Dohrn, Villa Comunale, 80121 Naples, Italy

* Correspondence: mscognamiglio@ice.mpg.de (M.S.); antonio.fiorentino@unicampania.it (A.F.); Tel.: +49-(0)-3641-5701609 (M.S.); +39-(0)-823-274576 (A.F.)

Received: 10 April 2019; Accepted: 1 May 2019; Published: 3 May 2019

Abstract: In several European countries, especially in Sweden, the seeds of the species *Astragalus boeticus* L. were widely used as coffee substitutes during the 19th century. Nonetheless, data regarding the phytochemistry and the pharmacological properties of this species are currently extremely limited. Conversely, other species belonging to the *Astragalus* genus have already been extensively investigated, as they were used for millennia for treating various diseases, including cancer. The current work was addressed to characterize cycloartane glycosides from *A. boeticus*, and to evaluate their cytotoxicity towards human colorectal cancer (CRC) cell lines. The isolation of the metabolites was performed by using different chromatographic techniques, while their chemical structures were elucidated by nuclear magnetic resonance (NMR) (1D and 2D techniques) and electrospray-ionization quadrupole time-of-flight (ESI-QTOF) mass spectrometry. The cytotoxic assessment was performed in vitro by 3-(4,5-dimethylthiazol-2-yl)-2,5-diphenyltetrazolium bromide (MTT) assays in Caco-2, HT-29 and HCT-116 CRC cells. As a result, the targeted phytochemical study of *A. boeticus* enabled the isolation of three new cycloartane glycosides, 6-*O*-acetyl-3-*O*-(4-*O*-malonyl)-β-D-xylopyranosylcycloastragenol (**1**), 3-*O*-(4-O-malonyl)-β-D-xylopyranosylcycloastragenol (**2**), 6-*O*-acetyl-25-*O*-β-D-glucopyranosyl-3-*O*-β-D-xylopyranosylcycloastragenol (**3**) along with two known compounds, 6-*O*-acetyl-3-*O*-β-D-xylopyranosylcycloastragenol (**4**) and 3-*O*-β-D-xylopyranosylcycloastragenol (**5**). Importantly, this work demonstrated that the acetylated cycloartane glycosides **1** and **4** might preferentially inhibit cell growth in the CRC cell model resistant to epidermal growth factor receptor (EGFR) inhibitors.

Keywords: *Astragalus boeticus* L.; spectroscopic analysis; cytotoxic activity; human colon cancer cell lines; acetylated astragalosides; Fabaceae

1. Introduction

Astragalus genus is the largest in the Fabaceae family and it is widely distributed throughout the cool, temperate, semiarid and arid regions of the world [1]. *Astragalus boeticus* L. is a Steno-Mediterranean species, which has represented an important cultivation in several countries of Europe, as its seeds have been widely used as coffee substitutes in times of poverty and coffee prohibition. In Sweden, during the 19th century, the monarchy introduced an extensive cultivation of the aforementioned species to produce the so-called Swedish coffee. After the beginning of the 20th century, its cultivation declined, and it was replaced by other substitutes [2]. In addition to this information, available literature data describing the phytochemistry and the bioactivities of *A. boeticus* are currently extremely limited.

On the contrary, a plethora of works regarding other species of the same genus exists. The *Astragalus* species were employed as forage for animals, albeit many species were found to be toxic, and responsible for causing locoism in cattle [3,4]. In both folk and modern medicine, several *Astragalus* spp. were considered medicinal plants of great importance, as these have been successfully used to cure a broad range of ailments [5]. In the Traditional Chinese Medicine "Astragali radix" (dried roots of *Astragalus membranaceus* Bunge and other *Astragalus* spp.) was a very well-known drug for its immune stimulant, hepato-protective, anti-diabetic, analgesic, expectorant and sedative properties [6].

Previous works investigated the chemical profile of *Astragalus* spp. in order to identify the active principles responsible for the bioactivity of the plant's crude extracts. Results from these studies described imidazoline alkaloids, nitro toxins and selenium derivatives as toxic compounds, while polysaccharides, phenols and saponins as biologically active constituents [6]. *Astragalus* saponins include both oleanane and cycloartane-type glycosides, yet the former occur far less in nature, thus the *Astragalus* genus was especially employed as an ideal source to find cycloartane saponins [7].

These compounds were the most extensively studied secondary metabolites from *Astragalus*, as they exhibited a wide range of biological and pharmacological properties. Indeed, these molecules were found to exert immunomodulatory, anti-cancer, anti-fungal, hepato-, kidney-, neuro- and vascular-protective activities [7–12]. So far, the most well-characterized biological effects were those related to their immune stimulant properties, which made these compounds ideal vaccine adjuvant candidates [13]. Alongside the capacity to modulate key immunity pathways, recent evidence supported the effectiveness of *Astragalus* saponins as anti-tumor compounds and/or as adjuvants in combination with orthodox chemotherapeutic agents [14,15].

The anti-cancer activities of these compounds have been evaluated towards a wide range of human malignancies, and a large part of these works evidenced the effectiveness of *Astragalus* saponins against gastric and colorectal cancers [16]. Consistent with this, our group recently demonstrated the anti-proliferative effects of *A. boeticus* in human colorectal cancer (CRC) cells [17].

Colorectal cancer is one of the most frequently-diagnosed malignant diseases in Europe, and one of the leading causes of cancer-related deaths worldwide [18]. Even if the outcome of patients with metastatic colorectal cancer (mCRC) has clearly improved during the last years, the current therapies are still not entirely efficient. Nowadays, resistance to both chemotherapy and molecularly-targeted therapies represents a major problem for setting up effective treatment. The EGFR, which was found overexpressed in 60% to 80% of colorectal cancers, is a transmembrane tyrosine kinase receptor that, once activated, triggers two main signaling pathways. These include the RAS-RAF-MAPK axis, which is mainly involved in cell proliferation, and the PI3KPTEN-AKT pathway, which is especially involved in cell survival and motility [19]. Thus, EGFR inhibitors, such as Cetuximab and Panitumumab, have been developed to block specifically the abnormal activation of those pathways in wild-type KRAS CRC patients [20].

In this study, we aimed at providing a detailed chemical characterization of cycloartane glycosides from *A. boeticus*, and at assessing their anti-proliferative activity towards human colorectal cancer cells endowed with diverse mutation profiles and drug sensitiveness. The ultimate goal of this research is to contribute to the search for new effective agents against refractory CRCs. As a result, we isolated and characterized five cycloartane glycosides (**1–5**), identifying compound **4** as a strong inhibitor of proliferation in CRC cell models resistant to anti-EGFR therapies.

2. Results and Discussion

2.1. Structural Elucidation of Cycloartane Glycosides from *Astragalus boeticus* L.

A crude hydro-alcoholic extract of *A. boeticus* leaves was partitioned between EtOAc and H_2O. The purification process, which was performed by using different chromatographic techniques, enabled the isolation of compounds 1, 2, 4 from the organic phase, while we also obtained 3 and 5 from the aqueous fraction (Figure 1). The structures of these metabolites were elucidated through a combination of NMR spectroscopy (1D and 2D techniques) and ESI-QTOF mass spectrometry.

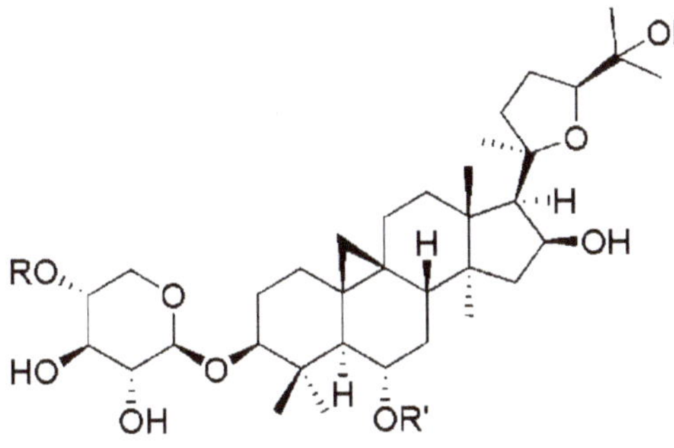

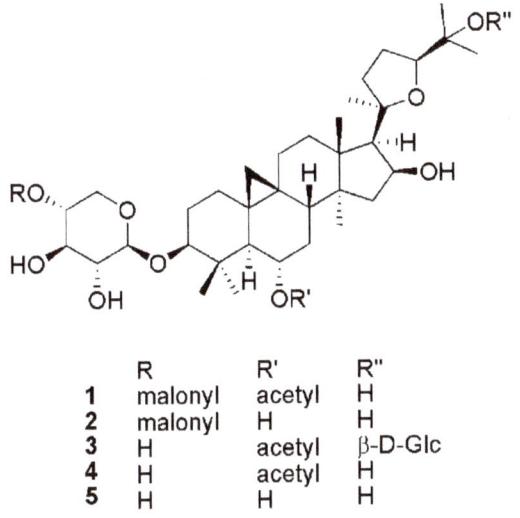

	R	R'	R"
1	malonyl	acetyl	H
2	malonyl	H	H
3	H	acetyl	β-D-Glc
4	H	acetyl	H
5	H	H	H

Figure 1. Structures of compounds **1–5**.

Compound **1** showed a molecular formula $C_{40}H_{62}O_{13}$ on the basis of the NMR data and ESI-QTOF mass spectrum. In fact, the ^{13}C NMR displayed 40 signals, which were identified using the HSQC experiment as eight methyls (—CH_3), eleven methylenes (=CH_2), eleven methines (=CH–), and ten quaternary carbons. The ESI-QTOF spectrum displayed the sodiated adduct of the quasimolecular ion at *m/z* 773.49, and a strong peak at *m/z* 687.46, which indicated the easy loss of an 86 Da fragment. In the ^{1}H NMR spectrum (Table 1), two methylene protons at δ_H 0.40 and δ_H 0.61 (δ_C 30.1), along with six singlet methyls at δ_H 0.98, 1.01, 1.05, 1.13, 1.22, 1.26, and 1.27 allowed compound **1** to be identified as a cycloartane triterpene. The doublet at δ_H 4.32 (δ_C 105.9), as well as other protons that resonated in the range between 3.18 and 4.85 ppm, suggested the presence of a sugar unit. Meanwhile, a methyl singlet at δ_H 1.99 supported the presence of an acetate group in the molecule. The above-mentioned methylene signals (δ_H 0.40 and δ_H 0.61) were assigned to H-19 protons; these, in the CIGAR-HMBC experiment (Figure 2), showed cross peaks with the C-9 (δ_C 21.8), C-10 (δ_C 29.6), C-1 (δ_C 32.8) C-11 (δ_C 26.8), C-5 (δ_C 51.2) and C-8 (δ_C 46.7). In the same experiment, the H-5 proton correlated with the C-1 methylene, the C-4 quaternary carbon at δ_C 42.8, and with two carbinols at δ_C 89.1 and δ_C 72.0. Thanks to the long-range heterocorrelations between the H-6 proton (δ_H 4.75) and the C-4, C-5, and C-8 carbons, it was feasible to assign the first carbinol to the C-3 methine, and then the second to the C-6 carbon. Moreover, the H-6 proton also had cross peaks with the carbonyl at δ_C 171.7, which in turn correlated with the methyl at δ_H 1.99. These data allowed the acetoxy (CH_3-COO-) group to be located at position 6. On the other hand, the H-3 proton correlated with the anomeric carbon at δ_C 105.9, suggesting that the glycosylation site was located on the hydroxyl at the C-3 carbon. Furthermore, the C-4 carbon showed correlations with the methyls at δ_H 0.98 and δ_H 1.05, values that were consequently assigned to the H-29 and H-28 protons, respectively. In addition, the methyls at δ_H 1.27 (δ_C 21.4) and 1.01 (δ_C 20.3) were attributed to the H-18 and H-30 protons, respectively, on the basis of the long range heterocorrelations between the C-18 carbon with the proton at δ_H 2.38 (H-17), which in turn correlated with the H-21 methyl at δH 1.22 (δ_C 28.4).

In the COSY experiment, the H-17 proton had cross peaks with a proton geminal to oxygen at δH 4.65 (H-16), which homocorrelated with the methylene protons at δ_H 1.87 and δ_H 1.45 (H-15), suggesting the presence of another hydroxyl at the C-16 carbon. Consequently, the remaining methyls at δ_H 1.13 and δ_H 1.26 were attributed to the H-26 and H-27 protons, respectively. In the CIGAR-HMBC experiment, these latter protons displayed heterocorrelations with a quaternary carbinol carbon at δ_C 71.2 (C-25), and with a carbinol methine at δ_C 82.6, which was bound to a proton at δ_H 3.76. This latter signal evidenced heterocorrelations with the diasterotopic protons at δ_H 2.02 and δ_H 1.73, while homocorrelations were with the methylene protons at δ_H 2.62 and 1.87 (δ_C 35.5). All these data supported the presence of a tetrahydrofuran moiety formed by an oxygen bridge among the C-20 and C-24 carbons of the side chain. Besides the ester carbonyl of the acetate group, two additional carbonyls at δ_C 170.6 and 171.7 were also evident in the ^{13}C NMR spectrum. In the CIGAR-HMBC experiment, both of them revealed cross peaks with the methylene at δ_H 3.69 (δ_H 51.8), while the carbon at δ_C 170.6 was further correlated with a proton at δ_C 4.72. These data were in agreement with the presence of a malonyl that was bound to the saccharide unit. In the HSQCTOXY experiment, the anomeric carbon at δ_C 105.9 showed cross peaks with the signals at δ_C 75.4, 75.2, 73.6 and δ_C 63.3. These carbons in the HSQC experiment correlated with the methines at δ_H 3.26, 3.57, 4.72 and to the methylene protons at δ_H 3.96 and 3.28, respectively. The H2BC experiment displayed the following correlations: Starting from the anomeric proton at δ_C 4.32 (H-1′)→75.4 (C-2′)→3.57 (H3′)→73.6 (C-4′)→3.96/3.28 (H-5′); starting from the anomeric carbon at δ_C 105.9 (C-1′)→3.26 (H-2′)→75.2 (C-3′)→4.72 (H-4′)→63.3 (C-5′). These data further supported the presence of a pentose that was bound to a malonyl group at the C-4′ carbon.

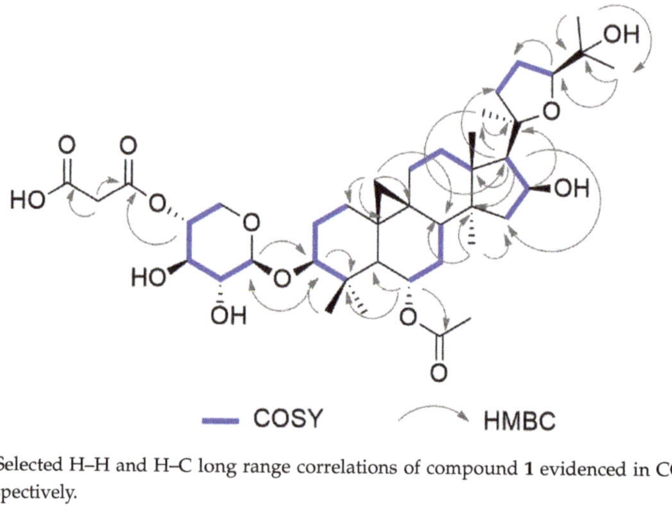

Figure 2. Selected H–H and H–C long range correlations of compound **1** evidenced in COSY and HMBC, respectively.

The stereostructure of the molecule was assigned on the basis of the nOe observed in the NOESY experiment (Figure 3). The sugar was identified as xylose by the GC-MS analysis of the acetylated alditol, which was obtained from the hydrolysis, reduction and acetylation of compound **1**. The coupling constant value of the anomeric proton allowed a β configuration for the anomeric carbon to be determined. The absolute configuration of the sugar was assigned by GC-MS, after a reaction of hydrolyzed saponins with L-cisteine methyl ester and acetylation [21].

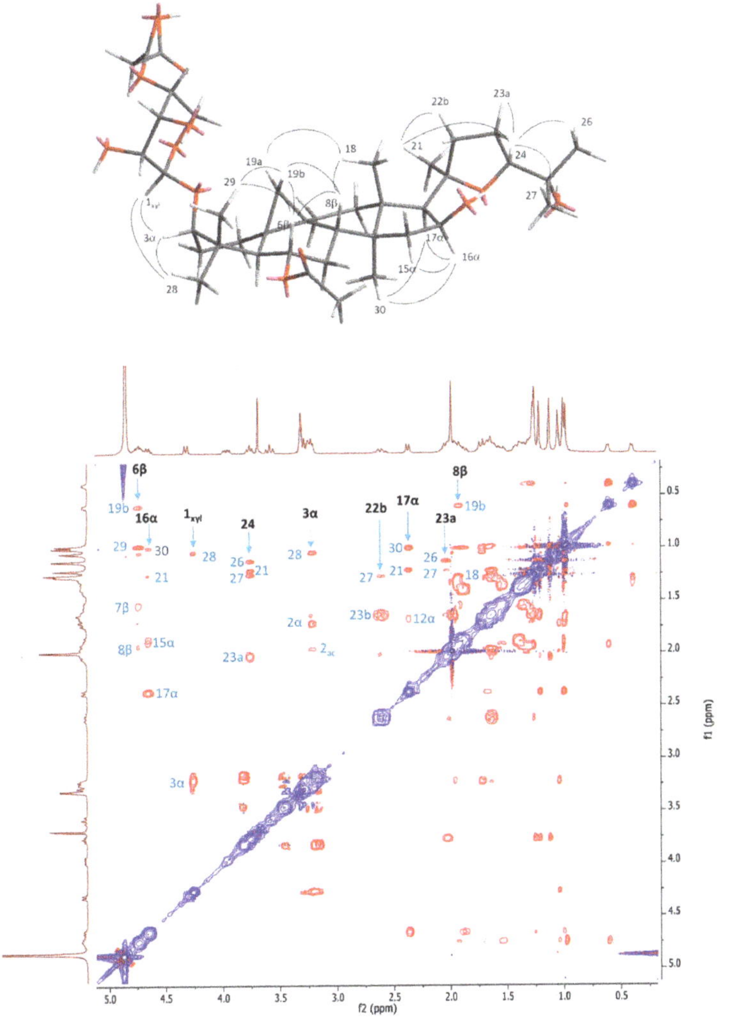

Figure 3. Key nOe correlation of compound **1** (top); NOESY experiment of compound **1** in CD_3OD (bottom).

The nOe evidenced in the NOESY experiments (Figure 3) allowed the configuration at the C-6 and C-16 carbons to be assigned. Based on these data, compound **1** was unequivocally identified as 6-*O*-acetyl-3-*O*-(4-*O*-malonyl)-β-D-xylopyranosylcycloastragenol (Figures S1–S9).

Compound **2** showed the molecular formula $C_{38}H_{60}O_{12}$ on the basis of the NMR data, and the presence of a quasimolecular peak at *m/z* 731.41 in the ESI-QTOF MS spectrum. The loss of an 86 Da fragment was demonstrated by the peak at *m/z* 645.39, indicating the presence of a malonyl moiety also in this molecule.

The ^1H NMR spectrum showed the H-19 protons at δ_H 0.37 and 0.53, and seven singlet methyls at δ_H 0.96 (H-30), 0.98 (H-28), 1.15 (H-26), 1.24 (H-27), 1.26 (H-29 and H-21). The absence of the characteristic signal associated with the methyl group of the acetate moiety demonstrated that compound **2** was the deacetylated form of compound **1**, and all the NMR data confirmed this hypothesis. In addition, the C3-sugar was characterized as xylose, and the malonyl was positioned to the C-4′ carbon of this saccharide moiety. Based on these data, compound **2** was unequivocally identified as 3-*O*-β-D (4-*O*-malonyl)xylopyranosylcycloastragenol.

Compound **3** showed the molecular formula $C_{43}H_{70}O_{15}$, calculated on the basis of its spectro-scopic features. In the ^{1}H-NMR spectrum, the signals of the aglycone, and those belonging to the C3-xylopyranose, were in good agreement with the previous metabolite. However, a further anomeric doublet at δ_C 4.51 suggested the presence of a second sugar. The heterocorrelation between this anomeric signal and the C-25 carbon at δ_H 79.9 allowed the second site of glycosylation to be located at position 25. The HSQCTOCSY experiment revealed the presence of an additional spin system due to this sugar, in which the anomeric proton (δ_C 4.51) correlated with the carbons at δc 99.6, 75.0, 78.2, 71.2, 77.5 and 62.7. These data were in agreement with the presence of a glucopyranose, a hypothesis that was confirmed by GC-MS analysis. Moreover, the coupling constant value indicated a β configuration for the anomeric carbon, while the D-series was established by GC-MS after the reaction of hydrolyzed saponins with L-cisteine methyl ester and acetylation. Based on these data, compound 3 was unequivocally identified as 6-*O*-acetyl-25-*O*-β-D-glucopyranosyl-3-*O*-β-D-xylo-pyranosylcycloastragenol.

Compound **4** showed a molecular formula $C_{37}H_{60}O_{10}$, calculated on the basis of its spectroscopic data. Of interest, this compound was also obtained by the mild acidic hydrolysis of compound **1**. In fact, when this compound was dissolved in water, after one day at room temperature, it was quantitatively converted in **4** by loss of the C4′-malonyl. All the NMR data confirmed this hypothesis, and allowed the identification of compound **4** as 6-*O*-acetyl-3-*O*-β-D-xylopyranosylcycloastragenol [22].

Compound **5** showed a molecular formula $C_{35}H_{58}O_9$, calculated on the basis of its spectroscopic data. The ^{1}H-NMR and ^{13}C-NMR signals of the aglycone and those belonging to the C3-xylopyranose were superimposable with the previous metabolites. Conversely, the lack of the singlet peak at δ_H 1.99 proved the absence of the C6-acetyl. All of these data enabled the identification of compound **5** as 3-*O*-β-D-xylopyranosylcycloastragenol [23].

2.2. *Cytotoxicity of Cycloartane Glycosides from Astragalus boeticus Against Human Colorectal Cancer Cells*

The cytotoxic activity of the isolated compounds (**1–5**) was assessed on three human colorectal cancer cell lines (Caco-2, HT-29 and HCT-116), using MTT (3-[4,5-dimethylthiazol-2-yl]-2,5-diphenyltetrazolium bromide) tetrazolium salt colorimetric assay (Figure 4). Results from these experiments demonstrated that cell proliferation was reduced by the treatment with compounds **1** and **4** in a dose-dependent manner, while **2**, **3** and **5** did not exert any significant effect. To our knowledge, no mechanistic studies regarding the proliferation reducing-effect of compounds **1** and **4** are available in literature. Yet, several previous works shed the light on the anticancer activity of other cycloartane glycosides (most of them isolated from *A. membranaceus*), which act by inducing apoptosis and modulating crucial cellular signaling pathways [24–27]. Importantly, a recent investigation pointed out that certain semisynthetic cycloastragenol derivatives impair inflammation-carcinogenesis by regulating the NF-KB signaling pathway [15].

Consistently, compound **4**, which has already been purified from the leaf extract of *A. membranaceus*, was described as a potentially anti-inflammatory molecule, because it was found to exert an inhibitory activity on the nitric oxide production in macrophages [21]. Recently, our group identified compound **4** as a metabolite responsible for the cytotoxicity of the *A. boeticus* extract. Here, this species underwent a further phytochemical investigation to understand whether analogues of compound **4** exert cytotoxicity as well. As it was already anticipated above, we demonstrated that compounds **1** and **4** were the active cycloartane glycosides isolated from *A. boeticus*.

In an attempt to further validate our findings, we compared the cytotoxicity of **4** (active compound) and **3** (inactive compound) with astragaloside IV (AS-IV), a commercially-available cycloartane glycoside extensively recognized as one of the main active components of several *Astragalus* spp.

Results from these experiments confirmed the notable cytotoxicity of compound **4**, while no effect was found for AS-IV, at least in our experimental conditions (Figure S10).

From a structural point of view, these insights proved that the C3-xylopyranosyl, along with the C6-acetoxy group and the C25-free hydroxyl function, were essential structural requirements for the cytotoxic activity of these triterpenoids. As already discussed, when compound **1** was in water solutions, such as a cellular environment, it converted into compound **4** by losing the C4′ malonyl. Thereby, it was demonstrated that compound **4** was the real bioactive structure. Compounds **2**, **3**, **5** and AS-IV present the C3-xylopyranosyl, while none of them has either the C6-acetoxy group or the C25-free hydroxyl function. In accordance with previous investigations, acylation of the C-3 and C-6 secondary alcohols of diverse cycloartane derivatives resulted in a higher cytotoxic activity. This evidence led researchers to hypotheses that acylated cycloartane glycosides could lose the acyl substituents to modify proteins that play a key role in cellular signaling, whose deregulation is involved in carcinogenesis. Specifically, the acyl groups can be covalently attached to the amino acid side chains regulating the protein functions and impairing cancer progression [15].

In our study, a detailed analysis of the cytotoxic effect unveiled a differential response of Caco-2, HT-29 and HCT-116 to the treatment with compound **4**. These insights could be interpreted by describing the human colon cancer cells employed in our experimental setting. Caco-2 cell line was the wild type for the KRAS, NRAS, BRAF, PIK3CA genes; thus representing an ideal cellular model to study metastatic CRCs sensitive to anti-EGFR agents. By contrast, HT-29 and HCT-116 harbored a BRAF and some KRAS/PIK3CA mutations, respectively—therefore identifying metastatic CRCs with intrinsic resistance to the anti-EGFR treatments [28,29].

Herein, the in vitro cytotoxic screening revealed as compound **4** was clearly more effective in treating HT-29 (3 μM) than HCT-116 (40 μM) and Caco-2 (50 μM) cell lines (Figure 4).

In clinics, the BRAF mutation status is a strong indicator of a very poor prognosis for mCRC patients; indeed, they showed a worse outcome for the therapies compared with those whose tumors were wild type [30–32]. Of interest, the inhibition of BRAF oncoprotein by the small-molecule drug PLX4032 (Vemurafenib) is highly effective in the treatment of melanoma [33], whilst metastatic CRC patients associated with the same mutation showed a very limited response to this drug [34]. In fact, Vemurafenib treatment induces EGFR feedback activation, causing continued proliferation in the presence of BRAF (V600E) inhibition. Unlike CRCs, melanomas express low levels of EGFR, and thus, they are not subject to this kind of feedback activation [35].

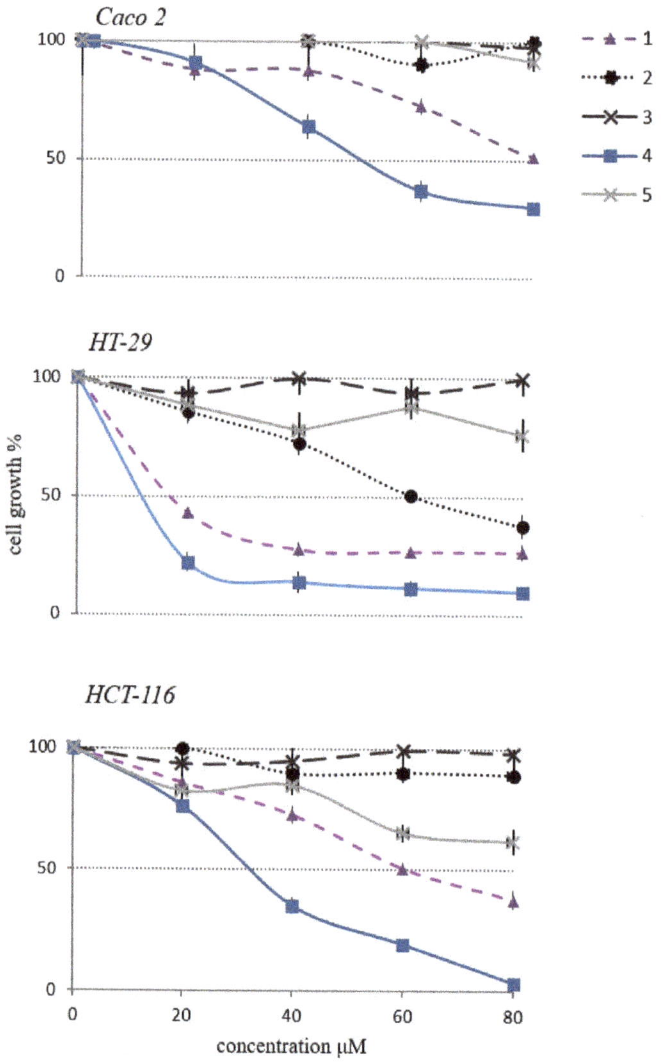

Figure 4. Cytotoxic activity of compounds **1–5** towards Caco-2, HT-29 and HCT-116 human colon cancer cell lines.

3. Materials and Methods

3.1. General Experimental Procedures

Analytical TLC was performed on Merck Kieselgel (Darmstadt, Germany) 60 F254 or RP-8 F254 plates with a 0.2 mm film thickness. Spots were visualized by UV light, or by spraying with H_2SO_4/AcOH/H_2O (1:20:4), and then heating at 120 °C for 5 min. Preparative TLC was performed on Merck Kieselgel 60 F254 plates with a 0.5 or 1.0 mm film thickness.

Column chromatography (CC) was performed on Fluka (Seelze, Germany) Amberlite XAD-4 and XAD-7, on Pharmacia (Stockholm, Sweden) Sephadex LH-20, on Merck Kieselgel 60 (70–240 mesh), or on Baker (Deventer, Netherlands) RP-8. Nuclear magnetic resonance (NMR) spectra were recorded at 300 (^1H) and 75 MHz (^{13}C) on a Varian Mercury 300 FT-NMR spectrometer in CD_3OD

or pyridine-d_5 solutions at 25 °C. Chemical shifts are reported in δ (ppm), and referenced to the residual solvent signal; J (coupling constant) are given in Hz. Standard pulse sequences and phase cycling from Varian library were used for ^{1}H, ^{13}C, DEPT, DQF-COSY, COSY, TOCSY, NOESY, HSQC, H2BC, HMBC and CIGAR–HMBC experiments. ^{1}H NMR spectra were acquired over a spectral window from 14 to −2 ppm, with 1.0 s relaxation delay, 1.70 s acquisition time (AQ), and 90° pulse width = 13.8 μs. The initial matrix was zero-filled to 64 K. ^{13}C NMR spectra were recorded in ^{1}H broadband decoupling mode, over a spectral window from 235 to −15 ppm, 1.5 s relaxation delay, 90° pulse width = 9.50 μs, and AQ = 0.9 s. The number of scans for both ^{1}H and ^{13}C NMR experiments were chosen, depending on the concentration of the samples. With regards to the homonuclear and heteronuclear 2D-NMR experiments, the data points, number of scans and increments were adjusted according to the sample concentrations. Correlation spectroscopy (COSY) and double quantum filtered COSY (DQF-COSY) spectra were recorded with gradient-enhanced sequence at spectral widths of 3000 Hz in both f2 and f1 domains; the relaxation delays were of 1.0 s. The total correlation spectroscopy (TOCSY) experiments were performed in the phase-sensitive mode with a mixing time of 90 ms. The spectral width was 3000 Hz. Nuclear Overhauser effect spectroscopy (NOESY) experiments were performed in the phase-sensitive mode. The mixing time was 500 ms, and the spectral width was 3000 Hz. For all the homonuclear experiments, the initial matrix of 512 × 512 data points was zero-filled to give a final matrix of 1 k × 1 k points. Proton-detected heteronuclear correlations were also measured. Heteronuclear single-quantum coherence (HSQC) experiments (optimized for $1J$(H,C) = 140 Hz) were performed in the phase sensitive mode with field gradient. The spectral width was 12,000 Hz in f1 (^{13}C) and 3000 Hz in f2 (1H) and 1.0 s of relaxation delay; the matrix of 1 k × 1 k data points was zero-filled to give a final matrix of 2 k × 2 k points. Heteronuclear 2 bond correlation (H2BC) spectra were obtained with T = 30.0 ms, and a relaxation delay of 1.0 s; the third order low-pass filter was set for 130 < $1J$(C,H) < 165 Hz. A heteronuclear multiple bond coherence (HMBC) experiment (optimized for $1J$(H,C) = 8 Hz) was performed in the absolute value mode with field gradient; typically, ^{1}H–^{13}C gHMBC were acquired with spectral width of 18,000 Hz in f1 (^{13}C) and 3000 Hz in f2 (1H) and 1.0 s of relaxation delay; the matrix of 1 k × 1 k data points was zero-filled to give a final matrix of 4 k × 4 k points. Constant time inverse-detected gradient accordion rescaled heteronuclear multiple bond correlation spectroscopy (CIGAR–HMBC) spectra (8 > nJ(H,C) > 5) were acquired with the same spectral width used for HMBC. Heteronuclear single quantum coherence-total correlation spectroscopy (HSQC-TOCSY) experiments were optimized for nJ(H,C) = 8 Hz, with a mixing time of 90 ms. For accurate mass measurements, the purified compounds were analyzed by an electrospray hybrid quadrupole orthogonal acceleration time-of-flight mass spectrometer (Q-TOF), fitted with a Z-spray electrospray ion source (Waters S.p.A.). All analyses were carried out in positive ion mode. The capillary source voltage and the cone voltage were set at 3500 V and 35 V, respectively. The source temperature was kept at 80 °C, and nitrogen was used as a drying gas (flow rate about 50 l/h). The time-of-flight analyzer of the mass spectrometer was externally calibrated, with GFP from *m*/*z* 50–1600. Accurate mass data were collected by directly infusing samples (1.5 pmol/μL in CH_3CN/H_2O, 1:1) into the system at a flow rate of 15 μL/min. The acquisition and processing of data were performed with the MassLynx 4.1 software (Waters S.p.A., Manchester, UK). GC-MS analyses were carried out using an HP 6890 GC instrument (Zebron ZB-5MS column, He flow 1.0 mL/min), coupled with a 5973 N mass spectrometer, equipped with an electron ionization source (EIMS), and operating with an electron energy of 70 eV. Full-scan mass spectra were collected between 0 and 600 amu at 2 scan/s. The MS was operated in the electron impact (EI) ionization mode, with an electron energy of 70 eV. The ion source and quadrupole temperatures were maintained at 230 and 150 °C, respectively. For the analyses of the acetylated alditols, the column head pressure was set at 7.41 p.s.i.

AS-IV was purchased from Shanghai Tauto Biotech Co., LTD. (Shanghai, China).

3.2. GC–MS Analysis of the Sugar Moieties

The GC-MS analysis of the sugar moieties has been previously described by Scognamiglio et al. [31]. Briefly, each metabolite (0.5 mg) was subjected to an acid hydrolysis with 2 N TFA (150 μL) at 120 °C for 1 h, obtaining the sugar moiety. This was dried under N2 flow, and reduced by adding MeOH (150 μL) and $NaBH_4$ (1.0 mg). The solution was incubated at room temperature for 1 h and then dried under N_2 flow after treatment with glacial AcOH and MeOH. The obtained alditol was acetylated by using anhydrous pyridine (200 μL) and Ac_2O (200 μL). This mixture was incubated for 20 min at 120 °C. Then, 500 μL of H_2O was added, and the product was extracted with CH_2Cl_2 (500 μL) following centrifugation at 3500 rpm for 5 min. The organic phase was dried under N_2 flow, dissolved in CH_2Cl_2 (500 μL) and analyzed by GC-MS. Temperature conditions were as follows: Injector port at 250 °C; the initial oven temperature was 160 °C for 50 s, then linearly increased to 200 °C at 10 °C/min. A further linear increase at 2.5 C/min was performed to 300 °C, and held for 40 min. Sample solutions were injected using the split mode.

3.3. Determination of Absolute Configuration of Monosaccharides of Compound **1** and **5**

Compound **1** and **5** (2 mg each) were hydrolyzed with 2 N TFA (250 μL) at 120 °C for 1 h. The reaction mixture was then dried under N_2 flow and dissolved in dry pyridine (100 μL). 100 μL of pyridine solution of L-cysteine methyl ester hydrochloride (0.06 mol/L) were added to pyridine solutions of the hydrolyzed compounds **1** and **5** and pure D-xylose, and L-xylose (0.04 mol/L). These mixtures were warmed at 60 °C for 1 h, afterwards, acetic anhydride (150 μL) was added at 120 °C for 20 min. The products were dried under N_2, dissolved in 500 μL of H_2O, and extracted with CH_2Cl_2 (500 μL) following centrifugation at 3500 rpm for 5 min. The organic phase was dried under N_2 flow, dissolved in CH_2Cl_2 (500 μL), and analyzed by GC-MS. Temperature conditions were as follows: Injector port at 250 °C; initial oven temperature 45 °C, then increased linearly to 300 °C at 20 °C/min, and then held for 25 min. Sample solutions were injected using the split mode. The retention times were: D-xylose 13.89 min, L-xylose 14.17 min.

3.4. Plant Material

Leaf samples of *A. boeticus* were collected at vegetative state, in April 2014 in "Castel Volturno Nature Reserve" (40°57.587′N, 14°00.105′E; southern Italy). Samples were harvested, frozen in liquid nitrogen and lyophilized. A Voucher specimen CE000016 has been deposited at the Herbarium of the Dipartimento di Scienze e Tecnologie Ambientali Biologiche e Farmaceutiche of Università degli Studi della Campania "Luigi Vanvitelli".

3.5. Extraction and Isolation of Compound **1–5**

Dried leaves (24.0 g) of *A. boeticus* were powdered, and underwent three cycles of an ultrasound-assisted extraction with an $MeOH/H_2O$ (1:1) solution (720 mL) [36], finally obtaining a crude extract (7.1 g). This was dissolved in H_2O and separated by liquid–liquid extraction, by using EtOAc as our extracting solvent. As a result, an organic and a water fraction were obtained. The former (1g) was chromatographed by SiO_2 CC, and eluted using a solution with an increasing degree of polarity ($CHCl_3$, $Me_2CO/CHCl_3$, $MeOH/CHCl_3$). Thus, 21 fractions have been collected. Of these, number 13 was chromatographed by C18 CC, and eluted with H_2O/MeOH (3:2) to give compound **1** (18.6 mg) and 2 (7.1 mg). Meanwhile, number 12 was purified by Flash-CC eluting with MeOH/ $CHCl_3$ (3:100) to obtain compound 4 (28 mg). On the other hand, the water fraction was chromatographed by XAD-4 (20–50 mesh; Fluka) and XAD-7 (20–50 mesh; Fluka) CC, obtaining an alcoholic eluate (900 mg) that was in turn purified by Sephadex LH-20. Subsequently, 17 fractions were given. Of these, fraction 13 was purified through RP-18 CC by using H_2O/MeOH (4:1) as the eluting system, consequently obtaining 30 fractions. One of these was chromatographed by TLC (0,5 mm), and eluted with the organic phase of $CHCl_3/MeOH/H_2O$ (13:7:2) to obtain compound **3** (11.8 mg). Finally, fraction 11 was chromatographed by TLC (0.5 mm) and eluted with the organic phase of $CHCl_3$/MeOH/H_2O (13:7:2) to give compound **5** (4.6 mg).

Compound **1**: 6-*O*-acetyl-3-*O*-(4-*O*-malonyl)-β-D-xylopyranosylcycloastragenol. $[\alpha]_D^{25}$ = +22.8 (c = 14.97 × 10^{-3}, MeOH). ^{1}H NMR (CD_3OD) and ^{13}C NMR (CD_3OD) see Table 1; ESI/Q-TOF: *m/z* 773.49 $[M + Na]^+$ (calcd.773.41 Da for $C_{40}H_{62}O_{13}Na$);

Compound **2**: 3-*O*-(4-*O*-malonyl)-β-D- xylopyranosylcycloastragenol. $[\alpha]_D^{25}$ = +9.70 (c = 2.06 × 10^{-3}, MeOH). ^{1}H NMR (CD_3OD) and ^{13}C NMR (CD_3OD) see Table 1; ESI/Q-TOF: *m/z* 731.41 [M+Na]+ (calcd. 731.40 Da for $C_{38}H_{60}O_{12}Na$);

Compound **3**: 6-*O*-acetyl-25-*O*-β-D-glucopyranosyl-3-*O*-β-D-xylopyranosylcycloastragenol. $[\alpha]_D^{25}$ = +13.7 (c= 6.06 × 10^{-3}, MeOH). ^{1}H NMR (CD_3OD) and ^{13}C NMR (CD_3OD) see Table 1; ESI/Q-TOF: *m/z* 849.46 $[M + Na]^+$ (calcd.849.43 Da for $C_{43}H_{70}O_{15}Na$);

Compound **4**: 6-acetyl-3-*O*-(4-*O*-malonyl)-β-D-xylopyranosylcycloastragenol. $[\alpha]_D^{25}$ = +7.65 (c = 5.1 × 10^{-3}, MeOH/H_2O, 2:1) [22];

Compound **5**: 3-*O*-β-D-xylopyranosylcycloastragenol. $[\alpha]_D^{25}$ = −340.1 (c = 3.74 × 10^{-3}) MeOH/H_2O, 1:1) [23].

Table 1. 1D and 2D nuclear magnetic resonance (NMR) data of compound **1–3** in CD_3OD.

	1				**2**				**3**			
Position	δ_C	**Type**	δ_H (*J* in Hz)	**HMBC**[a]	δ_C	**Type**	δ_H (*J* in Hz)	**HMBC**[a]	δ_C	**Type**	δ_H (*J* in Hz)	**HMBC**[a]
1	32.8	CH_2	1.85 *s* 1.67 *s*	2, 10 2, 10	32.3	CH_2	1.84 *s* 1.65 *s*	2, 10 2, 10	32.8	CH_2	1.29 s	
2	30.3	CH_2	1.98 *ov* 1.64 *ov*	3, 4 3, 4	30.0	CH_2	1.88 *ov* 1.69 *ov*	3, 4 3, 4	30.2	CH_2	1.99 ov	3, 4
3	89.1	CH	3.21 *d* (*J* = 1.8)	28, 29, 1_{xyl}	89.1	CH	3.29 *ov*	28, 29, 1_{xyl}	89.1	CH	3.21 *ov*	1_{xyl}
4	42.8	C			42.0	C			42.8	C		
5	51.2	CH	1.71 *s*	1, 4, 7, 10, 28, 29	53.9	CH	1.38 *s*	1, 4, 7, 10, 28, 29	51.3	CH	1.72 *s*	1, 4, 7, 10, 28, 29
6	72.0	CH	4.75 *ov*	4, 5, 7, 8, 1_{Ac}	68.5	CH	3.48 *ov*	4, 5, 7, 8	72.1	CH	4.75 *ov*	4, 5, 1_{ac}
7	34.0	CH_2	1.56 *ov*	5, 6	33.4	CH_2	1.46 *ov*	5, 6	34.1	CH_2	1.57	5, 6, 8, 9, 14
8	46.7	CH	1.95 *s*	6, 9, 10, 13, 14, 19, 30	48.0	CH	1.46 *s*	6, 9, 10, 13, 14, 19, 30	46.1	CH	1.94 *s*	6, 10, 13, 14, 15, 19
9	21.8	C			21.4	C			21.6	C		
10	29.6	C			29.2	C			29.2	C		
11	26.8	CH_2	1.97 *m*	8, 12, 19	26.4	CH_2	1.97 s	8, 12, 19	26.4	CH_2	1.97 *s*	12
12	34.1	CH_2	1.64 *ov* 1.56 *ov*	14, 18 14, 18	33.4	CH_2	1.54 *ov* 1.37 *ov*	14, 18 14, 18	34.1	CH_2	1.64 *ov* 1.56 *ov*	
13	47.0	C			44.7	C			46.9	C		
14	46.4	C			47.0	C			46.6	C		
15	46.2	CH_2	1.87 *d* (*J* = 8.0) 1.39 *d* (*J* = 8.0)	8, 13, 17, 30 8, 13, 17, 30	46.4	CH_2	1.98 *d* (*J* = 4.4) 1.32 *d* (*J* = 6.8)	8, 13, 17, 30 8, 13, 17, 30	46.0	CH_2	1.86 *d* (*J* = 6.0) 1.42 *d* (*J* = 6.4)	8, 13, 14, 17, 30 13, 14, 30
16	74.5	CH	4.65 *m*	13, 14, 15	73.9	CH	4.64 *m*	13, 14, 15	74.3	CH	4.65 *m*	13, 14, 15
17	58.9	CH	2.37 *d* (*J* = 7.8)	13, 14, 16, 20, 21, 22	58.2	CH	2.37 *d* (*J* = 7.7)	13, 14, 16, 20, 21, 22	58.7	CH	2.38 *d* (J=8.0)	13, 14, 16, 20, 21, 22
18	21.4	CH_3	1.27 *s*	12, 15, 17	21.4	CH_3	1.23 s	12, 15, 17	21.7	CH_3	1.27 s	12, 15, 17
19	30.1	CH_2	0.61 *s* 0.40 *s*	1, 5, 8, 9, 10 1, 5, 8, 9, 10, 11	31.4	CH_2	0.53 *s* 0.37 *s*	1, 5, 8, 9, 10 1, 5, 8, 9, 10, 11	30.2	CH_2	0.61 *s* 0.40 *s*	1, 5, 8, 9, 10,11 1, 5, 8, 9, 10, 11
20	88.3	C	-		88.2	C	-		88.3	C	-	
21	28.4	CH_3	1.22 *s*	17, 20, 22	28.1	CH_3	1.25 s	17, 20, 22	28.0	CH_3	1.24 s	
22	35.5	CH_2	2.62 *ov* 1.87 ov	17, 20, 21 17, 20, 21	34.9	CH_2	1.69 *ov*	17, 20, 21 17, 20, 21	35.6	CH_2	2.54 *ov* 1.84	17 17
23	26.8	CH_2	2.02 *ov* 1.73	20, 24, 25 17, 24, 25	26.4	CH_2	2.02 *ov*	20, 24, 25 17, 24, 25	26.8	CH_2	2.16 *ov* 1.72	24, 25 24, 25
24	82.6	CH	3.76 *m*	25	81.4	CH	3.80 *m*	25	83.0	CH	3.82 *m*	1_{glc}

Table 1. *Cont.*

	1				2				3			
Position	δ_C	Type	δ_H (J in Hz)	HMBC[a]	δ_C,	Type	δ_H (J in Hz)	HMBC[a]	δ_C,	Type	δ_H (J in Hz)	HMBC[a]
25	71.2	C	-		71.2	C	-		79.9	C	-	
26	26.6	CH_3	1.13 *s*	17, 24, 25	26.5	CH_3	1.15 *s*	17, 24, 25	23.2	CH_3	1.22 *s*	20, 23, 24, 25
27	27.6	CH_3	1.26 *s*	24, 25, 26	27.1	CH_3	1.24 *s*	24, 25, 26	25.3	CH_3	1.38 *s*	23, 24, 26
28	27.2	CH_3	1.05 *s*	3, 4, 5, 29	16.1	CH_3	0.98 *s*	3, 4, 5, 29	16.5	CH_3	0.98 *s*	3, 4, 5, 28
29	16.6	CH_3	0.98 *s*	3, 4, 5, 28	27.1	CH_3	1.25 *s*	3, 4, 5, 28	27.3	CH_3	1.04 *s*	3, 4, 5, 29
30	20.3	CH_3	1.01 *s*	9, 14, 15	20.9	CH_3	0.96 *s*	9, 14, 15	20.2	CH_3	0.99 *s*	14, 15
1_{xyl}	105.9	CH	4.32 *d* (J = 7.4)	3, 5_{xyl}	105.9	CH	4.43 *d* (J = 7.4)	3, 5_{xyl}	107.4	CH	4.26 *d* (J = 7.0)	3
2_{xyl}	75.4	CH	3.26 *ov*	4_{xyl}	75.4	CH	3.26 *ov*	4_{xyl}	75.5	CH	3.19 *ov*	
3_{xyl}	75.2	CH	3.57 *ov*	4_{xyl}, 5_{xyl}	75.2	CH	3.57 *ov*	4_{xyl}, 5_{xyl}	78.0	CH	3.29 *ov*	
4_{xyl}	73.6	CH	4.72 *m*	2_{xyl}, 3_{xyl}, 5_{xyl}, 2_{mal}	73.6	CH	4.72 *m*	2_{xyl}, 3_{xyl}, 5_{xyl}, 2_{mal}	71.2	CH	3.46 *m*	
5_{xyl}	63.3	CH_2	3.28 *ov* 3.96 *ov*	1_{xyl}, 3_{xyl}, 4_{xyl} 1_{xyl}, 3_{xyl}, 4_{xyl}	63.3	CH_2	3.28 *ov* 3.96 *ov*	1_{xyl}, 3_{xyl}, 4_{xyl} 1_{xyl}, 3_{xyl}, 4_{xyl}	66.7	CH_2	3.18 *ov* 3.82 *ov*	
1_{glc}	-	-	-		-		-		99.6	CH	4.51 *d* (J = 6.6)	25
2_{glc}	-	-	-		-		-		75.0	CH	3.18 *ov*	5_{glc}
3_{glc}	-	-	-		-		-		78.2	CH	3.32 *ov*	1_{glc}, 5_{glc}
4_{glc}	-	-	-		-		-		71.2	CH	3.31 *ov*	6_{glc}
5_{glc}	-	-	-		-		-		77.5	CH	3.24 *ov*	1_{glc}, 3_{glc}
6_{glc}	-	-	-		-		-		62.7	CH_2	3.65 *ov* 3.79 *ov*	4_{glc} 4_{glc}
1_{ac}	172.2	C	-		-		-		172.2	C		
2_{ac}	22.2	CH_3	1.99 *s*	1_{ac}	-		-		21.8	CH_3	1.99 *s*	1_{ac}
1_{mal}	170.6	C	-		170.6	C	-		-		-	
2_{mal}	51.8	CH_2	3.69 *s*	1_{mal}, 3_{mal}	51.8	CH_2	3.69 *s*	1_{mal}, 3_{mal}	-		-	
3_{mal}	171.7	C	-		171.7	C	-		-		-	

[a] HMBC correlations, optimized for 6 Hz, are from proton(s) stated to the indicated carbon; [b] obscured; *d* = doublet, *m* = multiplet, *ov* = overlapped, *s* = singlet, *t* = triplet.

3.6. Cell Lines

The human HCT-116, HT-29, Caco-2 colorectal cancer cell lines were obtained from the American Type Culture Collection (ATCC) (Manassas, VA). HCT-116, HT-29 cancer cells were cultured in RPMI 1640 medium (Lonza, Cologne, Germany) supplemented with 10% fetal bovine serum, 2 mM L-glutamine, 50 U/mL penicillin and 100 μg/mL streptomycin (Lonza, Cologne, Germany). The Caco-2 cell line was cultured in DMEM medium (Lonza, Cologne, Germany), supplemented with 10% fetal bovine serum, 2 mM L-glutamine, 1% non-essential amino acid, 50 U/mL penicillin and 100 μg/mL streptomycin (Lonza, Cologne, Germany).

3.7. Proliferation Assay

The cell proliferation assay was performed with a 3-(4,5-dimethylthiazol-2-yl)-2,5-diphenyl-tetrazolium bromide (MTT) assay. Briefly, cells in logarithmic growth phase were plated in 96-well plates and incubated for 24 h before exposure to increasing doses of DMSO-diluted compounds (20, 40, 60, and 80 μM). For compounds **1** and **4** that exerted a strong cytotoxic effect in the HT-29 cell line, a lower range of doses (2, 4, 6, and 10 μM) was also investigated. 48 h after treatment, 50 μL of 1 mg/mL (MTT) were mixed with 200 μL of medium and added to the well. 1 h after incubation at 37 °C, the medium was removed, and the purple formazan crystals produced in the viable cells were solubilized in 100 μL of dimethyl sulfoxide, and quantitated by measurement of absorbance at 570 nm with a plate reader. Results were reported as mean ± s.d. of % of cell growth, with respect to the control from six replicate analyses. The control was represented by a 0.08% DMSO treatment, which corresponded to the higher amount of DMSO used for the tests.

4. Conclusions

A plethora of previous investigation regarding the phytochemistry and the bioactive components of diverse species belonging to the *Astragalus* genus are available in literature. However, to our knowledge, there are no data regarding the phytochemical constituents of *A. boeticus*. In this study, we focused on the cycloartane derivatives present in *A. boeticus*, because of its putative cytotoxic activity.

Specifically, the targeted phytochemical study of *A. boeticus* led to the isolation of five cycloartane-type glycosides (**1–5**); of these, **1**, **2** and **3** were isolated and characterized for the first time. The cytotoxic activity of compounds **1–5** was evaluated in vitro, disclosing a strong proliferation-reducing effect of compound **4** in the HT-29 human colon cancer cell line, which was employed as a preclinical model to study refractory mCRCs that are resistant to anti-EGFR therapies, as well as other chemotherapeutic drugs currently used in the clinical setting. Our results therefore provide a small molecule scaffold that might be potentially important for the development of new agents effective against refractory mCRCs.

Indeed, these insights pave the way to further investigations aimed to figure out whether compound **4** acts on CRC cell models resistant to EGFR inhibitors with high selectivity, and if so, to elucidate the mechanism by which the anti-proliferative activity occurs.

On the other hand, as several limitations are intrinsically associated with our in vitro experimental system, future experiments shall also be addressed to evaluate the pharmacokinetic properties, and the bioavailability of the active molecule in animal models.

Supplementary Materials: The following are available online at http://www.mdpi.com/1420-3049/24/9/1725/s1, Figure S1: ^{1}H NMR spectrum of compound **1**. Figure S2: ^{13}C NMR spectrum of compound **1**. Figure S3: COSY spectrum of compound **1**. Figure S4: HSQC spectrum of compound **1**. Figure S5: CIGAR-HMBC spectrum of compound **1**. Figure S6: H2BC spectrum of compound **1**. Figure S7: HSQCTOCSY spectrum of compound **1**. Figure S8: ESI QTOF spectrum of compound **1**. Figure S9: ESI TOF MS/MS spectrum of compound **1**. Figure S10: cytotoxicity of AS-IV in comparison with compound **3** and **4**.

Author Contributions: V.G. and M.S. designed the experiments, discussed and interpreted the results. A.E. selected and identified the plant species. V.G. and M.S. carried out the experiments. A.C. and R.R. carried out the M.S. analyses. V.G. and M.S. wrote the manuscript. A.E., B.D.A. and F.C. analyzed the experimental data. A.E.,

B.D.A. interpreted the results. T.T., N.P., A.F. designed the experiments, discussed and interpreted the results and reviewed the manuscript. All authors revised the manuscript.

Funding: This work was funded by Regione Campania, "Technology Platform per la Lotta alle Patologie Oncologiche" Grant: iCURE (CUP B21C17000030007–SURF17061BP000000008).

Conflicts of Interest: The authors declare no conflict of interest.

References

1. Verotta, L.; El-Sebakhy, N. *Cycloartane and oleanane saponins from Astragalus sp. Studies in Natural Products Chemistry*; Elsevier: Amsterdam, The Netherlands, 2001; pp. 179–234.
2. Prohens, J.; Andújar, I.; Vilanova, S.; Plazas, M.; Gramazio, P.; Prohens, R.; Herraiz, F.J.; De Ron, A.M. Swedish coffee (Astragalus boeticus L.), a neglected coffee substitute with a past and a potential future. *Genet. Resour. Crop Evol.* **2013**, *61*, 287–297. [CrossRef]
3. Williams, M.C.; Davis, A.M. Nitro Compounds in Introduced Astragalus Species. *J. Range Manage.* **1982**, *35*. [CrossRef]
4. Cook, D.; Ralphs, M.H.; Welch, K.D.; Stegelmeier, B.L. Locoweed Poisoning in Livestock. *Rangelands* **2009**, *31*, 16–21. [CrossRef]
5. Ionkova, I.; Shkondrov, A.; Krasteva, I.; Ionkov, T. Recent progress in phytochemistry, pharmacology and biotechnology of Astragalus saponins. *Phytochem. Rev.* **2014**, *13*, 343–374. [CrossRef]
6. Rios, J.L.; Waterman, P.G. A review of the pharmacology and toxicology of Astragalus. *Phytother. Res.* **1997**, *11*, 411–418. [CrossRef]
7. Gülcemal, D.; Aslanipour, B.; Bedir, E. Secondary Metabolites from Turkish Astragalus Species. In *Plant and Human Health, Volume 2: Phytochemistry and Molecular Aspects*; Ozturk, M., Hakeem, K.R., Eds.; Springer International Publishing: Berlin, Germany, 2019; pp. 43–97.
8. Wang, Y.; Auyeung, K.K.; Zhang, X.; Ko, J.K. Astragalus saponins modulates colon cancer development by regulating calpain-mediated glucose-regulated protein expression. *BMC Complement. Altern. Med.* **2014**, *14*, 401. [CrossRef]
9. Yang, L.P.; Shen, J.G.; Xu, W.C.; Li, J.; Jiang, J.Q. Secondary metabolites of the genus Astragalus: Structure and biological-activity update. *Chem. Biodivers.* **2013**, *10*, 1004–1054. [CrossRef]
10. Shkondrov, A.; Krasteva, I.; Bucar, F.; Kunert, O.; Kondeva-Burdina, M.; Ionkova, I. A new tetracyclic saponin from Astragalus glycyphyllos L. and its neuroprotective and hMAO-B inhibiting activity. *Nat. Prod. Res.* **2018**, *23*, 1–7. [CrossRef]
11. Pistelli, L.; Bertoli, A.; Lepori, E.; Morelli, I.; Panizzi, L. Antimicrobial and antifungal activity of crude extracts and isolated saponins from Astragalus verrucosus. *Fitoterapia* **2002**, *73*, 336–339. [CrossRef]
12. Yin, X.; Zhang, Y.; Yu, J.; Zhang, P.; Shen, J.; Qiu, J.; Wu, H.; Zhu, X. The antioxidative effects of astragalus saponin I protect against development of early diabetic nephropathy. *J. Pharmacol. Sci.* **2006**, *101*, 166–173. [CrossRef]
13. Aslanipour, B.; Gulcemal, D.; Nalbantsoy, A.; Yusufoglu, H.; Bedir, E. Secondary metabolites from Astragalus karjaginii BORISS and the evaluation of their effects on cytokine release and hemolysis. *Fitoterapia* **2017**, *122*, 26–33. [CrossRef]
14. Auyeung, K.K.; Law, P.C.; Ko, J.K. Combined therapeutic effects of vinblastine and Astragalus saponins in human colon cancer cells and tumor xenograft via inhibition of tumor growth and proangiogenic factors. *Nutr. Cancer* **2014**, *66*, 662–674. [CrossRef] [PubMed]
15. Debelec-Butuner, B.; Ozturk, M.B.; Tag, O.; Akgun, I.H.; Yetik-Anacak, G.; Bedir, E.; Korkmaz, K.S. Cycloartane-type sapogenol derivatives inhibit NFkappaB activation as chemopreventive strategy for inflammation-induced prostate carcinogenesis. *Steroids* **2018**, *135*, 9–20. [CrossRef] [PubMed]
16. Auyeung, K.K.; Han, Q.B.; Ko, J.K. Astragalus membranaceus: A Review of its Protection Against Inflammation and Gastrointestinal Cancers. *Am. J. Chin. Med.* **2016**, *44*, 1–22. [CrossRef]
17. Graziani, V.; Scognamiglio, M.; Belli, V.; Esposito, A.; D'Abrosca, B.; Chambery, A.; Russo, R.; Panella, M.; Russo, A.; Ciardiello, F.; et al. Metabolomic approach for a rapid identification of natural products with cytotoxic activity against human colorectal cancer cells. *Sci. Rep.* **2018**, *8*, 5309. [CrossRef] [PubMed]

18. Malvezzi, M.; Carioli, G.; Bertuccio, P.; Rosso, T.; Boffetta, P.; Levi, F.; La Vecchia, C.; Negri, E. European cancer mortality predictions for the year 2016 with focus on leukaemias. *Ann. Oncol.* **2016**, *27*, 725–731. [CrossRef] [PubMed]
19. Baselga, J. The EGFR as a target for anticancer therapy - focus on cetuximab. *Eur. J. Cancer* **2001**, *37*, S16–S22. [CrossRef]
20. Ciardiello, F.; Tortora, G. EGFR antagonists in cancer treatment. *N. Engl. J. Med.* **2008**, *358*, 1160–1174. [CrossRef]
21. Scognamiglio, M.; D'Abrosca, B.; Fiumano, V.; Chambery, A.; Severino, V.; Tsafantakis, N.; Pacifico, S.; Esposito, A.; Fiorentino, A. Oleanane saponins from Bellis sylvestris Cyr. and evaluation of their phytotoxicity on Aegilops geniculata Roth. *Phytochemistry* **2012**, *84*, 125–134. [CrossRef]
22. Wang, Z.B.; Zhai, Y.D.; Ma, Z.P.; Yang, C.J.; Pan, R.; Yu, J.L.; Wang, Q.H.; Yang, B.Y.; Kuang, H.X. Triterpenoids and Flavonoids from the Leaves of Astragalus membranaceus and Their Inhibitory Effects on Nitric Oxide Production. *Chem. Biodivers.* **2015**, *12*, 1575–1584. [CrossRef]
23. Kitagawa, I.; Wang, H.; Saito, M.; Takagi, A.; Yoshikawa, M. Saponin and sapogenol. XXXV. Chemical constituents of astragali radix, the root of Astragalus membranaceus Bunge. (2). Astragalosides I, II and IV, acetylastragaloside I and isoastragalosides I and II. *Chem. Pharm. Bull.* **1983**, *31*, 698–708. [CrossRef]
24. Tin, M.M.; Cho, C.H.; Chan, K.; James, A.E.; Ko, J.K. Astragalus saponins induce growth inhibition and apoptosis in human colon cancer cells and tumor xenograft. *Carcinogenesis* **2007**, *28*, 1347–1355. [CrossRef] [PubMed]
25. Auyeung, K.K.; Cho, C.H.; Ko, J.K. A novel anticancer effect of Astragalus saponins: Transcriptional activation of NSAID-activated gene. *Int. J. Cancer* **2009**, *125*, 1082–1091. [CrossRef] [PubMed]
26. Ionkova, I.; Momekov, G.; Proksch, P. Effects of cycloartane saponins from hairy roots of Astragalus membranaceus Bge., on human tumor cell targets. *Fitoterapia* **2010**, *81*, 447–451. [CrossRef]
27. Auyeung, K.K.; Woo, P.K.; Law, P.C.; Ko, J.K. Astragalus saponins modulate cell invasiveness and angiogenesis in human gastric adenocarcinoma cells. *J. Ethnopharmacol.* **2012**, *141*, 635–641. [CrossRef] [PubMed]
28. Saif, M.W. Colorectal cancer in review: The role of the EGFR pathway. *Expert Opin Investig. Drugs* **2010**, *19*, 357–369. [CrossRef] [PubMed]
29. Veluchamy, J.P.; Spanholtz, J.; Tordoir, M.; Thijssen, V.L.; Heideman, D.A.; Verheul, H.M.; de Gruijl, T.D.; van der Vliet, H.J. Combination of NK Cells and Cetuximab to Enhance Anti-Tumor Responses in RAS Mutant Metastatic Colorectal Cancer. *PLoS ONE* **2016**, *11*, e0157830. [CrossRef] [PubMed]
30. Richman, S.D.; Seymour, M.T.; Chambers, P.; Elliott, F.; Daly, C.L.; Meade, A.M.; Taylor, G.; Barrett, J.H.; Quirke, P. KRAS and BRAF Mutations in Advanced Colorectal Cancer Are Associated With Poor Prognosis but Do Not Preclude Benefit From Oxaliplatin or Irinotecan: Results From the MRC FOCUS Trial. *J. Clin. Oncol.* **2009**, *27*, 5931–5937. [CrossRef]
31. Roth, A.D.; Tejpar, S.; Delorenzi, M.; Yan, P.; Fiocca, R.; Klingbiel, D.; Dietrich, D.; Biesmans, B.; Bodoky, G.; Barone, C.; et al. Prognostic role of KRAS and BRAF in stage II and III resected colon cancer: Results of the translational study on the PETACC-3, EORTC 40993, SAKK 60-00 trial. *J. Clin. Oncol.* **2010**, *28*, 466–474. [CrossRef]
32. Van Cutsem, E.; Kohne, C.H.; Lang, I.; Folprecht, G.; Nowacki, M.P.; Cascinu, S.; Shchepotin, I.; Maurel, J.; Cunningham, D.; Tejpar, S.; et al. Cetuximab plus irinotecan, fluorouracil, and leucovorin as first-line treatment for metastatic colorectal cancer: Updated analysis of overall survival according to tumor KRAS and BRAF mutation status. *J. Clin. Oncol.* **2011**, *29*, 2011–2019. [CrossRef]
33. Chapman, P.B.; Hauschild, A.; Robert, C.; Haanen, J.B.; Ascierto, P.; Larkin, J.; Dummer, R.; Garbe, C.; Testori, A.; Maio, M.; et al. Improved survival with vemurafenib in melanoma with BRAF V600E mutation. *N. Engl. J. Med.* **2011**, *364*, 2507–2516. [CrossRef] [PubMed]
34. Kopetz, S.; Desai, J.; Chan, E.; Hecht, J.R.; O'Dwyer, P.J.; Lee, R.J.; Nolop, K.B.; Saltz, L. PLX4032 in metastatic colorectal cancer patients with mutant BRAF tumors. *J. Clin. Oncol.* **2010**, *28*, 3534. [CrossRef]

35. Prahallad, A.; Sun, C.; Huang, S.D.; Di Nicolantonio, F.; Salazar, R.; Zecchin, D.; Beijersbergen, R.L.; Bardelli, A.; Bernards, R. Unresponsiveness of colon cancer to BRAF(V600E) inhibition through feedback activation of EGFR. *Nature* **2012**, *483*, 100–146. [CrossRef]
36. Scognamiglio, M.; Fiumano, V.; D'Abrosca, B.; Esposito, A.; Choi, Y.H.; Verpoorte, R.; Fiorentino, A. Chemical interactions between plants in Mediterranean vegetation: The influence of selected plant extracts on Aegilops geniculata metabolome. *Phytochemistry* **2014**, *106*, 69–85. [CrossRef] [PubMed]

Sample Availability: Samples of the compounds are not available from the authors.

molecules

MDPI

Article

Phenolic Compounds from *Humulus lupulus* as Natural Antimicrobial Products: New Weapons in the Fight against Methicillin Resistant *Staphylococcus aureus, Leishmania mexicana* and *Trypanosoma brucei* Strains

Laetitia Bocquet [1], Sevser Sahpaz [1], Natacha Bonneau [1], Claire Beaufay [2], Séverine Mahieux [3], Jennifer Samaillie [1], Vincent Roumy [1], Justine Jacquin [1], Simon Bordage [1], Thierry Hennebelle [1], Feng Chai [4], Joëlle Quetin-Leclercq [2], Christel Neut [3] and Céline Rivière [1,*]

1 EA 7394—ICV, Charles Viollette Research Institute, SFR Condorcet FR CNRS 3417, Univ. Lille, INRA, ISA-Yncréa, Univ. Artois, Univ. Littoral Côte d'Opale, 3 rue du Professeur Laguesse, 59000 Lille, France; laetitia.bocquet1309@gmail.com (L.B.); sevser.sahpaz@univ-lille.fr (S.S.); natacha.bonneau@univ-lille.fr (N.B.); jennifer.samaillie@univ-lille.fr (J.S.); vincent.roumy@univ-lille.fr (V.R.); justine.jacquin@yncrea.fr (J.J.); simon.bordage@univ-lille.fr (S.B.); thierry.hennebelle@univ-lille.fr (T.H.)
2 Pharmacognosy Research group, Louvain Drug Research Institute, Université Catholique de Louvain, 1200 Brussels, Belgium; claire.beaufay@uclouvain.be (C.B.); joelle.leclercq@uclouvain.be (J.Q.-L.)
3 U995—LIRIC, Lille Inflammation Research International Center, Univ. Lille, Inserm, CHU Lille, 59000 Lille, France; severine.mahieux@univ-lille.fr (S.M.); christel.neut@univ-lille.fr (C.N.)
4 U1008—Controlled Drug Delivery Systems and Biomaterials, Univ. Lille, Inserm, CHU Lille, 59000 Lille, France; feng.chai@univ-lille.fr
* Correspondence: celine.riviere@univ-lille.fr; Tel.: +33-3-20-96-40-41

Academic Editor: Pinarosa Avato
Received: 28 January 2019; Accepted: 10 March 2019; Published: 14 March 2019

Abstract: New anti-infective agents are urgently needed to fight microbial resistance. Methicillin-resistant *Staphylococcus aureus* (MRSA) strains are particularly responsible for complicated pathologies that are difficult to treat due to their virulence and the formation of persistent biofilms forming a complex protecting shell. Parasitic infections caused by *Trypanosoma brucei* and *Leishmania mexicana* are also of global concern, because of the mortality due to the low number of safe and effective treatments. Female inflorescences of hop produce specialized metabolites known for their antimicrobial effects but underexploited to fight against drug-resistant microorganisms. In this study, we assessed the antimicrobial potential of phenolic compounds against MRSA clinical isolates, *T. brucei* and *L. mexicana*. By fractionation process, we purified the major prenylated chalcones and acylphloroglucinols, which were quantified by UHPLC-UV in different plant parts, showing their higher content in the active flowers extract. Their potent antibacterial action (MIC < 1 μg/mL for the most active compound) was demonstrated against MRSA strains, through kill curves, post-antibiotic effects, anti-biofilm assays and synergy studies with antibiotics. An antiparasitic activity was also shown for some purified compounds, particularly on *T. brucei* (IC_{50} < 1 to 11 μg/mL). Their cytotoxic activity was assessed both on cancer and non-cancer human cell lines.

Keywords: *Humulus lupulus*; prenylated phenolic compounds; antimicrobial agents; methicillin-resistant *Staphylococcus aureus*; *Leishmania mexicana mexicana*; *Trypanosoma brucei brucei*

1. Introduction

Multidrug-resistant microorganisms are rapidly spreading throughout the world leading to treatment failures [1]. Antibacterial resistance in humans is affected by an inappropriate or excessive use of antibiotics in human health but is also partially affected by the use of antibiotics in animal-rearing. Some national action plans, such as restrictive measures of antibiotic use in human and animal health, are now imposed in all parts of the world but the problem of antimicrobial resistance is far from being solved [2,3]. Therefore, the discovery of new antimicrobial compounds is crucial.

Several plant-derived natural products, characterized by a huge structural diversity, including phenolic compounds, are cited as antimicrobial agents and resistance-modifying agents (RMAs) [4]. They could constitute a valuable interim solution, until new classes of antibiotics are discovered [5].

Methicillin-resistant *Staphylococcus aureus* (MRSA) strains are considered as a very urgent health problem because of their propagation in the last 15 years in the elderly and in immunocompromised patients, mainly due to their increasing implication in nosocomial infections and the lack of development of new antimicrobials. In 2016, the percentage of MRSA among all *S. aureus* isolates remained above 25% in several countries in Southern Europe and greater than 15% in France, especially for invasive isolates [6]. MRSA is also one of the principal multi-resistant bacterial pathogen responsible for complicated skin and hospital-acquired infections, associated with high mortality rates [7,8]. Furthermore, these strains are very often involved in infections of diabetic foot ulcers characterized by frequent complications and risks of lower-limb amputations [9]. *S. aureus* has the ability, like most Gram-positive organisms, to acquire resistance to practically all useful antibiotics. Several mechanisms can explain this resistance: modification of target sites, enzymatic degradation or structural modification of antibiotics and, expression of efflux pumps [5,10–12]. These bacteria also produce virulence factors involved in pathogenesis like adhesion and biofilm formation, which enhance bacterial resistance [13,14].

On the other hand, many parasitic infections deserve a special attention due to the lack of effective treatments. *Trypanosoma brucei* is a parasite conveyed by the tsetse fly and responsible for the Human African Trypanosomiasis (HAT) or sleeping sickness. This fatal disease if untreated leads to central nervous system disturbances, including sensory, motor and psychic troubles and neuroendocrine abnormalities [15,16]. Leishmaniasis, caused by different *Leishmania* species, is responsible for chronic skin and visceral diseases transmitted by sand-flies [17].

Hop (*Humulus lupulus* L.) is a climbing dioecious plant belonging to the Cannabaceae family. This species is cultivated worldwide for its female inflorescences (cones), usually called "hops", which are used in the brewing industry. The compounds sought by brewers are prenylated acylphloroglucinol derivatives, also called bitter acids and in particular α-acids (humulone derivatives) which are isomerized into iso-α-acids during the brewing process. These compounds confer some bitterness and antiseptic properties to beer [18]. This plant is also known to have many pharmacological activities, including sedative, oestrogenic, anti-inflammatory, chemopreventive and antimicrobial activities [19]. The antimicrobial activity is mainly attributed to prenylated acylphloroglucinols, in particular to α-acids and β-acids (lupulone derivatives) and to prenylated chalcones, including xanthohumol (Figure 1) [20–22]. Few studies, however, describe the activity of this plant and especially of its specialized metabolites against multidrug resistant strains [14,23] and parasites [24,25]. In addition, the mechanisms of the inhibitory activities observed are not really expanded upon now.

In this context, we studied the antimicrobial potential of hop phenolic compounds against MRSA strains, *Trypanosoma brucei brucei* (Tbb) and *Leishmania mexicana mexicana* (Lmm). We opted for a fractionation using Centrifugal Partition Chromatography (CPC) and preparative High-Performance Liquid Chromatography (HPLC) to purify the major antimicrobial phenolic compounds from the most active sub-extract of hop. Purified compounds were then quantified in hop extracts. Their antibacterial potential against MRSA clinical isolates was assessed. The most promising compounds were then selected for further experiments in order to strengthen our knowledge of their action on the bacterial strains, through kill curves, post-antibiotic effects, anti-biofilm and synergy assays. The antiparasitic activity of some chalcones and acylphloroglucinols against Tbb and Lmm was also evaluated. Their cytotoxicity activity was determined on various human cell lines.

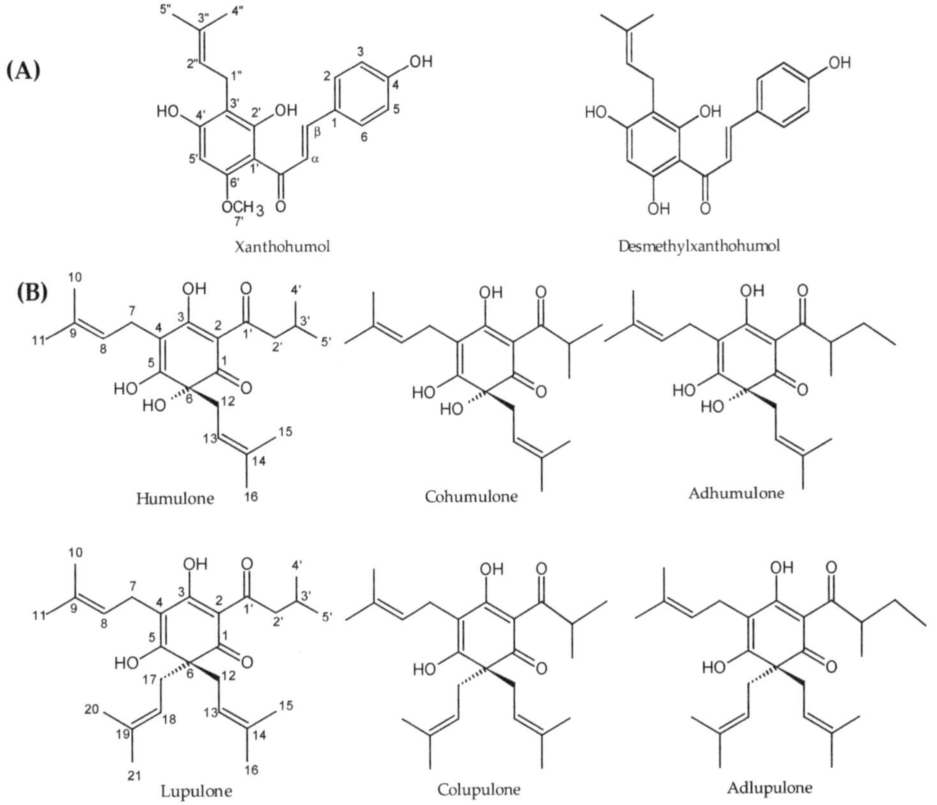

Figure 1. Structures of the main prenylated phenolic compounds from hops. (**A**) prenylated chalcones (**B**) acylphloroglucinol derivatives.

2. Results

2.1. Antimicrobial Activity of Hop Extracts and Sub-Extracts against Gram-Positive and Gram-Negative Bacteria and Parasites

We evaluated the antimicrobial activity of hop extracts and sub-extracts towards bacterial clinical isolates and parasites (Tbb and Lmm).

We first confirmed the antibacterial activity of the crude hydro-ethanolic extract of cones against Gram-positive bacteria, namely *Corynebacterium*, *Enterococcus*, *Mycobacterium*, *Staphylococcus* and *Streptococcus* strains, with MICs ranging from 39 to 156 μg/mL (Table 1). Some yeasts have also been studied. On the 36 *Candida albicans* strains tested (data not shown), only the two presented in Table 1 were susceptible to our extracts. Leaves, stems and rhizomes showed a weak antimicrobial activity. The liquid-liquid fractionation of the most active crude extract (cones) with dichloromethane (DCM) and water led to set up a second screening only focused on Gram-positive bacteria (Table 2). This partition also led us to direct the activity towards non-polar compounds as the non-polar sub-extract was indeed more active than the crude extract. Enterococci appeared less susceptible to the DCM sub-extract than staphylococci and streptococci. *S. aureus* strains were the most susceptible with MICs ranging from 9.8 to 19.5 μg/mL (Table 2). This non-polar fraction of hops is known to contain prenylated chalcones and acylphloroglucinol derivatives (Figure 1) which were further purified to analyze their activity.

Table 1. MIC (in µg/mL) of hop hydro-ethanolic crude extracts (Co: cones, Le: leaves, St: stems, Rh: rhizomes) against some human pathogenic bacteria with their corresponding antibiotic susceptibility (S: susceptible I: intermediate, R: resistant).

Bacterial Strains and Yeasts	MIC (µg/mL)				Antibiotic and Antifungal Susceptibility		
	Co	Le	St	Rh	GEN	VAN	AMX
Gram-positive							
Corynebacterium T25-17	39	NA	NA	NA	S	S	S
Enterococcus faecalis C159-6	39	NA	NA	NA	R	S	R
Enterococcus sp. 8153	156	NA	NA	NA	R	S	S
Mycobacterium smegmatis 5003	39	NA	NA	NA	S	S	S
Staphylococcus aureus 8146	39	NA	NA	NA	S	S	I
Staphylococcus aureus 8147	39	NA	NA	NA	S	S	S
Staphylococcus epidermidis 5001	39	NA	NA	NA	S	S	S
Staphylococcus epidermidis 10282	98	NA	NA	NA	S	S	S
Staphylococcus lugdunensis T26A3	156	NA	NA	625	S	S	S
Staphylococcus warneri T12A12	39	NA	NA	625	S	R	S
Streptococcus agalactiae T25-7	39	NA	NA	NA	R	S	S
Streptococcus agalactiae T53C2	78	NA	NA	NA	S	S	S
Streptococcus dysgalactiae T46C14	39	NA	NA	NA	S	S	S
Gram-negative							
Acinetobacter baumannii 9010	NA	NA	NA	NA	S	R	R
Acinetobacter baumannii 9011	NA	NA	NA	625	R	R	R
Citrobacter freundii 11041	NA	NA	NA	NA	S	R	S
Citrobacter freundii 11042	NA	NA	NA	NA	S	R	R
Enterobacter cloacae 11050	NA	NA	NA	NA	S	R	R
Enterobacter cloacae 11051	NA	NA	NA	NA	R	R	R
Enterobacter cloacae 11053	NA	NA	NA	NA	S	R	R
Escherichia coli 8138	NA	NA	NA	NA	S	R	R
Escherichia coli 8157	NA	NA	NA	NA	S	R	R
Escherichia coli ATCC 25922	NA	NA	NA	NA	S	R	I
Klebsiella pneumoniae 11016	NA	NA	NA	NA	S	R	R
Klebsiella pneumoniae 11017	NA	NA	NA	NA	S	R	R
Proteus mirabilis 11060	NA	NA	NA	NA	S	R	R
Providencia stuartii 11038	NA	NA	NA	NA	S	R	S
Pseudomonas aeruginosa 8131	NA	NA	NA	625	S	R	R
Pseudomonas aeruginosa ATCC 27583	NA	NA	NA	625	R	R	R
Salmonella sp. 11033	NA	NA	NA	NA	S	R	R
Serratia marcescens 11056	NA	NA	NA	NA	S	R	R
Serratia marcescens 11057	NA	NA	NA	NA	R	R	R
Stenotrophomonas maltophilia	NA	NA	NA	625	S	R	R
Yeasts					**AMB**	**FLC**	**VRC**
Candida albicans 13203	156	625	NA	NA	S	R	R
Candida albicans ATCC 10231	<39	NA	NA	NA	S	S	S

Gentamicin (GEN) S ≤ 4, R > 8; Vancomycin (VAN) S ≤ 4, R > 16; Amoxicillin (AMX) S ≤ 4, R > 16; Amphotericin B (AMB) S ≤ 1, R > 1; Fluconazole (FLC) S ≤ 2, R > 4; Voriconazole (VRC) S ≤ 0.12, R > 0.12. NA means not active, MIC ≥ 1250 µg/mL.

Table 2. MIC (in μg/mL) of the crude extract and the dichloromethane (DCM) sub-extract of cones against Gram-positive strains with their corresponding antibiotic susceptibility (S: susceptible, I: intermediate, R: resistant).

Gram-Positive Strains	MIC (μg/mL)		Antibiotic Susceptibility		
	Crude Extract	DCM	GEN	VAN	AMX
Corynebacterium T25-17	39	19.5	S	S	S
Enterococcus faecalis C159-6	156	78	R	R	R
Enterococcus faecalis T26-B7	313	156	R	S	S
Enterococcus faecalis T34-2	313	156	S	S	S
Enterococcus faecalis T37A4	156	156	R	S	S
Enterococcus faecalis T39-C11	156	156	S	S	S
Staphylococcus aureus 8146	19.5	9.8	S	S	S
Staphylococcus aureus 8147	19.5	9.8	S	S	S
Staphylococcus aureus CIP 224	39	19.5	S	S	S
Staphylococcus aureus T1.1	39	19.5	S	S	S
Staphylococcus aureus T25.10	39	19.5	S	S	R
Staphylococcus aureus T25.3	39	19.5	S	S	R
Staphylococcus aureus T25.9	39	19.5	S	S	R
Staphylococcus aureus T26A4	39	19.5	S	S	S
Staphylococcus aureus T28.1	19.5	9.8	S	S	R
Staphylococcus aureus T36B1	39	19.5	S	S	R
Staphylococcus aureus T47A12	39	19.5	S	S	R
Staphylococcus aureus T6.7	39	9.8	S	S	R
Staphylococcus epidermidis 5001	39	19.5	S	S	S
Staphylococcus warneri T12A12	78	19.5	S	S	S
Staphylococcus lugdunensis T26A3	39	19.5	S	S	S
Staphylococcus pettenkoferi T3.3	78	39	S	S	S
Staphylococcus saprophyticus 08237	39	9.8	S	S	S
Streptococcus agalactiae 13225	39	19.5	S	S	S
Streptococcus agalactiae 13226	39	19.5	S	S	S
Streptococcus agalactiae T25.7	39	19.5	I	S	S
Streptococcus agalactiae T38.2	39	19.5	S	S	S
Streptococcus agalactiae T40A2	39	19.5	S	S	S

Gentamicin (GEN) S ≤ 4, R > 8; Vancomycin (VAN) S ≤ 4, R > 16; Amoxicillin (AMX) S ≤ 4, R > 16. NA means not active, MIC ≥ 1250 μg/mL.

Extracts and sub-extracts were also tested for their antiparasitic effect. This activity was for the first-time described here on Tbb with respective IC_{50} of 7.8 and 4.6 μg/mL for the hydro-ethanolic crude extract and the DCM sub-extract of cones. Hops is less active against Lmm with IC_{50} of 29.0 and 28.2 μg/mL, respectively.

2.2. Purification of Hops Prenylated Chalcones and Acylphloroglucinols and Quantification in Hop Samples

Major prenylated chalcones (xanthohumol and desmethylxanthohumol) and prenylated acylphloroglucinols (cohumulone, humulone, colupulone and lupulone) were purified from the active DCM sub-extract of cones by centrifugal partition chromatography (CPC) and preparative high-performance liquid chromatography (HPLC) (Figure 1). Their structure was established by comparison with their spectral data, including NMR data and mass spectra, with reported values [26–29] (Supplementary Material, Tables S2–S4). These compounds were identified in the different plant crude extracts by UHPLC-UV-MS on the basis of their retention times and their mass spectrum (Figure 2 and Supplementary Material, Figures S1–S3). They were then used for quantification in different parts of the plant and for activities testing.

Quantification was performed on crude hydro-ethanolic extracts of the cultivar 'Nugget' used for bioassays. Concerning our method, good linearity was observed for each compound over the concentration range (Supplementary Material, Table S1). Evaluation of the method on the cones extract showed acceptable intra- and inter-day precisions for xanthohumol (RSD% = 10.6, 12.0), humulone (RSD% = 12.4, 13.8) and lupulone (RSD% = 10.3, 10.7).

The contents in prenylated phenolic compounds were much higher in the crude extract of cones than in stems, roots and leaves crude extracts (Figures 2 and 3). Only xanthohumol and humulone have been quantified in the stems extract. No prenylated phenolic compounds could be quantified in the rhizome extract. Interestingly, humulone was the main compound in cones extract (147 μg/mg), with a total alpha/beta acid (humulone/lupulone derivatives) ratio of 2.4, whereas lupulone was the most abundant compound in leaves extract, with a ratio of 0.5.

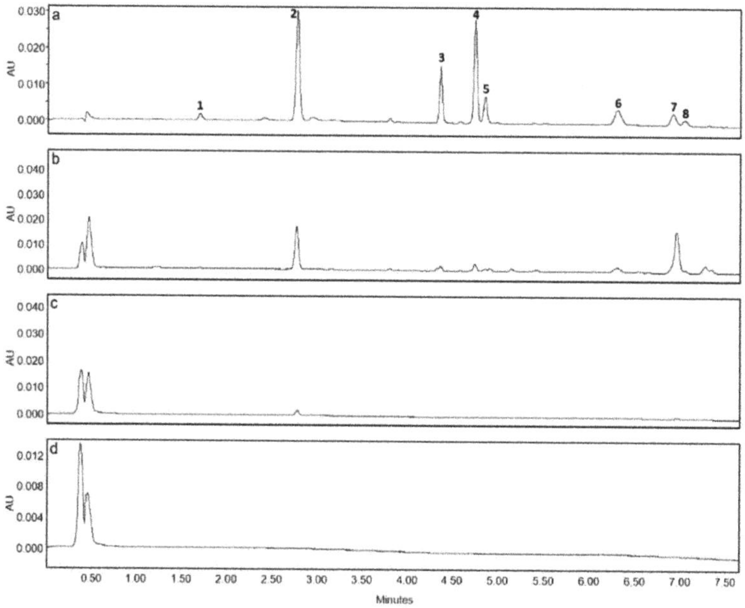

Figure 2. LC-UV chromatograms (370 nm) of crude extracts prepared at 100 μg/mL in MeOH for (**a**) cones and 1 mg/mL in MeOH for (**b**) leaves, (**c**) stems and (**d**) rhizomes. Compounds identified are as follows: desmethylxanthohumol (**1**) rt 1.70 min, xanthohumol (**2**) rt 2.78 min, cohumulone (**3**) rt 4.37 min, humulone (**4**) rt 4.75 min, adhumulone (**5**) rt 4.86 min, colupulone (**6**) rt 6.31 min, lupulone (**7**) rt 6.92 min, adlupulone (**8**) rt 7.05 min.

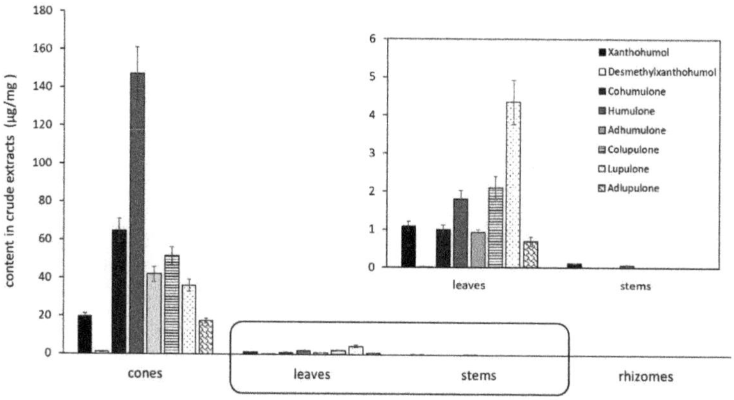

Figure 3. Content of prenylated chalcones and acylphloroglucinols in crude hydro-alcoholic extracts of different hop parts (in μg/mg) (n = 3, mean ± SD).

2.3. *Antibacterial Activity of Purified Prenylated Phenolic Compounds*

2.3.1. Antibacterial Activity of Purified Compounds against Selected MRSA and Methicillin-Sensitive *Staphylococcus aureus* (MSSA) Strains

All compounds tested were active against selected oxacillin susceptible and resistant *S. aureus* clinical isolates (Table 3). Indeed, methicillin resistance is routine researched by using oxacillin disks. The first strain (T28.1) was more intensively studied because it combined many pathologic features like isolation from a diabetic foot infection and harbouring genes implicated in antibiotic resistance, capsule formation and biofilm formation [30]. Lupulone was the most promising compound with MICs from 0.6 to 1.2 μg/mL towards MRSA strains. With the exception of lupulone, we demonstrated that xanthohumol and desmethylxanthohumol were more active than bitter acids, with MICs ranging from 9.8 to 19.5 and 19.5 to 39 μg/mL towards MRSA. However, desmethylxanthohumol was slightly less active than xanthohumol. MICs did not differ between MRSA and MSSA strains.

Table 3. MIC of hop chalcones and acylphloroglucinols against selected MRSA (T28.1 and T25.10) and MSSA (T26A4 and 08143) strains.

Bacteria MIC in μg/Ml (μM)	Chalcones		Acylphloroglucinols				OXA
	XN	DMX	Cohumulone	Humulone	Colupulone	Lupulone	
S. aureus T28.1	9.8 (27.7)	39 (114.7)	156 (448.3)	78 (215.5)	39 (97.5)	1.2 (2.9)	R
S. aureus T25.10	9.8 (27.7)	19.5 (57.3)	313 (899.4)	156 (430.9)	78 (195)	0.6 (1.45)	R
S. aureus T26A4	9.8 (27.7)	39 (114.7)	313 (899.4)	156 (430.9)	39 (97.5)	0.6 (1.45)	S
S. aureus 08143	19.5 (55)	39 (114.7)	313 (899.4)	156 (430.9)	78 (195)	1.2 (2.9)	S

XN: xanthohumol, DMX: desmethylxanthohumol. Positive control was oxacillin (OXA, S $\leq$ 2 μg/mL, R $\geq$ 4 μg/mL [31]).

Isoxanthohumol (Figure 4), a flavanone known to be a metabolite of xanthohumol, was also tested against the strain MRSA T28.1 and its MIC was found to be of similar activity as desmethylxanthohumol (MIC = 39 μg/mL).

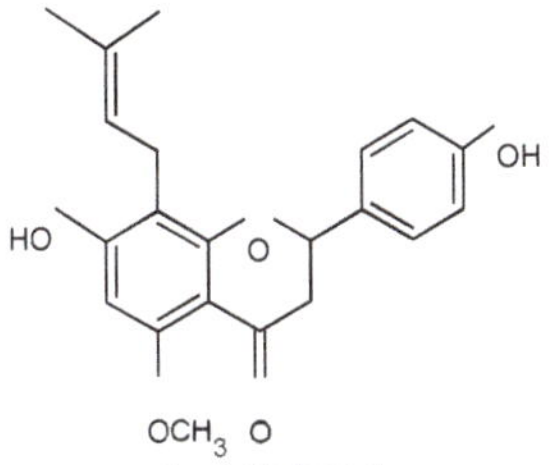

Figure 4. Structure of isoxanthohumol.

Xanthohumol, desmethylxanthohumol and lupulone were selected for further experiments on the *S. aureus* T28.1 clinical isolate, in order to better understand how they act on MRSA.

2.3.2. Further Experiments on MRSA T28.1 with the Most Promising Compounds Xanthohumol, Desmethylxanthohumol and Lupulone

Synergies Assessed by Checkerboard

One of the strategies employed to overcome resistant strains is the combination of current antibacterial agents with natural compounds. Hops phenolic compounds and selected antibiotics (ciprofloxacin, gentamicin, oxacillin and rifampicin) were combined using the checkerboard method, to establish the best combination of products for increasing the activity [32].

The antibacterial action of hops compounds can be enhanced by combining xanthohumol with desmethylxanthohumol or with lupulone, showing an additive effect (Table 4). In contrast, the combination of desmethylxanthohumol with lupulone was found to be antagonistic.

The combination of hops compounds with selected antibiotics highlighted interesting effects (Table 4). Xanthohumol was synergistic to additive with the four antibiotics. For example, rifampicin can be 8 times more active when combined with xanthohumol. Desmethylxanthohumol showed a synergistic activity with gentamicin, synergistic to additive with ciprofloxacin and additive with oxacillin, while sometimes antagonist effect was observed with rifampicin. The interaction of lupulone with ciprofloxacin was additive and this association was antagonist or indifferent with gentamicin and rifampicin.

Table 4. Effect of the combination of hops compounds between them and with selected antibiotics.

Association	FIC Index	Effect
XN-DMX	0.74–1	Additive
XN-Lupulone	0.75	Additive
DMX-Lupulone	5	Antagonist
CIP-XN	0.49–1	Synergistic to additive
CIP-DMX	0.38–1.5	Synergistic to indifferent
CIP-Lupulone	0.63–1	Additive
GEN-XN	0.14–1	Synergistic to additive
GEN-DMX	0.03–0.28	Synergistic
GEN-Lupulone	9	Antagonist
OXA-XN	0.28–0.75	Synergistic to additive
OXA-DMX	0.5–0.76	Additive
OXA-Lupulone	0.19–1.25	Synergistic to indifferent
RIF-XN	0.25–0.75	Synergistic to additive
RIF-DMX	1–5	Indifferent to antagonist
RIF-Lupulone	2.2–6	Indifferent to antagonist

Association can be synergistic (FIC < 0.5), additive ($0.5 \leq$ FIC ≤ 1), indifferent ($1 <$ FIC ≤ 4) or antagonist (FIC > 4). Ranges result from 3 independent experiments. XN: xanthohumol, DMX: desmethylxanthohumol, CIP: ciprofloxacin, GEN: gentamicin, OXA: oxacillin, RIF: rifampicin.

Kill Curve

Kill curves allowed the determination of time-dependent bacteriostatic and bactericidal concentrations of each product [33] (Figure 5).

Xanthohumol decreased the bacterial population by 0.5 log(CFU/mL) during the first 6 h at sub-inhibitory concentration (MIC/2) and by 2 log(CFU/mL) during 24 h at the MIC. It was bactericidal at 2xMIC, rapidly decreasing the bacterial population to around 3 log(CFU/mL) during the first 4 h which means that only 1 bacterium among 1000 initially present is still alive (Figure 5A).

Desmethylxanthohumol decreased the bacterial population during the first hours at the MIC. The bacteria grew back after 6 h of culture. However, it was bactericidal at 2 × MIC; reaching the detection threshold of 1 log(CFU/mL) after 24 h (Figure 5B).

Although lupulone was the most active compound (based on MIC of 1.2 μg/mL), it slightly decreased the bacterial population only at 4 × MIC. Lower concentrations just slowed down growth (Figure 5C) and a reduction between the control and 2 × MIC is about 3 log(CFU/mL).

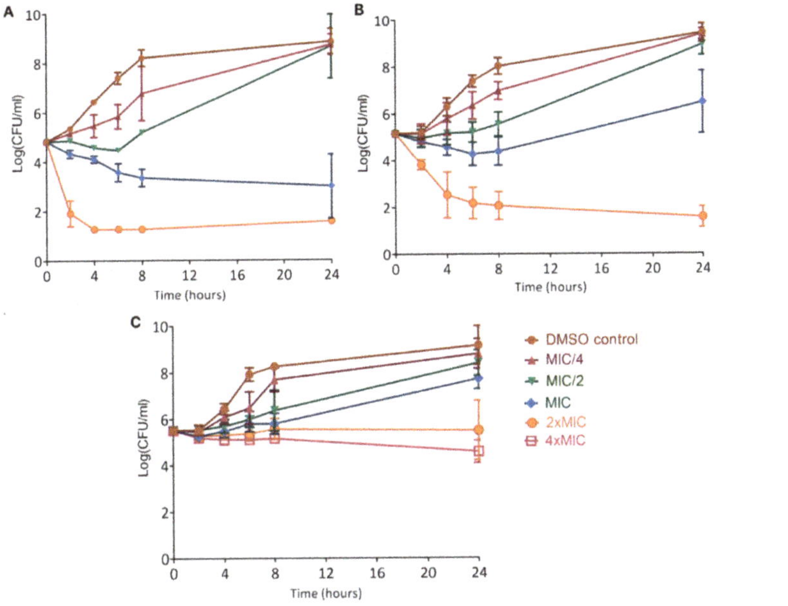

Figure 5. Kill curves showing the effect of xanthohumol (**A**), desmethylxanthohumol (**B**) and lupulone (**C**) on *S. aureus* T28.1 growing during 24 h. The detection threshold of the experiment is 1 log(CFU/mL).

Post-Antibiotic Effects

Post-antibiotic tests highlighted the fragility of the bacterial population after 2 h exposure to the active compounds followed by inactivation, which resulted in a delayed regrowth [33]. The growth retardation is quantified by the difference between the time necessary for each condition to grow from a log10 (T) and the corresponding time for the control (C). These parameters are graphically determined as shown in Figure 6.

The three compounds tested caused delayed growth at all concentrations evaluated (Table 5).

Here again, even if lupulone was the most active (based on MIC values), it caused a low effect after its inactivation with a maximum delay close to 55 min. In contrast, xanthohumol and desmethylxanthohumol caused a significant delay for regrowth. Desmethylxanthohumol inhibited bacterial regrowth for up to almost 2.5 h after pre-treatment at the MIC. Xanthohumol had the same effect at the MIC and it increased with the concentration, the delay reaching 3.29 h at 4 × MIC.

Table 5. Post-antibiotic effect on *S. aureus* T28.1 for each hops selected compound after 2 h exposure. Values are the maximum delayed growth retardation obtained after 3 independent experiments.

	Maximum Growth Retardation (h)			
	MIC/2	**MIC**	**2 × MIC**	**4 × MIC**
Xanthohumol	1.34	2.23	2.05	3.29
Desmethylxanthohumol	2.10	2.32	2.29	2.34
Lupulone	0.26	0.53	0.54	0.47

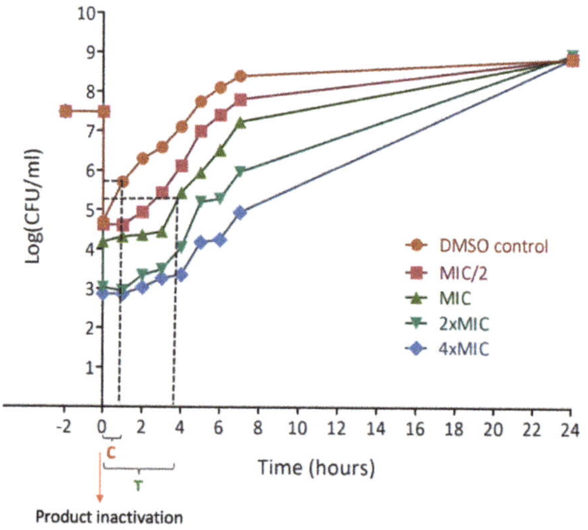

Figure 6. Post-antibiotic curve of xanthohumol indicating graphical determination of parameters for the determination of the growth delay. Time between −2 and 0 shows the pre-treatment with antibacterial product. Time 0 corresponds to the product inactivation. The growth retardation is quantified during the first hours of culture, comparing each condition with the control, using the formula: PAE = T − C. Where T is the time needed for the bacterial population to grow by 1 log10 (the present example is for the MIC) and C is the corresponding time for the control.

Anti-Biofilm Assays

Biofilms contribute to bacterial resistance, forming a complex protecting shell [34]. We initially considered the activity of hops compounds on artificial surfaces, which was confirmed on a bone substitute, the natural colonized substrate of the model strain *S. aureus* T28.1. The influence of the compounds was assessed both on the biofilm formation and on the destruction of preformed biofilms.

Xanthohumol totally inhibited the biofilm formation on artificial surface at the MIC (Figure 7A), which correlates with the bactericidal effect pointed out with kill curves (Figure 5A). Desmethylxanthohumol and lupulone showed a significant inhibition of biofilm formation at sub-inhibitory concentrations (Figure 7A). Thus, this effect seems independent of the bactericidal activity (Figure 5B,C). The same trend was observed on bone substitutes (Figure 7C). Even if the inhibition of the biofilm formation is found less intense in bone substitute, this potential remains very interesting, in particular for desmethylxanthohumol and lupulone. These last products showed a significant decrease of the biofilm formation on bone substitute discs at MIC (Figure 7C).

Hops compounds are also able to destroy the biofilm. Xanthohumol showed a non-dose-dependent activity at the MIC and above, which is similar to the inhibition dose for the biofilm formation (Figure 7B). As seen previously, desmethylxanthohumol and lupulone showed a greater anti-biofilm potential than xanthohumol. A significant biofilm destruction was also observed at sub-inhibitory concentrations, at MIC/4, with 81% and 62.8%, respectively.

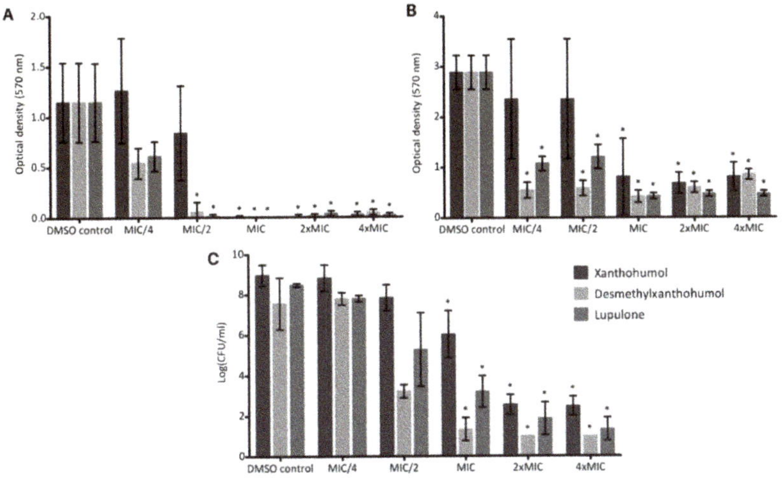

Figure 7. Effect of xanthohumol, desmethylxanthohumol and lupulone on the biofilm formation (**A**) of *S. aureus* T28.1 on artificial surface (**A**), on the biofilm destruction of *S. aureus* T28.1 on artificial surface (**B**) and on the biofilm formation of *S. aureus* T28.1 on bone substitute (**C**). According to Shapiro test, means tagged with * are significantly different from the control (p = 0.05) using Kruskal Wallis and Dunn's tests for (**A**) and for lupulone and desmethylxanthohumol for (**C**) or ANOVA and Tukey test for (**B**) and for xanthohumol for (**C**).

2.4. Antiparasitic Activity of Purified Prenylated Phenolic Compounds

The two chalcones, xanthohumol and desmethylxanthohumol, as well as two acylphloroglucinols, humulone and lupulone, were tested against the two parasites: *Trypanosoma brucei brucei* (Tbb) and *Leishmania mexicana mexicana* (Lmm) and were active. Lupulone is the most promising compound with IC_{50} of 0.9 and 4.7 µg/mL against Tbb and Lmm, respectively (Table 6). As for antibacterial activities, we demonstrated that xanthohumol and desmethylxanthohumol were more active than humulone on parasites, with IC_{50} from 2.4 to 6.1 and 7.7 to 26.2 µg/mL on both Tbb and Lmm.

Table 6. IC_{50} of hops chalcones and acylphloroglucinols against some *Trypanosoma brucei brucei* and *Leishmania mexicana mexicana* strains.

Parasites IC_{50} in µg/mL (µM)	XN	DMX	Humulone	Lupulone	SUR	PEN
Tbb	2.4 ± 0.2 (6.8)	7.7 ± 0.6 (22.6)	10.9 ± 0.8 (30.1)	0.9 ± 0.0 (2.2)	0.05 (0.038)	-
Lmm	6.1 ± 3.1 (17.2)	26.2 ± 1.8 (77)	28.8 ± 1.5 (77.9)	4.7 ± 0.1 (11.3)	-	0.07 (0.21)

XN: xanthohumol, DMX: desmethylxanthohumol. Positive controls were suramin (SUR) and pentamidine (PEN). ND: Not determined.

2.5. Cytotoxicity

We evaluated the antiproliferative activity of hops compounds on various cancer and non-cancer cell lines (Table 7). We showed that desmethylxanthohumol is the less toxic compound. Considering its moderate activity, active dose could be toxic. Active concentration of desmethylxanthohumol on Tbb is the only one lower than the cytotoxicity on the tested cell lines. Xanthohumol was also toxic at the antibacterial concentration on all the targeted cell lines. For both chalcones, selectivity indexes (cytotoxic IC_{50}/active IC_{50}) would be close to 1. A special attention has to be paid on lupulone, its pronounced antibacterial activity gives selectivity index > 4 compared to its cytotoxicity against MG-63 (Table 7). Antibacterial and anti-biofilm concentrations showed a cell viability close to 100%. These data make lupulone a very good candidate for a topical bone application.

Table 7. Cytotoxic activities of hops extracts and isolated compounds (chalcones and acylphloroglucinols) against WI-38, J774, Hep-G2 and MG-63 cell lines.

Cell Lines IC_{50} ± SD in µg/mL (µM)	Hydro-Alcoholic Crude Extract	MC Sub-Extract	XN	DMX	Humulone	Lupulone	CAMP
WI-38	7.6 ± 0.1	5.1 ± 1.0	6.9 ± 0.5 (19.5)	60.7 ± 2.5 (178.5)	10.5 ± 2.3 (29)	1.1 ± 0.0 (2.6)	0.06 ± 0.0 (0.17)
J774	19.7 ± 2.8	11.4 ± 2.1	3.4 ± 0.5 (9.6)	9.7 ± 1.0 (28.5)	11.5 ± 0.3 (31.7)	1.5 ± 0.1 (3.6)	0.01 ± 0.0 (0.03)
Hep-G2	6.8 ± 2.5	6.5 ± 2.1	2.5 ± 0.8 (7.1)	22.4 ± 2.9 (65.9)	ND	1.2 ± 0.5 (2.9)	0.4 ± 0.2 (1.15)
MG-63	31.4 ± 8.1	21.1 ± 0.4	10.4 ± 2.6 (29.4)	39.5 ± 3.3 (116.2)	ND	4.3 ± 0.4 (10.4)	4.4 ± 1.5 (12.6)

XN: xanthohumol, DMX: desmethylxanthohumol. Positive control was camptothecin (CAMP). ND: Not determined.

3. Discussion

Multi-drug resistance (MDR) bacteria, like methicillin-resistant *Staphylococcus aureus* (MRSA), present a major challenge for the medical community in the treatment of infections, such as diabetic foot infections [6,35]. The discovery of new antibiotics is not fast enough to offset the global spread of resistant pathogens. At the same time, we can observe a worrying emergence of resistance to some of the newer antibiotic agents [36–38]. Hence, the development of combination of current agents with other type of resistance-modifying agents, such as natural antibacterial agents, can be an alternative strategy to overcome MDR [39].

In this context, we evaluated the antibacterial potential of hop extracts and more particularly of three pure compounds isolated from hops (xanthohumol, desmethylxanthohumol and lupulone) towards MRSA, one of the most aggressive agents, with different approaches [33]. We began by a classical MIC determination, which is only an endpoint method, followed by kill-time curves assessing the time dependent effect and synergistic studies, in combination with antibiotics, giving more information on their resistance modifying potential. The checkerboard method is the preferred technique of choice to analyze these interactions, with however a certain variability in the methods of interpretation [32]. The study of a post-antibiotic effect (PAE), also applicable to substances other than antibiotics, made it possible to follow the regrowth of bacteria after inactivation of the antibacterial substance after a defined contact time at an active concentration. When damaged bacteria need some time to recover in comparison to the control, the regrowth will be lowered, which means in clinical situations that administration intervals of the antimicrobial substances can be delayed. Another innovative point is the effect on biofilms, concerning about 60% of infections. In biofilms, the bacteria are surrounded by a thick layer of extracellular polysaccharides which makes them inaccessible to antibiotics but also to defenses of the immune system. Furthermore, the lack of nutrients lowers dramatically the bacterial multiplication. As most of the antibiotics act on mechanisms implicated in multiplication, this is the second reason for their lack of action on biofilms. Influence on biofilms can be studied in two manners: destruction of established biofilms or inhibition of their formation. The first manner is more relevant for clinicians as at the time of diagnosis the biofilm is already established.

The antibacterial activity of hops has been known for many years [40,41] but has been poorly evaluated against resistant strains. We showed here their effects on *Corynebacterium*, *Enterococcus*, *Mycobacterium*, *Staphylococcus* and *Streptococcus* strains, some being resistant to antibiotics (Table 1). Their effect on *Bacillus*, *Streptomyces* and *Micrococcus* strains was previously underlined [22,41]. Hops extracts are also able to combat some human pathogenic bacteria found in food, such as *Clostridium perfringens* and *Listeria monocytogenes* [42,43]. The screening conducted on some *C. albicans* strains showed that the spectrum of activity of hops extracts against these yeasts is weak, only two strains were susceptible to our extracts. The *C. albicans* ATCC 10,231 reference strain was previously tested by Langezaal et al. [44] who also found an efficiency of cones extract. Other studies have demonstrated that hops extracts are more efficient on bacteria than yeasts, showing no effect of hops constituents on *Saccharomyces* strains [41]. Contrarily to Langezaal et al. [44] and Abram et al. [45]

who have detected a slight activity of cones extracts against *E. coli* strains, our extracts were inactive towards Gram-negative bacteria. Stems, leaves and rhizomes have been rarely studied. According to our results, their crude hydro-ethanolic extracts showed a weak antimicrobial activity in comparison with cones, as already highlighted for leaves against some bacteria [45]. Nevertheless, the rhizomes extract appeared to be more active than leaves and stems extracts (Table 1). Previous research on the quantification of the phenolic hop compounds in cones and leaves by LC-UV is reported in the literature [46]. With our method of quantification, no prenylated phenolic compounds could be quantified in the rhizome extract. Consequently, the activity of rhizomes could be related to the presence of other metabolites. The antibacterial activity of cones was mainly attributed to apolar compounds because the DCM sub-extract of cones was more active than the crude extract of the same plant part (Table 2). The content of phenolic compounds in hops is influenced in particular by the cultivar, the growth location, the field conditions, the climate, which may explain the differences in activities found in the literature [47,48].

Phenolic compounds are known to be an anti-staphylococcal class of metabolites. In our study, all purified hops prenylated chalcones and acylphloroglucinol derivatives showed an antibacterial activity towards selected *S. aureus* strains (Table 3). In the literature, the antibacterial activity of hops is mainly linked to acylphloroglucinol derivatives. This activity is enhanced by the degree of hydrophobicity of the compound [49]. The number and the length of the side chains, because of their interaction with the bacterial cell wall, is stated to influence positively the antibacterial action, so lupulone derivatives are more efficient than humulone derivatives [22,42], which is in accordance with our results. Lupulone is much more active than humulone with respective MICs ranging from 0.6 to 1.2 and 78 to 156 μg/mL towards MRSA strains (Table 3). With the exception of lupulone, we also demonstrated that xanthohumol and desmethylxanthohumol are more active than other bitter acids. Xanthohumol showed MIC ranging from 9.8 to 19.5 μg/mL against selected *S. aureus* strains. In comparison with one of the most studied promising antimicrobial chalcone, licochalcone A, which showed MIC ranging from 2 to 15 μg/mL against Gram-positive bacteria including *S. aureus* [50], the activity of xanthohumol is in the same range. Several studies have focused on the antibacterial potential of xanthohumol which showed various MICs from 2 to 125 μg/mL on *S. aureus*, depending on the strain's resistance profile and the compound's purity [14,22]. According to our results, desmethylxanthohumol was slightly less active than xanthohumol, with MICs ranging from 19.5 to 39 μg/mL against *S. aureus* strains (Table 3). The structural difference between the two molecules is the 6′-methoxyl group for xanthohumol replaced by a 6′-phenol group for desmethylxanthohumol (Figure 1). The 6′-phenol substituent is considered as a crucial group in the equilibrium chalcone-flavanone but is not expected to contribute to the activity [51]. According to Ávila et al. [51], the methylation of the 6-phenol group could lead to less active compounds, which is not the case in our study. Desmethylxanthohumol is known for its antioxidant and apoptotic activities [52] but to our knowledge, no antibacterial potential was highlighted. Olivella et al. [53] have demonstrated that chalcones have the most favorable structure for a bacteriostatic action, in comparison with flavanones. In rats, xanthohumol is partially absorbed by intestinal cells and transported in blood. The non-absorbed part of xanthohumol can be transformed into the corresponding flavanone, isoxanthohumol, by the intestinal microbiota [54]. The conversion of isoxanthohumol into 8-prenyl-naringenin occurs only in the colon and not in the stomach and small intestine [55,56]. In this context, we also tested the activity of isoxanthohumol (Figure 4) against the strain MRSA T28.1. This compound showed a MIC equal to 39 μg/mL. It is interesting to note that, even if isoxanthohumol is less active than xanthohumol, its MIC was found to be of similar than desmethylxanthohumol.

The antibacterial potential of xanthohumol, desmethylxanthohumol and lupulone against MRSA is therefore promising. Their MICs are in the same order of magnitude as those obtained for antibacterial phenolic compounds known for their important activity against MRSA strains, with MICs varying between 1.56 and 125 μg/mL [4]. Most of them are known to be antibacterial compounds but they are not used to combat strains resistant to antibiotics. Some hops metabolites also showed antibacterial activities against others strains such as: *Bacillus subtilis, Clostridium difficile, Enterococcus strains* and *Streptococcus strains* for the Gram-positive bacteria; *Bacteroides fragilis, Helicobacter pylori* and *Yersinia enterocolitica* for the Gram-negative bacteria [20].

To overcome bacterial resistance, one of the strategies employed is the use of a combination of drugs, such as antibiotics combined with natural products, which has already shown promising results [57]. The checkerboard is a method to establish the best combination of products increasing the activity [32,58]. The antibacterial action of hops compounds can be enhanced by combining concomitantly xanthohumol with desmethylxanthohumol or with lupulone. The effect is twice as intense because the MIC is divided by two. By contrast, the combination of desmethylxanthohumol with lupulone leads to an antagonist effect (Table 4). The combination of natural products with antibiotics may in some cases have a synergistic effect. Xanthohumol and rifampicin can be 8 times more active when they are combined. Furthermore, for both xanthohumol and lupulone, the MIC for oxacillin drops below the threshold concentration of 2 μg/mL for oxacillin resistance, which means that in the presence of these synergistic compounds the strains will no longer be classified as MRSA, so reverting their resistance. Desmethylxanthohumol has an additive effect with oxacillin but this interaction does not render the strain susceptible to this antibiotic. Desmethylxanthohumol also has a promising interaction with ciprofloxacin and gentamicin. Some authors have previously detected synergies of xanthohumol and lupulone with polymyxin, ciprofloxacin or tobramycin [59]; and of xanthohumol with oxacillin or linezolid [14].

Kill curves demonstrated a great bactericidal action of xanthohumol at the MIC, of desmethylxanthohumol from 2 × MIC, whereas lupulone is slightly bactericidal after 24 h only at 4 × MIC (Figure 5). Comparing the activity of the two chalcones, desmethylxanthohumol showed a lower bactericidal action at the MIC than xanthohumol, which is probably linked to the presence of the 6′-hydroxyl group (Figure 1). Post-antibiotic effect is a part of pharmacodynamic studies, showing that xanthohumol and desmethylxanthohumol cause a significant delay for regrowth (Table 6). It means that the bacterial growth remains inhibited even after the product has been inactivated or metabolized by the body. These data provide an indication of the delay between two applications in a clinical situation. This is the first time that PAE is analyzed for hop compounds. This effect underlines an important reduction time for recovery which means that in vivo models will have to be checked for delay in drug administration.

Xanthohumol, desmethylxanthohumol and lupulone showed an inhibition of the biofilm formation of the *S. aureus* model strain on abiotic surface, with a sub-inhibitory action for desmethylxanthohumol and lupulone (Figure 7). Rozalski et al. studied the anti-adherent potential of a hops extract enriched in xanthohumol, pure xanthohumol and a spent hops extract rich in various common flavonols and flavanols [14]. They demonstrated a potent effect of xanthohumol on the biofilm formation at the MIC with 86.5% of inhibition. In comparison, our results showed an inhibition close to 100% at the MIC for the selected MRSA clinical isolate. In addition, we have also demonstrated that a previous formation of the biofilm does not prevent hops compounds to act on bacteria. In both cases, desmethylxanthohumol and lupulone seem to be more effective than xanthohumol, with an inhibition of the biofilm formation and a biofilm destruction at sub-inhibitory concentrations (Figure 7). Bogdanova et al. [23] also showed an anti-biofilm potential of some hops compounds but lower than that of our study. This result could be related to a lower purity of their products (from 82 to 87% in Reference [23]). This potential has been confirmed on a synthetic bone substitute which is the natural colonized substrate of *S. aureus* T28.1 (Figure 7). Even if the inhibition of the biofilm formation is found somewhat less intense in bone substitute than on inert surface, this potential remains very interesting, in particular for desmethylxanthohumol and lupulone. Moreover, according to our results, the anti-biofilm effect for these two products seems to be independent of the bactericidal effect pointed out with kill curves (Figure 5). To our knowledge, the anti-biofilm effect has never been assessed for hops compounds on bone substitutes. These data confirmed the promising potential of hops compounds to tackle MRSA not only on planktonic cells (MIC, kill curves) but also on biofilms approaching clinical situations.

Diabetic foot infections (DFI) affect one ulcerated foot out of two and in many cases lead to serious complications [60]. About 50% of patients hospitalized for a DFI suffer from an osteomyelitis and the prevalence of MRSA is often associated [61]. Low diffusion in necrotic tissues emphasizes topical antibiotic therapy for the management of mildly to moderately infected diabetic foot ulcers which has shown satisfactory results in some cases, allowing high concentrations of antibiotics at the site of infection without potentially toxic systemic levels [62]. Some medical devices such as beads loaded with antibiotics can bring high concentrations of local antibiotics for a long time in the case of deep wounds [63,64]. In addition, some topical antimicrobial agents, such as impregnated wound dressings with antimicrobials, could be of interest in the prevention or possibly the treatment of mild infections [65]. DFI generates many problems in clinical practice in terms of both diagnosis and therapeutic care mainly due to formation of persistent biofilms. The anti-biofilm action of hops metabolites both on artificial surface and on a synthetic bone substitute could bring out a new perspective to treat infected diabetic foot ulcers, an emerging public health problem. Thus, hop phenolic compounds with their dual action, antibacterial and anti-biofilm, are potential agents in the treatment of infections due to MRSA. Their additive or synergistic action with antibiotics could render treatments more effective and thus could prevent potential systemic toxicity if used in topical application. In this context, we evaluated the antiproliferative activity of the three phenolic compounds on different human cell lines and in particular against the human osteoblasts MG-63 cell line. After 48 h exposure, we showed a toxicity of xanthohumol on the targeted cell line. In the literature, data on its cytotoxicity depend on the cell type used and is very variable. For example, Ho et al. and Yong et al. have determined respectively an IC_{50} of about 75 and 100 μg/mL against a human hepatocellular carcinoma [66] and a lung cell line [67]. These concentrations are higher than the active doses reported in our work. In vivo studies have also confirmed the good safety at approximately 1000 mg of xanthohumol/kg of body weight of mice [68] and up to 180 mg of compound in humans for a short intake [69]. According to our results, desmethylxanthohumol is the less toxic compound on the MG-63 osteoblastic cells. However, considering its moderate activity, bactericidal and anti-biofilm concentrations would be toxic. To our knowledge, there is no comparison data available in the literature. Special attention has to be paid on lupulone. Its very pronounced antibacterial activity makes it non-toxic at the active doses. Moreover, anti-biofilm concentrations (MIC/4 and MIC/2) lead to a cell viability close to 100%. Comparing with the literature, some authors have determined IC_{50} ranging from 3.7 to 4.4 μg/mL on prostate cancer cells, which is close to other results [70] and IC_{50} from 8.3 to 16.6 μg/mL on breast cancer cells [71]. IC_{50} values are always higher than the active doses we have identified. All these data make lupulone a very good candidate for a topical bone application. Further research could be done by combining xanthohumol or desmethylxanthohumol with antibiotics as it would reduce the dose and avoid toxicity.

In addition, we evaluated the antiparasitic activity of the main chalcones and the main acylphloroglucinols of hop against two parasites: *Trypanosoma brucei brucei* (Tbb) and *Leishmania mexicana mexicana* (Lmm). Human African trypanosomiasis and leishmaniasis are indeed two protozoan infections considered as neglected tropical diseases with a strong impact on human health because in particular fatal if untreated [16,17]. Lupulone was the most active compound and humulone the less active. The four compounds tested were more active against Tbb than against Lmm (Table 6). Data on the antiparasitic activities of hops compounds are quite limited and especially concern xanthohumol. This chalcone was active against *Plasmodium falciparum* [24] and against *Leishmania amazonensis* [72] with IC_{50} in the μM range.

4. Materials and Methods

4.1. Phytochemical Analysis

4.1.1. General Experimental Procedures

For extraction and fractionation, synthesis grade ethanol (EtOH) and dichloromethane (DCM) were furnished by VWR Prolabo® (Fontenay-sous-Bois, France). Water was bi-distilled. All organic solvents for Centrifugal Partition Chromatography (CPC) purification were High Pressure Liquid Chromatography (HPLC) grade except for the n-heptane which was synthesis grade (Carlo Erba Reagents®, Val-de-Reuil, France). Ethyl acetate (EtOAc) and methanol (MeOH) were purchased from Fisher Scientific® (Illkirch, France). Water was purified using Millipore Integral 5 (Merck®, Trosly-Breuil, France) water purification system with a resistivity of not less than 18 $M\Omega \cdot cm^{-1}$. For analyses, acetonitrile (LC-MS grade) was purchased in Carlo Erba Reagents® (Val de Reuil, France), whereas methanol (LC-MS grade) came from Fischer Scientific® (Illkirch, France). The chloroform-d6 ($CDCl_3$) and MeOD for Nuclear Magnetic Resonance (NMR) experiments was obtained from Euriso-Top® (Gif-sur-Yvette, France).

Analytical Thin Layer Chromatography (TLC) were performed on pre-coated silica gel 60 F (0.25 mm, Merck®, Darmstadt, Germany). Detection was achieved at 254 and 366 nm, then by spraying with the unspecific anisaldehyde sulphuric reagent and heating at 100 °C for 10 min.

Ultra-High Performance Liquid Chromatography (UHPLC) analyses and quantification were carried out using an Acquity UPLC® H-Class Waters® system (Waters, Guyancourt, France) equipped with a diode array detector (DAD) and an Acquity QDa ESI-Quadrupole Mass Spectrometer. The software used was Empower 3. The stationary phase was a Waters® Acquity BEH C18 column (2.1 × 50 mm, 1.7 μm) connected to a 0.2 μm in-line filter. Preparative HPLC was performed using a Shimadzu® HPLC system equipped with a LC-20AP binary high-pressure pump, a CBM-20A controller and a SPD-M20A diode array detector. The software used was LabSolution. The stationary phase was a VisionHT HL C18 (5 μm, 250 × 22 mm) column (Grace®, France).

CPC was performed using an Armen instrument 250 mL rotor (SCPC-250-L) provided by Gilson® (Saint-Avé, France). CPC analyses were monitored using Shimadzu® pump and detector.

Nuclear Magnetic Resonance (NMR) spectra were recorded on a Bruker® DPX-500 spectrometer. High Resolution Mass Spectrometry (HR-MS) analyses were carried out using a Thermo Fisher Scientific® Exactive Orbitrap Mass Spectrometer equipped with an electrospray ion source.

4.1.2. Plant Extract Preparation and Fractionation

Female hop plants (*Humulus lupulus* L., cultivar 'Nugget') were harvested at maturity stage at the Beck farm (Bailleul, Northern France), at the time of harvesting of hop by producers in September. A voucher specimen was kept at the Faculty of pharmacy in Lille (laboratory of pharmacognosy) under reference NugBeck2015. After drying for 10 days at room temperature, protected from light, rhizomes, stems, leaves and cones were powderized separately with a blender. Crude hydro-alcoholic extracts of each part were obtained after an ethanol/water (9:1; *v*/*v*; 15 mL/g) mixture-based extraction with three successive macerations of four hours and one overnight, stirring in the dark. The percentage yields (PY) on a dry weight basis of each crude extract were: 35.5% (cones), 20.3% (leaves), 21.1% (rhizomes) and 17.2% (stems). The crude extract of female cones was fractionated by a liquid-liquid separation using dichloromethane (DCM) and water to obtain two sub-extracts. The corresponding sub-extracts were obtained with percentages yields of 52% and 48% respectively

4.1.3. Purification of Phenolic Compounds

Xanthohumol, desmethylxanthohumol, humulone, cohumulone, lupulone, colupulone were purified from the DCM sub-extract of cones in several steps. A first fractionation was performed by CPC. Using the Arizona solvent system P: n-heptane/EtOAc/MeOH/water (6:5:6:5; *v*/*v*), the rotor was entirely filled at 30 mL/min with the aqueous stationary phase in the ascending mode with rotation (500 rpm). Then, the rotation speed was increased from 500 to 1600 rpm. The organic mobile phase was pumped into the column in ascending mode at a flow rate of 8 mL/min. DCM sub-extract (2 g), initially dissolved in 10 mL of the organic/aqueous phase mixture (1:1), was filtered with a Millipore (0.45 μm) syringe filter and was injected immediately after the displacement of stationary phase (approximatively 80 mL). Fractions of 8 mL were collected every min. The CPC was run in ascending mode for 60 min and then switched to extrusion mode (recovery of the stationary phase) for 10 additional minutes at 30 mL/min with the same rotor speed (1600 rpm). The content of the outgoing organic phase was monitored by online UV absorbance measurement at 254 nm and 370 nm. All the fractions were checked by TLC and developed with toluene/ethyl acetate/formic acid (73:18:9; *v*/*v*) in order to regroup 5 sub-fractions (MC1 to MC5) from ascendant mode and 3 sub-fractions (MC6 to MC8) from extrusion mode. This CPC method allowed us to purify, in one step, xanthohumol (Figure 1), with 98% purity from MC4. The other compounds were purified from other sub-fractions using preparative HPLC. The mobile phase was composed of water (solvent A) and acetonitrile (solvent B). The following proportions of solvent B were: 10–75% (0–5 min), 75% (5–30 min), 75–100% (30–35 min) and 100% (35–45 min) at 12 mL/min. Injections with 500 μL of a 60 mg/mL fraction solution in methanol were performed. This process allowed us to purify several acylphloroglucinol derivatives (α- and β-acids) from sub-fractions MC1 and MC2, as well as another chalcone, desmethylxanthohumol, from the sub-fraction MC7, with a purity greater than 95% (Figure 1). Throughout the process, we protected the samples of the light as much as possible.

4.1.4. UHPLC-UV-MS Analyses

The crude hydro-ethanolic extracts of hop parts (cones, leaves, stems and rhizomes) were analyzed by UHPLC-UV-MS. The mobile phase consisted of 0.1% formic acid in water and of 0.1% formic acid in acetonitrile. The gradient of acetonitrile was: 50% (0–1 min), 50–75% (1–3 min), 75% (3–5 min), 75–100% (5–7 min) and 100% (7–9,5 min) at 0.3 mL/min. Column temperature was set at 30 °C. Solutions of crude extracts were prepared in MeOH at 100 μg/mL for cones and 1 mg/mL for the other parts. Injection volume was 2 μL. The main chalcones and acylphloroglucinols were identified on the basis of the retention time of the purified standards and their mass spectra.

The ionization was performed in negative mode. Cone voltage was set at 10 V. Probe temperature was 600 °C. Capillary voltage was 0.8 kV. The MS-Scan mode was used from 100 to 1000 Da.

4.1.5. Quantification Using UHPLC-UV

The most abundant prenylated chalcones and acylphloroglucinol derivatives were quantified in hop crude hydro-ethanolic extracts (cones, leaves, stems and rhizomes), according to the international guidelines for analytical techniques for quality control of pharmaceuticals [73]. Quantification was performed in UV at 370 nm for chalcones and 330 nm for acylphloroglucinols. *Co*- and *ad*-acids were quantified from the respective calibration curves of the *n*-acids (humulone for alpha acids and lupulone for beta acids), using molecular weight ratio. Desmethylxanthohumol was quantified from xanthohumol calibration curve, using molecular weight ratio. Solutions of crude extracts were prepared in MeOH at 100 μg/mL for cones and 1 mg/mL for the other parts. Sample solutions were prepared in triplicate the same day. Aliquots of each solution (2 μL) were injected in triplicate.

Stock solutions of xanthohumol, humulone and lupulone, previously purified, were prepared at the concentration of 1 mg/mL in MeOH for quantification, then stored at −20 °C until use. Fifteen working solutions (100 μg/mL to 2.5 ng/mL) were daily prepared by dilutions. Three mixed solutions containing the three analytes were prepared at the concentrations of 100, 50 and 25 μg/mL from stock solutions. Then, lower concentrations were obtained from these intermediate solutions by successive dilutions in MeOH. Calibration curves were designed to cover the expected range of concentrations in samples after preliminary injection of crude extracts solutions. Nine, ten and twelve concentration levels were respectively used for calibration curves of lupulone, xanthohumol and humulone. They were built by plotting peak area (y) as a function of the nominal concentration for each calibration level (x) and then fitted by weighted ($1/x$) least square linear regression. Linearity and precision of the method, as well as the limit of detection (LOD) and the limit of quantification (LOQ) were reported in Table S1 (Supplementary Material). LOD was defined as the lowest concentration with a $S/N > 3$. LOQ was defined as the lowest concentration with a deviation <20% on back calculation. Intra and inter-day precisions were evaluated on cone sample solutions. They were prepared on three different days, in triplicate each day ($n = 3$, $k = 3$). 2 µL of each solution was injected 3 times.

4.1.6. Structural Elucidation

Structures of purified compounds were determined using NMR and HR-MS. Mono- (^1H and ^{13}C) and bi-dimensional (COSY, HSQC, HMBC) spectra were carried out for each compound. Prenylated chalcones were solubilized in deuterated methanol (MeOD) whereas acylphloroglucinol derivatives were solubilized in deuterated chloroform ($CDCl_3$). HR-MS analyses were carried out in positive mode with a range of m/z 100–1000 amu. Products were solubilized in methanol with a drop of DCM for the acylphloroglucinols.

4.2. Antimicrobial Bioassays

4.2.1. Antibacterial Screening of Extracts and Sub-Extracts Using Agar Dilution Method

Clinical bacterial isolates from human samples collected in Lille (France) and some collection strains were used. The first screening step on pathogenic bacteria was carried out with crude hydro-alcoholic extracts of different hop parts (Table 1). The second screening was performed using sub-extracts of cones on Gram-positive bacteria, including methicillin-sensitive *Staphylococcus aureus* (MSSA) and methicillin-resistant *Staphylococcus aureus* (MSSA) strains (Table 2). These tests were carried out on Petri dishes, Mueller-Hinton Agar (MHA) (Oxoid, UK) was mixed with the plant extract solution in MeOH at 5% (solvent control: 5% MeOH). Final extract concentrations in Petri dishes ranged from 1250 to 4.9 µg/mL. A multi-headed inoculator allowed spotting bacterial strains at 10^5 CFU/mL in cysteinated Ringer (CR) solution (Merck®, France). Minimal Inhibitory Concentrations (MICs) were visually determined after 24 h of incubation at 37 °C.

4.2.2. Antibacterial Susceptibility of Compounds Using Broth Microdilution Method

For bioassays, xanthohumol, desmethylxanthohumol, humulone, cohumulone, lupulone and colupulone were used had a minimum purity of 95% (HPLC-UV). The protocol employed was inspired by Abedini et al. [74] with some modifications. Products were solubilized in DMSO and serially diluted two-fold in MH medium. A bacterial suspension at 10^5 CFU/mL was added to obtain a final volume of 200 µL. Final phenolic product concentrations in wells ranged from 625 to 2.4 µg/mL (exception for lupulone for which dilutions were continued until 0.3 µg/mL). The susceptibility of the strain to DMSO has previously been assessed, the DMSO concentration in wells taken into account did not exceed 5% (concentration without effect on growth). Plates were incubated overnight with stirring (60 rpm) at 37 °C. The bacterial growth was indicated visually and by a developer of enzymatic activity (iodonitrotetrazolium chloride—INT, AppliChem, Germany) which reveals bacterial growth by a purple color after 15 min heating at 55 °C.

For the following experiments, the MRSA strain T28.1, isolated from a pathological sample of osteitis, was used. It was previously characterized by DNA biochips, which allowed highlighting some β-lactamases and the SCC-mec genes confirming the methicillin resistance [30]. Moreover, genes for enzymes and proteins involved in the capsule biosynthesis (capH5, capJ5 and capK5) and several intracellular adhesion proteins implicated in biofilm formation (icaA, icaC and icaD) were present.

The commercial product, isoxanthohumol, was also tested against *S. aureus* T28.1 (purity superior to 95%, Phytolab®, Germany).

4.2.3. Synergies with Selected Antibiotics (Checkerboard Method)

Checkerboard method was used to assess the potential co-action of xanthohumol, desmethylxanthohumol and lupulone between them or with some antibiotics [32,58]. Antibiotics were previously selected on the basis of a first screening using E-tests (BioMérieux®, France). They covered several classes and are currently used to treat either *S. aureus* infections or bone infections: oxacillin (purity 95%, Acros Organics, Belgium), ciprofloxacin, gentamicin and rifampicin (purity 99.9%, 65.7% and 99.2% respectively, PanReac AppliChem®, Germany). Each test was performed on a 96-well microplate using an 8-by-8 well configuration. Concentration of hops phenolic compounds and antibiotics tested ranged from MIC/4 to 4xMIC. Wells were filled with 100 μL of MH medium, 10 μL of each compound (DMSO for products and water for antibiotics) and 80 μL of a 10^5 CFU/mL bacterial suspension with appropriate solvent controls. Final concentration in DMSO was 5%, which did not affect the bacterial growth. The MIC of each product alone was checked at each test. Microplates were incubated overnight at 60 rpm and 37 °C. The bacterial growth was visually assessed and confirmed by revealing bacterial enzymatic activity by adding INT.

After visual analysis, the combination with the highest activity was determined by the calculation of the fractional inhibitory concentration (FIC) index [32], interpreted as synergistic (FIC < 0.5), additive ($0.5 \leq \text{FIC} \leq 1$), indifferent ($1 < \text{FIC} \leq 4$) or antagonist (FIC > 4).

$$\text{FIC index} = \frac{\text{MIC A with B}}{\text{MIC A alone}} + \frac{\text{MIC B with A}}{\text{MIC B alone}}$$

4.2.4. Kill Curves

This experiment allowed following in time the effect of the product on a growing bacterial population, highlighting the bactericidal or bacteriostatic effect [75]. Stock solutions of xanthohumol, desmethylxanthohumol and lupulone were prepared in DMSO 20 times more concentrated than the desired final concentrations (MIC/4 to 4xMIC). An aliquot of 0.5 mL of purified product in DMSO was added to 8.5 mL of brain heart infusion (BHI) medium (Oxoid, UK). 1 mL of bacterial suspension at 10^5 CFU/mL was then introduced to the culture tube. A 5% DMSO control served as a negative control and was performed at each test. Culture tubes were incubated at 37 °C for 24 h. Counts were made every 2 h until 8 h and at 24 h by plating aliquots of serial tenfold dilutions on MHA. The determined bacterial concentrations were then converted into log(CFU/mL) and were expressed as a function of time. The detection threshold of this method was 10 CFU/mL and 1 log(CFU/mL) on graphics.

4.2.5. Post-Antibiotic Effect (PAE)

This method allows quantifying the delayed regrowth of a bacterial population following exposure to an active compound [76]. Stock solutions of xanthohumol, desmethylxanthohumol and lupulone were prepared in DMSO 20 times more concentrated than the desired final concentrations (MIC/4 to $4 \times$ MIC). A 2 h pre-treatment with purified prenylated compounds was performed using 8.5 mL of BHI medium, 0.5 mL of purified product in DMSO and 1 mL of a bacterial suspension at 10^5 CFU/mL, incubated at 37 °C. Final concentrations in DMSO did not exceed 5%. The hop compound was then inactivated by a 1000-fold dilution. After inactivation, a growth curve was performed with counts at 30 min and every 2 h. The growth lag was quantified by comparison with the control, using the following formula:

$$\text{PAE} = \text{T} - \text{C}$$

T is the time needed for the bacterial population to grow by 1 log(CFU/mL) at the given concentration, C is the corresponding time for the control (Figure 5)

4.2.6. Anti-Biofilm Tests

These experiments were inspired and adapted from Liu et al. [77]. They were performed using a 96-well microplate with a flat bottom.

On Artificial Surface

First, the effect of xanthohumol, desmethylxanthohumol and lupulone was assessed on the biofilm formation: 180 µL of BHI medium containing glucose at 10 mg/mL was added to each well of a 96-well microplate with 10 µL of the product previously solubilized in DMSO and 10 µL of a 10^5 CFU/mL bacterial suspension. The maximum concentration in DMSO was 5%. Final concentrations of purified products were from MIC/4 to 4 × MIC. After 24 h incubation at 37 °C, wells were voided and washed 3 times with phosphate buffered saline solution (PBS, Sigma-Aldrich, Saint-Quentin Fallavier, France). Plates were then dried and 150 µL of crystal violet solution at 20 mg/mL in MeOH (Sigma-Aldrich®, Saint-Quentin Fallavier, France) were added for 15 min. After removing crystal violet, 150 µL of EtOH were added to solubilize crystal violet present in adherent bacteria. The optical density was read at 570 nm.

The effect was also evaluated after the biofilm formation in order to evaluate if the hop phenolic compounds are able to destroy it. A first culture of 24 h at 37 °C with 190 µL of BHI medium and 10 µL of a 10^5 CFU/mL bacterial suspension allowed producing the biofilm. Wells were voided and washed with PBS. The biofilm was then treated with xanthohumol, desmethylxanthohumol or lupulone diluted at 5% in the BHI medium to obtain a final volume of 200 µL. Plates were incubated for 24 h at 37 °C, then voided and colored with crystal violet as above.

On Synthetic Bone Substitute

β-Tricalcium phosphate discs (Cerasorb®, Curasan, Germany) were used as bone substitute. Non-glucose enriched BHI medium was used here, because the bacterial glucose metabolism causes an acidification of the culture medium which leads to the disintegration of the discs. Discs were introduced in a 24-well plate: 1.8 mL of BHI media were added with 0.1 mL of product in DMSO (5%) and 0.1 mL of a 10^5 CFU/mL bacterial suspension. Final concentrations of hop phenolic compounds were from MIC/4 to 4 × MIC. After 24 h at 37 °C, counts were performed in two steps. First, planktonic bacteria were counted from 100 µL of the culture supernatant by plating tenfold dilutions on MHA. Then, bacteria adhering to the discs were counted: discs were removed and washed with a CR solution, then, 10 mL of CR were added to each disk and treated 1 min by sonication (35 kHz) and 30 s by vortex. The obtained suspension was enumerated as previously. The detection threshold was also 1 log(CFU/mL).

4.2.7. Antiparasitic Activity of Hops Using Broth Microdilution Method

Tbb were cultivated in HMI9 medium containing 10% heat-inactivated foetal bovine serum (FBS) (Sigma-Aldrich), 150 mM L-cysteine and 20 mM beta-mercaptoethanol at 37 °C (CO_2 5%). Lmm (MHOM/BZ/84/BEL46) were cultivated in SDM-79 medium (Gibco) supplemented with 15% heat-inactivated FBS (Sigma-Aldrich) and 5 mg/L hemin at 28 °C (CO_2 5%). Antiparasitic bioassays were performed as described by Bero et al. [17]. Suramin (SUR) and pentamidine (PEN) were used as positive controls respectively. The hops compounds (xanthohumol, desmethylxanthohumol, humulone, lupulone) concentration that inhibits 50% of the cell viability (IC_{50}) was determined using GraphPad Prism, version 5.01 (GraphPad Software, San Diego, CA, USA).

4.3. Antiproliferative Effect of Purified Compounds on Human Cell Lines

Several human cell lines were used for the cytotoxic bioassays: non-cancer lung fibroblasts (WI-38), hepatocellular carcinoma (Hep-G2), osteosarcoma (MG-63) and the mouse monocyte macrophage J774. Cells were seeded into wells of a 96-well microplate in a Gibco™ Dulbecco's modified eagles medium (DMEM), except for MG-63 which were cultivated in a minimum essential medium (MEM) (ThermoFisher Scientific, Illkirch-Graffenstaden, France). Both media were enriched with 10% FBS (ThermoFisher Scientific, France) and some antibiotics (mixture penicillin/streptomycin 100 UI/mL, Sigma Aldrich). After one or two days at 37 °C (5% of CO_2), wells were emptied by suction. Cells were then treated with hops compounds (xanthohumol, desmethylxanthohumol, humulone, lupulone) in DMSO at 0.2% in the culture medium, to obtain a final volume of 100 μL in wells (negative control: 0.2% DMSO). Camptothecin was used as a positive control. After 48 to 72 h exposure, culture medium was replaced by 10% of Alamar blue or 3-(4,5-dimethylthiazol-2-yl)-2,5-diphenyltetrazolium bromide (MTT) in the medium (ThermoFisher Scientific®, Illkirch, France) and plates were incubated the time necessary to the reaction. Results were measured respectively by fluorescence (excitation 530 nm and emission 590 nm) or by optical density at 550 nm. The IC_{50} of each product was determined using GraphPad Prism (version 5.01).

4.4. Statistical Analyses

Statistical analyses were carried out using the software R, version 3.4.1 (The R Foundation for Statistical Computing, Vienna, Austria). Each experiment was performed in independent triplicates. For each distribution, the normality of the residues was assessed using Shapiro test. If the normality was accepted, an ANOVA and the Tukey HSD test were performed. If the normality was refused, Kruskal Wallis and Dunn's tests were used at a significance level of $p = 0.05$.

5. Conclusions

Xanthohumol, desmethylxanthohumol and lupulone from hops, with their dual antibacterial and anti-biofilm actions, are potential agents in the treatment of infections due to MRSA. Their additive or synergistic actions with antibiotics could render treatments more effective and thus could prevent toxicity at systemic level if used in topical application. Their chemical structures differ from current anti-staphylococcal agents and enable us to assume that they act on a different target site of action in *S. aureus*. The exact identification of this target is a future challenge. Moreover, for the first-time, activity of hops phenolic compounds was highlighted on the Tbb and Lmm parasites.

Supplementary Materials: The following are available online, Table S1. Linearity and sensitivity of the quantification method by UPLC-UV for xanthohumol, humulone and lupulone, Table S2. ^{1}H and ^{13}C NMR data for xanthohumol and desmethylxanthohumol in MeOD[a], Table S3. ^{1}H and ^{13}C NMR data for humulone and cohumulone in CDC13[a], Table S4. ^{1}H and ^{13}C NMR data for lupulone and colupulone in CDC13[a], Figure S1. Chromatograms at 370 nm of the crude hydro-ethanolic extract of cones and purified chalcones (desmethylxanthohumol and xanthohumol), Figure S2. Chromatograms at 330 nm of the crude hydro-ethanolic extract of cones and purified acylphloroglucinol derivatives (cohumulone, humulone, colupulone and lupulone), Figure S3. Total ion chromatogram of the crude hydro-ethanolic extract of cones in negative mode and selected ion recording of purified chalcones (desmethylxanthohumol and xanthohumol) and acylphloroglucinol derivatives (cohumulone, humulone, colupulone and lupulone).

Author Contributions: In this paper, L.B. (PhD student) performed the purification of hops phenolic compounds, all antibacterial bioassays and some cytotoxicity assays (Hep-G2). S.S. is one of the supervisors of L.B. and is head of the department of pharmacognosy. N.B. performed the quantification of compounds in different extracts and J.J. prepared the extracts. C.B. performed the antiparasitic bioassays and some cytotoxicity experiments (WI-38 and J774) and J.Q.-L. designed and supervised these bioassays. S.M. helped L.B. in the realization of antibacterial experiments and C.N. conceived and supervised these bioassays. V.R. supervised cytotoxicity assays against Hep-G2. S.B. and T.H. contributed in the realization of a few experiments. F.C. conceived and performed cytotoxicity experiments against MG-63. J.S. helped L.B. in the purification of compounds and the realization of some antibacterial bioassays. C.R. is the supervisor of L.B. and is at the origin of the project. She obtained the funding of the PhD fellowship of L.B. She designed the entire project and she mainly supervised the phytochemistry part. C.R., L.B., C.N., J.Q.-L. and N.B. contributed to the writing of the paper and all of the authors approved the manuscript.

Funding: This work was supported by the Region Hauts-de-France and the University of Lille 2 (PhD fellowship of L. Bocquet), as well as European Union, French State and the Region of Hauts-de-France (CPER/FEDER Alibiotech project).

Acknowledgments: The authors wish to thank Beck family (Bailleul, France) to supply hop samples each year. They are grateful to PSM (University of Lille, France, J.F. Goossens) and LARMN (University of Lille, France, N. Azaroual), as well as the laboratory of bacteriology (LIRIC, France) and the laboratory of toxicology (S. Anthérieu) for access to equipment. They also acknowledge Charlotte Maillet and Isabelle Houcke (LIRIC, France) and Maude Bourlet (UCL) for their skillful technical assistance. The authors wish to thank Eric Senneville (Centre Hospitalier Gustave Dron, Department of Infectious Diseases) for his helpful comments on the manuscript.

Conflicts of Interest: The authors declare no conflict of interest.

References

1. OMS. Global Action Plan on Antimicrobial Resistance. 2015. Available online: www.wpro.who.int/entity/drug_resistance/resources/global_action_plan_eng.pdf (accessed on 4 March 2019).
2. ANSES; ANSM; Santé Publique France. Consommation D'antibiotiques et Résistance aux Antibiotiques en France: Nécessité D'une Mobilisation Déterminée et Durable. 2016. Available online: http://invs.santepubliquefrance.fr/Publications-et-outils/Rapports-et-syntheses/Maladies-infectieuses/2016/Consommation-d-antibiotiques-et-resistance-aux-antibiotiques-en-France-necessite-d-une-mobilisation-determinee-et-durable (accessed on 4 March 2019).
3. Kavanagh, K.T.; Abusalaim, S.; Calderon, L.E. The incidence of MRSA infections in the United States: Is a more comprehensive tracking system needed? *Antimicrob. Resist. Infect. Control* **2017**, *6*, 34. [CrossRef] [PubMed]
4. Gibbons, S. Anti-staphylococcal plant natural products. *Nat. Prod. Rep.* **2004**, *21*, 263–277. [CrossRef] [PubMed]
5. Abreu, A.C.; McBain, A.J.; Simões, M. Plants as sources of new antimicrobials and resistance-modifying agents. *Nat. Prod. Rep.* **2012**, *29*, 1007–1021. [CrossRef] [PubMed]
6. European Centre for Disease Prevention and Control. *Surveillance of Antimicrobial Resistance in Europe 2016*; Annual Report of the European Antimicrobial Resistance Surveillance Network (EARS-Net); ECDC: Stockholm, Sweden, 2017.
7. Cosgrove, S.E.; Sakoulas, G.; Perencevich, E.N.; Schwaber, M.J.; Karchmer, A.W.; Carmeli, Y. Comparison of mortality associated with methicillin-resistant and methicillin-susceptible *Staphylococcus aureus* bacteremia: A meta-analysis. *Clin. Infect. Dis.* **2003**, *36*, 53–59. [CrossRef] [PubMed]
8. Hanberger, H.; Walther, S.; Leone, M.; Barie, P.S.; Rello, J.; Lipman, J.; Marshall, J.C.; Anzueto, A.; Sakr, Y.; Pickkers, P.; et al. Increased mortality associated with meticillin-resistant *Staphylococcus aureus* (MRSA) infection in the Intensive Care Unit: Results from the EPIC II study. *Int. J. Antimicrob. Agents* **2011**, *38*, 331–335. [CrossRef] [PubMed]
9. Dunyach-Remy, C.; Ngba Essebe, C.; Sotto, A.; Lavigne, J.P. *Staphylococcus aureus* Toxins and Diabetic Foot Ulcers: Role in Pathogenesis and Interest in Diagnosis. *Toxins* **2016**, *8*, 209. [CrossRef] [PubMed]
10. Stavri, M.; Piddock, L.J.; Gibbons, S. Bacterial efflux pump inhibitors from natural sources. *J. Antimicrob. Chemother.* **2007**, *59*, 1247–1260. [CrossRef] [PubMed]
11. Handzlik, J.; Matys, A.; Kieć-Kononowicz, K. Recent Advances in Multi-Drug Resistance (MDR) Efflux Pump Inhibitors of Gram-Positive Bacteria *S. aureus*. *Antibiotics* **2013**, *2*, 28–45. [CrossRef]
12. Brincat, J.P.; Broccatelli, F.; Sabatini, S.; Frosini, M.; Neri, A.; Kaatz, G.W.; Cruciani, G.; Carosati, E. Ligand Promiscuity between the Efflux Pumps Human P-Glycoprotein and *S. aureus* NorA. *ACS Med. Chem. Lett.* **2012**, *3*, 248–251. [CrossRef]
13. Gould, I.M.; David, M.Z.; Esposito, S.; Garau, J.; Lina, G.; Mazzei, T.; Peters, G. New insights into meticillin-resistant *Staphylococcus aureus* (MRSA) pathogenesis, treatment and resistance. *Int. J. Antimicrob. Agents* **2012**, *39*, 96–104. [CrossRef]
14. Rozalski, M.; Micota, B.; Sadowska, B.; Stochmal, A.; Jedrejek, D.; Wieckowska-Szakiel, M.; Rozalska, B. Antiadherent and Antibiofilm Activity of *Humulus lupulus* L. Derived Products: New Pharmacological Properties. *BioMed Res. Int.* **2013**, *2013*, 7. [CrossRef]
15. Keita, M.; Bouteille, B.; Enanga, B.; Vallat, J.M.; Dumas, M. *Trypanosoma brucei brucei*: A Long-Term Model of Human African Trypanosomiases in Mice, Meningo-Encaphalitis, Astrocytosis, and Neurological Disorders. *Exp. Parasitol.* **1997**, *85*, 183–192. [CrossRef]

16. Ponte-Sucre, A. An Overview of *Trypanosoma brucei* Infections: An Intense Host-Parasite Interaction. *Front. Microbiol.* **2016**, *7*, 2126. [CrossRef]
17. Bero, J.; Hannaert, V.; Chataigne, G.; Hérent, M.F.; Quetin-Leclercq, J. In vitro antitrypanosomal and antileishmanial activity of plants used in Benin in traditional medicine and bio-guided fractionation of the most active extract. *J. Ethnopharmacol.* **2011**, *137*, 998–1002. [CrossRef]
18. Steenackers, B.; De Cooman, L.; De Vos, D. Chemical transformations of characteristic hop secondary metabolites in relation to beer properties and the brewing process: A review. *Food Chem.* **2015**, *172*, 742–756. [CrossRef]
19. Bocquet, L.; Sahpaz, S.; Hilbert, J.L.; Rambaud, C.; Rivière, C. *Humulus lupulus* L., a very popular beer ingredient and medicinal plant: Overview of its phytochemistry, its bioactivity, and its biotechnology. *Phytochem. Rev.* **2018**, *17*, 1047–1090. [CrossRef]
20. Bocquet, L.; Sahpaz, S.; Rivière, C. An Overview of the Antimicrobial Properties of Hop. In *Natural Antimicrobial Agents*; Mérillon, J.M., Rivière, C., Eds.; Series Sustainable Development and Biodiversity; Springer International Publishing AG: Cham, Switzerland, 2018; Volume 19, pp. 31–54.
21. Teuber, M.; Schmalreck, A.F. Membrane leakage in *Bacillus subtilis* 168 induced by the hop constituents lupulone, humulone, isohumulone and humulinic acid. *Arch. Für Mikrobiol.* **1973**, *94*, 159–171. [CrossRef]
22. Gerhäuser, C. Broad spectrum anti-infective potential of xanthohumol from hop (*Humulus lupulus* L.) in comparison with activities of other hop constituents and xanthohumol metabolites. *Mol. Nutr. Food Res.* **2005**, *49*, 827–831. [CrossRef]
23. Bogdanova, K.; Röderova, M.; Kolar, M.; Langova, K.; Dusek, M.; Jost, P.; Kubelkova, K.; Bostik, P.; Olsovska, J. Antibiofilm activity of bioactive hop compounds humulone, lupulone and xanthohumol toward susceptible and resistant staphylococci. *Res. Microbiol.* **2018**, *169*, 127–134. [CrossRef]
24. Frölich, S.; Schubert, C.; Bienzle, U.; Jenett-Siems, K. In Vitro Antiplasmodial activity of prenylated chalcone derivatives of hops (*Humulus lupulus*) and their interaction with Haemin. *J. Antimicrob. Chemother.* **2005**, *55*, 883–887. [CrossRef]
25. Srinivasan, V.; Goldberg, D.; Haas, G.J. Contribution to the Antimicrobial Spectrum of Hop Constituents. *Econ. Bot.* **2004**, *58*, 230–238. [CrossRef]
26. Höltzel, A.; Schlotterbeck, G.; Albert, K.; Bayer, E. Separation and characterisation of hop bitter acids by HPLC-^{1}H NMR coupling. *Chromatographia* **1996**, *42*, 499–505. [CrossRef]
27. Zhang, X.; Liang, X.; Xiao, H.; Xu, Q. Direct characterization of bitter acids in a crude hop extract by liquid chromatography-atmospheric pressure chemical ionization mass spectrometry. *J. Am. Soc. Mass Spectrom.* **2004**, *15*, 180–187. [CrossRef] [PubMed]
28. Vogel, S.; Ohmayer, S.; Brunner, G.; Heilmann, J. Natural and non-natural prenylated chalcones: Synthesis, cytotoxicity and anti-oxidative activity. *Bioorg. Med. Chem.* **2008**, *16*, 4286–4293. [CrossRef]
29. Intelmann, D.; Haseleu, G.; Hofmann, T. LC-MS/MS quantitation of hop-derived bitter compounds in beer using the ECHO technique. *J. Agric. Food Chem.* **2009**, *57*, 1172–1182. [CrossRef] [PubMed]
30. Senneville, E.; Brière, M.; Neut, C.; Messad, N.; Lina, G.; Richard, J.L.; Sotto, A.; Lavigne, J.P.; The French Study Group on the Diabetic Foot. First report of the predominance of clonal complex 398 *Staphylococcus aureus* strains in osteomyelitis complicating diabetic foot ulcers: A national French study. *Clin. Microbiol. Infect.* **2014**, *20*, O274–O277. [CrossRef]
31. EUCAST, European Committee on Antimicrobial Susceptibility Testing. Comité de l'Antibiogramme de la Société Française de Microbiologie. Recommandations. 2019. Available online: File:///C:/Users/celine/Desktop/CASFM2019_V1.0.pdf (accessed on 4 March 2019).
32. Bonapace, C.R.; Bosso, J.A.; Friedrich, L.V.; White, R.L. Comparison of methods of interpretation of checkerboard synergy testing. *Diagn. Microbiol. Infect. Dis.* **2002**, *44*, 363–366. [CrossRef]
33. Mahieux, S.; Nieto-Bobadilla, M.S.; Houcke, I.; Neut, C. How to Study Antimicrobial Activities of Plant Extracts: A Critical Point of View. In *Natural Antimicrobial Agents*; Mérillon, J.M., Rivière, C., Eds.; Series Sustainable Development and Biodiversity; Springer International Publishing AG: Cham, Switzerland, 2018; Volume 19, pp. 55–71.
34. Stoodley, P.; Sauer, K.; Davies, D.G.; Costerton, J.W. Biofilms as Complex Differentiated Communities. *Annu. Rev. Microbiol.* **2002**, *56*, 187–209. [CrossRef] [PubMed]

35. Centers for Disease Control and Prevention. *Antibiotic Resistance Threats in the United States, 2013*; Centers for Disease Control and Prevention: Atlanta, GA, USA, 2013. Available online: http://www.cdc.gov/drugresistance/threat-report-2013/pdf/ar-threats-2013-508.pdf (accessed on 4 March 2019).
36. Tacconelli, E.; Carrara, E.; Savoldi, A.; Harbarth, S.; Mendelson, M.; Monnet, D.L.; Pulcini, C.; Kahlmeter, G.; Kluytmans, J.; Carmeli, Y.; et al. Discovery, research, and development of new antibiotics: The WHO priority list of antibiotic-resistant bacteria and tuberculosis. *Lancet. Infect. Dis.* **2018**, *18*, 318–327. [CrossRef]
37. Arias, C.A.; Murray, B.E. A New Antibiotic and the Evolution of Resistance. *N. Engl. J. Med.* **2015**, *372*, 1168–1170. [CrossRef]
38. Ventola, C.L. The Antibiotic Resistance Crisis. Part 1: Causes and Threats. *PT* **2015**, *40*, 277–283.
39. Bollenbach, T. Antimicrobial interactions: Mechanisms and implications for drug discovery and resistance evolution. *Curr. Opin. Microbiol.* **2015**, *27*, 1–9. [CrossRef]
40. Mizobuchi, S.; Sato, Y. Antifungal Activities of Hop Bitter Resins and Related Compounds. *Agric. Biol. Chem.* **1985**, *49*, 399–403.
41. Schmalreck, A.F.; Teuber, M. Structural features determining the antibiotic potencies of natural and synthetic hop bitter resins, their precursors and derivatives. *Can. J. Microbiol.* **1975**, *21*, 205–212. [CrossRef]
42. Larson, A.E.; Yu, R.R.Y.; Lee, O.A.; Price, S.; Haas, G.J.; Johnson, E.A. Antimicrobial activity of hop extracts against *Listeria monocytogenes* in media and in food. *Int. J. Food Microbiol.* **1996**, *33*, 195–207. [CrossRef]
43. Cermak, P.; Olsovska, J.; Mikyska, A.; Dusek, M.; Kadleckova, Z.; Vanicek, J.; Nyc, O.; Sigler, K.; Bostikova, V.; Bostik, P. Strong antimicrobial activity of xanthohumol and other derivatives from hops (*Humulus lupulus* L.) on gut anaerobic bacteria. *APMIS* **2017**, *125*, 1033–1038. [CrossRef]
44. Langezaal, C.R.; Chandra, A.; Scheffer, J.J.C. Antimicrobial screening of essential oils and extracts of some *Humulus lupulus* L. cultivars. *Pharmaceutisch Weekblad. Sci. Ed.* **1992**, *14*, 353–356. [CrossRef]
45. Abram, V.; Čeh, B.; Vidmar, M.; Hercezi, M.; Lazić, N.; Bucik, V.; Mozina, S.S.; Kosir, I.J.; Kac, M.; Demsar, L.; et al. A comparison of antioxidant and antimicrobial activity between hop leaves and hop cones. *Ind. Crops Prod.* **2015**, *64*, 124–134. [CrossRef]
46. Prencipe, F.P.; Brighenti, V.; Rodolfi, M.; Mongelli, A.; d'all'Asta, C.; Ganino, T.; Bruni, R.; Pellati, F. Development of a new high-performance liquid chromatography method with diode array and electrospray ionization-mass spectrometry detection for the metabolite fingerprinting of bioactive compounds in *Humulus lupulus* L. *J. Chromatogr. A* **2014**, *1349*, 50–59. [CrossRef]
47. Čeh, B.; Kač, M.; Košir, I.J.; Abram, V. Relationships between Xanthohumol and Polyphenol Content in Hop Leaves and Hop Cones with Regard to Water Supply and Cultivar. *Int. J. Mol. Sci.* **2007**, *8*, 989–1000. [CrossRef]
48. Farag, M.A.; Porzel, A.; Schmidt, J.; Wessjohann, L.A. Metabolite profiling and fingerprinting of commercial cultivars of *Humulus lupulus* L. (hop): A comparison of MS and NMR methods in metabolomics. *Metabolomics* **2012**, *8*, 492–507. [CrossRef]
49. Simpson, W.J.; Smith, A.R. Factors affecting antibacterial activity of hop compounds and their derivatives. *J. Appl. Bacteriol.* **1992**, *72*, 327–334. [CrossRef]
50. Tsukiyama, R.I.; Katsura, H.; Tokuriki, N.; Kobayashi, M. Antibacterial activity of licochalcone A against spore-forming bacteria. *Antimicrob. Agents Chemother.* **2002**, *46*, 1226–1230. [CrossRef]
51. Ávila, H.P.; Smânia, E.F.; Monache, F.D.; Smânia, A., Jr. Structure-activity relationship of antibacterial chalcones. *Bioorg. Med. Chem.* **2008**, *16*, 9790–9794. [CrossRef]
52. Teng, Y.; Li, X.; Yang, K.; Li, X.; Zhang, Z.; Wang, L.; Deng, Z.; Song, B.; Yan, Z.; Zhang, Y.; et al. Synthesis and antioxidant evaluation of desmethylxanthohumol analogs and their dimers. *Eur. J. Med. Chem.* **2017**, *125*, 335–345. [CrossRef]
53. Olivella, M.S.; Zarelli, V.E.P.; Pappano, N.B.; Debattista, N.B. A comparative study of bacteriostatic activity of synthetic hydroxylated flavonoids. *Braz. J. Microbiol.* **2001**, *32*, 229–232. [CrossRef]
54. Legette, L.; Ma, L.; Reed, R.L.; Miranda, C.L.; Christensen, J.M.; Rodriguez-Proteau, R.; Stevens, J.F. Pharmacokinetics of xanthohumol and metabolites in rats after oral and intravenous administration. *Mol. Nutr. Food Res.* **2012**, *56*, 466–474. [CrossRef]
55. Żołnierczyk, A.K.; Mączka, W.K.; Grabarczyk, M.; Wińska, K.; Woźniak, E.; Anioł, M. Isoxanthohumol—Biologically active hop flavonoid. *Fitoterapia* **2015**, *103*, 71–82. [CrossRef]

56. Possemiers, S.; Bolca, S.; Grootaert, C.; Heyerick, A.; Decroos, K.; Dhooge, W.; De Keukeleire, D.; Rabot, S.; Verstraete, W.; Van de Wiele, T. The prenylflavonoid isoxanthohumol from hops (*Humulus lupulus* L.) is activated into the potent phytoestrogen 8-prenylnaringenin in vitro and in the human intestine. *J. Nutr.* **2006**, *136*, 1862–1867. [CrossRef]
57. Hemaiswarya, S.; Kruthiventi, A.K.; Doble, M. Synergism between natural products and antibiotics against infectious diseases. *Phytomedicine* **2008**, *15*, 639–652. [CrossRef]
58. Hsieh, M.H.; Yu, C.M.; Yu, V.L.; Chow, J.W. Synergy assessed by checkerboard a critical analysis. *Diagn. Microbiol. Infect. Dis.* **1993**, *16*, 343–349. [CrossRef]
59. Natarajan, P.; Katta, S.; Andrei, I.; Babu Rao Ambati, V.; Leonida, M.; Haas, G.J. Positive antibacterial co-action between hop (*Humulus lupulus*) constituents and selected antibiotics. *Phytomedicine* **2008**, *15*, 194–201. [CrossRef]
60. Lipsky, B.A.; Peters, E.J.; Senneville, E.; Berendt, A.R.; Embil, J.M.; Lavery, L.A.; Urbančič-Rovan, V.; Jeffcoate, W.J. Expert opinion on the management of infections in the diabetic foot. *Diabetes Metab. Res. Rev.* **2012**, *1*, 163–178. [CrossRef] [PubMed]
61. Nicodème, J.D.; Nicodème Paulin, E.; Zingg, M.; Uçkay, I.; Malacarne, S.; Suva, D. Pied diabétique infecté: Du diagnostic à la prise en charge. *Rev. Méd. Suisse* **2015**, *11*, 1238–1241.
62. Lipsky, B.A.; Hoey, C. Topical Antimicrobial Therapy for Treating Chronic Wounds. *Clin. Infect. Dis.* **2009**, *49*, 1541–1549. [CrossRef] [PubMed]
63. Barth, R.E.; Vogely, H.C.; Hoepelman, A.I.; Peters, E.J.; Peters, E.J. To bead or not to bead? Treatment of osteomyelitis and prosthetic joint associated infections with gentamicin bead chains. *Int. J. Antimicrob. Agents* **2011**, *38*, 371–375. [CrossRef]
64. Roeder, B.; Van Gils, C.C.; Maling, S. Antibiotic beads in the treatment of diabetic pedal osteomyelitis. *J. Foot Ankle Surg.* **2000**, *39*, 124–130. [CrossRef]
65. O' Meara, S.M.; Cullum, N.A.; Majid, M.; Sheldon, T.A. Systematic review of antimicrobial agents used for chronic wounds. *Br. J. Surg.* **2001**, *88*, 4–21. [CrossRef]
66. Ho, Y.C.; Liu, C.H.; Chen, C.N.; Duan, K.J.; Lin, M.T. Inhibitory effects of xanthohumol from hops (*Humulus lupulus* L.) on human hepatocellular carcinoma cell lines. *Phytother. Res.* **2008**, *22*, 1465–1468. [CrossRef]
67. Yong, W.K.; Ho, Y.F.; Malek, S.N. Xanthohumol induces apoptosis and S phase cell cycle arrest in A549 non-small cell lung cancer cells. *Pharmacogn. Mag.* **2015**, *11*, 275–283.
68. Dorn, C.; Bataille, F.; Gaebele, E.; Heilmann, J.; Hellerbrand, C. Xanthohumol feeding deas not impair organ function and homeostasis in mice. *Food Chem. Toxicol.* **2010**, *48*, 1890–1897. [CrossRef] [PubMed]
69. Legette, L.C.; Karnpracha, C.; Reed, R.L.; Choi, J.; Bobe, G.; Christensen, J.M.; Rodriguez-Proteau, R.; Purnell, J.; Stevens, J.F. Human pharmacokinetics of xanthohumol, an anti-hyperglycemic flavonoid from hops. *Mol. Nutr. Food Res.* **2014**, *58*, 248–255. [CrossRef]
70. Mouratidis, P.X.E.; Colston, K.W.; Tucknott, M.L.; Tyrrell, E.; Pirianov, G. An Investigation into the Anticancer Effects and Mechanism of Action of Hop β-Acid Lupulone and Its Natural and Synthetic Derivatives in Prostate Cancer Cells. *Nutr. Cancer* **2013**, *65*, 1086–1092. [CrossRef] [PubMed]
71. Tyrrell, E.; Archer, R.; Tucknott, M.; Colston, K.; Pirianov, G.; Ramanthan, D.; Dhillon, R.; Sinclair, A.; Skinner, G.A. The synthesis and anticancer effects of a range of natural and unnatural hop β-acids on breast cancer cells. *Phytochem. Lett.* **2012**, *5*, 144–149. [CrossRef]
72. Monzote, L.; Lackova, A.; Staniek, K.; Steinbauer, S.; Pichler, G.; Jäger, W.; Gille, L. The antileishmanial activity of xanthohumol is mediated by mitochondrial inhibition. *Parasitology* **2017**, *144*, 747–759. [CrossRef]
73. *International Conference on Harmonization of Technical Requirements for the Registration of Pharmaceuticals for Human Use (ICH), Guideline Q2(R1)-Validation of Analytical Procedures: Text and Methodology*; ICH Secretariat, c/o; IFPMA: Geneva, Switzerland, 2005.
74. Abedini, A.; Roumy, V.; Mahieux, S.; Biabiany, M.; Standaert-Vitse, A.; Rivière, C.; Sahpaz, S.; Bailleul, F.; Neut, C.; Hennebelle, T. Rosmarinic Acid and Its Methyl Ester as Antimicrobial Components of the Hydromethanolic Extract of *Hyptis atrorubens* Poit. (Lamiaceae). *Evid. Based Complement. Altern. Med.* **2013**, *2013*, 1–11. [CrossRef]
75. Zwietering, M.H.; Jongenburger, I.; Rombouts, F.M.; van't Riet, K. Modeling of the Bacterial Growth Curve. *Appl. Environ. Microbiol.* **1990**, *56*, 1875–1881.

76. MacKenzie, F.M.; Gould, I.M. The post-antibiotic effect. *J. Antimicrob. Chemother.* **1993**, *32*, 519–537. [CrossRef] [PubMed]
77. Liu, H.; Zhao, Y.; Zhao, D.; Gong, T.; Wu, Y.; Han, H.; Xu, T.; Peschel, A.; Han, S.; Qu, D. Antibacterial and anti-biofilm activities of thiazolidione derivatives against clinical Staphylococcus strains. *Emerg. Microbes Infect.* **2015**, *4*, e1.

Sample Availability: Samples of the compounds are available from the authors.

molecules

MDPI

Article

Identification of Phytoconstituents in *Leea indica* (Burm. F.) Merr. Leaves by High Performance Liquid Chromatography Micro Time-of-Flight Mass Spectrometry

Deepika Singh *, Yin-Yin Siew, Teck-Ian Chong, Hui-Chuing Yew, Samuel Shan-Wei Ho, Claire Sophie En-Shen Lim, Wei-Xun Tan, Soek-Ying Neo and Hwee-Ling Koh *

Department of Pharmacy, Faculty of Science, National University of Singapore, 18 Science Drive 4, Singapore 117543, Singapore; yindividual@hotmail.com (Y.-Y.S.); TI_Chong90@gmail.com (T.-I.C.); youyiting1979@yahoo.com.sg (H.-C.Y.); samuel.ho.s.w@icloud.com (S.S.-W.H.); clairesophie1992@yahoo.com.sg (C.S.E.-S.L.); tweixun07@hotmail.com (W.-X.T.); phansy@nus.edu.sg (S.-Y.N.)

* Correspondence: phads@nus.edu.sg (D.S.); phakohhl@nus.edu.sg (H.-L.K.); Tel.: +65-65163120 (H.-L.K.)

Academic Editor: Pinarosa Avato
Received: 24 January 2019; Accepted: 15 February 2019; Published: 16 February 2019

Abstract: *Leea indica* (Vitaceae) is a Southeast Asian medicinal plant. In this study, an ethyl acetate fraction of *L. indica* leaves was studied for its phytoconstituents using high-performance liquid chromatography-electrospray ionization-mass spectrometry (HPLC-ESI-microTOF-Q-MS/MS) analysis. A total of 31 compounds of different classes, including benzoic acid derivatives, phenolics, flavonoids, catechins, dihydrochalcones, coumarins, megastigmanes, and oxylipins were identified using LC-MS/MS. Among them, six compounds including gallic acid, methyl gallate, (−)-epigallocatechin-3-*O*-gallate, myricetin-3-*O*-rhamnoside, quercetin-3-*O*-rhamnoside, and 4′,6′-dihydroxy-4-methoxydihydrochalcone 2′-*O*-β-D-glucopyranoside were isolated and identified by NMR analysis. The LC-MS/MS analysis led to the tentative identification of three novel dihydrochalcones namely 4′,6′-dihydroxy-4-methoxydihydrochalcone 2′-*O*-rutinoside, 4′,6′-dihydroxy-4-methoxydihydrochalcone 2′-*O*-glucosylpentoside and 4′,6′-dihydroxy-4-methoxydihydrochalcone 2′-*O*-(3″-*O*-galloyl)-β-D-glucopyranoside. The structural identification of novel dihydrochalcones was based on the basic skeleton of the isolated dihydrochalcone, 4′,6′-dihydroxy-4-methoxydihydrochalcone 2′-*O*-β-D-glucopyranoside and characteristic LC-MS/MS fragmentation patterns. This is the first comprehensive analysis for the identification of compounds from *L. indica* using LC-MS. A total 24 compounds including three new dihydrochalcones were identified for the first time from the genus *Leea*.

Keywords: *Leea indica*; HPLC-ESI-microTOF-Q-MS/MS; phenolics; dihydrochalcones

1. Introduction

Leea indica (Burm. f.) Merr. (Vitaceae), commonly known as Bandicoot berry, is an evergreen perennial shrub or a small tree of 2 to 16 m in height. It is distributed throughout Bangladesh, China, India, Malaysia, Singapore, North Australia, Thailand, and Vietnam [1–3]. Traditionally, *L. indica* is used as a remedy during pregnancy, for birth control, body pain, skin problems, and relief from dizziness [4,5]. *L. indica* is reported to possess various pharmacological activities, e.g., analgesic, anti-angiogenesis, anti-oxidant, anti-inflammatory, anti-microbial, anti-proliferative, hepatoprotective, sedative, and anxiolytic activities [3,5–12]. The plant contains different classes of compounds including phenolics, terpenoids, phthalic acid derivatives, and steroids [13–15]. Currently, there are very few reports available on the phytochemistry of *L. indica*.

The objective of the present study was to isolate and identify chemical constituents from an ethyl acetate fraction of *L. indica* leaves. The comprehensive chemical identification was carried out by high performance liquid chromatography coupled to electrospray ionization and quadrupole time-of-flight mass spectrometry (HPLC-ESI-microTOF-Q-MS) analysis along with the isolation of compounds **1**, **5**, **10**, **14**, **18**, and **27** from ethyl acetate fraction. The structures of the isolated compounds were identified using NMR and MS analyses. A total of 31 compounds belonging to different classes including benzoic acid derivatives, flavonoids, coumarins, megastigmanes, catechins, dihydrochalcones, and oxylipins were identified. Here we report the identification of three novel dihydrochalcones along with 28 known compounds from the ethyl acetate fraction of *L. indica* leaves. In total, 24 compounds, including three novel dihydrochalcones, are reported for the first time in the genus *Leea*.

2. Results and Discussion

2.1. Isolation and Identification of Compounds

The methanolic extract of *L. indica* leaves was fractionated with hexane, dichloromethane and ethyl acetate. The dried yields were 0.005%, 0.027% and 1.32% respectively. Purification of the major organic ethyl acetate fraction by repeated column chromatography led to the isolation of compounds **1**, **5**, **10**, **14**, **18**, and **27**. The compounds were identified as gallic acid (**1**) [16], methyl gallate (**5**) [17], epigallocatechin-3-*O*-gallate (**10**) [18], myricetin-3-*O*-rhamnoside (**14**) [19], quercetin-3-*O*-rhamnoside (**18**), [19] and 4′,6′-dihydroxy-4-methoxydihydrochalcone 2′-*O*-β-D-glucopyranoside (**27**) [20] by comparing their analytical data (^{1}H, ^{13}C and 2D-NMR, and LC-MS) with those reported in the literature [16–20].

2.2. Identification of Dihydrochalcones by LC-ESI-MS/MS Analysis

The ethyl acetate fraction of *L. indica* leaves was analyzed by the LC-ESI-MS/MS method. Figure 1 shows the base peak chromatogram (BPC) of the ethyl acetate fraction of *L. indica* leaves at 254 nm. Figure 2 shows the structures of the 31 compounds identified. In total, 31 compounds were identified of which ten compounds (**1**, **4**, **5**, **8**, **9**, **10**, **14**, **15**, **18** and **21**) were verified by comparison with reference standards. Seven compounds were tentatively identified as dihydrochalcone derivatives: 3-hydroxyphloridzin **17**, phloridzin **21**, 4′,6′-dihydroxy-4-methoxydihydrochalcone 2′-*O*-rutinoside **25** (m/z 595), 4′,6′-dihydroxy-4-methoxydihydrochalcone 2′-*O*-glucosyl pentoside **26** (m/z 581), 4′,6′-dihydroxy-4-methoxydihydrochalcone 2′-*O*-β-D-glucopyranoside **27**, 4′,6′-dihydroxy-4-methoxydihydrochalcone 2′-*O*-(6″-*O*-galloyl)-β-D-glucopyranoside **29** (m/z 601) and 2′,4′,6′-trihydroxy-4-methoxydihydrochalcone (3-methylphloretin) **31**. Compounds **25**, **26** and **29** are reported for the first time. While dihydrochalcone phloridzin has been previously reported in *L. indica* [13], the other six dihydrochalcone derivatives have not been previously reported in the same plant species. The observed MS peaks including retention time, observed mass, calculated mass, molecular formula, ppm error, and MS/MS data are presented in Table 1.

Table 1. Identification of compounds from ethyl acetate fraction of *L. indica* by HPLC-ESI-microTOF-Q-MS/MS at 254 nm in negative ionization mode.

Peak no.	RT (min)	Observed $[M-H]^-$	Calculated $[M-H]^-$	Error (ppm)	Molecular Formula	Fragment Ions (m/z)	Identified Compound
1	10.9	169.0146	169.0142	−2.2	$C_7H_6O_5$	125.0444	Gallic acid
2	15.9	305.0668	305.0667	−0.4	$C_{15}H_{14}O_7$	261.0623, 219.0682, 179.0279, 167.0371, 165.0179, 151.1024	Gallocatechin †
3	20.6	327.0726	327.0722	−1.4	$C_{14}H_{16}O_9$	312.0487, 234.0173, 207.0298, 206.0222, 192.0079	Bergenin

Table 1. *Cont.*

Peak no.	RT (min)	Observed $[M-H]^-$	Calculated $[M-H]^-$	Error (ppm)	Molecular Formula	Fragment Ions (*m/z*)	Identified Compound
4	21.4	305.0668	305.0667	−0.4	$C_{15}H_{14}O_7$	287.059, 261.076, 219.0694, 221.0473, 179.0362, 167.0387, 165.0199	Epigallocatechin †
5	24.5	183.0304	183.0299	−2.7	$C_8H_8O_5$	169.0107	Methyl gallate †
6	26.3	913.1455	913.1469	1.6	$C_{44}H_{34}O_{22}$	761.1369, 743.1264, 609.1287, 591.1153, 573.1038, 447.0733, 423.0709, 285.0410, 169.0143	Theasinensin A (isomer 1) †
7	27.0	913.1471	913.1469	−0.2	$C_{44}H_{34}O_{22}$	761.131, 743.1255, 609.1205, 591.1148, 573.1104, 447.0721, 423.0752, 285.0422, 169.0178	Theasinensin A (isomer 2) †
8	28.5	285.0399	285.0405	2.1	$C_{15}H_{10}O_6$	243.0291, 217.0528, 199.0420, 175.047	Kaempferol
9	28.8	289.0721	289.0718	−1.0	$C_{15}H_{14}O_6$	221.0795, 203.0724, 175.0323	Epicatechin
10	29.8	457.0784	457.0776	−1.6	$C_{22}H_{18}O_{11}$	305.0660, 261.0803, 219.0637, 169.0142	Epigallocatechin-3- *O*-gallate †
11	31.0	911.1315	911.1312	−0.2	$C_{44}H_{32}O_{22}$	759.1258, 741.1135, 589.1027, 571.0861, 441.0556, 423.0727, 305.0618, 301.0453, 285.0431, 169.0135	Theasinensin A quinone †
12	32.2	897.1515	897.1520	0.5	$C_{44}H_{34}O_{21}$	745.1526, 727.1485, 575.1195, 557.1, 449.0938, 423.0693, 287.0576, 269.0482, 169.0127	Theasinensin F †
13	33.7	177.0191	177.0193	1.2	$C_9H_6O_4$	148.9428, 132.9003, 105.9031	Esculetin †
14	36.4	463.0886	463.0882	−0.8	$C_{21}H_{20}O_{12}$	317.029, 316.0226, 287.0199, 271.0247, 179.0012, 135.8248	Myricetin 3-*O*-rhamnoside (myricitrin)
15	36.9	300.9989	300.9990	0.2	$C_{14}H_6O_8$	283.9927, 245.0151, 229.0091, 201.0309, 200.0171, 173.0194	Ellagic acid †
16	38.3	441.0831	441.0827	−0.9	$C_{22}H_{18}O_{10}$	289.0701, 271.06, 245.9752, 169.0132	Catechin gallate (isomer) †
17	41.2	451.1254	451.1246	−1.7	$C_{21}H_{24}O_{11}$	289.0724, 271.1548, 167.0353	3-Hydroxyphloridzin †
18	41.7	447.0931	447.0933	0.4	$C_{21}H_{20}O_{11}$	301.0325, 300.0271, 255.0296, 179.0009	Quercetin 3-*O*-rhamnoside (Quercitrin)
19	43.2	417.0833	417.0827	−0.6	$C_{20}H_{18}O_{10}$	284.0316, 257.0446, 255.0304, 227.0339	Kaempferol 3-*O*-arabinoside †
20	45.0	615.1001	615.0992	−1.5	$C_{28}H_{24}O_{16}$	463.0903, 317.0319, 297.0616, 178.9989, 169.0188	Myricetin-*O*-(*O*-galloyl)-3-rhamnopyranoside (isomer 1) †
21	46.0	435.1299	435.1297	−0.5	$C_{21}H_{24}O_{10}$	273.0758, 167.0349	Phloridzin
22	46.5	615.0988	615.0992	0.6	$C_{28}H_{24}O_{16}$	463.0817, 317.0332, 297.0677, 178.9976, 169.011	Myricetin-*O*-(*O*-galloyl)-3-rhamnopyranoside (isomer 2) †
23	46.8	315.0146	315.0146	0.1	$C_{15}H_8O_8$	299.9902, 270.9912, 243.9987, 151.0037	Methyl-*O*-ellagic acid †
24	50.4	599.1048	599.1042	−1.0	$C_{28}H_{24}O_{15}$	447.0893, 301.0369, 169.0125, 151.8637	Quercitrin 2″-*O*-gallate †
25	51.4	595.2031	595.2032	0.2	$C_{28}H_{36}O_{14}$	433.1347, 329.1078, 308.2508, 287.0929, 167.0376	4′,6′-Dihydroxy-4-methoxy dihydrochalcone 2′-*O*-rutinoside †

Table 1. *Cont.*

Peak no.	RT (min)	Observed $[M-H]^-$	Calculated $[M-H]^-$	Error (ppm)	Molecular Formula	Fragment Ions (*m/z*)	Identified Compound
26	52.1	581.1889	581.1876	−0.5	$C_{27}H_{34}O_{14}$	419.1210, 329.102, 311.0951, 293.0907, 287.0926, 273.0953, 243.1026, 167.0355	4′,6′-Dihydroxy-4-methoxy dihydrochalcone 2′-*O*-glucosylpentoside †
27	53.6	449.1452	449.1453	0.4	$C_{22}H_{26}O_{10}$	329.1080, 287.0921, 273.0744, 272.0683, 243.1032, 181.017, 167.0298, 166.0275, 151.0067	4′,6′-Dihydroxy-4-methoxy dihydrochalcone 2′-*O*-β-D-glucopyranoside †
28	54.5	327.2171	327.2177	1.8	$C_{18}H_{32}O_5$	309.2164, 298.9867, 291.1998, 239.1283, 229.1447, 211.1327, 183.0131, 171.103	9,12,13-Trihydroxy octadecadienoic acid †
29	55.0	601.1595	601.1563	−5.3	$C_{29}H_{30}O_{14}$	439.0901, 329.1098, 313.0559, 287.0914, 271.0502, 243.1106, 211.0199, 169.0167	4′,6′-Dihydroxy-4-methoxy dihydrochalcone 2′-*O*-(3″-*O*-galloyl)-β-D-glucopyranoside †
30	57.7	221.1186	221.1183	−1.4	$C_{13}H_{18}O_3$	149.0978	Dehydrovomifoliol †
31	58.6	287.0926	287.0925	−0.2	$C_{16}H_{16}O_5$	243.1034, 167.037, 151.0043	2′,4′,6′-Trihydroxy-4-methoxy dihydrochalcone (3-Methylphloretin) †

† Compounds identified for the first time in the genus *Leea*.

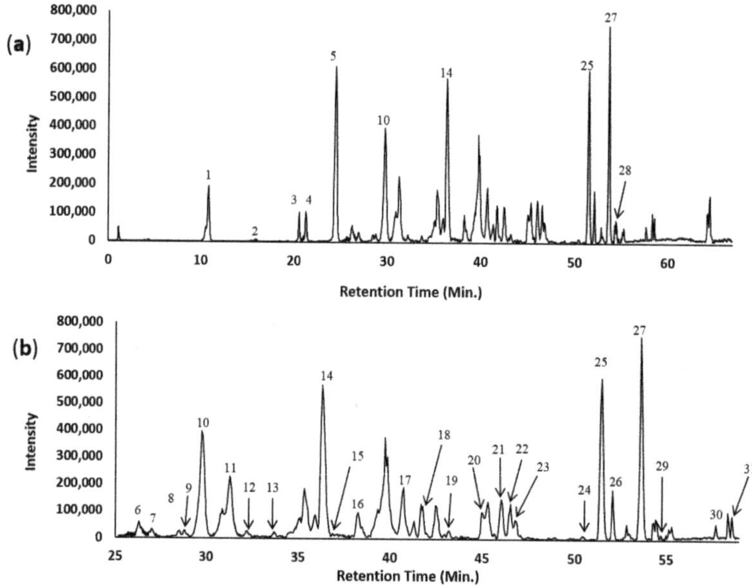

Figure 1. (**a**) Base peak chromatogram (BPC) of *L. indica* ethyl acetate fraction by HPLC-ESI-MS in negative ionization mode; (**b**) Expanded BPC. Peak labeling represents the compounds identified.

The structural identification of three new dihydrochalcones **25**, **26** and **29** was based on the relevance of the LC-MS/MS fragmentation patterns with the isolated compound 4′,6′-dihydroxy-4-methoxy dihydrochalcone 2′-*O*-β-D-glucopyranoside **27**. The MS/MS spectra of compounds **25**, **26**, **27** and **29**, showed a common base ion peak at *m*/*z* 287 for 2′,4′,6′-trihydroxy-4-methoxydihydrochalcone, which is a characteristic ion formed by the loss of glycoside(s) and/or galloyl glycoside moieties.

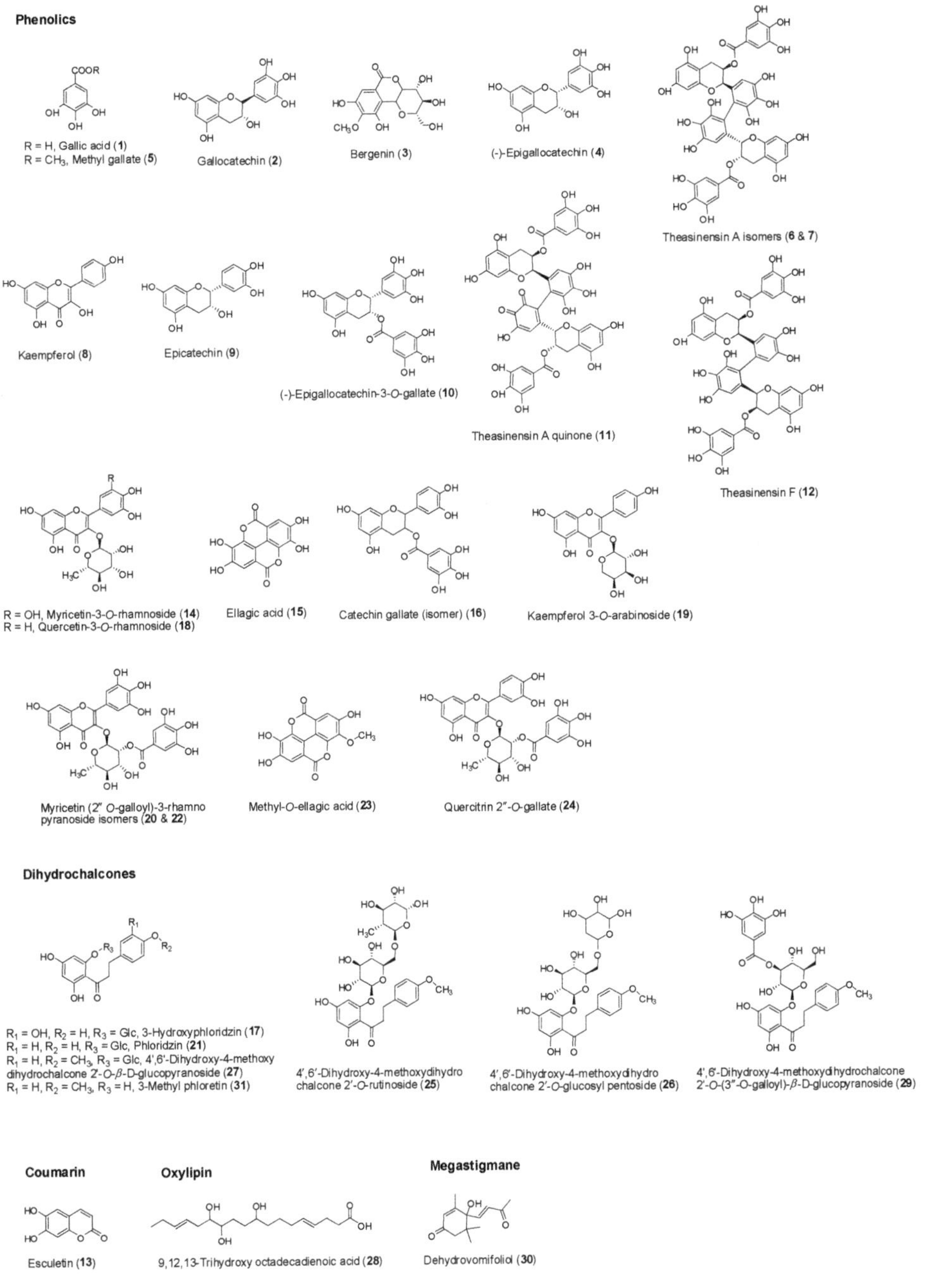

Figure 2. Structures of compounds identified in *L. indica* according to their chemical classes.

In LC-MS spectra, peaks **25**, **26** and **29** eluted at retention times (RT) 51.4, 52.1 and 55.0 min, and showed precursor ions $[M-H]^-$ at m/z 595.2031, 581.1889 and 601.1595, respectively. Peaks **25** (m/z 595) and **26** (m/z 581) showed a mass difference of 146 Da (rhamnose) and 132 Da (arabinose/xylose) respectively compared to the isolated dihydrochalcone **27** (m/z 449).

Also, peak **26** (*m*/*z* 581) was found to be 14 Da lighter than peak **25** (*m*/*z* 595), indicating the presence of a pentose sugar. In agreement with mass analysis data, peaks **25** and **26** were tentatively characterized as 4′,6′-dihydroxy-4-methoxydihydrochalcone 2′-*O*-rutinoside (*m*/*z* 595) and 4′,6′-dihydroxy-4-methoxydihydrochalcone 2′-*O*-glucosylpentoside (*m*/*z* 581) respectively.

Peak **25** displayed a molecular ion $[M - H]^-$ at *m*/*z* 595.2031 ($C_{28}H_{36}O_{14}$) and fragment ions at *m*/*z* 433, 329 and 287 (Scheme 1 and Figure S1). In the MS/MS spectrum, a characteristic fragment ion at *m*/*z* 287 as base peak suggested that this compound corresponded to a 2′,4′,6′-trihydroxy-4-methoxydihydrochalcone linked to a rutinose moiety, where the neutral loss of 308 Da is characteristic of the loss of a rutinose moiety [21]. The fragments at *m*/*z* 433 $[M - C_{10}H_{10}O_2 - H]^-$ and 329 $[M - C_{10}H_{18}O_8 - H]^-$ were obtained by the cleavage of the C-C bond of chalcone and sugar moiety respectively (Scheme 1). The fragment ion at *m*/*z* 329 $[M - H - C_9H_{13}O_7 - H_2O - CH_3]^-$ was obtained by the cleavage of a glucose moiety, with the loss of a water molecule and further by losing a methyl group. Based on these deductions, peak **25** was tentatively identified as 4′,6′-dihydroxy-4-methoxydihydrochalcone 2′-*O*-rutinoside, a new dihydrochalcone.

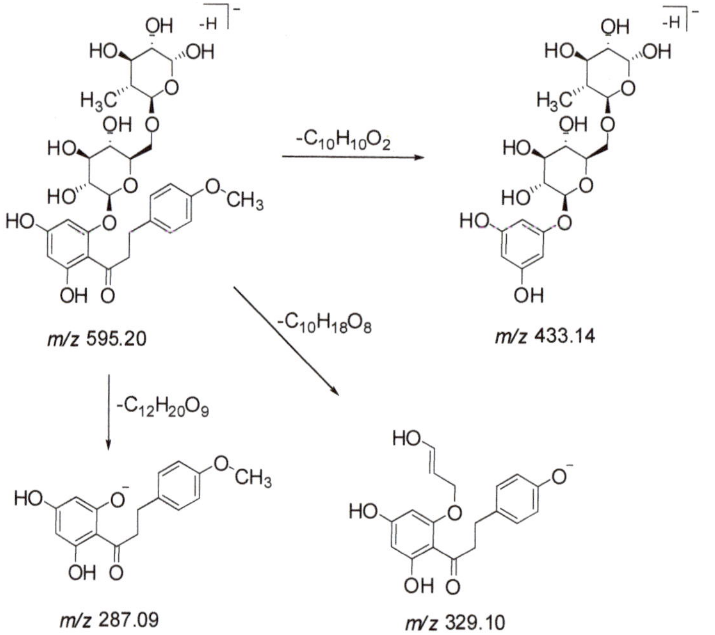

Scheme 1. Proposed MS/MS fragmentation of compound **25**.

Peak **26** exhibited a precursor ion $[M - H]^-$ at *m*/*z* 581.1889 ($C_{27}H_{34}O_{14}$) and fragment ions at *m*/*z* 419, 311, 293, and 243 (Scheme 2 and Figure S2). The MS/MS spectrum showed product ion at *m*/*z* 287 ($C_{16}H_{16}O_5$) $[M - H - 162\ Da - 132\ Da]^-$ as base peak by the loss of a glucosylpentoside moiety, suggesting to possess a basic skeleton of isolated dihydrochalcone **27**. The cleavage of a C-C bond gave a fragment ion at *m*/*z* 419 due to the loss of a $C_{10}H_{10}O_2$ moiety. The neutral loss of 312 Da showed the presence of a glucosyl pentoside moiety, losing a molecule of water to generate a product ion at *m*/*z* 293 (Scheme 3). Therefore, compound **26** was plausibly identified as 4′,6′-dihydroxy-4-methoxydihydrochalcone 2′-*O*-glucosylpentoside and found as first occurrence in nature.

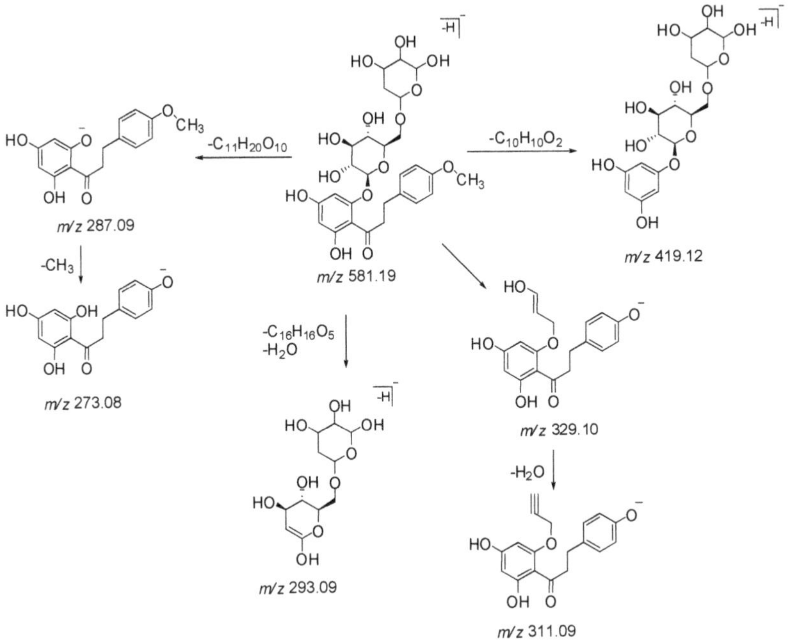

Scheme 2. Proposed MS/MS fragmentation of compound **26**.

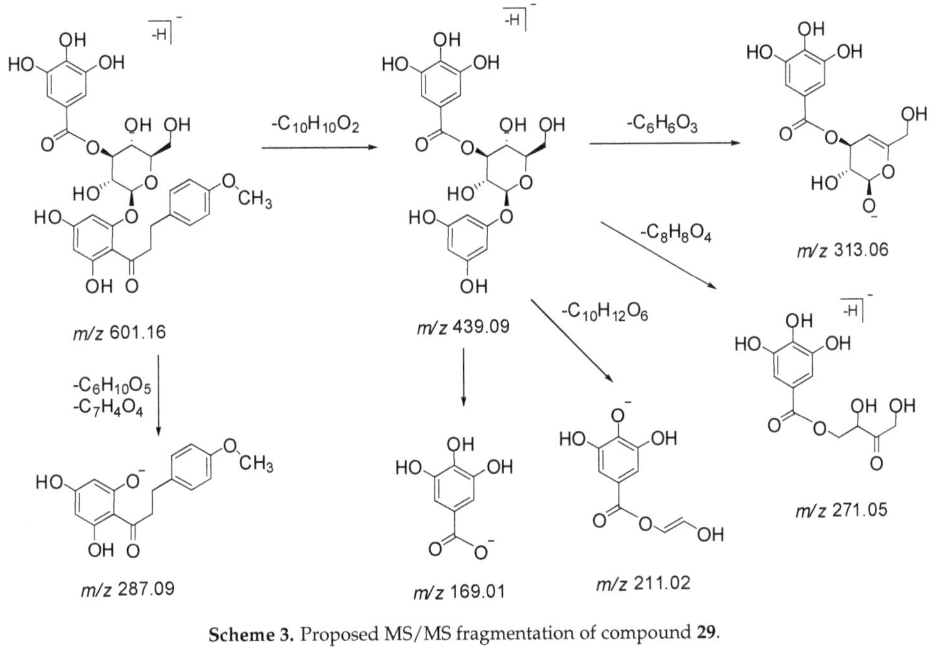

Scheme 3. Proposed MS/MS fragmentation of compound **29**.

Peak **29** showed a precursor ion $[M - H]^-$ at m/z 601.1595 ($C_{29}H_{30}O_{14}$) and fragment ions at m/z 439, 313, 287, 271, 211, and 169 in the MS/MS spectrum. A base ion peak at m/z 287 $[M - C_6H_{10}O_5 - C_7H_4O_4 - H]^-$ was observed due to the loss of glucose (162 Da) and galloyl (153 Da) moieties. Fragment ions at m/z 169 and m/z 313 indicate the presence of a galloyl and a galloylglucose moiety respectively. Monogalloylglucose can exist as five possible isomers namely, 1-*O*-galloylglucose, 2-*O*-galloylglucose, 3-*O*-galloylglucose, 4-*O*-galloylglucose, and 6-*O*-galloylglucose [22]. The characteristic fragment ions at m/z 271 and 211 suggest that the substitution of the galloyl group could be at the C-3 position of the glucose moiety (Scheme 3 and Figure S3). Product ion detected at m/z 439 suggested the cleavage of the C-C bond (loss of $C_{10}H_{10}O_2$ moiety) in the MS/MS spectrum. Thus, the compound corresponding to peak **29** was tentatively identified as a new dihydrochalcone 4′,6′-dihydroxy-4-methoxydihydrochalcone 2′-*O*-(3″-*O*-galloyl)-β-D-glucopyranoside. It is also a gallic acid derivative of the isolated dihydrochalcone **27**.

The isolated dihydrochalcone **27** exhibited a precursor ion $[M - H]^-$ at m/z 449.1452 ($C_{22}H_{26}O_{10}$). The MS/MS spectrum showed product ions at m/z 287 $[M - C_6H_{10}O_5 - H]^-$ and 273 $[M - C_6H_{10}O_5 - CH_3 - H]^-$ due to the loss of glucose (162 Da) and methyl groups (15 Da) (Figure S4). Compound **27** was isolated and identified as 4′,6′-dihydroxy-4-methoxydihydrochalcone 2′-*O*-β-D-glucopyranoside.

The LC-MS fragmentation patterns of the three novel dihydrochalcones (**25**, **26** and **29**) were compared to the isolated dihydrochalcone (**27**), and we noted that the observed HR-MS data were in good agreement with the calculated masses. Further isolation of the peaks **25**, **26** and **29** and spectroscopic analyses would be required to unambiguously confirm the proposed structures of these dihydrochalcones.

3. Materials and Methods

3.1. Plant Materials

Fresh ground leaves of *L. indica* were collected in Singapore. A voucher specimen (no. LI-0109) was deposited at the herbarium of the National University of Singapore (NUS) Medicinal Plant Research Group.

3.2. Chemicals and Reagents

Standards gallic acid, methyl gallate, myricitrin, quercitrin, epigallocatechin-3-*O*-gallate, ellagic acid, epicatechin, and kaempferol were purchased from Sigma-Aldrich (St. Louis, MO, USA). Phloridzin and epigallocatechin were purchased from TCI Co. Ltd. (Tokyo, Japan). LC-MS grade solvents (acetonitrile, methanol and formic acid) were purchased from MERCK (Darmstadt, Germany) and water used in LC analysis was obtained using Milli-Q advanced system (Millipore, Milford, MA, USA).

3.3. Extraction and Isolation

The fresh ground leaves of *L. indica* (2.8 kg) were macerated with 70% v/v MeOH at room temperature. The extract was filtered and concentrated under vacuum, yielding a crude methanolic extract. The dried methanolic extract was dissolved in water and partitioned with different solvents, concentrated under vacuum to give hexane (0.005%), dichloromethane (0.027%) and ethyl acetate (1.32%) fractions.

The ethyl acetate fraction (37.0 g) was chromatographed over silica gel using 25% EtOAc–hexane as eluent, yielding a white solid, which was recrystallized in $CHCl_3$-MeOH as white needles of methyl gallate (60 mg). Fractions obtained from repeated silica gel column chromatography of EtOAc fraction using 6–10% MeOH-$CHCl_3$ as eluent were further purified by Sephadex (LH-20) and reversed phase cartridge yielding two compounds gallic acid (140 mg) and 4′,6′-dihydroxy-4-methoxydihydrochalcone 2′-*O*-β-D-glucopyranoside (12 mg). The estimated concentration of gallic acid in the fresh leaves was 0.005–0.011% w/w. Pooled fractions obtained from silica gel column chromatography of the EtOAc fraction using 10–20% MeOH-$CHCl_3$ were further subjected to Sephadex (LH-20) column chromatography. At an eluent concentration of 50% MeOH-water, a mixture of two compounds was obtained. It was further purified by silica gel column chromatography eluting with 8% MeOH-$CHCl_3$

and 10–12% MeOH-$CHCl_3$ to yield quercetin-3-*O*-rhamnoside (5 mg) and myricetin-3-*O*-rhamnoside (650 mg) respectively. Epigallocatechin-3-*O*-gallate (64 mg) was obtained from the silica gel column chromatography using 2–5% methanol in dichloromethane. The structures of isolated compounds **1**, **5**, **10**, **14**, **18**, and **27** were confirmed by NMR and LC-MS analyses.

3.4. General Information

NMR spectra were recorded on a Bruker Avance-400 Spectrometer (Fallanden, Switzerland), ^{1}H at 400 MHz and ^{13}C at 100 MHz in deuterated solvents using tetramethylsilane (TMS) as an internal reference. Deuterated solvents, methanol-d_4 and dimethyl sulfoxide-d_6 for NMR were purchased from Sigma-Aldrich (USA).

Silica-gel (60–120, 100–200, 70–230 mesh; Merck, Germany), Sephadex LH-20 (Sigma, Uppsala, Sweden) and reversed phase C18 (77.9 μm) cartridge column from Waters (Ireland) were used for chromatographic separation. Thin layer chromatography was performed on pre-coated Si-gel 60 F_{254} plates (Merck, Germany) using a visualizing reagent.

The LC-MS analysis was carried out using a Dionex Ultimate 3000 VWD system coupled with a VWD and a micro-TOF-Q mass detector (Bruker Daltonics Inc., Billerica, MA, USA). Chromatographic separation was performed on an RP-C_{18} column (3.0 × 150 mm; particle size 2.7 μM; Agilent Poroshell 120, New Castle, DE, USA), operated at 25 °C. Analysis was carried out using a gradient elution program of 0.1% formic acid in water (A) and 0.1% formic acid in acetonitrile (B) as a mobile phase at a flow rate of 0.5 mL/min. The following gradient system was used: 0–45 min, 5–30% B; 45–60 min 30–100% B and 60–65 min 100% B. UV detection was performed by scanning the samples at 210, 254, 280, and 360 nm. Electrospray ionization mass spectra (ESI-MS) were recorded in negative ionization mode. The mass range of m/z 50–2000 was scanned. For MS/MS analysis, collision energies were set automatically.

4. Conclusions

This study presents the comprehensive identification of chemical constituents of an ethyl acetate fraction of *L. indica* leaves using HPLC-ESI-microTOF-Q-MS/MS analysis. Here we identified 31 compounds, among them six phenolic compounds were isolated by column chromatography. Three novel dihydrochalcones derivatives were tentatively identified as 4′,6′-dihydroxy-4-methoxydihydrochalcone 2′-*O*-rutinoside, 4′,6′-dihydroxy-4-methoxydihydro chalcone 2′-*O*-glucosylpentoside and 4′,6′-dihydroxy-4-methoxydihydrochalcone 2′-*O*-(3″-*O*-galloyl)-β-D-glucopyranoside. A total of 24 compounds are reported for the first time in the genus *Leea*. Our results indicated that *L. indica* is a good source of diverse phenolic contents including phenolic acids (gallic acid and methyl gallate), polyphenolic (ellagic acid), flavan-3-ols (gallocatechin, epigallocatechin and epigallocatechin-3-*O*-gallate), flavonoids/flavonoid glycosides (kaempferol, quercitrin, myricitrin), dihydrochalcones (phloridzin and its derivatives), and dimeric catechins (theasinensin A dimers and theasinensin F). The wide range of potential bioactive compounds supports the diverse pharmacological activities of *L. indica*. Further research to identify and develop useful therapeutics and health supplements from *L. indica* is warranted.

Supplementary Materials: Supplementary materials are available online. Figure S1: MS^2 spectrum and proposed fragmentation pattern of compound **25**; Figure S2: MS^2 spectrum and proposed fragmentation pattern of compound **26**; Figure S3: MS^2 spectrum and proposed fragmentation pattern **29**; Figure S4: MS^2 spectrum and proposed fragmentation pattern of compound **27**.

Author Contributions: D.S.: isolation and identification of compounds, data analysis, preparation and correction of manuscript; Y.-Y.S., T.-I.C.: extraction of plant materials, isolation and identification of compounds; H.-C.Y., S.S.-W.H., C.S.E.-S.L. and W.-X.T.: extraction of plant materials; S.-Y.N.: correction of manuscript; H.-L.K.: conception of study and correction of manuscript.

Funding: This work is supported by the National University of Singapore-Leeward Pacific Pte Ltd research collaboration grant (R-148-000-172-592) to H.-L.K. and the National University of Singapore Provost Industrial PhD Programme Research Scholarship to Y.-Y.S.

Acknowledgments: The authors are grateful to Steven Yuan Cheng Hui, Dept. of Chemistry, NUS for technical support and Kim-Chuan Ng of the Nanyang Technological University Community Herb Garden, Singapore for his kind support.

Conflicts of Interest: The authors declare no conflict of interest.

References

1. Ridsdale, C.E. Leeaceae. In *Flora Malesiana, Series I—Spermatophyta Flowering Plants*; Noordhoff International Publishing: Leiden, The Netherlands, 1976; Volume 7, pp. 755–782.
2. The Angiosperm Phylogeny Group. An update of the Angiosperm Phylogeny Group classification for the orders and families plants: APG III. *Bot. J. Linn. Soc.* **2009**, *161*, 105–121. [CrossRef]
3. Siew, Y.Y.; Yew, H.C.; Neo, S.Y.; Seow, S.V.; Lew, S.M.; Lim, S.W.; Lim, C.S.E.S.; Ng, Y.C.; Seetoh, W.G.; Ali, A.; et al. Evaluation of anti-proliferative activity of medicinal plants used in Asian Traditional Medicine to treat cancer. *J. Ethnopharmacol.* **2019**, *235*, 75–87. [CrossRef] [PubMed]
4. Bourdy, G.; Walter, A. Maternity and medicinal plants in Vanuatu I. The cycle of reproduction. *J. Ethnopharmacol.* **1992**, *37*, 179–196. [CrossRef]
5. Singh, D.; Siew, Y.Y.; Yew, H.C.; Neo, S.Y.; Koh, H.L. Botany, phytochemistry and pharmacological activities of *Leea* species. In *Medicinal Plants: Chemistry, Pharmacology, and Therapeutic Applications*; Swamy, M.K., Patra, J.K., Rudramurthy, G.R., Eds.; CRC Press Taylor & Francis Group: Boca Raton, FL, USA, 2019; in press.
6. Wiart, C.; Mogana, S.; Khalifah, S.; Mahan, M.; Ismail, S.; Buckle, M.; Narayana, A.K.; Sulaiman, M. Antimicrobial screening of plants used for traditional medicine in the state of Perak, Peninsular Malaysia. *Fitoterapia* **2004**, *75*, 68–73. [CrossRef] [PubMed]
7. Raihan, M.O.; Habib, M.R.; Brishti, A.; Rahman, M.M.; Saleheen, M.M.; Manna, M. Sedative and anxiolytic effects of the methanolic extract of *Leea indica* (Burm. f.) Merr. Leaf. *Drug Discov. Ther.* **2011**, *5*, 185–189. [CrossRef] [PubMed]
8. Wong, Y.H.; Kadir, H.A. *Leea indica* ethyl acetate fraction induces growth-inhibitory effect in various cancer cell lines and apoptosis in Ca Ski human cervical epidermoid carcinoma cells. *Evid. Based Complement Alternat. Med.* **2011**. Available online: http://dx.doi.org/10.1155/2011/293060 (accessed on 18 January 2019).
9. Reddy, N.S.; Navanesan, S.; Sinniah, S.K.; Wahab, N.A.; Sim, K.S. Phenolic content, antioxidant effect and cytotoxic activity of *Leea indica* leaves. *BMC Complement Altern. Med.* **2012**, *12*, 128. Available online: http://dx.doi.org./10.1186/1472-6882-12-128 (accessed on 18 January 2019). [CrossRef] [PubMed]
10. Rahman, M.A.; Imran, T.B.; Islam, S. Antioxidative, antimicrobial and cytotoxic effects of the phenolics of *Leea indica* leaf extract. *Saudi J. Biol. Sci.* **2013**, *20*, 213–225. [CrossRef] [PubMed]
11. Avin, B.R.V.; Thirusangu, P.; Ramesh, C.K.; Vigneswarana, V.; Kumar, M.V.P.; Mahmood, R.; Prabhakar, B.T. Screening for the modulation of neovessel formation in non-tumorigenic and tumorigenic conditions using three different plants native to Western ghats of India. *Biomed. Aging Pathol.* **2014**, *4*, 343–348. [CrossRef]
12. Mishra, G.; Khosa, R.L.; Singh, P.; Jha, K.K. Hepatoprotective activity of ethanolic extract of *Leea indica* (Burm. f.) Merr. (Leeaceae) stem bark against paracetamol induced liver toxicity in rats. *Niger. J. Exp. Clin. Biosci.* **2014**, *2*, 59–63. [CrossRef]
13. Saha, K.; Shaari, K.; Lajis, N.H. Phytochemical study on *Leea indica* (Burm. F.) Merr. (Leeaceae). *J. Bangladesh Chem. Soc.* **2007**, *20*, 139–147.
14. Srinivasan, G.V.; Ranjith, C.; Vijayan, K.K. Identification of chemical compounds from the leaves of *Leea indica*. *Acta Pharm.* **2008**, *58*, 207–214. [CrossRef] [PubMed]
15. Wong, Y.H.; Kadir, H.A.; Ling, S.K. Bioassay-guided isolation of cytotoxic cycloartane triterpenoid glycosides from the traditionally used medicinal plant *Leea indica*. *Evid. Based Complement Alternat. Med.* **2012**. Available online: http://dx.doi.org/10.1155/2012/164689 (accessed on 18 January 2019).
16. Liu, J.X.; Di, D.L.; Shi, Y.P. Diversity of chemical constituents from *Saxifraga montana* H. *J. Chinese Chem. Soc.* **2008**, *55*, 863–870. [CrossRef]
17. Ekaprasada, M.T.; Nurdin, H.; Ibrahim, S.; Dachriyanus, H. Antioxidant activity of methyl gallate isolated from the leaves of *Toona sureni*. *Indones. J. Chem.* **2009**, *9*, 457–460. [CrossRef]
18. Zhong, Y.; Shahidi, F. Lipophilized epigallocatechin gallate (EGCG) derivatives as novel antioxidants. *J. Agric. Food Chem.* **2011**, *59*, 6526–6533. [CrossRef]

19. Aderogba, M.A.; Ndhlala, A.R.; Rengasamy, K.R.R. Antimicrobial and selected in vitro enzyme inhibitory effects of leaf extracts, flavonols and indole alkaloids isolated from *Croton menyharthii*. *Molecules* **2013**, *18*, 12633–12644. [CrossRef]
20. Silva, D.H.S.; Yoshida, M.; Kato, M.J. Flavonoids from *Iryanthera sagotiana*. *Phytochemistry* **1997**, *46*, 579–582. [CrossRef]
21. Zhang, M.; Duan, C.; Zang, Y.; Huang, Z.; Liu, G. The flavonoid composition of flavedo and juice from the pummel cultivar (*Citrus grandis* (L.) Osbeck) and the grapefruit cultivar (*Citrus paradise*). *Food Chem.* **2011**, *129*, 1530–1536. [CrossRef]
22. Fathoni, A.; Saepudin, A.; Cahyanal, H.; Rahayu, D.U.C.; Haib, J. Identification of nonvolatile compounds in clove (*Syzygium aromaticum*) from Manado. *AIP Conf. Proc.* **2017**, *1862*. [CrossRef]

Sample Availability: Samples are not available from the authors.

molecules

MDPI

Article

Phenolic Content and Antioxidant Activity in *Trifolium* Germplasm from Different Environments

Aldo Tava [1,*], Łukasz Pecio [2], Roberto Lo Scalzo [3], Anna Stochmal [2] and Luciano Pecetti [1]

1 CREA Research Centre for Animal Production and Aquaculture, viale Piacenza 29, 26900 Lodi, Italy; luciano.pecetti@crea.gov.it
2 Department of Biochemistry and Crop Quality, Institute of Soil Science and Plant Cultivation, State Research Institute, ul. Czartoryskich 8, 24-100 Pulawy, Poland; lpecio@iung.pulawy.pl (Ł.P.); asf@iung.pulawy.pl (A.S.)
3 CREA Research Centre for Engineering and Agro-Food Processing, via G. Venezian 26, 20133 Milano, Italy; roberto.loscalzo@crea.gov.it
* Correspondence: aldo.tava@crea.gov.it; Tel.: +39-0371-40471

Academic Editor: Pinarosa Avato
Received: 19 December 2018; Accepted: 14 January 2019; Published: 15 January 2019

Abstract: Phenolics are important mediators in plant-environment interactions. The presence and concentration of phenolic compounds and their antioxidant activity were evaluated in leaves and flowers of a set of *Trifolium* species originating from contrasting environments encompassing lowland and mountain sites. The current germplasm proved a great reservoir of phenolic compounds, with different chemical structure and, possibly, diversified biological activity. Germplasm groups with specific phenolic composition were observed. In some cases, different patterns bore a taxonomic meaning. Lowland germplasm showed higher concentration of total phenolics in leaves than mountain accessions (50.30 vs. 34.19 mg/g dry matter (DM)), while the latter had higher concentration in flowers (114.16 vs. 57.44 mg/g DM). Outstanding concentration of isoflavones was observed in leaves of lowland germplasm (24.19 mg/g DM), and of both proanthocyanidins and flavonoids in flowers of mountain germplasm (53.81 and 56.62 mg/g DM, respectively). The pattern of phenolic composition in lowland and mountain germplasm was suggestive of different adaptive strategies. Three assays of antioxidant activity were tested, which were characterised by rather different reactivity towards phenolic composition. The scavenging activity was higher for leaf extracts of lowland germplasm, and for flower extracts of mountain germplasm. Besides identifying germplasm of interest, this study also suggested possible links between environmental factors and concentration and composition of phenolic compounds.

Keywords: antioxidant activity; flavonoids; isoflavones; phenolics; proanthocyanidins; *Trifolium*

1. Introduction

The genus *Trifolium* includes a large array of species. Some of them represent very important forage crops worldwide, such as white clover (*T. repens* L.), and red clover (*T. pratense* L.) [1,2]. Other species have an agronomic relevance in specific areas, such as berseem clover (*T. alexandrinum* L.) and subterranean clover (*T. subterraneum* L.) in Mediterranean environments [3]. Wild forms of these and other cultivated species, as well as populations of many other *Trifolium* species occur in natural grasslands of diversified environments, where they can represent valuable feed resources [4–6].

Besides being rich in proteins, *Trifolium* species have been reported to contain a wealth of biologically active secondary metabolites [7], of which phenolic compounds are one of the main classes. Phenolic compounds have a wide range of structures, but they generally share a remarkable antioxidant activity [8]. Flavonoids are an important class of phenolics that includes compound groups such as flavones, flavonols and isoflavones, all characterized by a phenylbenzopyran chemical structure [8].

In recent decades, there has been an increasing interest on flavonoids in medical research owing to their useful properties, such as anti-inflammatory, estrogenic, antimicrobial, antiallergenic and antitumor activities [9]. The antioxidant activity, determined by their ability of decreasing free radical formation and scavenging free radicals and reactive oxygen species (ROS), is an asset of major interest for flavonoids [10,11].

The role of flavonoids and other phenolic compounds as protective dietary constituents (nutraceuticals) with their antioxidant capacity has also become an increasingly important area of research [12]. The potential benefit that a dietary intake of phenolics may produce in the prevention or reduction of degenerative diseases such as cardiovascular diseases and cancer has been reported [13,14]. Isoflavones are a group of flavonoids typical of some legume species only. They exhibit estrogenic activity and represent the main phytoestrogens of current interest as nutraceuticals and dietary supplements [15,16]. An antioxidant activity of possible physiological relevance was also reported for isoflavones such as genistein and daidzein [17].

Phenolic compounds, including flavonoids, have often been used as chemotaxonomic markers in plants [18]. These compounds were also examined in the genus *Trifolium*. Oleszek et al. [19] characterized the phenolic composition of over 50 *Trifolium* species, emphasizing similarities and differences among taxa for the concentration pattern of the main groups of phenolics. More recently, the isoflavone prunetin was proposed as a possible chemotaxonomic marker in snow clover (*T. pratense* L. subsp. *nivale* (Koch) Arcang.) [20].

Phenolics play a fundamental role in the interaction of plants with the environment, including their defense mechanisms against biotic and abiotic stresses and other adaptation processes [21,22]. It is well known that the presence of phenolics in plants and the subsequent antioxidant capacity can also be subjected to significant variation due to environmental conditions and to biotic and abiotic stresses [23,24]. Hence, the current study evaluated the presence and concentration of phenolic compounds, as well as their antioxidant activity in a set of *Trifolium* species originating from different Italian environments. The main objectives of this investigation were to identify germplasm of interest as potential source of phenolic metabolites, also in view of their possible exploitation for medical/nutraceutical purposes, and to assess any possible role of the environment on the phenolic composition of the species.

2. Results

2.1. *Germplasm Collection and Identification of Phenolics*

The list of *Trifolium* species used in this investigation is reported in Table 1. Both cultivated and natural populations from different environments (lowlands and mountains) were analyzed for their phenolic content. Phenolics occurring in the extract of the 14 *Trifolium* samples under investigation were separated by UPLC method (see Materials and Methods) and UV spectra were obtained using a photo diode array detector. As an example, the UPLC chromatogram of leaf and flower extracts of *T. repens* var. *sylvestre* is shown in Figure 1. Six groups of phenolics were identified based on their characteristic absorption spectra (Figure 2), namely: phenolic acids (Figure 2A), clovamides (Figure 2B), flavanols (Figure 2C), flavones (Figure 2D), flavonols (Figure 2E) and isoflavones (Figure 2F).

A comparison was made of their retention times and mass spectral data obtained in positive and negative mode with those of standard compounds or with compounds previously reported in literature for *Trifolium* spp. [19,20,25–28]. A tentative identification of phenolics was performed based on key fragment ions and other MS observations. For flavonoids and their glycosyl derivatives the loss of 162 *m/z* was indicative of hexose (glucose or galactose), the loss of 146 *m/z* was indicative of rhamnose, the loss of 132 *m/z* was indicative of pentose (xylose or arabinose). Moreover, the loss of 44 *m/z* in the negative ion mode and the loss of 86 *m/z* were indicative of the presence of a malonate.

Table 1. List of *Trifolium* germplasm evaluated for the concentration of phenolic compounds and antioxidant activity.

#	Species	Common Name	Germplasm Type	Name/Origin	Adaptation to/Origin From
1	*T. alexandrinum*	Berseem clover	Experimental cultivar	Sintetica E/Italy	Lowlands
2	*T. pratense*	Red clover	Cultivar	Aiace/Italy	Lowlands
3	*T. pratense* subsp. *nivale*	Snow clover	Natural population	Rhaetian Alps	Mountains*
4	*T. repens*	White clover (non-Ladino large-leaved type)	Cultivar	Regal/USA	Lowlands
5	*T. subterraneum*	Subterranean clover	Natural population	Sardinia	Lowlands
6	*T. subterraneum*	Subterranean clover	Natural population	Sardinia	Lowlands
7	*T. pratense*	Red clover	Natural population	Po Valley	Lowlands
8	*T. repens* var. *giganteum*	White clover (Ladino type)	Natural population	Po Valley	Lowlands
9	*T. alpinum*	Alpine clover	Natural population	Graian Alps	Mountains
10	*T. badium*	Brown clover	Natural population	Graian Alps	Mountains
11	*T. ochroleucum*	Sulphur clover	Natural population	Cottian Alps	Mountains
12	*T. pratense* subsp. *nivale*	Snow clover	Natural population	Graian Alps	Mountains
13	*T. repens* var. *sylvestre*	White clover (small-leaved type)	Natural population	Graian Alps	Mountains
14	*T. thalii*	Thal clover	Natural population	Graian Alps	Mountains

* Collected as seed in a mountain area and grown *ex-situ* in a lowland site.

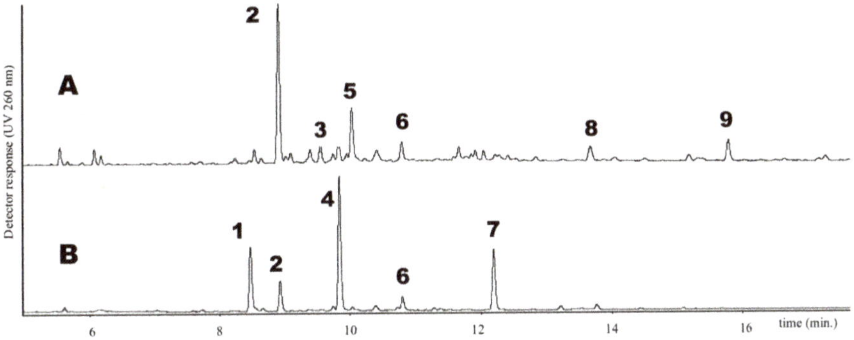

Figure 1. UPLC chromatogram of extracts from (**A**) leaves and (**B**) flowers of *T. repens* var. *sylvestre* (#13). **1**: myricetin-3-*O*-galactoside; **2**: quercetin-3-*O*-[xylosyl-(1→2)-galactoside]; **3**: kaempferol-3-*O*-[rhamnosyl-(1→6)-xylosyl-(1→2)-galactoside]; **4**: quercetin-3-*O*-galactoside; **5**: kaempferol-3-*O*-[xylosyl-(1→2)-galactoside]; **6**: kaempferol-3-*O*-galactoside; **7**: quercetin-3-*O*-galactoside-6′′-*O*-acetate; **8**: formononetin-7-*O*-glucoside; **9**: formononetin-7-*O*-glucoside-6′′-*O*-malonate.

Branched *C*-glycosides were also investigated by the presence of characteristic ions $[M - H - 60]^-$, $[M - H - 90]^-$, and $[M - H - 120]^-$ [25–29].

Along with clovamide (*N*-caffeoyl-L-DOPA), phenolic acids were detected in almost all *Trifolium* extracts in low amount and were mostly constituted by glycosyl derivatives of caffeic acid, ferulic acid and coumaric acid.

Flavanols were identified in very low amount (< 0.3 mg g^{-1} dry matter) in some extracts, and identified as catechin/epicatechin and a catechin dimer. Flavones, flavonols and isoflavones represented the main bulk of flavonoid constituents of the extracts. The most abundant, tentatively identified, flavonoids in the 14 *Trifolium* samples are reported in Table 2 where their percentage amount in the whole extracts is indicated. All the identified compounds were quantitatively evaluated by appropriate standards (see Experimental).

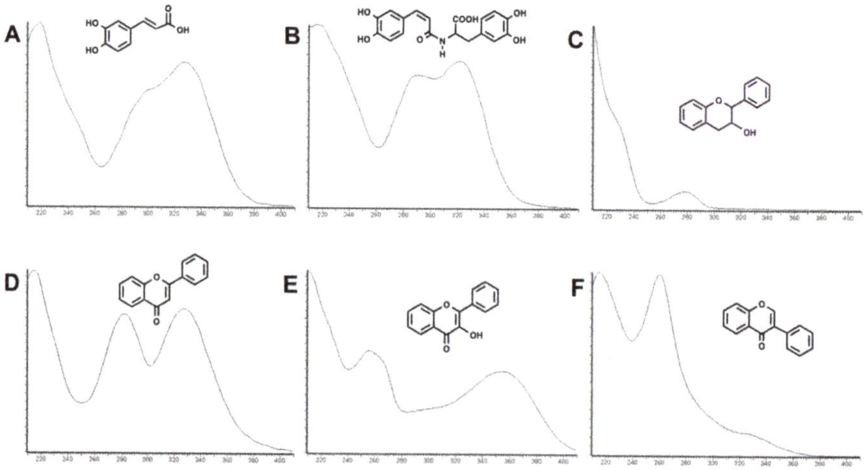

Figure 2. Characteristic UV spectra of the six groups of phenolics identified in *Trifolium* spp. **A**: phenolic acid; **B**: clovamide; **C**: flavanol; **D**: flavone, **E**: flavonol; **F**: isoflavone.

Glycosyl and glycosyl malonate derivative of luteolin, together with lower amount of derivatives of apigenin and of the isoflavone biochanin A, were the most abundant compounds identified in *T. alexandrinum* (#1) extracts. In flowers, large amounts of quercetin galactoside and quercetin glucoside were also detected. All these compounds were previously reported in the species [30–32]. High amounts of glycosyl and glycosyl malonate derivative of flavones (quercetin in leaves and quercetin and kaempferol in flowers) and isoflavones (biochanin A and formononetin in leaves and flowers) were detected in red clover (#2 and #7), as previously reported in this widely investigated *Trifolium* species [19,20,33–36]. In snow clover (#3 and #12) extracts, glycosyl and glycosyl malonate derivative of flavones (quercetin) and isoflavones (formononetin and prunetin) were detected in large amounts in both leaves and flowers. The abundant presence of prunetin was reported to be a characteristic feature of this clover species [20]. Leaf extracts of *T. repens* (#4, #8 and #13, see Figure 1) featured high content of di- and trisaccharide derivative of flavonols quercetin and kaempferol, together with other minor compounds, as already reported [37–40]. Flowers were characterized instead by high amount of quercetin galactoside and its acetyl derivative, together with lower content of myricetin galactoside. Subterranean clover (#5 and #6) leaves and flowers confirmed the large presence of isoflavones biochanin A, genistein and formononetin glycosides and glycosyl malonate derivatives [28]. *T. alpinum* (#9) extracts showed a complex mixture of flavonoids. In leaves, they were mainly constituted by mono and diglycosides of quercetin, while kaempferol glycosides were detected in flowers. The presence of glycosides of a quercetin isomer (MW=302) was also detected. The very low amount of isoflavones assessed in this *Trifolium* species was inconsistent with previous results [26]. Di- and tri-saccharide derivatives of quercetin were observed in *T. badium* (#10) extracts. An unidentified flavonoid (MW = 462) was abundant in leaves, while a monoglycoside of luteolin/luteolin isomer (MW = 286) was detected in large amount in flowers.

Leaves of *T. ochroleucum* (#11) mainly comprised mono- and di-saccharides of quercetin and, to a lesser extent, kaempferol. Quercetin and kaempferol glycosyl malonates were detected as the main constituents of flower extracts. Higher flavonoid content had been previously reported in *T. ochroleucum* leaves [19]. Quercetin and kaempferol diglycosides were abundant in *T. thalii* (#14) leaf extract, while the flower extract largely contained myricetin and quercetin glycosides. The isoflavone formononetin glycoside and its malonyl derivative were also detected in leaves.

Table 2. The most abundant, tentatively identified flavonoids in the 14 *Trifolium* samples and their quantitative evaluation (% dry matter, $n = 3$, mean value ± standard deviation) in leaves and flowers. See Table 1 for taxonomic classification, origin and adaptation of each sample.

#	UV λ_{max} (nm)	$[M + H]^+$ (*m/z*)	$[M - H]^-$ (*m/z*)	MW	Compound	Leaves	Flowers
1	253, 354	465, 303	463, 301	464	quercetin-3-*O*-galactoside	-	8.9 ± 0.5
	254, 354	465, 303	463, 301	464	quercetin-3-*O*-glucoside	-	10.2 ± 0.4
	255, 346	449, 287	447, 285	448	luteolin-7-*O*-glucoside	24.8 ± 1.6	8.7 ± 0.2
	266, 432	433, 271	431, 269	432	apigenin-7-*O*-glucoside	4.5 ± 0.3	0.5 ± 0.1
	254, 346	535, 449$[M - 86]^+$, 287	533, 489$[M - 44]^-$, 285	534	luteolin-7-*O*-glucoside-6″-*O*-malonate	17.8 ± 0.6	30.4 ± 0.9
	266, 337	519, 433$[M - 86]^+$, 271	517, 473$[M - 44]^-$, 269	518	apigein-7-*O*-glucoside-6″-*O*-malonate	3.8 ± 0.3	2.6 ± 0.4
	254, 344	287	285	286	luteolin	15.3 ± 0.2	3.7 ± 0.9
	260, 324	533, 285	531, 487$[M - 44]^-$, 283	532	biochanin A-7-*O*-glucoside-6″-*O*-malonate	7.4 ± 0.7	6.8 ± 0.9
2	253, 354	465, 303	463, 301	464	quercetin-3-*O*-galactoside	6.5 ± 0.2	5.5 ± 0.8
	256, 354	551, 303	549, 505$[M - 44]^-$, 301	550	quercetin-3-*O*-glucoside-6′′- *O*-malonate	6.2 ± 0.2	14.7 ± 0.5
	265, 344	535, 287	533, 489$[M - 44]^-$, 285	534	kaempferol-3-*O*-galactoside-6′′-*O*-malonate	-	11.7 ± 1.3
	251, 300	517, 269	515, 471$[M - 44]^-$, 267	516	formononetin-7-*O*-glucoside-6′′-*O*-malonate	14.5 ± 0.8	7.9 ± 0.7
	260, 324	533, 285	531, 487$[M - 44]^-$, 283	532	biochanin A-7-*O*-glucoside-6′′-*O*-malonate	20.9 ± 1.6	18.0 ± 1.7
3	253, 354	465, 303	463, 301	464	quercetin-3-*O*-galactoside	11.1 ± 0.4	15.1 ± 1.2
	256, 354	551, 303	549, 505$[M - 44]^-$, 301	550	quercetin-3-*O*-glucoside-6′′-O-malonate	9.0 ± 0.3	26.3 ± 1.4
	251, 300	431, 269	429, 267	430	formononetin-7-*O*-glucoside	3.1 ± 0.4	1.5 ± 0.2
	251, 300	517, 269	515, 471$[M - 44]^-$, 267	516	formononetin-7-*O*-glucoside-6′′-*O*-malonate	3.7 ± 0.1	1.7 ± 0.1
	260, 325	447, 285	445, 283	446	prunetin-4′-*O*-glucoside	7.6 ± 1.5	2.3 ± 0.9
	260, 325	355, 285	531, 487$[M - 44]^-$, 283	532	prunetin-4′-*O*-glucoside-6′′-O-malonate	20.0 ± 0.2	9.5 ± 1.2
4	266, 337	481, 319	479, 317	480	myricetin-3-*O*-galactoside	-	10.9 ± 0.2
	256, 347	743, 597, 303	741, 301	742	quercetin-3-*O*-{[rhamnosyl-(1→6)]-[xylosyl-(1→2)-galactoside]}	6.4 ± 0.6	2.0 ± 0.1
	256, 354	597, 465, 303	595, 301	596	quercetin-3-*O*-[xylosyl-(1→2)-galactoside]	22.6 ± 2.2	6.8 ± 0.1
	256, 344	727, 581, 449, 287	725, 285	742	kaempferol-3-*O*-{[rhamnosyl-(1→6)]-[xylosyl-(1→2)-galactoside]}	6.3 ± 0.4	1.1 ± 0.1
	253, 354	465, 303	463, 301	464	quercetin-3-*O*-galactoside	3.0 ± 0.2	24.5 ± 0.9
	265, 346	581, 449, 287	579, 285	580	kaempferol-3-*O*-[xylosyl-(1→2)-galactoside]	10.6 ± 0.7	1.5 ± 0.1
	256, 355	507, 303	505, 301	506	quercetin-3-*O*-galactoside-6′′-*O*-acetate	0.9 ± 0.1	23.0 ± 0.3
5	259, 325	433, 271	431, 269	432	genistein-7-*O*-glucoside	14.4 ± 0.7	
	265, 344	535, 287	533, 489$[M - 44]^-$, 285	534	orobol-7-*O*-glucoside-6′′-*O*-malonate	4.2 ± 0.1	
	259, 325	519, 271	517, 473$[M - 44]^-$, 269	518	genistein-7-*O*-glucoside-6′′-*O*-malonate	13.2 ± 0.2	
	260, 325	447, 285	445, 283	446	biochanin A-7-*O*-glucoside	13.5 ± 1.0	
	260, 325	533, 285	531, 487$[M - 44]^-$, 283	532	biochanin A-7-*O*-glucoside-6′′-*O*-malonate	35.8 ± 1.9	
6	259, 325	433, 271	431, 269	432	genistein-7-*O*-glucoside	11.4 ± 1.3	4.2 ± 0.8
	259, 325	519, 271	517, 473$[M - 44]^-$, 269	518	genistein-7-*O*-glucoside-6′′-*O*-malonate	13.6 ± 0.4	6.0 ± 0.4
	251, 300	431, 269	429, 267	430	formononetin-7-*O*-glucoside	4.9 ± 0.7	7.9 ± 1.8
	251, 300	517, 269	515, 471$[M - 44]^-$, 267	516	formononetin-7-*O*-glucoside-6′′-*O*-malonate	12.9 ± 0.4	25.5 ± 3.0
	260, 325	447, 285	445, 283	446	biochanin A-7-*O*-glucoside	8.3 ± 0.6	6.7 ± 1.2
	260, 325	533, 285	531, 487$[M - 44]^-$, 283	532	biochanin A-7-*O*-glucoside-6′′-*O*-malonate	23.9 ± 2.3	24.8 ± 2.7

Table 2. *Cont.*

7	253, 354	465, 303	463, 301	464	quercetin-3-*O*-galactoside	8.7 ± 0.5	8.5 ± 1.2
	256, 354	551, 303	549, 505$[M - 44]^-$, 301	550	quercetin-3-*O*-glucoside-6′′-*O*-malonate	8.9 ± 0.2	21.1 ± 0.3
	265, 344	535, 287	533, 489$[M - 44]^-$, 285	534	kaempferol-3-*O*-galactoside-6′′-*O*-malonate	-	14.1 ± 2.4
	251, 300	517, 269	515, 471$[M - 44]^-$, 267	516	formononetin-7-*O*-glucoside-6′′-*O*-malonate	8.3 ± 0.5	4.7 ± 0.6
	260, 324	533, 285	531, 487$[M - 44]^-$, 283	532	biochanin A-7-*O*-glucoside-6′′-*O*-malonate	18.9 ± 1.0	9.4 ± 0.9
8	266, 337	481, 319	479, 317	480	myricetin-3-*O*-galactoside	-	13.5 ± 0.6
	256, 347	743, 597, 303	741, 301	742	quercetin-3-*O*-{[rhamnosyl-(1→6)]-[xylosyl-(1→2)-galactoside]}	5.7 ± 0.5	2.1 ± 0.1
	256, 354	597, 465, 303	595, 301	596	quercetin-3-*O*-[xylosyl-(1→2)-galactoside]	22.3 ± 0.6	8.8 ± 0.3
	256, 344	727, 581, 449, 287	725, 285	742	kaempferol-3-*O*-{[rhamnosyl-(1→6)]-[xylosyl-(1→2)-galactoside]}	4.0 ± 0.3	1.3 ± 0.1
	253, 354	465, 303	463, 301	464	quercetin-3-*O*-galactoside	2.5 ± 0.3	29.9 ± 0.5
	256, 355	507, 303	505, 301	506	quercetin-3-*O*-galactoside-6′′-*O*-acetate	1.3 ± 0.1	21.7 ± 0.3
9	256, 354	627, 465, 303	625, 301	626	quercetin-hexose-hexose	11.4 ± 0.1	16.6 ± 0.4
	265, 344	611, 449, 287	609, 447, 285	610	kaempferol-hexose-hexose	-	3.6 ± 0.0
	255, 332	949, 625, 463, 303	947	948	302-hexose-hexose-hexose-hexose	10.1 ± 01	1.7 ± 0.1
	256, 355	465, 303	463, 301	464	quercetin-3-*O*-galactoside	0.7 ± 0.0	9.1 ± 0.1
	256, 355	465, 303	463, 301	464	quercetin-3-*O*-glucoside	1.3 ± 0.1	18.9 ± 0.1
	254, 332	833, 303	831, 301	832	302-hexose-hexose-hexose-acetate	6.0 ± 0.2	1.0 ± 0.0
	265, 341	449, 287	447, 285	448	kaempferol-3-*O*-glucoside	-	3.9 ± 0.1
10	256, 354	759	757, 595, 462, 301	758	quercetin-hexose-hexose-pentose	5.0 ± 0.1	-
	256, 354	773, 303	771, 609, 462, 301	772	quercetin-hexose-hexose-rhamnose	8.8 ± 0.2	1.0 ± 0.1
	282, 332	463	461, 285	462	unidentified	18.2 ± 0.7	-
	265, 348	449, 287	447, 285	448	luteolin-hexose	6.7 ± 0.4	60.1 ± 0.4
	256, 349	595	593, 447, 285	594	luteolin-rhamnose-hexose	8.7 ± 0.2	8.6 ± 0.1
11	256, 354	773, 611, 465, 303	771, 301	772	quercetin-hexose-hexose-rhamnose	3.9 ± 0.1	0.9 ± 0.1
	256, 354	627, 465, 303	625, 301	626	quercetin-hexose-hexose	5.8 ± 0.2	0.3 ± 0.0
	256, 354	611, 449, 303	609, 447, 301	610	quercetin-hexose-rhamnose	6.5 ± 0.2	0.9 ± 0.1
	256, 356	757, 611, 465, 303	755, 301	756	quercetin-hexose-rhamnose-rhamnose	26.7 ± 0.2	10.8 ± 0.5
	256, 355	465, 303	463, 301	464	quercetin-3-*O*-galactoside	8.9 ± 0.2	12.1 ± 0.8
	265, 344	741, 595, 449, 287	739, 593, 447, 285	740	kaempferol-hexose-rhamnose-rhamnose	9.6 ± 0.1	10.5 ± 0.2
	256, 354	551, 303	549, 505$[M - 44]^-$, 301	550	quercetin-3-*O*-glucoside-6′′-*O*-malonate	2.4 ± 0.1	26.1 ± 0.1
	265, 344	535, 287	533, 489$[M - 44]^-$, 285	534	kaempferol-3-*O*-galactoside-6′′-*O*-malonate	-	16.8 ± 1.9
12	253, 354	465, 303	463, 301	464	quercetin-3-*O*-galactoside	4.5 ± 0.3	21.6 ± 1.9
	256, 355	465, 303	463, 301	464	quercetin-3-*O*-glucoside	10.1 ± 2.0	1.1 ± 0.3
	256, 354	551, 303	549, 505$[M - 44]^-$, 301	550	quercetin-3-*O*-glucoside-6′′-O-malonate	27.2 ± 2.1	44.6 ± 2.6
	251, 300	431, 269	429, 267	430	formononetin-7-*O*-glucoside	1.8 ± 0.6	-
	260, 325	447, 285	445, 283	446	prunetin-4′-*O*-glucoside	8.7 ± 1.9	0.5 ± 0.0
	260, 325	355, 285	531, 487$[M - 44]^-$, 283	532	prunetin-4′-*O*-glucoside-6′′-O-malonate	17.4 ± 1.2	1.9 ± 0.1

Table 2. *Cont.*

	266, 337	481, 319	479, 317	480	myricetin-3-*O*-galactoside	-	18.9 ± 0.2
	256, 354	597, 465, 303	595, 301	596	quercetin-3-*O*-[xylosyl-(1→2)-galactoside]	29.1 ± 0.3	8.1 ± 0.2
	256, 344	727, 581, 449, 287	725, 285	742	kaempferol-3-*O*-{[rhamnosyl-(1→6)]-[xylosyl-(1→2)-galactoside]}	3.3 ± 0.1	0.4 ± 0.1
13	253, 354	465, 303	463, 301	464	quercetin-3-*O*-galactoside	3.9 ± 0.1	36.4 ± 0.4
	265, 346	581, 449, 287	579, 285	580	kaempferol-3-*O*-[xylosyl-(1→2)-galactoside]	11.0 ± 1.2	1.1 ± 0.2
	263, 351	449, 287	447, 285	448	kaempferol-3-*O*-galactoside	3.8 ± 0.5	6.3 ± 0.1
	256, 355	507, 303	505, 301	506	quercetin-3-*O*-galactoside-6′′-*O*-acetate	1.5 ± 0.3	17.8 ± 0.3
	266, 337	481, 319	479, 317	480	myricetin-3-*O*-galactoside	-	23.4 ± 0.2
	256, 354	597, 465, 303	595, 301	596	quercetin-3-*O*-[xylosyl-(1→2)-galactoside]	46.2 ± 0.3	10.8 ± 0.3
	253, 354	465, 303	463, 301	464	quercetin-3-*O*-galactoside	4.2 ± 0.2	46.3 ± 0.6
14	265, 346	581, 449, 287	579, 285	580	kaempferol-3-*O*-[xylosyl-(1→2)-galactoside]	9.6 ± 0.3	1.2 ± 0.1
	256, 355	523, 319	521, 317	522	myricetin-3-*O*-galactoside-6″-*O*-acetate	-	5.2 ± 0.1
	251, 300	431, 269	429, 267	430	formononetin-7-*O*-glucoside	4.8 ± 0.8	-
	251, 300	517, 269	515, 471[M − 44]$^-$, 267	516	formononetin-7-*O*-glucoside-6′′-*O*-malonate	6.0 ± 1.5	-

2.2. Evaluation of Phenolic Compounds in the *Trifolium* Species in Relation to Their Antioxidant Activities

To facilitate the assessment of the biological activity of the different *Trifolium* extracts and to evaluate their antioxidant properties in relation to the phytocomplex (whole extract), the detected compounds were grouped into four distinct classes based on their chemical structure and biological properties, namely, phenolic acids, clovamides, isoflavones, and other flavonoids, this latter including flavanols, flavonols, and flavones. The presence of a fifth group of phenolic compounds, namely proanthocyanidins (or condensed tannins) was assessed by the butanol/HCl method [41], and evaluated with pelargonidin as a standard. Although with some limitations, this method was reported to allow for the most effective detection of proanthocyanidins [42–44]. Pelargonidin was selected as a standard because of its presence in all samples among anthocyanidins obtained from the acid-catalysed cleavage of the condensed tannins. Preliminary investigation performed by a cellulose bidimensional thin layer chromatography (2D TLC) of the obtained anthocyanidin (data not reported), showed the presence of pelargonidin, cyanidin and delfinidin. In all the analyzed samples, variation was observed for these compounds, with pelargonidin being one of the most detected compounds.

Results of the quantitative evaluation of different phenolics in leaves and flowers of the 14 samples of clover under investigation are reported in Tables 3–5.

Flower tissues featured higher concentration of total phenolics compared to leaves across all accessions (Table 3). However, differences between plant organs for individual phenolic group concentrations were not consistent, with no difference for phenolic acids and clovamides, higher concentration in leaves for isoflavones, and higher concentration in flowers for other flavonoids and for proanthocyanidins. The antioxidant activity was higher in flower than in leaf extracts according to each of the three applied assays.

It is widely accepted that leaves have higher amount of phenolic compounds than flowers, owing to the abundance of pathway precursors in leaves due to photosynthesis [45,46]. However, the current result of higher concentration of total phenolics in flowers than in leaves had several precedents in different folk-medicine species, such as yarrow, *Achillea millefolium* L. [47], pomegranate, *Punica granatum* L. [48], or white-weed, *Ageratum conyzoides* L. [49]. The facts that pigments are composed of flavonoids in most flowers, and that proanthocyanidins are produced by closely related branches of the flavonoid pathway using the same metabolic intermediates, make of no surprise the finding that flowers in our germplasm collection were particularly rich in these groups of phenolics. Abeynayake et al. [50] reported that white clover plants accumulate higher level of proanthocyanidins in flowers than in vegetative tissues. In addition to a possible ultraviolet (UV)-screening effect exerted by phenolics [22], a role for flavonoids was reported in the development of functional pollen [51], which may also explain the abundance of these compounds in flower tissues. Total phenolic concentration in flowers, especially as proanthocyanidins, fully supported higher antioxidant activity of flower compared to leaf extracts, no matter the applied scavenging assay. Nonetheless, greater sensitivity of the peroxyl radical scavenging for proanthocyanidins was evident, confirming the results in Jayaprakasha et al. [52], thus accounting for the current outstanding difference between leaf and flower extracts for this assay.

The 14 *Trifolium* samples differed significantly ($P < 0.05$) for leaf phenolic concentrations and antioxidant activity according to ANOVA (Table 4). The red clover cultivar Aiace (#2) was rich in phenolic acids, followed by the snow clover population #3 and the berseem clover experimental cultivar #1. Clovamides were found in highest concentration in red clover samples (#2 and #7) and they were also present in the snow clover populations #3 and #12 and the berseem cultivar #1.

Table 3. Comparison between leaves and flowers (mean values across the 14 *Trifolium* samples reported in Table 1) for concentration of phenolic groups and antioxidant activity.

	Phenolic Group Concentration (mg/g Dry Matter)						Antioxidant Activity Assay		
Sample	Phenolic Acids	Clovamides	Isoflavones	Other Flavonoids	Proanthocyanidins	Total Phenolics	Fremy's Salt Scavenging *	Superoxide Anion Scavenging *	Peroxyl Radical Scavenging **
leaves	2.13 a	5.23 a	14.51 a	20.83 b	1.12 b	43.83 b	4.94 b	2.03 b	44.93 b
flowers	1.33 a	3.12 a	2.23 b	34.90 a	40.84 a	82.42 a	11.06 a	4.61 a	489.29 a

In each column, mean values followed by different letters (a or b) are different at $P < 0.05$ according to analysis of variance. * µmol gallic acid equivalents (GAE)/100 g freeze-dried matter;.** mmol Trolox equivalents (TE)/100 g freeze-dried matter.

Table 4. Concentration of phenolic groups and antioxidant activity determined on leaves of 14 *Trifolium* samples. See Table 1 for taxonomic classification.

	Phenolic Group Concentration (mg/g Dry Matter)						Antioxidant Activity Assay		
#	Phenolic acids	Clovamides	Isoflavones	Other Flavonoids	Proanthocyanidins	Total Phenolics	Fremy's Salt Scavenging *	Superoxide Anion Scavenging *	Peroxyl Radical Scavenging **
1	4.66	8.53	4.20	41.15	4.10	62.65	5.37	2.12	28.00
2	5.94	29.86	22.63	13.78	0.66	72.89	15.40	4.07	88.25
3	4.68	8.64	16.55	16.88	0.14	46.90	6.08	2.19	21.60
4	1.40	-	0.31	9.19	0.05	10.96	3.18	2.13	10.05
5	2.00	-	70.03	7.55	0.06	79.64	1.47	1.82	137.50
6	1.87	-	48.00	7.94	0.03	57.84	2.15	0.61	8.85
7	2.85	22.33	22.72	21.08	0.12	69.11	9.40	1.92	130.00
8	1.27	-	0.70	6.18	0.25	8.42	3.27	0.60	3.70
9	-	-	0.38	27.68	0.37	28.44	4.49	0.88	16.80
10	-	-	0.17	34.70	8.58	43.45	3.24	5.86	24.30
11	2.42	-	0.54	44.14	0.39	47.51	3.63	2.19	24.10
12	1.71	3.89	14.56	28.54	0.32	49.02	5.54	1.58	110.85
13	-	-	0.56	14.39	0.04	14.95	3.37	0.93	2.55
14	1.02	-	0.79	18.50	0.47	21.79	2.59	1.43	22.45
$LSD_{(P = 0.05)}$	1.17	0.48	2.72	2.79	0.18	4.18	2.43	1.60	30.04

* µmol gallic acid equivalents (GAE)/100 g freeze-dried matter; ** mmol Trolox equivalents (TE)/100 g freeze-dried matter.

Table 5. Concentration of phenolic groups and antioxidant activity determined on flowers of 13 *Trifolium* samples. See Table 1 for taxonomic classification.

	Phenolic Group Concentration (mg/g Dry Matter)						Antioxidant Activity Assay		
#	Phenolic Acids	Clovamides	Isoflavones	Other Flavonoids	Proanthocyanidins	Total Phenolics	Fremy's Salt Scavenging *	Superoxide Anion Scavenging *	Peroxyl Radical Scavenging **
1	2.23	6.88	1.15	19.12	29.14	58.53	5.04	4.41	46.30
2	2.63	11.99	10.91	23.70	42.94	92.18	6.20	1.13	423.40
3	2.83	7.29	5.17	22.58	39.03	76.90	5.06	1.00	394.40
4	0.85	-	0.14	15.47	24.10	40.82	9.96	2.69	436.80
6	0.46	-	4.57	0.74	4.96	10.73	2.35	0.76	4.10
7	2.89	10.50	5.44	25.58	37.39	81.81	6.37	1.92	190.00
8	0.44	-	0.08	21.21	30.53	52.27	11.35	1.72	34.60
9	-	-	0.22	27.81	33.31	61.51	8.56	5.48	150.20
10	-	-	-	80.29	81.28	161.57	16.75	9.93	696.00
11	2.56	-	-	44.12	30.30	76.99	7.42	5.31	1065.20
12	1.13	1.29	1.29	54.01	56.88	117.17	9.87	3.67	603.00
13	1.28	-	-	55.60	54.95	111.83	27.19	9.90	940.60
14	-	-	-	63.46	66.11	129.57	27.61	12.01	1376.50
$LSD_{(P = 0.05)}$	0.62	0.62	0.62	6.77	3.23	8.93	2.33	2.51	253.37

* µmol gallic acid equivalents (GAE)/100 g freeze-dried matter; ** mmol Trolox equivalents (TE)/100 g freeze-dried matter.

The subterranean clover populations #5 and #6 showed the highest concentration of isoflavones, followed by the two red clover samples (#2 and #7) and the two snow clover populations (#3 and #12). Three mountain species, namely, sulphur clover (#11), brown clover (#10) and alpine clover (#9) featured the highest concentration of other flavonoids, together with the berseem clover (#1). The two white clover accessions from lowlands (#4 and #8) and the two subterranean clover populations (#5 and #6) were characterized by the lowest concentration of other flavonoids. Proanthocyanidins were abundant in leaves of brown clover (#10) and berseem clover (#1) only. The leaf concentration of total phenolics exceeded the level of 60 mg g^{-1} dry matter in the two red clover accessions (#2 and #7), the subterranean clover population #5 and the berseem clover #1, while barely reaching the level of 10 mg g^{-1} dry matter in the two lowland white clover samples (#8 and #4).

Just as for the leaf samples, there was significant variation among accessions ($P < 0.05$) according to ANOVA for the flower phenolic concentrations and antioxidant activity (Table 5). However, accession patterns of phenolic concentrations were largely different in flowers compared to leaves. Only clovamides showed an outstanding consistency between flowers and leaves of exclusive presence in red clover (#2 and #7), snow clover (#3 and #12) and berseem clover (#1) germplasm (Tables 4 and 5). Concentration of phenolic acids was highest in flowers of the red clover samples (#2 and #7), the snow clover population #3, the sulphur clover population #11 and the berseem clover cultivar #1. Isoflavone concentration (much lower in flowers than in leaves, see Table 3) was highest in the red clover accessions (#2 and #7), the snow clover population #3 and the subterranean clover population #6. The subterranean clover population #5, featuring the highest isoflavone concentration in leaves, was missing in the flower analysis, owing to too few flowers to be used in the chemical determinations. The brown clover population #10 showed the highest concentration of other flavonoids, followed by the Thal clover population #14, while the subterranean clover population #6 had remarkably low concentration of these compounds. Somewhat similar was the pattern of proanthocyanidin concentration, with highest values in mountain accessions (brown clover #10, Thal clover #14, snow clover #12, and white clover #13) and lowest one in the subterranean clover #6. The very high concentration of proanthocyanidins in the mentioned mountain accessions clearly contributed to their highest concentrations of flower total phenolics, with values exceeding 100 mg/g dry matter, while the subterranean clover population #6 was bottom ranking for flower total phenolics with a concentration of about 10 mg/g dry matter (Table 5).

Oleszek et al. [19] partitioned their *Trifolium* collection into groups according to the patterns of leaf phenolic composition. The present germplasm also featured accession groups with specific phenolic composition. In some cases, these patterns bore a taxonomic meaning. *T. subterraneum* and *T. pratense* (the latter, both as red clover and as snow clover subspecies) were characterized by high leaf concentration of isoflavones. Clovamides were restricted to red clover and, to a lesser extent, snow clover and berseem clover. Most alpine species and berseem clover were rich in flavonoids other than isoflavones. White clover (across the three evaluated taxonomic forms) featured the lowest leaf phenolic concentration.

The richness of leaf isoflavones in subterranean clover confirms previous results on this species [28]. Red clover isoflavone extracts are commercially available as nutraceuticals and they have been proposed as an alternative to hormone-replacement therapy [53]. Subterranean clover may represent an interesting new source of isoflavones, with higher concentration of these compounds and more diverse pattern of isoflavone composition compared to red clover [28].

As emphasized [19], attention should be paid for exploitation to those species comprising good concentration of different phenolic groups, as the presence of these groups may provide synergistic health effects of plant extracts.

Accession rankings for the antioxidant activity of leaf extracts according to the three assays were quite inconsistent (Table 4). The highest activity was observed in the two red clover samples (#2 and #7) for the Fremy's salt scavenging, in the subterranean clover population #5, the red clover population #7 and the snow clover population #12 for the peroxyl radical scavenging, and in the brown clover population #10 and the red clover cultivar #2 for the superoxide anion scavenging. The inconsistency of accession ranking for the three assays was confirmed by the lack of significant pairwise correlation between assays based on leaf accession values (data not reported).

Unlike for the data on leaf extracts, there was some consistency of accession ranking between assays for the antioxidant activity of flower extracts (Table 5). In particular, the Thal clover population #14 and the subterranean clover population #6 were always top- and bottom-ranking, respectively, regardless of the scavenging assay. The mountain white clover population #13 also featured rather high antioxidant activity of flower extract with all three assays. Overall, there were moderately high positive pairwise correlations between scavenging assays, ranging from $r = 0.74$, $P < 0.01$ (Fremy's salt vs. peroxyl radical) to $r = 0.87$, $P < 0.01$ (Fremy's salt vs. superoxide anion).

The presence of diversified patterns of phytochemical composition, and the contemporary presence of structurally different groups of phenolics, such as isoflavones, other flavonoids and proanthocyanidins, that were likely to determine different responses to the antioxidant assays [54], justified the choice of three methods of antioxidant measurements. These assays were characterised, indeed, by rather different reactivity towards distinct free radical molecular probes, as successively confirmed by the results of the regression analysis described below.

Lowland accessions had higher concentration of phenolic acids, clovamides and isoflavones, and lower concentration of other flavonoids and proanthocyanidins, than mountain accessions consistently in leaves and flowers. However, lowland germplasm showed higher concentration of total phenolics in leaves, while mountain accessions had higher concentration of total phenolics in flowers (Table 6). This inconsistency was mostly due to outstanding concentration of isoflavones in leaves of lowland germplasm, and of both proanthocyanidins and flavonoids other than isoflavones in flowers of mountain germplasm. An inconsistency of rankings between germplasm provenances was also largely observed for the antioxidant activity. Lowland accessions had, on average, higher scavenging activity of leaf extracts in two assays out of three, whereas the scavenging activity of flower samples was higher in mountain than in lowland germplasm regardless of the assay (Table 6).

As already anticipated, the high concentration of flavonoids (other than isoflavones) and proanthocyanidins, associated with higher antioxidant capacities, in flower tissues of mountain germplasm can be a hint of the photoprotection effect recognized to flavonoids and other phenolics [55], possibly exerted on the sensitive reproductive system [23]. It is indeed well known that UV levels increase with altitude, and mountain species must be provided with adequate protection. Accumulation of flavonoids in response to UV-B exposition was reported in silver birch, *Betula pendula* Roth [56], while UV-stress-adapted germplasm displayed particularly high constitutive or elicited levels of flavonoids and other phenolics in *Arabidopsis thaliana* (L.) Heynh. [57] and in white clover [38]. UV absorption is one of the UV-protective properties ascribed to flavonoids, which also include energy dissipation and antioxidant activities [55]. A role of free-radical scavenging in response to UV exposure can be postulated [58].

The pattern of phenolic composition in lowland germplasm was suggestive of different adaptive strategies. The abundance of isoflavones in lowland leaves, in particular, may indicate natural selection to decreased palatability for herbivores, or increased defence systems against invertebrate pests [59].

Table 7 summarizes the best linear models predicted for leaf and flower samples from the multiple regression analysis of the antioxidant activity on mean concentrations of groups of phenolic compounds within the *Trifolium* germplasm. The concentration of 'other flavonoids' and that of 'proanthocyanidins' consistently proved affected by multicollinearity in flowers, and for that reason only the former was retained in the regressions on flower data. Regardless of the scavenging assay and the plant organ, the adjusted R^2 of the models was only moderate at most, with the exception of the good prediction of the Fremy's salt scavenging in leaves ($R^2 = 0.934$, $P < 0.001$). In both leaves and flowers, the peroxyl radical scavenging had a complex best fitting model, including most of the phenolic groups as regressors, whereas the Fremy's salt and the superoxide anion scavenging showed simpler models for both plant organ extracts.

Table 6. Mean values of concentration of phenolic groups and antioxidant activity in leaves and flowers of *Trifolium* samples originating from, and sampled in, either lowland. (#1, 2, 4, 5, 6, 7 and 8 in Table 1) or mountain areas (# 9, 10, 11, 12, 13 and 14 in Table 1).

Area of Germplasm Origin and Sampling	Phenolic Group Concentration (mg/g Dry Matter)						Antioxidant Activity Assay		
	Phenolic Acids	Clovamides	Isoflavones	Other Flavonoids	Proanthocyanidins	Total Phenolics	Fremy's Salt Scavenging *	Superoxide Anion Scavenging *	Peroxyl Radical Scavenging **
Leaves									
Lowlands	2.86 a	7.62 a	24.19 a	14.82 b	0.75 b	50.30 a	5.75 a	1.90 a	58.05 a
Mountains	0.86 b	0.65 b	3.00 b	27.99 a	1.70 a	34.19 b	3.81 b	2.15 a	33.51 b
Flowers									
Lowlands	1.65 a	5.34 a	4.04 a	11.84 b	28.18 b	57.44 b	6.88 b	2.11 b	189.18 b
Mountains	0.90 b	0.70 b	0.25 b	56.62 a	53.81 a	114.16 a	16.24 a	7.72 a	805.23 a

In each column within each plant organ, mean values followed by different letters (a or b) are different at $P < 0.05$ according to analysis of variance. * μmol gallic acid equivalents (GAE)/100 g freeze-dried matter; ** mmol Trolox equivalents (TE)/100 g freeze-dried matter.

Table 7. Prediction of antioxidant activity in leaves and flowers of *Trifolium* germplasm, based on multiple regression analysis of accession mean values of each antioxidant assay on accession mean concentrations of groups of phenolic compounds. Group concentrations in the models (in parentheses) are expressed as mg g^{-1} dry matter.

Antioxidant Activity Assay	Best Linear Model	Model F Probability	Adjusted R^2
Leaves			
Fremy's salt scavenging *	3.368 + 0.373 *(clovamides) − 0.026 *(isoflavones)	< 0.001	0.934
Superoxid anion scavenging *	1.194 + 0.059 *(clovamides) + 0.468 *(proanthocyanidins)	< 0.001	0.685
Peroxyl radical scavenging * *	−2.217 − 12.624 *(phenolic acids) + 4.012 *(clovamides) + 1.317 *(other flavonoids) + 1.765 *(isoflavones)	< 0.05	0.554
Flowers			
Fremy's salt scavenging *	5.444 − 1.886 *(phenolic acids) + 0.233 *(other flavonoids)	< 0.001	0.524
Superoxid anion scavenging *	0.887 − 0.230 *(clovamides) + 0.127 *(other flavonoids)	< 0.001	0.728
Peroxyl radical scavenging **	−242.1 + 217.8 *(phenolic acids) − 80.8 *(clovamides) + 16.5 *(other flavonoids) + 52.5 *(isoflavones)	< 0.05	0.601

* μmol gallic acid equivalents (GAE)/100 g freeze-dried matter; ** mmol Trolox equivalents (TE)/100 g freeze-dried matter

The concentration of clovamides had a consistent, positive regression coefficient in the three best models predicted for the antioxidant activity in leaves. Similarly, the concentration of the group of flavonoids other than isoflavones contributed positively to predicting the antioxidant activity with all assays in flowers (Table 7).

The multicollinearity between the concentrations of flavonoids and proanthocyanidins prevented their simultaneous assessment as regressors in the prediction of the antioxidant activity. However, when taken individually in a simple correlation analysis with the three scavenging assays, the mean flower concentration of proanthocyanidins also proved positively correlated with the antioxidant activity, with correlation ranging between $r = 0.63$ ($P < 0.05$) with the peroxyl radical and $r = 0.73$ ($P < 0.01$) with the superoxide anion scavenging.

Although claimed as interesting antioxidant compounds, clovamides proved to be important but not critical for the antioxidant activity in cocoa, *Theobroma cacao* L. [60]. Subsequent findings indicated them as potent bioactive compounds with anti-inflammatory activity in human cells [61]. In the current study, clovamides appeared to have a conditional, positive role in determining the antioxidant activity of leaf extracts in the genus *Trifolium*. Our results are in line with those by Kolodziejczyk et al. [62], who reported that clovamide-rich extract from *T. pallidum* reduced the damage induced by oxidative stress to blood platelets and plasma.

A key role in determining the antioxidant activity in flowers of *Trifolium* germplasm was exerted instead by the classes of flavonoids (isoflavones excluded) and proanthocyanidins, which was fully justified by the strong antioxidant properties reported for these compounds [11,52,63]. As already mentioned, flower pigmentation and UV screening contribute to the abundance of flavonoids and proanthocyanidins in flower tissues.

This investigation confirmed the genus *Trifolium* as a great reservoir of phenolic compounds, with different chemical structure and, possibly, largely diversified biological activity. Such a wealth of potentially important metabolites is available for clinical and nutraceutical utilization. It is worth reminding that, unlike other species claimed for extraction of biologically active compounds, most *Trifolium* species have a well-established agronomic technique for their cultivation. This study also suggested possible links between environmental factors (stresses, in particular) and concentration and composition of phenolic compounds.

3. Materials and Methods

3.1. Plant Material

Swards of red clover, white clover, subterranean clover, berseem clover and snow clover were sampled in the lowland site of Lodi [45°19′ N, 9°30′ E, 81 m above sea level (asl)], in the Po Valley plain, northern Italy (Table 1). Some of the materials belonging to these taxa were grown in plots at the experimental station of the Research Centre for Animal Production and Aquaculture (CREA-ZA). In particular, the red clover cultivar Aiace, the white clover cultivar Regal (a non-Ladino large-leaved type of *T. repens*) and one snow clover natural population from the Rhaetian Alps were sampled from one-year-old sown swards. Aiace and Regal are cultivars selected in Italy and the USA, respectively, and both are adapted to temperate, favorable climatic conditions, such as those experienced under the sub-continental climate of Lodi (847 mm long-term average annual rainfall, 12.2 °C average annual mean daily temperature, −1.3 °C average minimum daily temperature of the coldest month). Seed of the snow clover population from the Rhaetian Alps was collected at 1850 m asl and it was sown in the lowland site as part of a trial carried out in altitude-contrasting environments. Germplasm of the annual species berseem clover (the experimental cultivar Sintetica-E) and subterranean clover (two natural populations whose seed was originally collected in Sardinia) were sown at CREA-ZA for this study. As both species are specifically adapted to Mediterranean conditions, they were sown in Lodi at the end of the winter preceding the sampling season to avoid possible frost damages. Besides the plot-grown materials, two more populations were sampled from a century-old grassland in Lodi, belonging to locally-adapted ecotypes of red clover and Ladino white clover (*T. repens* L. var. *giganteum* Lagr.-Foss.), respectively. Other natural populations used in this investigation were identified and sampled in the Alpine region (Table 1). They included one small-leaved population of white clover (*T. repens* var. *sylvestre*), which encompassed, therefore, three different types in the study, and one population each of snow clover, alpine clover (*T. alpinum* L.), brown clover (*T. badium* Schreb.), sulphur clover (*T. ochroleucum* Huds.) and Thal clover (*T. thalii* Vill.). Identification of different taxa was made according to reference guides on the Alpine flora [64]. All the mountain populations except the sulphur clover were sampled in the Graian Alps above 1900 m asl. The sulphur clover population was sampled in the Cottian Alps at 1250 m asl.

All the materials were sampled at the same phenological stage of full bloom. This stage occurred in spring (May) in the lowland site of Lodi, and in summer (July) in the mountain locations. Two samples of leaves and flowers were collected, respectively, from each sward, refrigerated and immediately brought to the laboratory. Leaf and flower samples were separately freeze-dried, finely powdered, defatted with chloroform and then used for the subsequent extractions.

3.2. Extraction and Purification of Total Phenolics

Samples (100 mg) were extracted with 80% MeOH (10 mL) at 50 °C using an automated accelerated solvent extractor ASE 200 (Dionex, Sunnyvale, CA, USA) at a working pressure of 1500 psi. Extracts were evaporated to dryness under reduced pressure at 40 °C, re-dissolved in 5 mL of Milli-Q water (Millipore Corp., Billerica, MA, USA) and purified using a C18 Sep-Pak (360 mg, 55–105 μm) cartridge (Waters Associates, Milford, MA, USA) preconditioned with water. The cartridge was washed first with water (5 mL) to remove sugars and other water-soluble compounds, then with 80% MeOH (5 mL) to elute phenolics. Extracts were evaporated to dryness under reduced pressure at 40 °C, re-dissolved in 2 mL of 80% MeOH and then used for analysis. Three independent extraction and purification procedures were performed on each replicated sample, and the extracts were properly diluted before analysis. A portion of the extracts was also freeze-dried for subsequent antioxidant activity assays.

3.3. Determination and Quantitation of Phenolic Composition

A Waters ACQUITY UPLC system equipped with a binary pump system, sample manager, column manager, photo diode array (PDA) detector (Waters Corp.) and coupled to a Waters ACQUITY TQD (tandem quadrupole mass detector) with an electrospray ionization (ESI) source was used. All data were acquired and processed using Waters MassLynx 4.1 and QuanLynx software. Chromatographic runs were carried out with a Waters BEH C18 column (100 mm × 1.0 mm i.d., 1.7 μm particles, 13 nm pore size) under a linear gradient of solvent A (H_2O/0.1% HCOOH) and solvent B (CH_3CN/0.1% HCOOH) as follows: 0.0–0.5 min (7% B), 8.0 min (25% B), 11.5 min (60% B), 12.0 min (80% B), 20 min (80% B). The flow rate was 0.19 mL/min, and the column temperature was 50 °C. A sample of 0.5 μL was injected for analysis. For MS detection, positive and negative ESI were used as ionization modes. Nitrogen was used as the desolvation and cone gas with flow rates of 800 L/h and 80 L/h, respectively. Argon was used as the collision gas at a flow rate of 2 mL/min. The MS parameters were as follows: Capillary 2.8 kV; extractor and radiofrequency voltage fixed at 3.0 V and 0.1 V, respectively; source and desolvation temperatures of 140 °C and 350 °C, respectively [20,28].

Phenolic compounds were identified by comparison of their UV absorption spectra, retention times and mass spectral data (positive and negative mode) with those of standard compounds, as well as with previously identified phenolic constituents of *Trifolium* spp. reported in the literature [19,20,25–28]. Individual compounds were quantified against reference standards at 260 nm. Astragalin, hyperoside, cymaroside, isoquercitrin, genistin, ononin, sissotrin, kaempferol, quercetin, apigenin, luteolin, myricetin, genistein, biochanin A, formononetin catechin, epicatechin were from Sigma-Aldrich (Milano, Italy). Concentration of glycoside malonates and acetates were calculated using the standard curves of the corresponding glycosides. Concentration of isoflavonoids without standards were calculated using the standard curves of ononin, while the concentration of other flavonoids was calculated using the calibration curves of isoquercitrin. Chlorogenic acid from Sigma-Aldrich was used to quantify clovamides and phenolic acids. For calibration curves, all standards were injected in triplicate in the range from 4.5 to 300 ng injection.

Proanthocyanidins (condensed tannins) were assessed by the butanol/HCl method [41], and evaluated with pelargonidin hydrochloride from Sigma-Aldrich as a standard.

All samples were extracted in triplicate and results expressed in mg g^{-1} dry matter as mean of three independent analyses ± standard deviation. As an indication of the relative abundance of the main tentatively identified compounds, the percentage values of their content in the whole extracts were reported in Table 2.

3.4. *Antioxidant Activity*

The purified freeze-dried extracts were subsequently treated at room temperature with 2.5 mL MeOH, 2.5 mL water, and acidified with 0.05 mL of 1N HCl. The mixture was vortexed for 60 s and centrifuged (5000× *g*, 5 min) and the supernatant directly used for antioxidant assays. The antioxidant activity was assessed by three different methods, aimed at understanding the potential action of the different groups of antioxidant compounds isolated and thoroughly characterized in *Trifolium* extracts. The three methods, described as follows, were the Fremy's salt scavenging and the superoxide anion scavenging, both carried out by Electron Paramagnetic Resonance (EPR), and the scavenging of peroxyl radicals, performed with a spectrophotometric approach.

3.4.1. Fremy's Salt Scavenging

This EPR assay was performed using Fremy's salt, potassium nitrosodisulfonate [$(KSO_3)_2NO$], a persistent water-soluble free radical that was successfully used in previous experiments investigating the antioxidant potential of fruit juices [65]. The reaction mixture contained 380 µL of 0.1 M acetate buffer, pH 4.5, and 100 µL of plant extract with 20 µL of 5.96 mM Fremy's salt solution dissolved in acetate buffer, final concentration 0.24 mM. Blank reaction was composed as before, by replacing the plant extract by the pure extracting solution. The mixture was stirred and transferred into a 100-µL glass capillary tube, and the EPR spectra were recorded after 3 min at 25 °C using a MS 200 EPR spectrometer (Miniscope, Berlin, Germany) operating on the X-band. The instrument settings were the following: field modulation 100 KHz, modulation amplitude 1500 mG, field constant 60 s, center field 3350 G, sweep width 99.70 G, X-band frequency 9.64 GHz, MW attenuation 7 dB, and gain 5. Under these conditions, the typical triplet Fremy's salt spectrum (1:1:1) was observed. The intensity of the EPR signal was measured at the height of the first line, with the resonance at 3336.6 G. The system was calibrated with solutions of gallic acid at known concentrations, hence the results were given as µmol of gallic acid equivalents (GAE)/100 g dried extract.

3.4.2. Superoxide Anion Scavenging

The antioxidant potential towards $O_2^{-\bullet}$ was based on the spin trapping of the radical generated by potassium superoxide (KO_2) in dimethyl sulfoxide (DMSO) with the addition of 18-crown-6 ether to complex K^+, using the previously performed and validated method by Picchi et al. [66], with some modifications. The spin trap reagent was 5,5-dimethylpyrroline-N-oxide (DMPO). Under these conditions, a typical DMPO-OOH adduct (1:1:1:1) was observed. The scavenging reaction mixture was 18-crown-6 ether/KO_2 (1:1, 20 mM) dissolved in DMSO. A blank solution contained 100 µL of a 100 mM DMPO phosphate buffer solution 0.1 M, pH 7.4, 130 µL of superoxide solution and 10 µL of extracting solution. The solution with the scavenging compound was composed exactly as the blank, by replacing 10 µL of extracting solution with the equivalent volume of the *Trifolium* extract. The reaction time was 60 sec at 25 °C. EPR recording conditions were as follows: field set, 3350 G; scan range, 70 G; scan time, 120 s; modulation amplitude, 1200 mG; microwave attenuation, 5 dB; receiver gain, 8 × 100. The intensity of the EPR signal was measured at the height of the first spectrum line, with the resonance at 3326.1 G. The system was calibrated with solutions of gallic acid at known concentrations, hence the results were given as mmol of gallic acid equivalents (GAE)/100 g dried extract.

3.4.3. Peroxyl Radical by Enzymatic Degradation of Linoleic Acid

In this method, the enzymatic peroxidation of linoleic acid, generating peroxyl radicals, was obtained by the addition of lipoxygenase (EC 1.13.11.12) with some modifications of the method described by Grossman and Zakut [67], successively checked and validated by Lo Scalzo et al. [68]. The peroxidation of linoleic acid was analyzed in the absence (blank) and presence (sample) of the assayed extracts by recording the increase in absorbance at 234 nm over 2 min at 25 °C after a 30 sec delay. The substrate was prepared by dissolving 40 µL of linoleic acid in 2 mL of absolute ethanol under nitrogen, followed by the addition of 10 µL of Tween 20. The solution was slowly mixed, then 40 mL of 0.05 M K_2HPO_4 were added, and the pH was adjusted to 9.0 with 0.05 M NaOH, the final substrate concentration resulting 3.21 mM. The lipoxygenase solution was freshly prepared by dissolving 11 mg of a lipoxygenase standard soybean extract (Sigma, St. Louis, MO, USA) in 16 mL of 0.1 M phosphate buffer (pH 7.0). In the sample test, the reaction solution was composed of 2.0 mL of 0.1 M phosphate buffer (pH 7.0), 0.2 mL of substrate (0.27 mM final concentration), 0.15 mL of scavenging solution, and 0.05 mL of lipoxygenase solution. In the blank test, the scavenging solution was substituted by 0.15 mL of pure extracting solution. The reaction was spectrophotometrically monitored at 234 nm to follow peroxyl radical conjugate diene formation. The antioxidant activity of enzymatically mediated linoleic acid peroxidation (LIPOX–LINOL) was expressed as the protection percentage monitored by the absorbance at 234 nm, by interpolating the data with those of a calibration curve obtained from standard solutions of Trolox (6-hydroxy-2,5,7,8-tetramethylchromane-2-carboxylic acid). The results were thus reported as mmol of Trolox equivalents (TE)/100 g dried extract.

3.5. Statistical Analyses

The general term 'accession' commonly used in germplasm collections was adopted throughout this work to equally indicate cultivated forms (cultivars), ecotypes, or natural populations of any evaluated species. Each replication of leaf and flower samples represented the basic experimental unit of each accession.

An analysis of variance (ANOVA) tested the differences between leaves and flowers (across all accessions and replications) for the mean concentration of each of the five groups of phenolics identified in this study and their total, and the mean antioxidant activity determined by three assays (Fremy's salt scavenging, superoxide anion scavenging and peroxyl radical scavenging). A second ANOVA assessed the differences among the 14 accessions (phenolic concentrations and antioxidant activity assays) for leaves and flowers, individually using the accession × replication variance as the error term. Differences between the areas of origin/sampling of the germplasm (lowlands vs. mountains) were assessed by another ANOVA for leaves and flowers, individually, testing the variance of the 'area' factor over the pooled variance of the nested factor 'accession within area'. In this analysis, the snow clover population #3, originating from the Alps but sampled in the lowland site, was excluded.

Given the diverse range of *Trifolium* taxa encompassed by the current germplasm, an attempt was made to predict by multiple regression the antioxidant activity in the genus based on the recorded concentrations of phenolic groups. Accession mean values of each of the three antioxidant assays and of the five groups of phenolics were used as dependent variable and independent variables, respectively, in the regressions separately run for leaf and flower data. Prior to the choice of the best predicting models, the presence of multicollinearity between regressors was verified by different indexes, namely, the variance inflation factor, the condition number and the eigenvalues [69]. The choice of the best predicting regression model for each antioxidant assay in leaves and flowers was made examining different methods, namely, the stepwise procedure, the adjusted R^2, the C(p) index and the Press number, and choosing the most consistent model accordingly [69]. All statistical analyses were carried out using the Proc GLM and Proc Reg of the SAS software.

Author Contributions: A.T. and L.P. (Luciano Pecetti) designed the experiment, analysed the data, wrote and revised the paper; A.T., Ł.P. (Łucas Pecio) and R.L.S. performed the analyses; A.S. commented the data and the draft manuscript. All authors have red and approved the manuscript.

Funding: This work was financially supported by a fellowship (to A.T.) of 'Consiglio per la ricerca in agricoltura e l'analisi dell'economia agraria'

Acknowledgments: Technical support from A. Ursino and B. Pintus of CREA-ZA Lodi, Italy, is gratefully acknowledged.

Conflicts of Interest: The authors declare no competing financial interest.

References

1. Abberton, M.T.; Marshall, A.H. White clover. In *Fodder Cops and Amenity Grasses*; Handbook of Plant Breeding Series; Volume 5, Boller, B., Posselt, U.K., Veronesi, F., Eds.; Springer: New York, NY, USA, 2010; pp. 457–476.
2. Boller, B.; Schubiger, F.X.; Kölliker, R. Red clover. In *Fodder Cops and Amenity Grasses*; Handbook of Plant Breeding Series; Volume 5, Boller, B., Posselt, U.K., Veronesi, F., Eds.; Springer: New York, NY, USA, 2010; pp. 439–456.
3. Piano, E.; Pecetti, L. Minor legume species. In *Fodder Cops and Amenity Grasses*; Handbook of Plant Breeding Series; Volume 5, Boller, B., Posselt, U.K., Veronesi, F., Eds.; Springer: New York, NY, USA, 2010; pp. 477–500.
4. Woodgate, K.; Maxted, N.; Bennet, S. A generic conspectus for the forage legumes of the Mediterranean basin. In *Genetic Resources of Mediterranean Pasture and Forage Legumes*; Bennett, S.J., Cocks, P.S., Eds.; Kluwer Academic Publishers: Dordrecht, The Netherlands, 1999; pp. 182–226.
5. Cavallero, A.; Aceto, P.; Gorlier, A.; Lombardi, G.; Lonati, M.; Martinasso, B.; Tagliatori, C. *I Tipi Pastorali delle Alpi Piemontesi*; Alberto Perdisa Editore: Bologna, Italy, 2007.
6. Rognli, O.A.; Fjellheim, S.; Pecetti, L.; Boller, B. Semi-natural grasslands as a source of genetic diversity. In *The Role of Grasslands in a Green Future. Grasslands Science in Europe*; Algadóttir, Á., Hopkins, A., Eds.; Prentsmiđjan Oddi: Reykjavík, Iceland, 2013; Volume 18, pp. 303–313.
7. Sabudak, T.; Guler, N. *Trifolium* L.—A review on its phytochemical and pharmacological profile. *Phytoter. Res.* **2009**, *23*, 439–446. [CrossRef]
8. Pereira, D.M.; Valentão, P.; Pereira, J.A.; Andrade, P.B. Phenolics: From chemistry to biology. *Molecules* **2009**, *14*, 2202–2211. [CrossRef]
9. Tapas, A.R.; Sakarkar, D.M.; Kakde, R.B. Flavonoids as nutraceuticals: A review. *Tropic. J. Pharm. Res.* **2008**, *7*, 1089–1099. [CrossRef]
10. Wang, H.; Cao, R.L.; Prior, J. Total Antioxidant Capacity of Fruits. *J. Agric. Food Chem.* **1996**, *44*, 701–705. [CrossRef]
11. Pietta, P.G. Flavonoids as antioxidants. *J. Nat. Prod.* **2000**, *63*, 1035–1042. [CrossRef] [PubMed]
12. Dillard, C.J.; German, J.B. Phytochemicals: Nutraceuticals and human health. *J. Sci. Food Agric.* **2000**, *80*, 1744–1756. [CrossRef]
13. Hertog, M.G.; Feskens, E.J.; Hallman, P.C.; Katan, M.B.; Kromhout, D. Dietary antioxidant flavonoids and risk of coronary heart disease: The Zutphen Elderly Study. *Lancet* **1993**, *342*, 1007–1011. [CrossRef]
14. Bobe, G.; Weinstein, S.J.; Albanes, D.; Hirvonen, T.; Ashby, J.; Taylor, P.R.; Virtamo, J.; Stolzenberg-Solomon, R.Z. Flavonoid intake and risk of pancreatic cancer in male smokers (Finland). *Cancer Epidemiol. Biomark. Prev.* **2008**, *17*, 553–562. [CrossRef] [PubMed]
15. Cornwell, T.; Cohick, W.; Raskin, I. Dietary phytoestrogen and health. *Phytochemistry* **2004**, *65*, 995–1016. [CrossRef] [PubMed]
16. Hidalgo, L.A.; Chedraui, P.A.; Morocho, N.; Ros, S.; San Miguel, G. The effect of red clover isoflavones on menopausal symptoms, lipid and vaginal cytology in menopausal women: A randomized, double-blind, placebo-controlled study. *Gynecol. Endocrinol.* **2005**, *21*, 257–264. [CrossRef]
17. Rüfer, C.E.; Kulling, S.E. Antioxidant activity of isoflavones and their major metabolites using different in vitro assays. *J. Agric. Food Chem.* **2006**, *54*, 2926–2931. [CrossRef] [PubMed]
18. McRae, J.M.; Yang, Q.; Crawford, R.J.; Palombo, E.A. Chemotaxonomic applications of flavonoids. In *Nutrition and Diet Research Progress Series: Flavonoids: Biosynthesis, Biological Effects and Dietary Sources*; Keller, R.B., Ed.; Nova Science Publisher: Hauppauge, NY, USA, 2009; Chapter 11; pp. 291–299.
19. Oleszek, W.; Stochmal, A.; Janda, B. Concentration of isoflavones and other phenolics in the aerial parts of *Trifolium* species. *J. Agric. Food Chem.* **2007**, *55*, 8095–8100. [CrossRef] [PubMed]

20. Tava, A.; Pecio, Ł.; Stochmal, A.; Pecetti, L. Clovamide and flavonoids from leaves of *Trifolium pratense* and *T. pratense* subsp. *nivale* grown in Italy. *Nat. Prod. Comm.* **2015**, *10*, 933–936.
21. Di Ferdinando, M.; Brunetti, C.; Fini, A.; Tattini, M. Flavonoids as antioxidants in plants under abiotic stresses. In *Abiotic Stress Responses in Plants: Metabolism, Productivity and Sustainability*; Ahmad, P., Prasad, M.N.V., Eds.; Springer Science+Business Media, LLC: New York, NY, USA, 2012; pp. 159–180.
22. Cheynier, V.; Comte, G.; Davies, K.M.; Lattanzio, V.; Martens, S. Plant phenolics: Recent advances on their biosynthesis, genetics, and ecophysiology. *Plant Physiol. Biochem.* **2013**, *72*, 1–20. [CrossRef] [PubMed]
23. Winkel-Shirley, B. Biosynthesis of flavonoids and effect of stress. *Curr. Opin. Plant Biol.* **2002**, *5*, 218–223. [CrossRef]
24. Blokhina, O.; Virolainen, E.; Fagerstedt, K.V. Antioxidants, oxidative damage and oxygen deprivation stress: A review. *Ann. Bot.* **2003**, *91*, 179–194. [CrossRef]
25. de Rijke, E.; Out, P.; Niessen, W.M.A.; Ariese, F.; Gooijer, C.; Brinkman, U.A.T. Analytical separation and detection methods for flavonoids. *J. Chromatogr. A* **2006**, *1112*, 31–63. [CrossRef]
26. Polasek, J.; Queiroz, E.F.; Hostettmann, K. On-line identification of phenolic compounds of *Trifolium* species using HPLC-UV-MS and post-column UV-derivatization. *Phytochem. Anal.* **2007**, *18*, 13–23. [CrossRef]
27. Kowalska, I.; Jedrejek, D.; Ciesla, L.; Pecio, L.; Masullo, M.; Piacente, S.; Oleszek, W.; Stochmal, A. Isolation, chemical and free radical scavenging characterization of phenolics from *Trifolium scabrum* L. aerial parts. *J. Agric. Food Chem.* **2013**, *61*, 4417–4423. [CrossRef]
28. Tava, A.; Stochmal, A.; Pecetti, L. Isoflavone content in subterranean clover germplasm from Sardinia. *Chem. Biodiv.* **2016**, *13*, 1038–1045. [CrossRef]
29. Stobiecki, M.; Kachlicki, P.; Wojakowska, A.; Marczak, L. Application of LC/MS systems to structural characterization of flavonoid glycoconjugates. *Phytochem. Lett.* **2015**, *11*, 358–367. [CrossRef]
30. Shehata, M.N.; Hassan, A.; El-Shazly, K. Identification of the oestrogenic isoflavones in fresh and fermented berseem clover (*Trifolium alexandrinum*). *Aust. J. Agric. Res.* **1982**, *33*, 951–956. [CrossRef]
31. Ahmed, Q.U.; Kaleem, M.; Parveen, N.; Khan, N.U. Phytochemical and pharmacological investigations of Egyptian colver, *Trifolium alexandrinum* L. Sustainable Management and Utilization of Medicinal Plant Resources. In Proceedings of the International Conference Medicinal Plants, Kuala Lumpur, Malaysia, 5–7 December 2005; pp. 219–226.
32. Sharaf, M. Chemical constituents from the seeds of *Trifolium alexandrinum*. *Nat. Prod. Res.* **2008**, *22*, 1620–1623. [CrossRef] [PubMed]
33. Lin, L.Z.; He, X.G.; Lindenmaier, M.; Yang, J.; Cleary, M.; Qui, S.X.; Cordell, G.A. LC-ESI-MS study of the flavonoid glycoside malonates of red clover (*Trifolium pratense*). *J. Agric. Food Chem.* **2000**, *48*, 354–365. [CrossRef] [PubMed]
34. Klejdus, B.; Vitamvasova-Sterbova, D.; Kuban, V. Identification of isoflavone conjugates in red clover (*Trifolium pratense*) by liquid chromatography-mass spectrometry after two-dimensional solid-phase extraction. *Anal. Chim. Acta* **2001**, *450*, 81–97. [CrossRef]
35. Tsao, R.; Papadopoulos, Y.; Yang, R.; Young, J.C.; McRae, K. Isoflavone profiles of red clovers and their distribution in different parts harvested at different growing stages. *J. Agric. Food Chem.* **2006**, *54*, 5797–5805. [CrossRef] [PubMed]
36. Saviranta, N.M.M.; Julkunen-Tiitto, R.; Oksanen, E.; Karjalainen, R.O. Leaf phenolic compounds in red clover (*Trifolium pratense* L.) induced by exposure to moderately elevated ozone. *Environ. Poll.* **2010**, *158*, 440–446. [CrossRef] [PubMed]
37. Foo, L.Y.; Lu, Y.; Molan, A.L.; Woodfield, D.R.; McNabb, W.C. The phenols and prodelphinidins of white clover flowers. *Phytochemistry* **2000**, *54*, 539–548. [CrossRef]
38. Hofmann, R.W.; Swinny, E.E.; Bloor, S.J.; Markham, K.R.; Ryan, K.G.; Campbell, B.D.; Jordan, B.R.; Fountain, D.W. Responses of nine *Trifolium repens* L. populations to ultraviolet-B radiation: Differential flavonol glycoside accumulation and biomass production. *Ann. Bot.* **2000**, *86*, 527–537. [CrossRef]
39. Carlsen, S.C.K.; Mortensen, A.G.; Oleszek, W.; Piacente, S.; Stochmal, A.; Fomsgaard, S. Variation in flavonoids in leaves, stem and flowers of white clover cultivars. *Nat. Prod. Comm.* **2008**, *3*, 1299–1306.
40. Kicel, A.; Wolbis, M. Study of the phenolic constituents of the lowes and leaves of *Trifolium repens* L. *Nat. Prod. Res.* **2012**, *26*, 2050–2054. [CrossRef] [PubMed]
41. Porter, L.J.; Hrstich, L.N.; Chan, B.G. The conversion of procyanidins and prodelphinidins to cyanidin and delphinidin. *Phytochemistry* **1986**, *25*, 223–230. [CrossRef]

42. Schofield, P.; Mbugua, D.M.; Pell, A.N. Analysis of condensed tannins: A review. *Anim. Feed Sci. Technol.* **2001**, *91*, 21–40. [CrossRef]
43. Wolfe, R.M.; Terrill, T.H.; Muir, J.P. Drying method and origin of standard affect condensed tannin (CT) concentrations in perennial herbaceous legumes using simplified butanol-HCl CT analysis. *J. Sci. Food Agric.* **2008**, *88*, 1060–1067. [CrossRef]
44. Kardel, M.; Taube, F.M.; Schulz, H.; Schütze, W.; Gierus, M. Different approaches to evaluate tannin content and structure of selected plant extracts—Review and new aspects. *J. Appl. Bot. Food Qual.* **2013**, *86*, 154–166.
45. Davies, K.M.; Schwinn, K.E. Molecular biology and biotechnology of flavonoids. In *Flavonoids Chemistry, Biochemistry and Applications*; Andersen, O.M., Markham, K.R., Eds.; CRC Press, Tylor & Francis Group: Boca Raton, FL, USA, 2006; Chapter 3; pp. 143–218.
46. Saboonchian, F.; Jamedi, R.; Sarghein, S.H. Phenolic and flavonoid content of *Elaeagnus angustifolia* L. (leaf and flower). *Avic. J. Phytomed.* **2014**, *4*, 231–238.
47. Dokhani, S.; Cottrell, T.; Khajeddin, J.; Mazza, G. Analysis of aroma and phenolic components of selected Achillea species. *Plant Food Hum. Nutr.* **2005**, *60*, 55–62. [CrossRef]
48. Mekni, M.; Azez, R.; Tekaya, M.; Mechri, B.; Hammami, M. Phenolic, non-phenolic compounds and antioxidant activity of pomegranate flower, leaf and bark extracts of Tunisian cultivars. *J. Med. Plants Res.* **2013**, *7*, 1100–1107.
49. Dores, R.G.R.; Guimaraes, S.F.; Braga, T.V.; Fonseca, M.C.M.; Martinus, P.M.; Ferreira, T.C. Phenolic compounds, flavonoids and antioxidant activity of leaves, flowers and roots of white-weed. *Hortic. Brasil.* **2014**, *32*, 486–490. [CrossRef]
50. Abeynayake, S.W.; Panter, S.; Chapman, R.; Webster, T.; Rochfort, S.; Mouradov, A.; Spangenberg, G. Biosynthesis of proanthocyanidins in white clover flowers: Cross talk within the flavonoid pathway. *Plant Physiol.* **2012**, *158*, 666–678. [CrossRef]
51. van der Meer, I.M.; Stam, M.E.; van Tunen, A.J.; Mol, J.N.M.; Stuitje, A.R. Antisense inhibition of flavonoid biosynthesis in petunia anthers results in male sterility. *Plant Cell* **1992**, *4*, 253–262. [CrossRef] [PubMed]
52. Jayaprakasha, G.K.; Singh, R.P.; Sakariah, K.K. Antioxidant activity of grape seed (*Vitis vinifera*) extracts on peroxidation models in vitro. *Food Chem.* **2001**, *73*, 285–290. [CrossRef]
53. Beck, V.; Rohr, U.; Jungbauer, A. Phytoestrogen derived from red clover: An alternative to estrogen replacement therapy? *J. Steroid Biochem. Mol. Biol.* **2005**, *94*, 499–518. [CrossRef] [PubMed]
54. Cao, G.; Sofic, E.; Prior, R.L. Antioxidant and prooxidant behavior of flavonoids: Structure-activity relationship. *Free Radic. Biol. Med.* **1997**, *22*, 749–760. [CrossRef]
55. Agati, G.; Brunetti, C.; Di Ferdinando, M.; Ferrini, F.; Pollastri, S.; Tattini, M. Funcional roles of flavonoids in photoprotection: New evidence, lessons from the past. *Plant Physiol. Biochem.* **2013**, *72*, 35–45. [CrossRef]
56. Morales, L.O.; Tegelberg, R.; Brosché, M.; Keinänen, M.; Lindfors, A.; Aphalo, P.J. Effects of solar UV-A and UV-B radiation on gene expression and phenolic accumulation in *Betula pendula* leaves. *Tree Physiol.* **2010**, *30*, 923–934. [CrossRef]
57. Bieza, K.; Lois, R. An *Arabidopsis* mutant tolerant to lethal ultraviolet-B levels shows constitutively elevated accumulation of flavonoids and other phenolics. *Plant Physiol.* **2001**, *126*, 1105–1115. [CrossRef]
58. Jansen, M.A.K.; Gaba, V.; Greenberg, B.M. Higher plants and UV-B radiation: Balancing damage, repair and acclimatation. *Trends Plant Sci.* **1998**, *3*, 131–135. [CrossRef]
59. Nichols, P.G.H.; Foster, K.J.; Piano, E.; Kaur, P.; Ghamkhar, K.; Pecetti, L.; Collins, W.J. Genetic improvement of subterranean clover (*Trifolium subterraneum* L.). 1. Germplasm, traits and future prospects. *Crop Pasture Sci.* **2013**, *64*, 312–346. [CrossRef]
60. Arlorio, M.; Locatelli, M.; Travaglia, F.; Coisson, J.D.; Del Grosso, E.; Minassi, A.; Appendino, G.; Martelli, A. Roasting impact on the contents of clovamide (*N*-caffeoyl-*L*-DOPA) and the antioxidant activity of cocoa beans (*Theobroma cacao* L.). *Food Chem.* **2008**, *106*, 967–975. [CrossRef]
61. Zeng, H.; Locatelli, M.; Bardelli, C.; Amoroso, A.; Coïsson, J.D.; Travaglia, F.; Arlorio, M.; Brunelleschi, S. Anti-inflammatory properties of clovamide and *Theobroma cacao* phenolic extracts in human monocytes: Evaluation of respiratory burst, cytokine release, NF-κB activation, and PPARγ modulation. *J. Agric. Food Chem.* **2011**, *59*, 5342–5350. [CrossRef] [PubMed]
62. Kolodziejczyk, J.; Olas, B.; Wachowicz, B.; Szajwaj, B.; Stochmal, A.; Oleszek, W. Clovamide-rich extract from *Trifolium pallidum* reduces oxidative stress-induced damage to blood platelets and plasma. *J. Physiol. Biochem.* **2011**, *67*, 391–399. [CrossRef] [PubMed]

63. Bagchi, D.; Bagchi, M.; Stohs, S.J.; Das, D.K.; Ray, S.D.; Kuszynski, C.A.; Joshi, S.S.; Pruess, H.G. Free radical and grape seed proanthocyanidin extract: Importance in human health and disease prevention. *Toxicology* **2000**, *148*, 187–197. [CrossRef]
64. Pignatti, S. *Flora d'Italia*; Edagricole: Bologna, Italy, 1982.
65. Gardner, P.T.; White, T.A.C.; McPhail, D.B. The relative contribution of vitamin C, carotenoid and phenolics to the antioxidant potential of fruit juices. *Food Chem.* **2000**, *68*, 471–474. [CrossRef]
66. Picchi, V.; Migliori, C.; Lo Scalzo, R.; Campanelli, G.; Ferrari, V.; Di Cesare, L.F. Phytochemical content in organic and conventionally grown Italian cauliflower. *Food Chem.* **2012**, *130*, 501–509. [CrossRef]
67. Grossman, S.; Zakut, R. Determination of the activity of lipoxygenase. In *Method of Biochemical Analysis*; Glick, D., Ed.; Wiley-Interscience: New York, NY, USA, 1979; pp. 313–316.
68. Lo Scalzo, R.; Todaro, A.; Rapisarda, P. Methods used to evaluate the peroxyl (ROO·) radical scavenging capacities of four common antioxidants. *Eur. Food Res. Technol.* **2012**, *235*, 1141–1148. [CrossRef]
69. Donatelli, M.; Annicchiarico, P. *Nota Sull'analisi di Dati Sperimentali in Agricoltura Tramite il SAS (Statistical Analysis System)*, Seconda edizione; ISCI e ISCF: Bologna, Italy, 1999.

Sample Availability: Samples of the compounds are not available from the authors.

molecules

MDPI

Article

Studies on the Design and Synthesis of Marine Peptide Analogues and Their Ability to Promote Proliferation in HUVECs and Zebrafish

Yinglin Zheng, Yichen Tong, Xinfeng Wang, Jiebin Zhou and Jiyan Pang *

School of Chemistry, Sun Yat-Sen University, Guangzhou 510275, China; zhengylin6@mail2.sysu.edu.cn (Y.Z.); tongych3@mail2.sysu.edu.cn (Y.T.); tomorrow1996@163.com (X.W.); sysuzhoujieb@163.com (J.Z.)

* Correspondence: cespjy@mail.sysu.edu.cn; Tel.: +86-208-403-6554

Academic Editor: Pinarosa Avato

Received: 30 November 2018; Accepted: 17 December 2018; Published: 25 December 2018

Abstract: In our previous studies, tripeptide **1** was found to induce angiogenesis in zebrafish embryos and in HUVECs. Based on the lead compound **1**, seven new marine tripeptide analogues **2–8** have been designed and synthesized in this paper to evaluate the effects on promoting cellular proliferation in human endothelial cells (HUVECs) and zebrafish. Among them, compounds **5–7** possessed more remarkable increasing proliferation effects than other compounds, and the EC_{50} values of these and the leading compound **1** were 1.0 ± 0.002 μM, 1.0 ± 0.0005 μM, 0.88 ± 0.0972 μM, and 1.31 ± 0.0926 μM, respectively. Furthermore, **5–7** could enhance migrations (58.5%, 80.66% and 60.71% increment after culturing 48 h, respectively) and invasions (49.08%, 47.24% and 56.24% increase, respectively) in HUVECs compared with the vehicle control. The results revealed that the tripeptide including L-Tyrosine or D-Proline fragments instead of L-Alanine of leading compound **1** would contribute to HUVECs' proliferation. Taking the place of the original (L-Lys-L-Ala) segment of leading compound **1**, a new fragment (L-Arg-D-Val) expressed higher performance in bioactivity in HUVECs. In addition, compound **7** could promote angiogenesis in zebrafish assay and it was more interesting that it also could repair damaged blood vessels in PTK787-induced zebrafish at a low concentration. The above data indicate that these peptides have potential implications for further evaluation in cytothesis studies.

Keywords: marine peptides; proliferation; migration; angiogenesis; zebrafish

1. Introduction

Marine peptides are mainly obtained from diverse marine organisms. Marine organisms play an important role as sources of nitrogen and amino acids, which have numerous potential physiological functions [1]. Because of their special marine environment, marine peptides have unique structures, such as rare coded amino acids, special connection bonds and highly modified amino acid residues. The structural diversity of marine peptides results in various bioactivities, such as neurotoxicity [2], anticancer [3], antivirus [4], antimicrobial [5], and antioxidant [6] effects.

Cellular proliferation is not only one of the most indispensable characteristics of the cell cycle, but the foundation of organism growth, inheritance and evolution. Proliferation plays an important role in physiology and pathology. It is a tightly regulated process and a normal occurrence in numerous biological processes, such as embryogenesis, tissue remodeling, bone development, the ovarian cycle and wound healing [7]. Over the past few years, researchers have started to focus more on cellular proliferation, which has a prominent role to play in the treatment of common diseases. For example, acute dermal wounds heal quickly in healthy individuals but turn into deep sores in diabetics, leading to severe infections in underlying tissues. Therefore, it is vital for promoting faster cellular proliferation and wound healing [8]. In bone repair and regeneration, osteogenic growth peptide (OGP) is a biologically active peptide that affects immune functions, proliferation and differentiation [9]. Furthermore, the significance of promoting proliferation has focused on therapeutic angiogenesis in recent years. Therapeutic angiogenesis, which can re-establish blood perfusion and rescue ischemic tissue, is used to treat ischemic diseases such as peripheral vascular occlusive disease (PVOD), a common manifestation of atherosclerosis with a high rate of morbidity [10]. Zebrafish embryo are recognized as a suitable model to explore the formation of blood vessel because their vascular system can be easily described in the developing embryo. Numerous pathways involved in angiogenesis in mammals are highly conserved in this model.

In our earlier work, novel marine cyclopeptide analogue xyloallenoide A (Figure 1) was isolated from the mangrove fungus *Xylaria* sp. 2508 in the South China Sea [11]. According to the structure of xyloallenoide A, a *t*-Butyloxy carbonyl (Boc)-protected cyclotripeptide (X-13) was synthesized [12], and it could dose-dependently induce angiogenesis in zebrafish embryos and human umbilical vein endothelial cells (HUVECs), which consisted of Boc-L-Lys, D-N-MeVal and D-N-MeAla. The compound X-13 expressed potent angiogenic properties and is very promising for development as a novel class of pro-angiogenic agents for angiotherapy [13]. Considering the complex structure and hard synthesis of cyclopeptides, a series of linepeptides were designed and synthesized [13]. Among them, tripeptide **1** with the group of D-Val, Boc-L-Lys and L-Ala had the strongest induced angiogenesis effect, both in vivo and in vitro. The effect of tripeptide **1** on angiogenesis wasmore significant than that of the compound X-13 [14]. Previous structure–activity relationship (SAR) analysis revealed that linear tripeptides and tetrapeptides, including Val, Lys and Ala amino acid segments, displayed favorable activities.

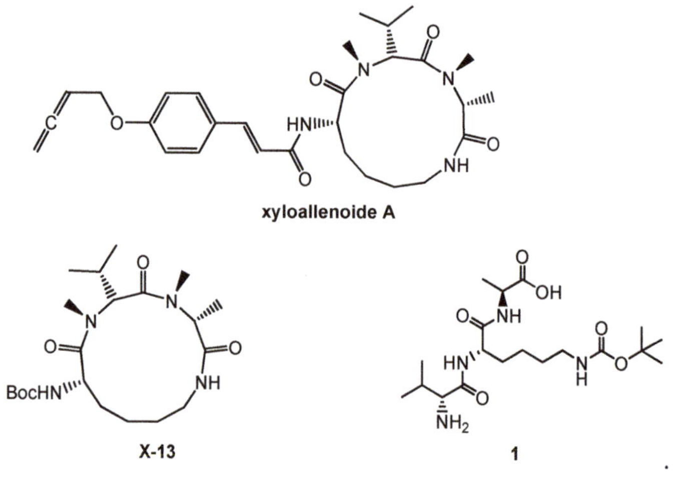

Figure 1. The structures of xyloallenoide A, X-13 and **1**.

In this paper, to explore more leading bioactive compounds resembling compound **1**, we designed a series of new tripeptides. Based on lead compound **1**, more tripeptides **2**–**8** (Figure 2), including a variety of different amino acids and substituents, were synthesized. Further promoting cellular proliferations were performed on HUVECs to identify more new candidate drugs and discuss the SAR. Moreover, the further proliferative and angiogenesis effects of selected compound were evaluated on normal and damaged zebrafish models.

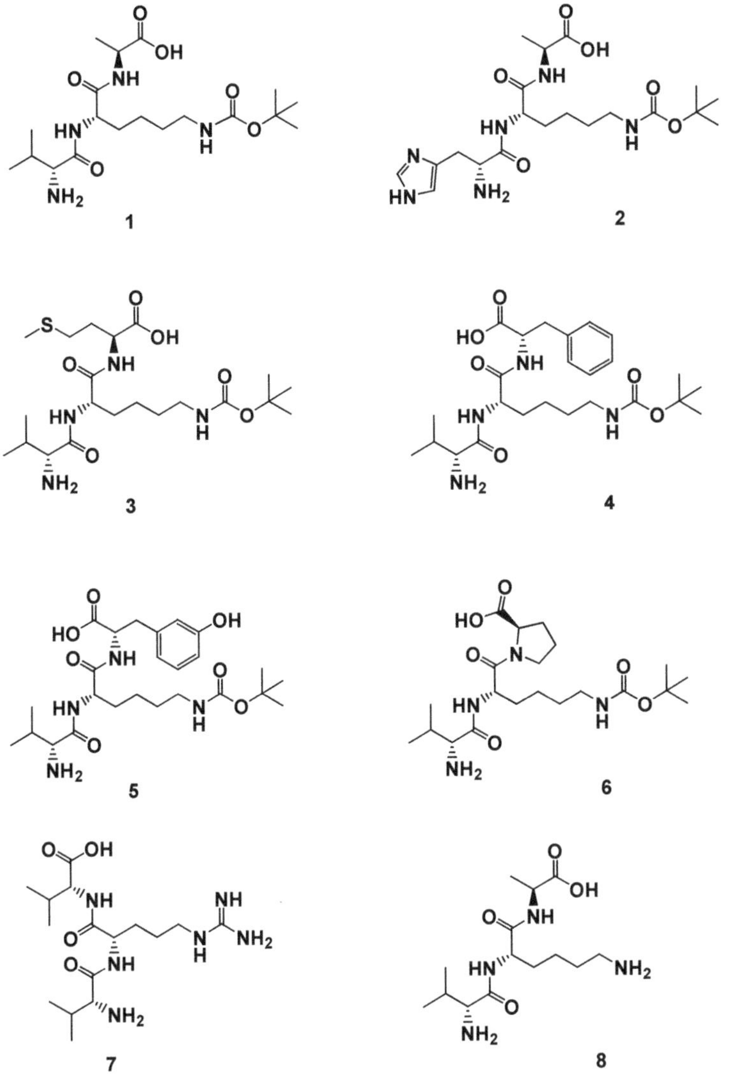

Figure 2. The structures of derivatives **1–8**. H-D-Val-L-Lys(Boc)-L-Ala-OH (**1**); H-D-His-L-Lys(Boc)-L-Ala-OH (**2**); H-D-Val-L-Lys(Boc)-L-Met-OH (**3**); H-D-Val-L-Lys(Boc)-L-Phe-OH (**4**); H-D-Val-L-Lys(Boc)-L-Tyr-OH (**5**); H-D-Val-L-Lys(Boc)-D-Pro-OH (**6**); H-D-Val-L-Arg-D-Val-OH (**7**); H-D-Val-L-Lys-L-Ala-OH (**8**).

2. Results and Discussion

2.1. Chemistry

To assess the cellular bioactivities of different modifications of compound **1**, a series of analogues **2–8** were designed, with modification focused on the different amino acids and the lipophilic/hydrophilic and acidity/alkaline properties of compounds. With the aim of studying the steric effect, compounds **4** and **8** were designed. Compound **2** was synthesized to explore the bioactivity of unsaturated alkaline amino acid, with D-Histidine instead of D-Valine. Compounds **3** and

6 were focused on the effect of the structure of the methylthio group and tetrahydropyrrole on cellular bioactivities. Furthermore, acidity and hydrophily are probably related to activity, so compound **5** was designed. Due to the Arg-Gly-Asp (RGD) sequence relating to angiogenesis [15], compound **7** containing an RGD moiety was synthesized.

The line peptide compounds **1–8** were prepared by our previous method [12] (Scheme 1). Generally, Cbz-D-Val-OH, Cbz-D-His-OH, H-L-Lys(Boc)-OMe and H-L-Arg(Pbf)-OMe were used as starting materials and coupled with another amino acid by coupling reagents (HOBt, HBTU and DIEA) to obtain the corresponding dipeptide and tripeptide. The dipeptide and tripeptide were demethylated using LiOH in THF/H_2O. All Cbz-groups were removed by H_2 with Pd/C-catalyzed. All the target molecules were purified through flash column chromatography, and the structures were fully characterized by ^{1}H NMR, ^{13}C NMR and HR-EI-MS. The purity of all target compounds was ≥95% as determined by HPLC analysis.

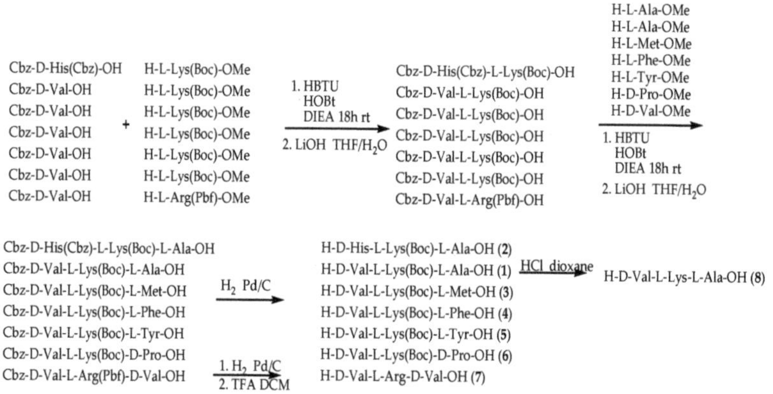

Scheme 1. Synthetic route of compounds **1–8**. All peptides were synthesis by HBTU, HOBt and DIEA as coupling reagents at room temperature 18 h. The dipeptide and tripeptide were demethylated using LiOH in THF/H_2O. All Cbz-groups were removed by H_2 with Pd/C-catalyzed.

2.2. *Effects of Compounds* **1–8** *on HUVEC Proliferation*

The endothelial cell's proliferation is an important phase in the process of normal life. Human umbilical vein endothelial cells (HUVECs) are frequently used to measure the angiogenic property in vitro. HUVECs are usually used as a laboratory model system for the study of the function and pathology of endothelial cells such as angiogenesis [16] and hypertension [17]. Like human umbilical artery endothelial cells, they exhibit a cobblestone phenotype when lining vessel walls. To evaluate the cellular bioactivity in vitro, compounds **1–8** were studied on the HUVECs with different concentrations: 0.0625 μM, 0.125 μM, 0.25 μM, 0.5 μM, 1 μM, 2 μM, 5 μM, 10 μM, and 50 μM. A quantity of 20 ng/mL VEGF was used as a positive control. The results are shown in Figure 3 and Table 1.

Lead compound **1** clearly showed a notable proliferative effect on HUVECs with EC_{50} value of 1.3 ± 0.0926 μM in a concentration-dependent manner. Compounds **5–7** possessed better proliferation effects with respect to HUVECs than other compounds, and the EC_{50} values were 1.0 ± 0.002 μM, 1.0 ± 0.0005 μM and 0.88 ± 0.0972 μM, respectively.

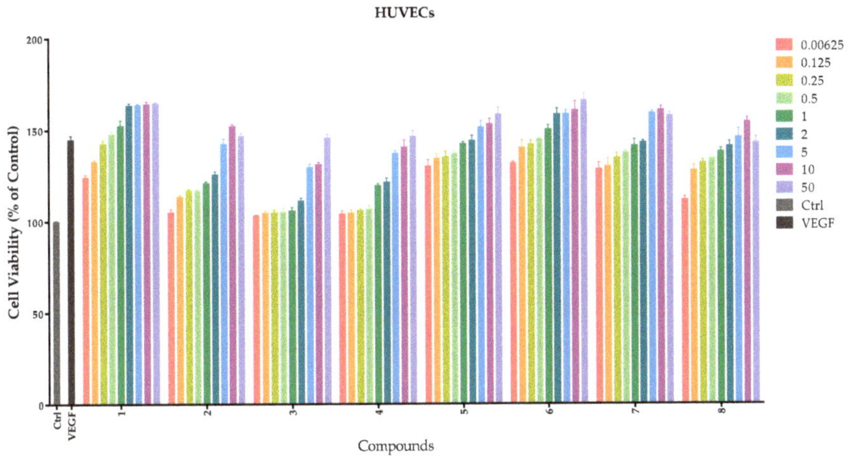

Figure 3. Effects of compounds **1–8** on proliferation of HUVECs. HUVECs were cultured with different concentrations (0–50 μM) of compounds. Cellular proliferation was assessed using the thiazolyl blue tetrazolium bromide (MTT) assay after 48 h. Data are expressed as the mean ± SEM (n = 4) of three individual experiments. The x-axis represents different compounds and the y-axis represents the cell viability (the control as 100%); different column colors represent different concentrations from 0.0625 μM to 50 μM.

Table 1. Values EC_{50} (μM) of compounds with respect to HUVEC proliferation.

Compounds	EC_{50} (μM)
1	1.31 ± 0.0926
2	57.55 ± 6.10
3	>200.00
4	76.02 ± 0.205
5	1.00 ± 0.002
6	1.00 ± 0.0005
7	0.88 ± 0.0972
8	1.33 ± 0.201

In view of the assays of promoting proliferation, the SAR analysis revealed that:

(a) the D-histidine fragment of compound **2** replaced the D-valine of compound 1, or L-methionine fragment of compound **3** replaced the L-alanine fragment of compound 1; both reduced cellular bioactivity, which might indicate that cellular proliferation was depressed due to steric hindrance of the substrates;

(b) secondly, the L-Tyrosine with phenol group (compound **5**) or D-proline with tetrahydropyrrole fragment (compound **6**) substituting for L-alanine also increased proliferation in HUVECs probably through hydrogen-bonding interaction;

(c) to our surprise, compound **7** exerted strong effects on HUVECs, which revealed that the L-Arg-D-Val fragment resembles the Lys(Boc)-L-Ala-OH in cytoactive terms;

(d) compared with compound **1** and **8**, we found that the *t*-Butyloxy carbonyl group was not a determinant factor in increasing cellular proliferation of HUVECs.

2.3. Migration Assays–Wound Healing of Compounds 5–7

Cellular migration is a central process in the development of multicellular organisms. The wound healing method was used to evaluate the effects of compounds on HUVEC migration. Based on the results of proliferative assay on HUVECs, compounds **1** and **5–7** were chosen to evaluate the effects of reconstruction and migration at 50 μM. DMSO served as a control. The states of cellular growth at 0 h, 12 h, 24 h, 36 h and 48 h are presented in Figure 4. No significant endothelial cellular migrations were found in compound-treated groups and the vehicle control HUVEC before 12 h. However, compounds **1**, **5**, **6** and **7** treated groups all showed an increase in migration (58.5%, 80.66%, 60.71%, and 80.63% increment, respectively) after 48 h when compared with the vehicle control.

(A)

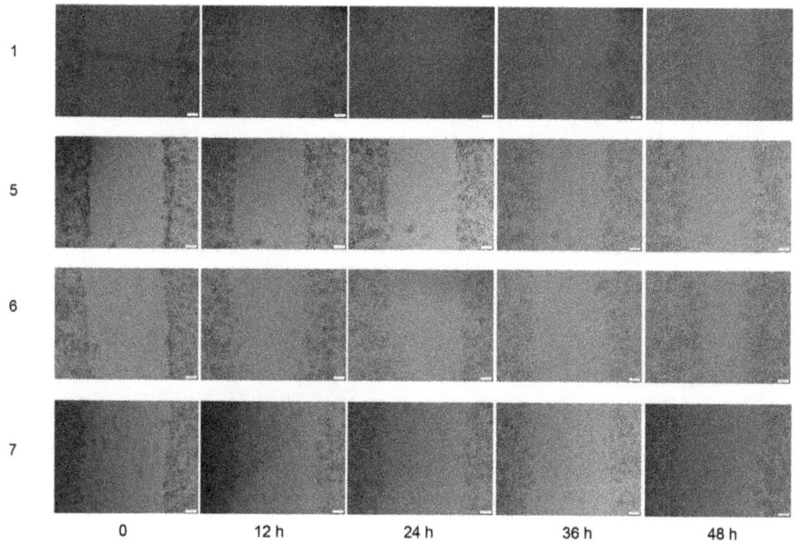

(B)

Compounds	Cellular Migration %				
	0 h	**12 h**	**24 h**	**36 h**	**48 h**
Control	0	12.12 ± 2.64	17.67 ± 1.92	23.76 ± 0.41	32.10 ± 1.23
1	0	33.55 ± 1.05	47.78 ± 1.01	70.48 ± 1.14	80.63 ± 0.54*
5	0	18.19 ± 0.90	23.56 ± 1.27	30.83 ± 0.43	58.53 ± 1.21*
6	0	27.46 ± 1.80	34.76 ± 1.22	38.86 ± 3.77	80.66 ± 0.68*
7	0	15.33 ± 1.51	25.23 ± 2.77	31.45 ± 1.03	60.71 ± 1.87*

(C)

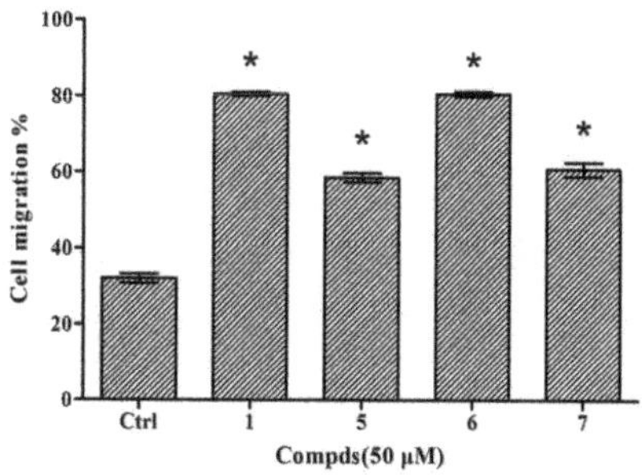

Figure 4. Effects of compounds **1** and **5**–**7** on HUVEC migration. (**A**) Observation of the effect of compounds on HUVEC migration; (**B**) The values of the compound-induced HUVEC migration at 0–48 h post-wounding; (**C**) Quantitative evaluation of the migration of HUVECs. Cellular migration was assessed at 48 h post-wounding. Data are expressed as the mean ± SEM (n = 4) of three individual experiments. Values vs control group: * $p < 0.01$ versus control.

2.4. *Invasion Assays of Compounds* **5–7** *in HUVECs*

Cellular proliferation, migration and invasion are clear characteristics of cytothesis in organisms. Therefore, transwell assays were utilized to determine the invasion of compounds **1** and **5–7** in HUVECs. There were 49.08%, 47.24%, 56.24%, and 53.17% increases in the invasion of HUVECs treated with compound **1** and **5–7** at 50 μM, respectively (Figure 5). The results indicated that compounds **5–7** were capable of inducing HUVEC migration similar to compound **1**. The above results suggest that these three tripeptides possess potential in the application of cytothesis studies.

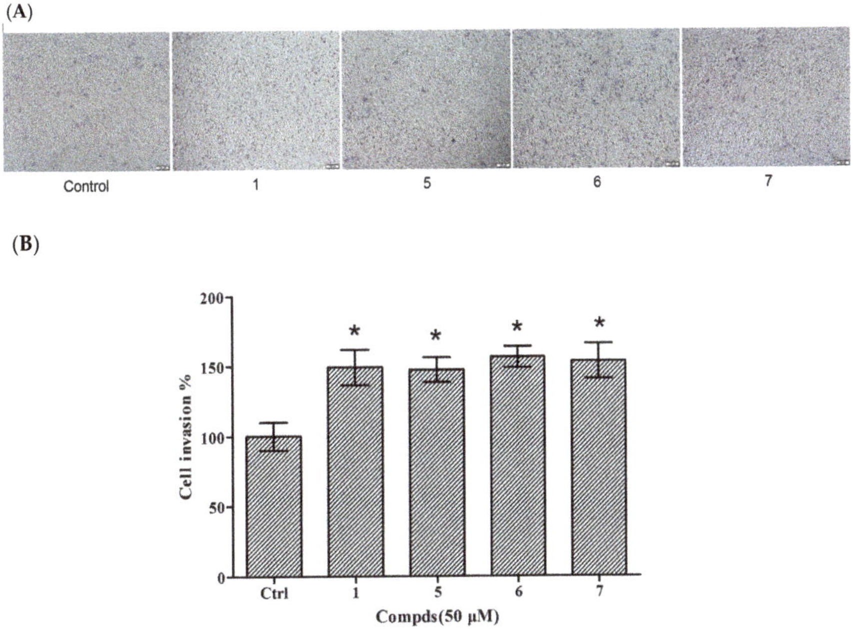

Figure 5. Effects of compounds **1** and **5–7** on HUVEC invasion. (**A**) Observation of the effect of compounds on HUVEC invasion; (**B**) Quantitative evaluation of the compound-induced HUVEC invasion. Cellular invasion was assessed at 24 h. Data are expressed as the mean ± SEM (n = 3) of three individual experiments. Values vs control group: * $p < 0.01$ versus control.

2.5. *The Angiogenic Activity of Compound* **6** *in Zebrafish*

It is meaningful to explore new candidate drugs for angiogenic therapy. An increasing number of studies are now available on the zebrafish model due to its short life cycle, availability and low cost. Based on the above assays, the proliferative effect of compound **7** was the most of significant on HUVEC proliferation. To further explore the effect of angiogenesis and restoration of blood vessel injury of compound **7**, the zebrafish assay was performed. The angiogenesis effects of compound **7** on normal zebrafish and PTK787-induced zebrafish blood vessel injury are presented in Figures 6 and 7, respectively. The results indicated that compound **7** could promote angiogenesis in zebrafish. It was more interesting that compound **7** could relieve the injuries of damaged sub-intestinal vein (SIV) on PTK787-induced zebrafish at a low concentration at 5 μM ($p < 0.05$), indicating that it can repair damaged blood vessels.

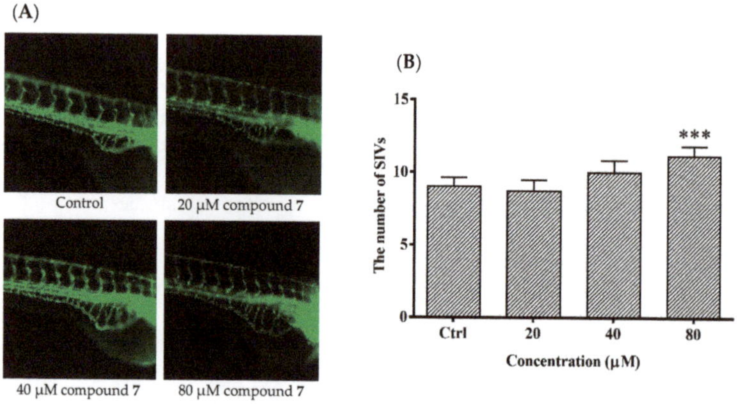

Figure 6. The effects of compound **7** on the angiogenesis formation in transgenic Tg (fli1: EGFP) zebrafish. Zebrafish embryos (24 hpf) were treated with test solution for 48 h and were evaluated using a microscope. (**A**) Representative images of blood vessel formation of zebrafish larvae at 72 hpf; (**B**) Quantitative analysis of the number of subintestinal vessel plexus (SIVs). Data are expressed as the means ± SEM (n = 10), and statistical significance was assessed by one-way ANOVA. Values vs control group: *** $p < 0.001$.

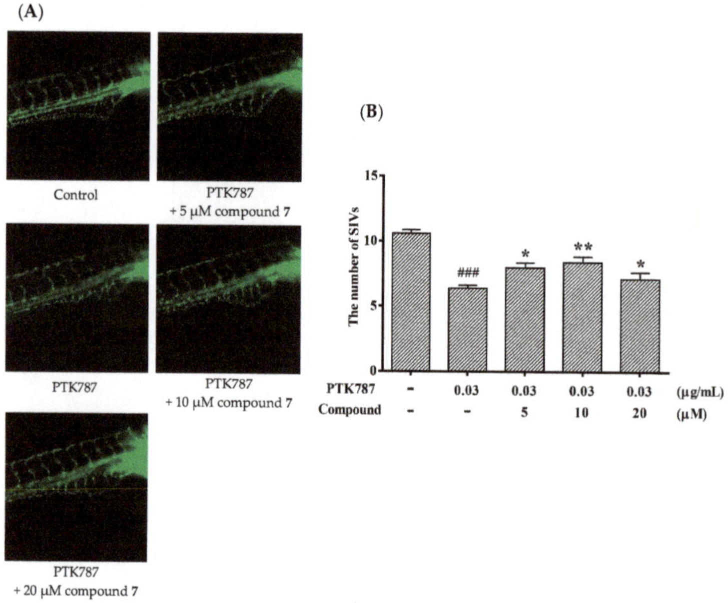

Figure 7. Compound **7** relieved the injuries of damaged SIVs in zebrafish. Zebrafish embryos (24 hpf) were treated with PTK787 for 24 h, then continually incubated with mixed solution of PTK787 and compound until 72 hpf. Zebrafish embryos were evaluated using a microscope. (**A**) Representative images of blood vessel formation of zebrafish larvae at 72 hpf; (**B**) Quantitative analysis of the regenerating caudal fin. Data are plotted as the mean ± SEM (n = 20), and statistical significance was assessed by one-way ANOVA. Values vs control group: ### $p < 0.001$; values vs model group: * $p < 0.05$ and ** $p < 0.01$.

3. Experimental Section

3.1. Chemistry

All reagents and solvents were of commercial quality. NMR data were recorded in methanol or DMSO, using TMS as an internal reference on a Varian Inova 500 MB NMR spectrometer (^{1}H, 500 MHz; ^{13}C, 125 MHz, Varian Medical Systems, Inc., Palo Alto, CA, USA), Bruker Avance 400 MB NMR spectrometer (^{1}H, 400 MHz; ^{13}C, 101 MHz, Bruker Corporation, Billerica, MA, USA). HREIMS were measured using Thermo MAT95XP High Resolution mass spectrometry (Thermo Fisher Scientific Inc. Waltham, MA, USA). EI were recorded on a Thermo DSQ EI-mass spectrometer. Column chromatography was carried out on silica gel (200–300 mesh, Qingdao Haiyang Chemical Co. Ltd., Qingdao, China). High-performance liquid chromatography (HPLC) was performed on a, Shimadzu LC-2010c (Shimadzu Corporation, Kyoto, Japan) equipped with UV detector. The purity of all compounds synthesized in this study was ≥95% as determined by HPLC analysis. Compounds **2–8** were first reported. The HPLC of compounds were shown in the Supplementary Flies (Tables S1–S9).

3.2. General Procedure for the Synthesis of Compounds 1–8

All the tested compounds were synthesized according to the literature [12]. Generally, amino acids Cbz-D-Val-OH and H-L-Lys(Boc)-OMe were used to starting materials and HBTU, HOBt and DIEA as coupling reagents. The mixtures were dissolved in DCM and stirred for 18 h at room temperature, followed by demethylation to form Cbz-D-Val-L-Lys(Boc)-OH. Coupling Cbz-D-Val-L-Lys(Boc)-OH and the O-methylation of L-alanie, L-methionine, L-phenylanaline, L-typrosine, and D-proline, respectively, in the same way and then demethylating with LiOH in THF/H_2O to form compounds **1**, **3**, **4**, **5** and **6**. Tripeptide **8** was obtained by removal of the Boc group of compound **1** in HCl/dioxane. Similarly, tripeptide **2** was obtained by coupling Cbz-D-His(Cbz)-OH, H-L-Lys(Boc)-OMe and H-L-Ala-OMe. Compound **7** was prepared by coupling Cbz-D-Val-OH, H-L-Arg(Pbf)-OMe and H-D-Val-OMe. The intermediate was then stirred in TFA/DCM to remove the Pbf-group to yield tripeptide 7. The NMR spectrum of compounds were shown in the Supplementary Flies (Figures S1–S15).

H-D-Val-L-Lys(Boc)-L-Ala-OH (**1**). White solid. ^{1}H NMR (500 MHz, MeOD) δ 8.54 (d, J = 8.2 Hz, 1H), 8.37 (d, J = 7.3 Hz, 1H), 6.68 (s, J = 8.4, 5.5 Hz, 1H), 4.21 (p, J = 7.4 Hz, 1H), 3.68 (d, J = 5.2 Hz, 1H), 2.88 (dd, J = 13.1, 6.7 Hz, 2H), 2.51 (dt, J = 3.6, 1.8 Hz, 7H), 2.18–1.98 (m, 1H), 1.73–1.45 (m, 2H), 1.30 (s, 11H), 1.29 (d, J = 7.3 Hz, 4H), 0.94 (dd, J = 11.8,6.9 Hz, 6H). ^{13}C NMR (125 MHz, MeOD) δ 174.26, 171.33, 168.10, 156.00, 77.81, 57.78, 52.63, 47.88, 30.35, 29.52, 28.74, 22.94, 18.86, 17.82, 17.52. EI-MS: m/z 417.5 (M^+); HR-EI-MS calcd. for $C_{19}H_{36}O_6N_4$: 417.5257 (M^+), found: 417.5228.

H-D-His-L-Lys(Boc)-L-Ala-OH (**2**). White solid. ^{1}H NMR (500 MHz, MeOD) δ 8.72 (s, 1H), 7.38 (s, 1H), 4.42–4.34 (m, 1H), 4.31 (dd, J = 8.7,5.3 Hz, 1H), 4.17 (t, J = 7.1 Hz, 1H), 3.25 (m, J = 15.0, 6.6 Hz, 1H), 3.00 (t, J = 7.2 Hz, 2H), 1.77 (dt, J = 13.8, 7.4 Hz, 1H), 1.69–1.58 (m, 1H), 1.40 (d, J = 7.3 Hz, 4H). ^{13}C NMR (125 MHz, MeOD) δ 174.25, 172.15, 167.32, 161.62, 157.30, 134.85, 128.41, 117.50, 110.01, 53.35, 52.24, 39.74, 31.43, 29.22, 27.38, 26.83, 22.58, 16.05. EI-MS: m/z 455.10 (M^+); HR-EI-MS calcd. for $C_{20}H_{35}O_6N_6$: 455.2612 (M^+), found: 455.2611.

H-D-Val-L-Lys(Boc)-L-Met-OH (**3**). White solid. ^{1}H NMR (500 MHz, MeOD) δ 4.59 (dd, J = 9.5, 4.3 Hz, 1H), 4.34 (dd, J = 9.0, 5.2 Hz, 1H), 3.82 (d, J = 3.6 Hz, 2H), 3.80 (d, J = 3.5 Hz, 3H), 3.77 (d, J = 7.8 Hz, 5H), 3.73–3.67 (m, 5H), 3.67–3.56 (m, 6H), 3.10–2.98 (m, 2H), 2.63 (ddd, J = 13.5, 8.5, 5.0 Hz, 1H), 2.53 (dt, J = 13.5, 7.9 Hz, 1H),2.23–2.13 (m, 2H), 2.09 (s, 4H), 1.96 (ddd, J = 14.2, 8.8, 4.3 Hz, 1H), 1.87 (dt, J = 12.7, 6.1 Hz, 1H), 1.77–1.63 (m, 1H), 1.45 (m, J = 55.4, 14.3, 7.2 Hz, 16H), 1.06 (dd, J = 6.8, 5.1 Hz, 7H). ^{13}C NMR (125 MHz, MeOD) δ 174.81, 174.47, 169.67, 158.59, 79.93, 73.03, 71.40, 65.15, 59.87, 54.90, 52.21, 32.76, 32.19, 31.42, 31.18, 30.54, 28.79, 24.25, 19.03, 18.03, 15.11. EI-MS: m/z 477.05 (M^+); HR-EI-MS calcd. for $C_{21}H_{39}O_6N_4S$: 475.2595 (M^-), found: 475.2597.

H-D-*Val*-L-*Lys(Boc)*-L-*Phe-OH* (**4**). White solid. ^{1}H NMR (500 MHz, MeOD) δ 7.32–7.24 (m, 1H), 7.23–7.14 (m, 1H), 4.63 (dd, J = 8.2, 5.2 Hz, 1H), 4.34 (dd, J = 9.1, 4.8 Hz, 1H), 3.63 (d, J = 6.2 Hz, 1H), 3.19 (dd, J = 14.0, 5.3 Hz, 1H), 3.02 (ddd, J = 8.4, 7.4, 4.4 Hz, 1H), 2.17 (dq, J = 13.6, 6.8 Hz, 1H), 1.8 (ddd, J = 14.3, 10.8, 5.9 Hz, 1H), 1.73–1.60 (m, 1H), 1.51–1.32 (m, 3H), 1.05 (t, J = 7.4 Hz, 1H). ^{13}C NMR (125 MHz, MeOD) δ 173.14, 172.67, 168.12, 157.18, 136.98, 128.98, 128.05, 126.39, 78.51, 88.49, 53.99, 53.38, 39.66, 36.85, 31.57, 29.99,29.12, 27.38, 22.84, 17.65, 16.55. EI-MS: m/z 493.10 (M$^+$); HR-EI-MS calcd. for $C_{25}H_{39}O_6N_4$: 491.2875 (M$^-$), found: 491.2877.

H-D-*Val*-L-*Lys(Boc)*-L-*Tyr-OH* (**5**). White solid. ^{1}H NMR (500 MHz, MeOD) δ 7.07 (d, J = 8.5 Hz, 1H), 4.56 (dd, J = 8.0, 5.1 Hz, 1H), 4.34 (dd, J = 9.0, 4.5 Hz, 1H), 3.86–3.73 (m, 9H), 3.73–3.67 (m, 4H), 3.66–3.57 (m, 5H), 3.14–2.80 (m, 2H), 2.17 (dd, J = 13.4, 6.7 Hz, 1H), 1.80 (dd, J = 14.3, 8.2 Hz, 1H), 1.72–1.61 (m, 1H), 1.05 (dd, J = 8.3, 7.1 Hz, 3H). ^{13}C NMR (125 MHz, MeOD) δ 155.92, 150.16, 129.99, 114.80, 71.63, 70.00, 63.75, 58.50, 54.25, 53.39, 36.11, 31.59, 29.99, 29.13, 27.38, 22.84, 17.66, 16.54. EI-MS: m/z 509.05 (M$^+$); HR-EI-MS calcd. for $C_{25}H_{39}O_7N_4$: 507.2824 (M$^-$), found: 507.2825.

H-D-*Val*-L-*Lys(Boc)*-D-*Pro-OH* (**6**). White solid. ^{1}H NMR (500 MHz, MeOD) δ 5.05 (t, J = 5.5 Hz, 1H), 4.71 (dd, J = 8.9, 4.9 Hz, 2H), 4.47–4.39 (m, 2H), 4.35 (dd, J = 9.7, 4.2 Hz, 1H), 3.91 (dd, J = 10.8, 6.0 Hz, 2H), 3.64 (dt, J = 9.5, 4.7 Hz, 4H), 3.49 (ddd, J = 19.1, 11.3, 6.0 Hz, 1H), 3.10–2.95 (m, 4H), 2.32–2.24 (m, 2H), 2.22–2.14 (m, 2H), 2.11–2.00 (m,5H), 1.94 (dd, J = 15.0, 7.6 Hz, 1H), 1.8 (dd, J = 16.2, 7.0 Hz, 2H), 1.67 (ddd, J = 14.0, 11.6, 6.8 Hz, 2H), 1.13 0 0.97 (m, 14H). ^{13}C NMR (125 MHz, MeOD) δ 173.93, 171.00, 167.96, 157.19, 78.48, 59.62, 59.22, 58.49, 58.31, 39.50, 30.57, 29.14, 28.83, 27.38, 24.20, 22.74, 22.03, 17.69, 16.54. EI-MS: m/z 443.05 (M$^+$); HR-EI-MS calcd. for $C_{21}H_{37}O_6N_4$: 441.2718 (M$^-$), found: 441.2720.

H-D-*Val*-L-*Arg*-D-*Val-OH* (**7**). White solid. ^{1}H NMR (500 MHz, MeOD) δ 4.58 (dd, J = 7.9, 6.0 Hz, 1H), 4.32 (d, J = 5.6 Hz, 1H), 3.85–3.77 (m, 2H), 3.77 (s, 1H), 3.69 (q, J = 5.7 Hz, 2H), 3.63 (dd, J = 11.1, 5.9 Hz, 1H), 3.26–3.14 (m, 3H), 2.19 (dqd, J = 13.7, 6.9, 4.0 Hz, 2H), 1.94–1.81 (m, 1H), 1.81–1.53 (m, 4H), 1.06 (dd, J = 8.6, 7.0 Hz, 7H), 0.98 (dd, J = 6.8, 4.2 Hz, 8H). ^{13}C NMR (125 MHz, MeOD) δ 171.95, 168.26, 157.24, 71.63, 70.01, 63.75, 58.43, 57.90, 40.56, 30.39, 30.03, 29.42, 25.21, 16.29, 17.60, 16.54. EI-MS: m/z 373.10 (M$^+$); HR-EI-MS calcd. for $C_{16}H_{33}O_4N_6$: 373.2557 (M$^+$), found: 373.2557.

H-D-*Val*-L-*Lys*-L-*Ala-OH* (**8**). White solid. ^{1}H NMR (400 MHz, MeOD) δ 4.41 (dd, J = 11.8, 6.0 Hz, 1H), 3.71 (d, J = 6.2 Hz, 1H),2.92 (t, J = 7.5 Hz, 1H), 2.20 (dq, J = 13.4, 6.6 Hz, 1H), 1.90 (tq, J = 14.0, 7.4 Hz, 1H), 1.74 (ddd, J = 23.2, 15.0, 7.8 Hz, 2H), 1.54 (dd, J = 15.0, 7.5 Hz, 1H), 1.39 (dd, J = 36.4, 19.5 Hz, 2H), 1.16–0.97 (m, 3H). EI-MS: m/z 317.20 (M$^+$); HR-EI-MS calcd. for $C_{14}H_{29}O_4N_4$: 317.2183 (M$^+$), found: 317.2178.

3.3. Cellular Culture and Drug Treatment

Human umbilical vein endothelial cellular (HUVEC) cells were obtained from ScienCell Research Laboratories, Inc. (San Diego, CA, USA). (CAT. 8000). HUVECs were cultured in M199 medium with 100 µg/mL penicillin-streptomycin, 30 µg/mL endothelial cellular growth supplement and 10% FBS in 75 cm^2 tissue culture flasks at 37 °C in a humidified atmosphere of 5% CO_2. Compounds were dissolved in DMSO to make a 200 µM stock solution and were then diluted to different concentrations as needed.

3.4. Proliferative Assays

HUVECs were seeded onto 96-well gelatin coated plates at a density of 10^4 cells/well. In order to achieve a quiescent state, complete medium was replaced after 24 h incubation with low serum (0.5% FBS) medium and re-incubated for 24 h. After this, the medium was replaced with various drug treatments diluted in low serum (0.5% FBS) medium. DMSO (0.1%) and VEGF (20 ng/mL) served as negative and positive controls, respectively. In accordance with the manufacturer's protocol, plates were incubated for an additional 48 h and cellular proliferation was assessed by the MTT, which is widely used to observe the growth of cell. The spectrophotometric absorbance of each well was measured. The wavelengths used to measure absorbance of the formazan product were 570 nm and 630 nm. The results were expressed as the percentage of proliferating cells.

3.5. Migration Assays

HUVEC migration assays were performed using the wound healing method. The HUVECs (3×10^5 cells) were seeded into each well of a 24-well plate and incubated with complete medium at 37 °C and 5% CO_2. After 24 h of incubation, cells were starved for additional 24 h by low serum (0.5% FBS) medium. The HUVECs were then scraped away horizontally in each well using a P100 pipette tip. Three randomly selected views along the scraped line were photographed on each well using an Olympus ix53 microscope (Olympus, Tokyo, Japan) and the CCD camera attached to the microscope at 10× magnification. The medium was then changed to fresh low serum (1% FBS) medium with compounds **1** and **5–7** (50 μM) or with DMSO. After incubation (0 h, 12 h, 24 h, 36 h and 48 h), another set of images were taken by the same method. Image analysis for signs of migration was performed by Metamorph Imaging Series (Molecular Devices, LLC., San Jose, CA, USA). The average scraped area of each well under each condition was measured and subtracted from that of the before-treatment condition. Data are expressed as percentage wound closure relative to the wound closure area in the control medium. The wound closure area of the control cells was set at 100%.

3.6. Invasion Assay

HUVEC invasion assay was carried out following previous methods [13]. Briefly, the effect of compounds **1** and **5–7** on HUVEC invasion was measured using the 10 mm tissue culture insert (transwell permeable supports, Corning Incorporated, Tewksbury, MA, USA) with polycabonate membarane (8 mm pores) and 24-well companion plate. The upper side and lower side of the membrane were pre-coated with 1:30 (*v/v*) of Matrigel (Corning Incorporated, Tewksbury, MA, USA). The HUVECs were resuspended in low serum (1% FBS) medium and seeded onto the culture inserts at 5×10^4 cells per insert in triplicate. They were then deposited into the 24-well companion plate with 500 μL of low serum (1% FBS) medium containing compounds (50 μM) in the presence. In addition, the wells of the companion plate, containing DMSO (0.1%), served as a vehicle control. The inserts were removed after 8 h of incubation and were then washed with PBS. Non-invasive cells on the upper surface of the membrane were removed by wiping with cotton swabs. The inserts were fixed in paraformaldehyate, stained with DAPI and mounted on a microscope and a CCD camera. Following this, HUVECs per insert were examined with the software Metamorph Imaging Series (Molecular Devices, Tokyo, Japan).

3.7. Zebrafish Assay of Compound 7

Zebrafish embryos were used to examine the effect of different compounds on embryonic angiogenesis. Compound **7** was added to embryo water from 24 hpf. Zebrafish embryos were generated by natural pairwise mating and raised at 28.5 °C in embryo water. Embryos were maintained in embryo water at 28 °C. Three embryos were placed into each well of a 96-well plate containing 200 μL embryo water with or without the drug. The blood vessel development using an inverted Olympus DP70 epifluorescence microscope (Olympus, Tokyo, Japan). Because the fish embryo receives nourishment from an attached yolk ball for the duration of the experiment, no additional maintenance was required during the duration of the experiments. After 72 hpf, the embryos were anesthetized using 0.05% 2-phenoxyethanol in embryo water, and each embryo was examined for the presence of ectopic vessels in the subintestinal vessel plexus (SIV). The experiments of zebrafish were conducted according to the guidelines for animal care and use of China and were approved by the animal ethics committee of the Chinese Academy of Medical Science (Beijing, China).

PTK787 is frequently used as angiogenesis inhibitors [18]. In order to test the effect of compound **7** on damaged zebrafish, we evaluated a quantitative assay in transgenic zebrafish using angiogenesis inhibitor PTK787. The 24 hpf embryos were cultured and collected. The inhibitor, PTK787 (0.03 μg/mL) was added into embryo water and the embryo were cultured 24 h. Subsequently, compound **7** was added into embryo water afer removing the PTK787 and cultured for 24 h. After 72 hpf, the embryos were anesthetized using 0.05% 2-phenoxyethanol in embryo water, and each embryo was examined for the presence of ectopic vessels in the subintestinal vessel plexus (SIV).

3.8. Statistical Analysis

Statistical analysis was performed using SPSS Statistics 21 software (IBM corporation, Armonk, NY, USA). Survival curves were analyzed by the life table method and evaluation of the effects of compounds on the mean survival time was done by the Wilcoxon rank sum test. All the curves and column diagrams were drawn using GraphPad Prism 6 software (GraphPad Software, Inc., San Diego, CA, USA). Data are expressed as the mean ± SEM. Statistical comparisons between groups were performed using one-way ANOVA followed by Dunnett's *t*-test using non-treatment as the control group. $p < 0.05$ was considered statistically significant.

4. Conclusions

In summary, seven compounds have been designed and synthesized to evaluate the proliferation, migration and invasion of HUVECs by MTT assays, based on the lead compound **1**, which was demonstrated significantly stimulate angiogenesis both in vivo and in vitro. Among these analogues, compounds **5–7** possess remarkable proliferations, migrations and invasions of HUVECs compared with the lead compound 1. The results show that hydrophilic, alkaline group, L-Tyrosine and D-Proline fragment substituting for L-alanine may greatly contribute to proliferation of HUVECs. To our surprise, compound **7** exerted a significant effect on HUVECs, which revealed that the L-Arg-D-Val fragment resembles Lys(Boc)-L-Ala-OH in terms of cytoactivity. With its good proliferation, compound **7** can promote angiogenesis in zebrafish and can repair blood vessels in PTK787-induced zebrafish at a low concentration. These small molecular peptides could be easily prepared compared the macromolecule proteins. Because of the briefness of their strutures, they would eventually develop into a promising drug candidate for the treatment of damage repair and related diseases.

Supplementary Materials: The following are available online, Figure S1: ^{1}H NMR (MeOD, 500 MHz) of Compound **1**, Figure S2: ^{13}C NMR (MeOD, 125 MHz) of Compound **1**, Figure S3: ^{1}H NMR (MeOD, 500 MHz) of Compound **2**, Figure S4: ^{13}C NMR (MeOD, 125 MHz) of Compound **2**, Figure S5: ^{1}H NMR (MeOD, 500 MHz) of Compound **3**, Figure S6: ^{13}C NMR (MeOD, 125 MHz) of Compound **3**, Figure S7: ^{1}H NMR (MeOD, 500 MHz) of Compound **4**, Figure S8: ^{13}C NMR (MeOD, 125 MHz) of Compound **4**, Figure S9: ^{1}H NMR (MeOD, 500 MHz) of Compound **5**, Figure S10: ^{13}C NMR (MeOD, 125 MHz) of Compound **5**, Figure S11: ^{1}H NMR (MeOD, 500 MHz) of Compound **6**, Figure S12: ^{13}C NMR (MeOD, 125 MHz) of Compound **6**, Figure S13: ^{1}H NMR (MeOD, 500 MHz) of Compound **7**, Figure S14: ^{13}C NMR (MeOD, 125 MHz) of Compound **7**, Figure S15: ^{1}H NMR (MeOD, 400 MHz) of Compound **8**, Table S1: Purities and retention times of all tested compounds, Table S2: HPLC chromatography of compound **1**, Table S3: HPLC chromatography of compound **2**, Table S4: HPLC chromatography of compound **3**, Table S5: HPLC chromatography of compound **4**, Table S6: HPLC chromatography of compound **5**, Table S7: HPLC chromatography of compound **6**, Table S8: HPLC chromatography of compound **7**, Table S9: HPLC chromatography of compound **8**.

Author Contributions: Conceptualization, Y.P. and Y.Z.; methodology, Y.Z. and X.W.; software, J.Z.; validation, J.P., Y.Z. and Y.C.; formal analysis, Y.Z.; investigation, Y.Z. and Y.T.; resources, X.W.; data curation, Y.T.; writing—original draft preparation, Y.Z.; writing—review and editing, J.P.; visualization, Y.Z.; supervision, J.P.; project administration, J.P.; funding acquisition, J.P.

Funding: This research received no external funding.

Acknowledgments: This work was supported by the National Natural Science Foundation of China (21172271), the Natural Science Foundation of Guangdong Province, China (Grant No. S2011020001231 and 2017A030313064) and the Major Scientific and Technological Special Project of Administration of Ocean and Fisheries of Guangdong Province (GDME-2018C013).

Conflicts of Interest: The authors declare no conflict of interest. The funders had no role in the design of the study; in the collection, analyses, or interpretation of data; in the writing of the manuscript, or in the decision to publish the results.

References

1. Zhou, X.; Liu, J.; Yang, B.; Lin, X.; Yang, X.W.; Liu, Y. Marine natural products with anti-HIV activities in the last decade. *Curr. Med. Chem.* **2013**, *20*, 953–973. [PubMed]
2. Edwards, D.J.; Marquez, B.L.; Nogle, L.M. Structure and biosynthesis of the jamaicamides, new mixed polyketide-peptide neurotoxins from the marine cyanobacterium *Lyngbya majuscula*. *Am. Math. Soc.* **2004**, *11*, 817–833. [CrossRef] [PubMed]
3. Huang, H.N.; Rajanbabu, V.; Pan, C.Y. A cancer vaccine based on the marine antimicrobial peptide pardaxin (GE33) for control of bladder-associated tumors. *Biomaterials* **2013**, *34*, 10151–10159. [CrossRef] [PubMed]
4. Jang, I.S.; Sun, J.P. Hydroxyproline-containing collagen peptide derived from the skin of the Alaska pollack inhibits HIV-1 infection. *Mol. Med. Rep.* **2016**, *14*, 5489–5494. [CrossRef] [PubMed]
5. Chopra, L.; Singh, G.; Choudhary, V. Sonorensin: An antimicrobial peptide, belonging to the heterocycloanthracin subfamily of bacteriocins, from a new marine isolate, *Bacillus sonorensis* MT93. *Appl. Environ. Microbiol.* **2014**, *80*. [CrossRef] [PubMed]
6. Ko, S.C.; Kim, D.; Jeon, Y.J. Protective effect of a novel antioxidative peptide purified from a marine Chlorella ellipsoidea protein against free radical-induced oxidative stress. *Food Chem. Toxicol.* **2012**, *50*, 2294–2302. [CrossRef] [PubMed]
7. Hyder, S.M.; Stancel, G.M. Regulation of angiogenic growth factors in the female reproductive tract by estrogens and progestins. *Mol. Endocrinol.* **1999**, *13*, 806–811. [CrossRef] [PubMed]
8. Singla, R.; Soni, S.; Patial, V. Cytocompatible anti-microbial dressings of *Syzygium cumini* cellulose nanocrystals decorated with silver nanoparticles accelerate acute and diabetic wound healing. *Sci. Rep.* **2017**, *7*. [CrossRef]
9. Suzane, C.P.; Marcell, C.M.; Sybele, S.; Joni, A.C.; Raquel, M.S.C. Role of osteogenic growth peptide (OGP) and OGP (10-14) in bone regeneration: A review. *Mol. Sci.* **2016**, *17*. [CrossRef]
10. Guo, D.; Murdoch, C.E.; Xu, H. Vascular endothelial growth factor signaling requires glycine to promote angiogenesis. *Sci. Rep.* **2017**, *7*. [CrossRef] [PubMed]
11. Lin, Y.; Wu, X.; Feng, S.; Jiang, G.; Zhou, S.; Vrijmoedb, L.L.P.; Gareth Jonesb, E.B. A novel N-cinnamoylcyclopeptide containing an allenic ether from the fungus *Xylaria* sp. (strain #2508) from the South China Sea. *Tetrahedron. Lett.* **2001**, *42*, 449–451.
12. Wang, S.Y.; Xu, Z.L.; Wang, H.; Li, C.R.; Fu, L.W.; Pang, J.Y.; Li, J.; She, Z.G.; Lin, Y.C. Total Synthesis, absolute configuration, and biological activity of xyloallenoide A. *Helv. Chim. Acta* **2012**, *95*, 973–982. [CrossRef]
13. Lu, X.L.; Xu, Z.L.; Yao, X.L. Marine cyclotripeptide X-13 promotes angiogenesis in zebrafish and human endothelial cells via PI3K/Akt/eNOS signaling pathways. *Mar. Drugs* **2012**, *10*, 1307–1320. [CrossRef] [PubMed]
14. Li, J.; Lu, X.; Wu, Q.; Yu, G.; Xu, Z.; Qiu, L.; Pei, Z.; Lin, Y.; Pang, J. Design, SAR, angiogenic activities evaluation and pro-angiogenic mechanism of new marine cyclopeptide analogs. *Curr. Med. Chem.* **2013**, *20*, 1183–1194. [CrossRef] [PubMed]
15. Byung, C.L.; Hyun, J.S.; Ji, S.K.; Kyung-Ho, J.; Yearn, S.C.; Kyung-Han, L.; Dae, Y.C. Synthesis of Tc-99m labeled glucos amino-Asp-cyclic (Arg-Gly-Asp-D-Phe-Lys) as a potential angiogenesis imaging agent. *Bioorg. Med. Chem.* **2007**, *15*, 7755–7764.
16. Park, H.J.; Zhang, Y.; Georgescu, S.P.; Johnson, K.L.; Kong, D.; Galper, J.B. Human umbilical vein endothelial cells and human dermal microvascular endothelial cells offer new insights into the relationship between lipid metabolism and angiogenesis. *Stem Cell Rev.* **2006**, *2*, 93–102. [CrossRef] [PubMed]
17. Yi, F.; Hao, Y.; Chong, X. Overexpression of microRNA-506-3p aggravates the injury of vascular endothelial cells in patients with hypertension by downregulating Beclin1 expression. *Exp. Ther. Med.* **2018**, *15*, 2844–2850. [CrossRef] [PubMed]
18. Tal, T.L.; Mccollum, C.W.; Harris, P.S. Immediate and long-term consequences of vascular toxicity during zebrafish development. *Reprod. Toxicol.* **2014**, *48*, 51–61. [CrossRef] [PubMed]

Sample Availability: Samples of the compounds **1–8** are available from the authors.

molecules

MDPI

Article

Ethanolic Extract of Folium Sennae Mediates the Glucose Uptake of L6 Cells by GLUT4 and Ca^{2+}

Ping Zhao [1,2,*], Qian Ming [1], Junying Qiu [1], Di Tian [1], Jia Liu [1], Jinhua Shen [1], Qing-Hua Liu [1] and Xinzhou Yang [2,3,*]

1 Institute for Medical Biology & Hubei Provincial Key Laboratory for Protection and Application of Special Plants in the Wuling Area of China, College of Life Sciences, South-Central University for Nationalities, Wuhan 430074, China; 18062196191@163.com (Q.M.); qiu927633@163.com (J.Q.); tiandi_2983@126.com (D.T.); 13512566172@163.com (J.L.); shenjinhua2013@163.com (J.S.); qinghualiu95@163.com (Q.-H.L.)

2 National Demonstration Center for Experimental Ethnopharmacology Education, South-Central University for Nationalities, Wuhan 430074, China

3 School of Pharmaceutical Sciences, South-Central University for Nationalities, 182 Min-Zu Road, Wuhan 430074, China

* Correspondence: p.zhao@scuec.edu.cn (P.Z.); xzyang@mail.scuec.edu.cn (X.Y.); Tel.: +86-027-67842576 (P.Z.)

Academic Editor: Pinarosa Avato

Received: 29 September 2018; Accepted: 8 November 2018; Published: 9 November 2018

Abstract: In today's world, diabetes mellitus (DM) is on the rise, especially type 2 diabetes mellitus (T2DM), which is characterized by insulin resistance. T2DM has high morbidity, and therapies with natural products have attracted much attention in the recent past. In this paper, we aimed to study the hypoglycemic effect and the mechanism of an ethanolic extract of Folium Sennae (FSE) on L6 cells. The glucose uptake of L6 cells was investigated using a glucose assay kit. We studied glucose transporter 4 (GLUT4) expression and AMP-activated protein kinase (AMPK), protein kinase B (PKB/Akt), and protein kinase C (PKC) phosphorylation levels using western blot analysis. GLUT4 trafficking and intracellular Ca^{2+} levels were monitored by laser confocal microscopy in L6 cells stably expressing IRAP-mOrange. GLUT4 fusion with plasma membrane (PM) was observed by myc-GLUT4-mOrange. FSE stimulated glucose uptake; GLUT4 expression and translocation; PM fusion; intracellular Ca^{2+} elevation; and the phosphorylation of AMPK, Akt, and PKC in L6 cells. GLUT4 translocation was weakened by the AMPK inhibitor compound C, PI3K inhibitor Wortmannin, PKC inhibitor Gö6983, G protein inhibitor PTX/Gallein, and PLC inhibitor U73122. Similarly, in addition to PTX/Gallein and U73122, the IP3R inhibitor 2-APB and a 0 mM Ca^{2+}-EGTA solution partially inhibited the elevation of intracellular Ca^{2+} levels. BAPTA-AM had a significant inhibitory effect on FSE-mediated GLUT4 activities. In summary, FSE regulates GLUT4 expression and translocation by activating the AMPK, PI3K/Akt, and G protein–PLC–PKC pathways. FSE causes increasing Ca^{2+} concentration to complete the fusion of GLUT4 vesicles with PM, allowing glucose uptake. Therefore, FSE may be a potential drug for improving T2DM.

Keywords: FSE; T2DM; GLUT4; Ca^{2+}; L6 cell

1. Introduction

Diabetes mellitus (DM) is a chronic metabolic disorder resulting from insufficient insulin secretion or insulin dysfunction. It may lead to a series of complications such as renal failure, cardiovascular disease, blindness, hypertension, non-alcoholic fatty liver disease (NAFLD), and obesity [1,2]. The global prevalence of DM is on the rise, especially in developing countries [3]. T2DM is the most prevalent form of DM and accounts for more than 90% of the cases of DM [4]. Insulin resistance is the typical feature of T2DM, which causes cells to stop responding adequately to the standard role of insulin. While the body continues to produce insulin, the cells in the body become resistant to its effects. Therefore, cells cannot effectively process insulin, resulting in hyperglycemia [5–7].

Blood glucose influx into cells requires glucose transporter family proteins (GLUTs) [1]. With the onset of hyperglycemia, the glucose uptake in the adipose tissue and muscles is mostly mediated by GLUT4, an isoform of a family of sugar transporter proteins (encoded on the SLC2A4 gene) containing 12 transmembrane domains. GLUT4 continuously recycles between intracellular vessels and the plasma membrane (PM) [8,9]. After insulin stimulation, GLUT4 proteins are mobilized to PM immediately, which enhances the rate of exocytosis and their fusion with PM (this process is synonymous with GLUT4 translocation). The increase in PM GLUT4 leads to glucose uptake [10]. Previous studies have reported that defective GLUT4 translocation is a feature of insulin resistance and an essential precursor of T2DM [4,7,11]. Thus, GLUT4 as a key regulatory target for glucose homeostasis is widely used in antidiabetic drug research.

Intracellular cytosolic free Ca^{2+} comes from both extracellular Ca^{2+} influx and Ca^{2+} release from intracellular stores (including sarcoplasmic reticulum, lysosomes, and mitochondria). As an important second messenger, it participates in many physiological activities of cells. Numerous studies have highlighted the role of cytosolic Ca^{2+} in GLUT4 synthesis, GLUT4 traffic (endocytosis and exocytosis), and glucose uptake. Wright reported that the treatment of L6 muscle cells with agents that increase Ca^{2+} leads to an increase in the GLUT4 protein content [12]. Li et al. found that Ca^{2+} signals promote GLUT4 exocytosis and reduce its endocytosis in muscle cells [13]. Johanna et al. described the role of Ca^{2+} influx for insulin-mediated glucose uptake in skeletal muscles [14]. Contreras-Ferrat et al. clearly showed that an inositol 1,4,5-triphosphate (IP3)-dependent Ca^{2+} release pathway is required for insulin-stimulated GLUT4 translocation and glucose uptake in cardiomyocytes [15]. Similarly, it has been reported that the AMPK, PKC, and insulin-dependent pathways were relatively independent of Ca^{2+}-regulated GLUT4 traffic [16–19]. Furthermore, increases in intracellular Ca^{2+} levels, even at concentrations too low to induce contractions, provide the signal to activate GLUT4 translocation in skeletal muscles [17].

Because of serious economic burdens and side effects of chemical agent-based DM treatment strategies [7,20,21], natural drug products are gaining popularity because of their various advantages, such as fewer side effects, better patient tolerance, relatively lower cost, and acceptance due to the long history of use. An important cause of these products' efficacy is that, unlike a single chemical entity aimed at a specific single target, many Chinese herbal medicines (such as the multi-flavonoid-rich plant extracts) are thought to alleviate the disorder of diabetes mellitus through an integrated effect upon multitarget sites [22,23]. Current studies have shown that phytochemicals, polysaccharides, flavonoids, terpenoids, tannins, steroids, and other chemicals naturally found in plants possess antidiabetic activity [8,24,25]. The two main antidiabetic agents represented by metformin and flavonoids were derived from medicinal plants. Folium Sennae, also called the senna leaf, is derived from the dried leaflets of *Cassia angustifolia Vahl* or *Cassia acutifolia Delile*, and belongs to the dicotyledonous leguminous family. It is native to India and Egypt, and is widely distributed in the Taiwan, Guangdong, Guangxi, and Yunnan provinces of China [26]. The Chinese Pharmacopoeia (2010) and Chinese Materia Medica state that senna leaves contain four sennosides (A, B, C, and D), rhein, emodin, chrysophanol, aloe-emodin, physcion, tinnevellin glucoside, kaempferol, phytosterol and its glycosides, pine camphor, salicylic acid, and several other ingredients. In addition to being well known as a natural laxative [27], the senna leaf has been found to exhibit antioxidant [28], antibacterial [29], anti-inflammatory [30], antitumor [31], analgesic [32], antimalarial [33], and antidiabetic [34] activities. Ayinla et al. reported that the ethanolic leaf extract of Senna fistula improved hematologic parameters, lipid profiles, and oxidative stress in alloxan-induced diabetic rats [35]. Thilagam et al. discovered that the ethanolic leaf extract of Senna surattensis inhibited the carbohydrate digestive enzymes and increased the peripheral glucose uptake in the isolated rat hemidiaphragm model [34]. Malematja et al. showed that Senna italica leaf acetone extract promoted glucose uptake and anti-obesity through the PI3K-dependent pathway [36]. However, only a few studies have assessed the possible hypoglycemic properties and hypoglycemic mechanisms of Folium Sennae (FSE).

In the present study, we observed that FSE displayed a strong effect in promoting glucose uptake, GLUT4 expression and translocation, and cytosolic Ca^{2+} levels in L6 rat skeletal muscle cells. We observed that FSE induced GLUT4 expression and translocation through the AMPK, PI3K/Akt, and PKC signaling pathways. FSE also increased cytosolic Ca^{2+} concentration by extracellular Ca^{2+} influx or/and intracellular Ca^{2+} release of G protein-IP3-IP3R signals, which assisted GLUT4 movement and stimulated glucose uptake. We elucidated the mechanism of action and validated the beneficial effects of FSE as an antidiabetic agent.

2. Results

2.1. FSE Increases GLUT4 Expression Levels and Glucose Uptake in L6 Cells

To confirm the possible hypoglycemic activity of FSE, we first studied its glucose uptake effect. As shown in Figure 1A, L6 cells were serum-deprived and then incubated with 100 nM insulin or different concentrations of FSE for 1 h. When compared with the control group, insulin (positive control) and 30, 60, and 120 μg/mL of FSE significantly promoted the glucose uptake of cells by 2.04-fold, 1.87-fold, 1.95-fold, and 1.68-fold, respectively. This result was based on the corresponding MTT assay after drug treatment. MTT results showed that neither FSE nor insulin caused toxicity to L6 cells (Figure S1). In the next step, we chose 60 μg/mL as the best concentration of FSE. To understand whether FSE affected the expression of the glucose regulator GLUT4, the total protein and mRNA of GLUT4 and the mRNA of IRAP in L6 cells were extracted after stimulation with insulin or FSE. The results showed that 100 nM insulin and 60 μg/mL FSE increased the protein expression of GLUT4 by 2.13-fold and 1.89-fold, respectively (Figure 1B). The fold increases of GLUT4 mRNA levels were even more prominent, at 4.13-fold with insulin and 2.8-fold with FSE (Figure 1C). In addition, as a resident protein of GLUT4 storage vesicles, insulin-regulated aminopeptidase (IRAP) also changed at the mRNA level, with 1.46-fold from insulin treatment and 1.70-fold from FSE treatment (Figure 1D).

2.2. FSE Stimulates GLUT4 Translocation and Increases Intracellular Ca^{2+} Levels

Since intracellular GLUT4 translocation to the cell surface can exert glucose uptake function, we further analyzed GLUT4 translocation in L6 cells under FSE treatment. L6 cells stably expressing IRAP-mOrange (L6-mOrange-IRAP) were transfected with red fluorescent protein (mOrange)-tagged IRAP. IRAP was initially found in specialized vesicles containing GLUT4, which immediately migrated to the cell surface along with GLUT4 after receiving insulin [37]. Some evidences proved that IRAP was highly co-localized with GLUT4 [38,39]. We used Fluo-4 AM fluorescent dyes during loading of cells with Ca^{2+} and monitored the translocation of GLUT4 and intracellular Ca^{2+} changes in live cells by real-time fluorescence microscopy. As a comparative insulin treatment, the image showed that the intracellular IRAP-mOrange signal was enhanced and signal accumulation appeared in adjacent PM region. Green fluorescence was significantly brightened after 100 nM insulin treatment in intracellular Ca^{2+} detection (Figure S2). Similarly, the IRAP fluorescence intensity in cytoplasm was obviously raised after the addition of 60 μg/mL FSE, and a substantial amount of red fluorescence accumulated at the cell periphery as revealed by IRAP-mOrange signals. Meanwhile, the green fluorescence of Ca^{2+} was densely distributed in the cells (Figure 2A). The fold growth curve increased with IRAP level at the PM region or with intracellular Ca^{2+}, and it increased in a time-dependent manner (Figure 2B). Our studies suggested that FSE promoted glucose uptake not only by stimulating GLUT4 expression and translocation but also by increasing intracellular Ca^{2+} levels.

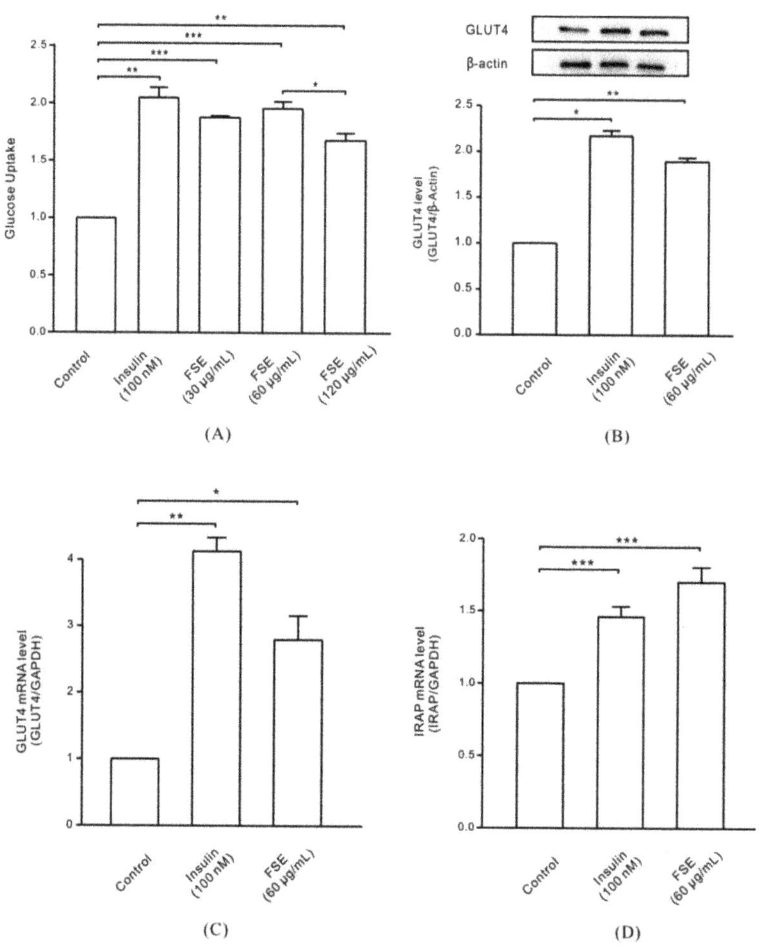

Figure 1. Enhancing the effects of Folium Sennae (FSE) on glucose uptake and GLUT4 expression in L6 cells. Insulin as a positive control. (**A**) Cells were incubated with 100 nM insulin or 30, 60, and 120 μg/mL FSE for 1 h, and glucose uptake was measured using a glucose assay kit. (**B**) Cells were stimulated with 100 nM insulin or 60 μg/mL FSE for 30 min. Whole cell lysates were subjected to western blot analysis for GLUT4, and the protein expression level was normalized against β-actin. (**C**) Cells were treated with 100 nM insulin or 60 μg/mL FSE for 30 min. GAPDH was used to normalize the mRNA level, and the relative expression of GLUT4 mRNA was investigated by real-time PCR. (**D**) Cells were treated with 100 nM insulin or 60 μg/mL FSE for 30 min. GAPDH was used to normalize the mRNA level, and the relative expression of IRAP mRNA was investigated by real-time PCR. The data were obtained from three independent repeated experiments. Significance analysis: * $p < 0.05$; ** $p < 0.01$; *** $p < 0.001$.

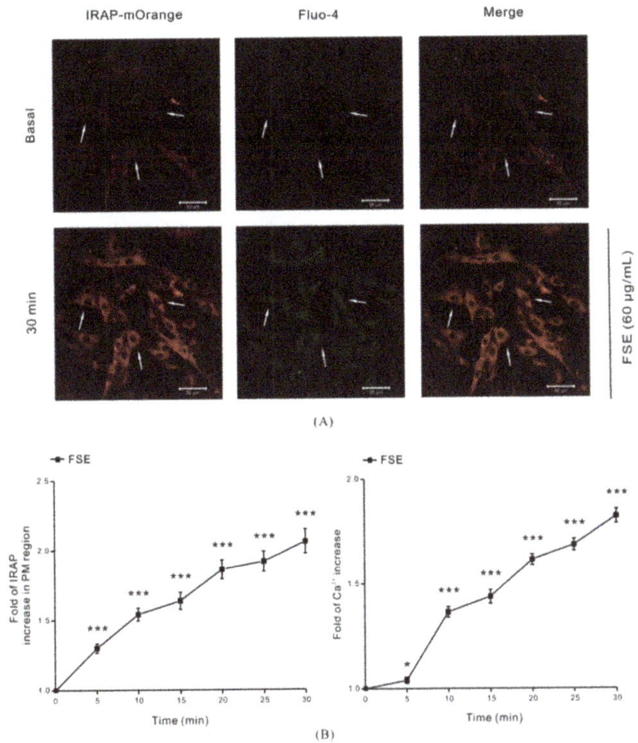

Figure 2. Stimulating effects of FSE on GLUT4 translocation and intracellular Ca^{2+} level. The red fluorescence of IRAP-mOrange stably expressed in L6 cells and the green fluorescence of Ca^{2+} were simultaneously observed by confocal microscope. Scale bar = 50 μm. (**A**) Intracellular Ca^{2+} was stained with Flou-4 AM for 20 min, followed by stimulation with 60 μg/mL FSE for 30 min. IRAP-mOrange fluorescence intensity and intracellular Ca^{2+} fluorescence concentration were detected at excitation wavelengths of 555 nm and 488 nm, respectively, and fluorescence superposition displayed specific positioning. (**B**) The cell images were recorded over 30 min, and the red fluorescence from the outside edges of cells and the green fluorescence of the whole cells were collected. Fluorescence quantization was done with Zeiss 2010 software. Significance analysis: * $p < 0.05$; *** $p < 0.001$.

2.3. The Role of Cytosolic Ca^{2+} in FSE-Mediated GLUT4 Translocation

In order to determine whether the increase of intracellular Ca^{2+} concentration after FSE stimulation was related to GLUT4 translocation, we blocked the different sources of intracellular Ca^{2+} before treatment with 60 μg/mL FSE to observe the GLUT4 translocation. FSE-induced increase of intracellular Ca^{2+} was partially inhibited with the removal of extracellular Ca^{2+}, but the FSE-mediated increase of IRAP fluorescence in the PM region remained unchanged (Figure 3A). This phenomenon can be explained by the observation that for FSE to evoke the rise of intracellular Ca^{2+}, it needs at least to mobilize extracellular Ca^{2+} influx. In addition, when 0 mM extracellular Ca^{2+}+BAPTA-AM was used to chelate cytosolic Ca^{2+}, the FSE-induced increase of intracellular Ca^{2+} was completely inhibited, and the increase of IRAP fluorescence in the PM region was also obviously blocked (Figure 3B). These findings supported the idea that cytosolic Ca^{2+} plays an important role in the process of FSE-induced GLUT4 translocation to the PM.

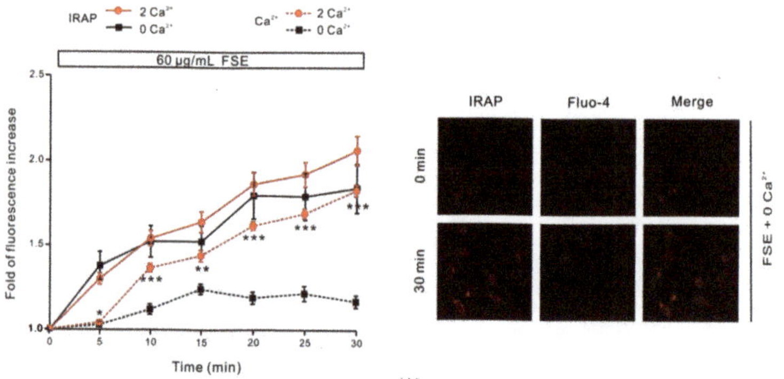

(A)

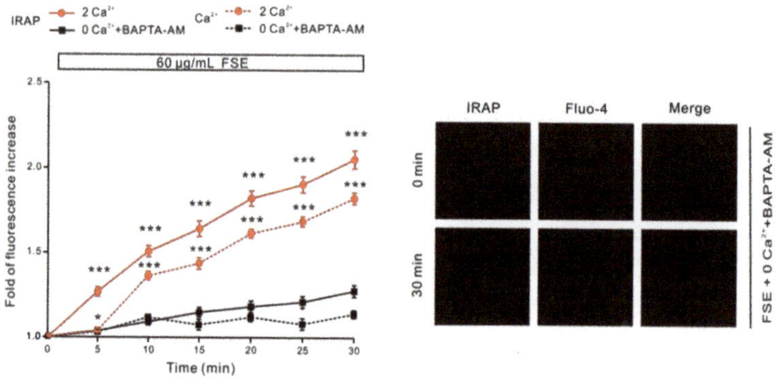

(B)

Figure 3. Role of intracellular Ca^{2+} on FSE-induced GLUT4 translocation. (**A**) After intracellular Ca^{2+} was loaded with Fluo-4 AM, cells were treated with 60 μg/mL FSE for 30 min under 0 mM extracellular Ca^{2+} conditions. * $p < 0.05$; ** $p < 0.01$; *** $p < 0.001$. (**B**) Cells were incubated for 30 min under the condition of 0 mM extracellular Ca^{2+} + 10 μM BAPTA-AM chelated intracellular Ca^{2+}, followed by stimulation with 60 μg/mL FSE for 30 min to quantify IRAP-mOrange fluorescence in the PM region and intracellular Ca^{2+} levels. Significance analysis: * $p < 0.05$; ** $p < 0.01$; *** $p < 0.001$.

2.4. FSE Enhances GLUT4 Translocation and Expression through the AMPK, PI3K/Akt, and PKC Pathways

Next, we attempted to shed light on some of the signaling pathways involved in GLUT4 translocation and expression. After treatment with AMPK inhibitor Compound C (10 μM, 30 min), PI3K inhibitor Wortmannin (100 nM, 30 min), or PKC inhibitor Gö6983 (10 μM, 30 min), the increase of IRAP fluorescence in the PM region induced by 60 μg/mL FSE was inhibited (Figure 4A), and the inhibition from compound C (Figure 4A, left) and Gö6983 (Figure 4A, right) was stronger than that from Wortmannin (Figure 4A, middle). This indicated that AMPK, PI3K/Akt, and PKC may be involved in FSE-mediated GLUT4 expression and translocation. Following this, we used western blot analysis to verify our conjecture. Compared with the control group, the expression levels of GLUT4 protein in L6 cells were increased by 1.87-fold (FSE), 1.33-fold (FSE+Compound C), 1.63-fold (FSE+Wortmannin), and 1.35-fold (FSE+Gö6983) after treatment with FSE and/or these different inhibitors (Figure 4B). Consistent with Figure 4, the three inhibitors also exhibited their inhibitory effects on FSE-mediated GLUT4 protein expression (vs. FSE). Western blotting of the signaling pathway-related proteins revealed that the phosphorylation levels of AMPK, Akt, and PKC in L6 cells after treatment with 60 μg/mL FSE were upregulated by 1.36-fold, 1.72-fold, and 1.92-fold, respectively. Also, FSE's effects were slightly lower than 1.54-fold of what was seen with 100 μg/mL metformin, 1.94-fold of what was seen with 100 nM insulin, and 2.74-fold of what was seen with 200 nM phorbol ester (PMA) in the positive control groups (Figure 4C–E). The above results showed that the increase in FSE-induced GLUT4 expression was dependent on AMPK, Akt, and PKC activities, and the FSE-promoted GLUT4 translocation also occurred through the AMPK, PI3K/Akt, and PKC pathways.

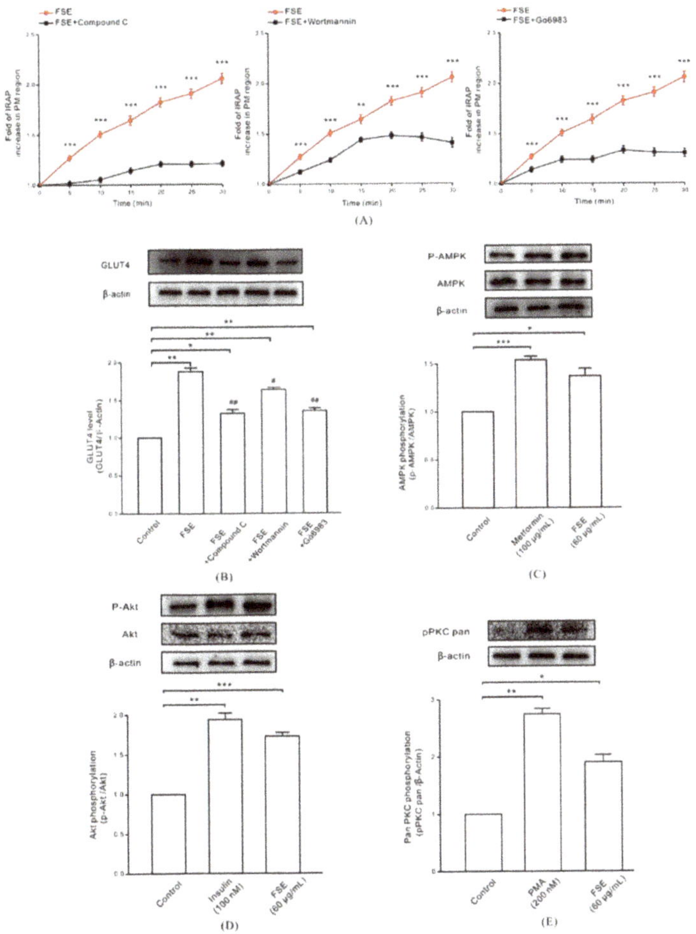

Figure 4. Effect of FSE on the AMPK, PI3K/Akt, and PKC signaling pathways and related proteins. (**A**) Cells were incubated with 10 μM compound C (AMPK inhibitor), 100 nM Wortmannin (PI3K inhibitor), or 10 μM Gö6983 (PKC inhibitor) for 30 min, and then treated with 60 μg/mL FSE. We calculated the fold of IRAP fluorescence increases in the PM region. * $p < 0.05$; ** $p < 0.01$; *** $p < 0.001$. (**B**) Cells were incubated with 10 μM compound C, 100 nM Wortmannin, or 10 μM Gö6983 inhibitor for 30 min and then were stimulated with 60 μg/mL FSE for 30 min. Whole cell lysates were subjected to western blot analysis for GLUT4 protein expression levels. * $p < 0.05$; ** $p < 0.01$, vs control group; # $p < 0.05$; ## $p < 0.01$, vs. FSE group. (**C**) L6 cells were treated with 100 μg/mL metformin (overnight) or 60 μg/mL FSE (30 min) and then analyzed for phosphorylated-AMPK, total AMPK, and β-actin protein level by western blot analysis. * $p < 0.05$; *** $p < 0.001$. (**D**) Cells were treated with 100 nM insulin or 60 μg/mL FSE for 30 min, followed by western blot analysis of phosphorylated Akt, total Akt, and β-actin. ** $p < 0.01$; *** $p < 0.001$. (**E**) Cells were treated with 200 nM PMA (4 h) or 60 μg/mL FSE (30 min), and western blot was used to analyze the phosphorylated protein level of PKC in L6 cells. Data were from three independent repeated experiments. * $p < 0.05$; ** $p < 0.01$.

2.5. G Protein and PLC Regulate FSE-Mediated Intracellular Ca^{2+} Increases and GLUT4 Translocation

G protein and PLC are upstream of the PKC pathway, and IP3R is one of the major receptors that trigger intracellular Ca^{2+} release. We investigated how G protein and PLC regulate FSE-induced Ca^{2+} increase and GLUT4 translocation. Cells treated with the Gβγ protein inhibitor 100 μM Gallein or Gα protein inhibitor 100 μM PTX for 6–8 h, or PLC inhibitor 2 μM U73122 for 30 min, significantly inhibited FSE-induced IRAP fluorescence intensity and intracellular Ca^{2+} elevation (Figure 5A–C). The results implied that FSE enhanced GLUT4 translocation via the G protein-PLC-PKC signaling pathway.

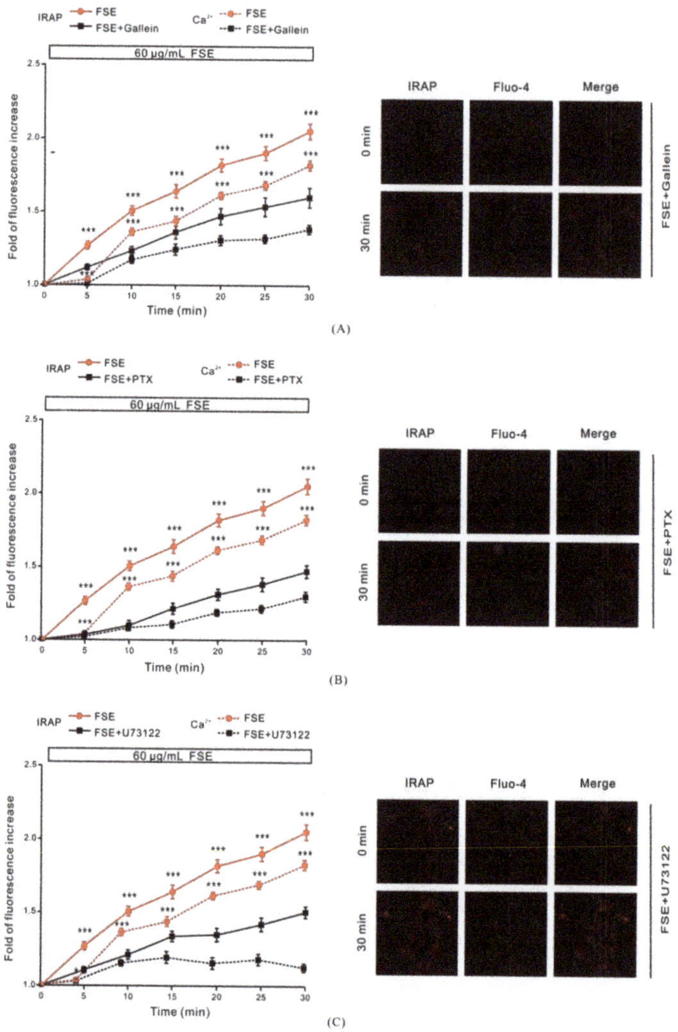

Figure 5. G protein-PLC signaling regulated FSE-mediated GLUT4 translocation and intracellular Ca^{2+} increase. (**A**) Cells were incubated for 6–8 h with 100 μM Gallein (Gβγ protein inhibitor) and then treated with 60 μg/mL FSE. * $p < 0.05$; *** $p < 0.001$. (**B**) Cells were incubated for 6–8 h with 100 μM PTX (Gα protein inhibitor), followed by the addition of 60 μg/mL FSE. *** $p < 0.001$. (**C**) Cells were treated with 2 μM U73122 (PLC inhibitor) for 30 min and were then stimulated by 60 μg/mL FSE. The IRAP-mOrange fluorescence in the PM region and the intracellular Ca^{2+} levels were quantified by Zeiss 2010 software. Significance analysis: * $p < 0.05$; *** $p < 0.001$.

2.6. IP3R Is Involved in FSE-Triggered Intracellular Ca^{2+} Release

The result shown in Figure 3 suggested the potential impact of intracellular Ca^{2+} release in the process of FSE-mediated GLUT4 translocation and the increase in intracellular Ca^{2+} levels. To support this hypothesis, we used 100 μM 2-APB to block IP3R-regulated intracellular Ca^{2+} release. We found that 2-APB had no effect on FSE-mediated GLUT4 translocation under 2 mM extracellular Ca^{2+}, but it evidently inhibited FSE-triggered Ca^{2+} release (Figure 6A). The ryanodine receptor (RyR), another channel that releases Ca^{2+} in the sarcoplasmic reticulum (SR)/endoplasmic reticulum (ER) [40], has attracted much attention due to its manipulation of intracellular Ca^{2+} output. Inhibition of RyR with 30 μM ryanodine had no effect on either GLUT4 translocation or intracellular Ca^{2+} increase mediated by FSE (Figure 6B). These findings indicated that IP3R, rather than RyR, was involved in the FSE-triggered increases of intracellular Ca^{2+}.

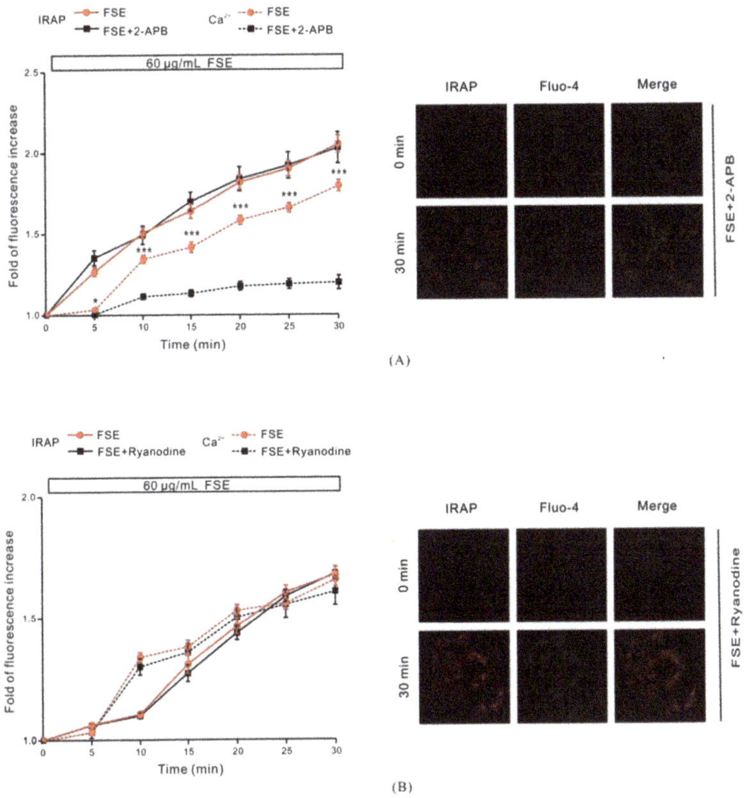

Figure 6. The IP3R receptor is involved in FSE-stimulated intracellular Ca^{2+} release. (**A**) Under extracellular 2 mM Ca^{2+}, cells were treated with 100 μM 2-APB (IP3RS blocker) for 30 min and then treated with 60 μg/mL FSE. (**B**) Under extracellular 2 mM Ca^{2+}, cells were incubated with 30 μM Ryanodine (RyR blocker) for 30 min, and the changes of IRAP-mOrange in the PM area and intracellular Ca^{2+} were measured after stimulation with 60 μg/mL FSE. Significance analysis: * $p < 0.05$; ** $p < 0.01$; *** $p < 0.001$.

2.7. Ca^{2+} Is Required for GLUT4 Insertion into the PM

Some studies have shown that Ca^{2+}-assisted binding of GLUT4 to the PM is involved in preparation for glucose uptake by cells [41,42]. In our study, myc-labeled GLUT4 was used to observe the fusion of GLUT4 vesicles with the PM in L6 cells stably expressing myc-GLUT4-mOrange. Fluorescence imaging revealed that FITC labeling for anti-myc antibody was not detected on the cell surface in the absence of drug stimulation. When we treated the cells for 30 min with 100 nM insulin and 60 μg/mL FSE, we observed significant increases of FITC fluorescence signals on the cell surfaces (Figure 7A). However, the FSE-induced FITC fluorescence signal on the cell surface was seriously suppressed under the condition of 0 mM extracellular Ca^{2+}/0 mM extracellular Ca^{2+} + 10 μM BAPTA-AM. On the other hand, the proportion of FITC-positive cells in the total number of mOrange cells showed (Figure 7B) that 0 mM Ca^{2+} + 10 μM BAPTA-AM had stronger inhibitory effects on FSE-mediated GLUT4 fusion with PM than the 0 mM Ca^{2+} group.

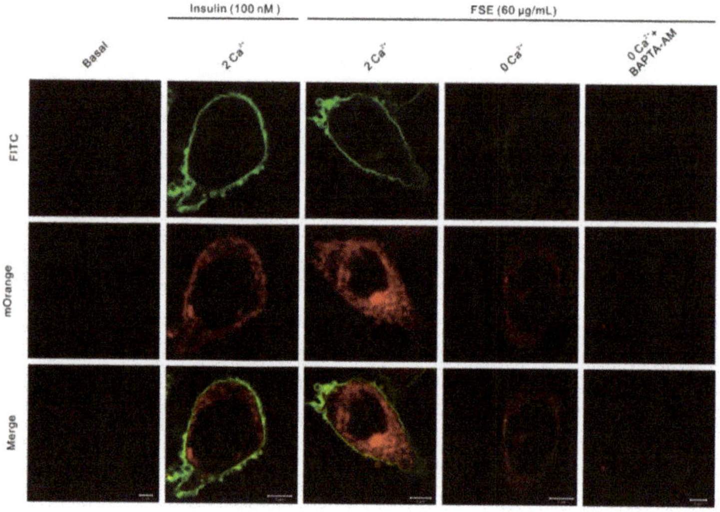

(A)

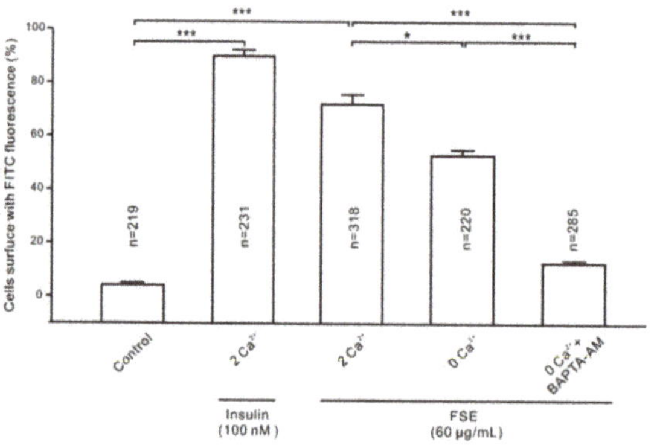

(B)

Figure 7. Involvement of Ca^{2+} in the fusion of GLUT4 and PM induced by FSE. (**A**) L6 cells transfected with plasmid GV348-myc-GLUT4-mOrange encoding an mOrange fusion protein with myc epitope-tagged GLUT4 (myc-GLUT4-FITC). Cells were stimulated with 100 nM insulin or 60 μg/mL FSE under 2 mM extracellular Ca^{2+}, 0 mM Ca^{2+}, and 0 mM Ca^{2+}+BAPTA-AM conditions. Then, cells were fixed and subjected to specific immunofluorescence antibody staining. The mOrange red fluorescence and FITC green fluorescence were detected by confocal microscopy at 555 nm and 488 nm excitation wavelengths, respectively. Scale bar = 5 μm. (**B**) The percentage of FITC-positive cells in the total mOrange cell population was counted. The results shown were from three independent replicate experiments. Significance analysis: * $p < 0.05$; ** $p < 0.01$; *** $p < 0.001$.

2.8. FSE-Induced Ca^{2+} Increases Improve Glucose Uptake in L6 Cells

To clarify the relationship between FSE-mediated glucose uptake and Ca^{2+}, a glucose uptake experiment was performed under various Ca^{2+} conditions. Results demonstrated that there was no significant difference in the glucose uptake between the groups in the absence of FSE or in the insulin-positive control group, whereas glucose uptake by cells was remarkably increased by 1.58-fold after the addition of FSE for 1 h in the culture medium with 2 mM extracellular Ca^{2+}. Similarly, insulin treatment showed a 1.68-fold increase in glucose uptake. To a certain extent, 0 mM extracellular Ca^{2+} inhibited the effect of FSE by 1.3-fold or the effect of insulin by 1.28-fold. Meanwhile, insulin or FSE-mediated glucose uptake was completely blocked under 0 mM Ca^{2+}+BAPTA-AM, which indicated that Ca^{2+} plays a crucial role in the FSE-induced glucose uptake process (Figure 8).

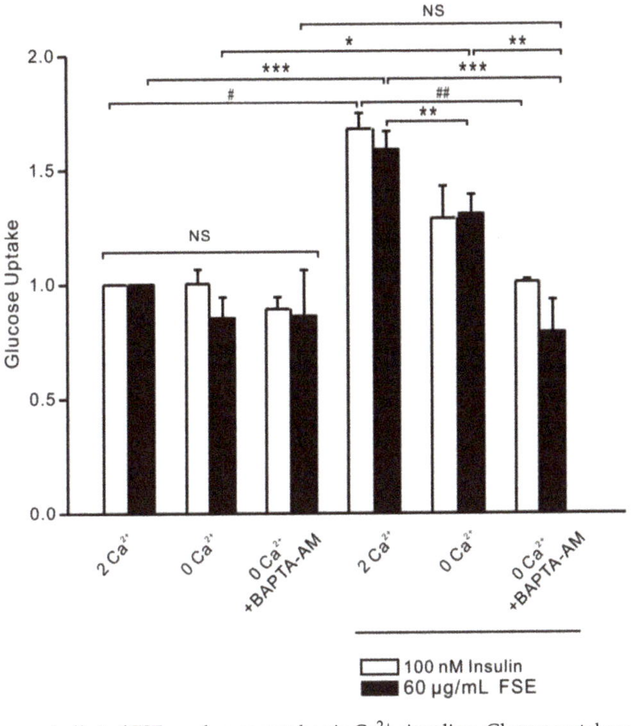

Figure 8. Increased effect of FSE on glucose uptake via Ca^{2+} signaling. Glucose uptake was measured using a glucose assay kit. L6 cells were serum-deprived for 2 h and incubated in 2 mM extracellular Ca^{2+}, 0 mM extracellular Ca^{2+}, or 0 mM extracellular Ca^{2+} + 10 μM BAPTA-AM chelated intracellular Ca^{2+} conditions. Cells were stimulated with vehicle, 60 μg/mL FSE, or 100 nM insulin for 1 h, and then the glucose uptake was measured. The experimental data are from six independent repeated experiments. Significant analysis: FSE group, * $p < 0.05$; ** $p < 0.01$; *** $p < 0.001$. Insulin group, # $p < 0.05$; ## $p < 0.01$.

3. Discussion

Diabetes has long been a global health problem. In particular, the high proportion of T2DM characterized by insulin resistance in DM has become the focus of DM research [43]. Skeletal muscle is the primary tissue for insulin-stimulated glucose uptake in the body. It consumes glucose and is responsible for approximately 80% of the postprandial glucose intake and consumption, and is therefore recognized as an important therapeutic target tissue for insulin resistance [11,44]. GLUT4 plays a crucial role in maintaining systemic glucose homeostasis. It is mostly intracellular in the unstimulated state but is acutely redistributed to the PM in response to insulin, contraction, and other stimuli [9]. The amount of glucose uptake is determined by the number of GLUT4 molecules on the muscle cell membranes [36,45]. Relevant studies reported that GLUT4 translocation and fusion with PM were the main rate-limiting steps for glucose disposal [46,47]. The existing synthetic antidiabetic drugs often exhibit side effects or resistance that pose a huge challenge to managing diabetes [43]. It is, therefore, necessary to find better medicines from herbs or natural products. Consequently, we extracted the effective products from the natural medicinal plant Folium Sennae. We investigated the potential activity of FSE on glucose uptake in L6 rat skeletal muscle cells in regard to GLUT4 expression, translocation, and fusion with PM and the participation of Ca^{2+} in this process.

It has been reported that an ethanolic extract of the leaves of *Senna surattensis* increased glucose uptake in an isolated rat hemidiaphragm model [34]. However, little is known about how FSE exerts its hypoglycemic mechanism in vivo. In this study, we first investigated the effect of FSE on the glucose uptake of L6 cells. Consistent with the reported results, FSE significantly increased glucose uptake in L6 cells. We also discovered that FSE upregulated GLUT4 mRNA and protein expression in GLUT4 molecular assays. The results suggested that there was some connection between FSE-induced glucose uptake and intracellular GLUT4 and IRAP motion (Figure 1).

Next, in order to observe the translocation of GLUT4 caused by FSE, we studied L6-IRAP-mOrange cells under confocal microscopy. Due to the high colocalization of intracellular IRAP and GLUT4 [48], IRAP was used as a reporter molecule to track and quantify dynamic information about GLUT4 in real time. Our results showed that FSE promoted the increase in IRAP expression in cytosol. By collecting red fluorescence in the periphery of the cells, we found marked increases in IRAP in the PM region, which indicated that FSE promoted GLUT4 translocation (Figure 2A,B). In this way, FSE-mediated increases in GLUT4 transcription and translation are able to provide more GLUT4 traffic to the PM, triggering glucose uptake in L6 cells. Previous studies have shown that increasing intracellular cytosolic Ca^{2+} concentration increases cell surface GLUT4 levels [19]. We observed that upon intracellular Ca^{2+} loading, the fluorescent indicator also increased almost synchronously with GLUT4. This phenomenon implied that FSE-enhanced GLUT4 translocation may mobilize intracellular Ca^{2+}.

We then sought to search for the signal transduction pathways by which FSE stimulates GLUT4 expression and translocation. There are various signaling pathways which are involved in GLUT4 translocation and/or expression, such as the AMPK pathway, the PI3K/Akt pathway, and the PKC pathway. AMPK, a key signaling molecule stimulated by muscle contraction, activates to cause GLUT4 translocation [45]. GLUT4 is a member of the glycolytic enzyme genes. Its expression was activated under the effect of the AMPK agonist AICAR [49]. PI3K can catalyze the phosphorylation of phosphatidylinositol 4,5-diphosphate (PIP2) to PIP3, activating the downstream signaling factor Akt by phosphorylation, thereby promoting GLUT4 translocation to the PM to absorb glucose into the muscle [44,50]. The PKCα inhibitor dioleoyl phosphoethanolamine retained cell surface GLUT4 by inhibiting PKCα-driven internalization in adipocytes. PKC β and λ were involved in the insulin signaling cascade causing PKC-meditated GLUT4 traffic in skeletal muscle cells [19,51]. When we studied which of the three signaling pathways was/were involved in FSE-mediated glucose uptake, we found that both Compound C and Gö6983 remarkably inhibited the promotion by FSE of GLUT4 translocation and expression, but the inhibition effect of Wortmannin was relatively weak (Figure 4A,B). This suggested that the PI3K/Akt pathway was not dominant in the process of FSE-mediated GLUT4 translocation. Furthermore, the observation that FSE increased the phosphorylation of AMPK, Akt, and PKC proteins in L6 cells further conjectured that FSE-induced glucose uptake was associated with the AMPK, Akt, and PKC signaling pathways (Figure 4C–E).

To study the relationship between FSE-mediated GLUT4 translocation and Ca^{2+}, we partially removed Ca^{2+} and found that 0 mM extracellular Ca^{2+} partially inhibited FSE-induced Ca^{2+} elevation but did not affect GLUT4 translocation (Figure 3A). While the intracellular and extracellular Ca^{2+} were all chelated, the FSE-induced Ca^{2+} increase was almost completely blocked and the GLUT4 translocation was also severely inhibited (Figure 3B), and it was certified that cytosolic Ca^{2+}

participated in FSE-induced GLUT4 translocation. In order to examine the source of cytosolic Ca^{2+}, internal Ca^{2+} release was also studied, in addition to external Ca^{2+} influx. IP3R and RyR are two important barriers to the release of Ca^{2+} from intracellular Ca^{2+} stores, controlling the output of internal Ca^{2+} [18]. Similar to 0 mM Ca^{2+}, FSE-mediated Ca^{2+} increase was obviously inhibited after 2-APB blocking IP3R. Nevertheless, GLUT4 translocation was not altered (Figure 6A). However, the inhibition of RyR did not have any impact on FSE-triggered Ca^{2+} elevation or GLUT4 translocation. These results showed that FSE-induced Ca^{2+} elevation may be related to IP3R (Figure 6B). To explain why simply blocking the external or internal Ca^{2+} source to reduce cytosolic Ca^{2+} concentration does not inhibit GLUT4 translocation of FSE, we propose that the lower Ca^{2+} concentration can cause the GLUT4 translocation process via FSE while Ca^{2+} can be obtained from another source, even if one of the sources was blocked.

G protein and PLC are upstream of the PKC signaling pathway and IP3R [52]. This provides a potential breakthrough point for simultaneously refining the pathway of FSE-regulated intracellular Ca^{2+} release and GLUT4 translocation. We found that G protein and PLC inhibitors disrupted the FSE-induced Ca^{2+} increase and displayed varying degrees of suppression efficacy. This was demonstrated by the observation that FSE induced intracellular Ca^{2+} release through the G protein-PLC-IP3-IP3R pathway. Regarding the partial inhibition of G protein and PLC inhibitors of GLUT4 translocation, we concluded that FSE-regulated GLUT4 translocation not only depends on one pathway, but may involve two or more signaling pathways (Figure 5A–C).

In addition, our studies testified that FSE increases Ca^{2+} to enhance GLUT4 insertion into the PM and increases glucose uptake. GLUT4 fusion is the last step in glucose uptake and several studies have reported a key role for Ca^{2+}/calmodulin in the late stages of GLUT4 vesicle docking/fusion [53,54]. As shown in Figures 7 and 8, both FSE-mediated GLUT4-PM fusion and glucose uptake were somewhat attenuated under conditions of abolishment of extracellular Ca^{2+}. When free Ca^{2+} ions were fully chelated by EGTA and BAPTA-AM, FSE-induced membrane fusion and especially glucose uptake were also seriously diminished. It can be seen that FSE-mediated membrane fusion and glucose uptake require Ca^{2+}, which makes Ca^{2+} indispensable in these steps.

Throughout the course of this research, the signaling pathways induced by FSE-mediated glucose uptake were found to be quite diverse. This diversity may be attributed to the differences in the active ingredients of FSE. Based on the components of FSE as described above, many interesting results have been found. For example, through inhibiting mitochondrial complex I activity, emodin increases cellular ROS and Ca^{2+} influx to activate AMPK, causing GLUT4 translocation and glucose uptake [55]. Emodin significantly improved the blood glucose of diabetic rats by activating the PI3K/Akt/GSK-3β signaling pathway [56]. Isolated chrysophanol from rhubarb rhizome increased tyrosine phosphorylation of the insulin receptor (IR) and accelerated GLUT4 mRNA expression [57]. Aloe-emodin glycosides stimulated glucose transport and glycogen storage through PI3K-dependent mechanisms in L6 myotubes [58]. Long-term dietary supplementation of kaempferol promoted the expression of AMPK and GLUT4 in skeletal muscles, thereby preventing hyperglycemia in middle-aged obese mice [59]. These statements implied that the FSE-regulated glucose pathway is a complex and vast network. Our study shows for the first time that FSE regulates glucose metabolism through the PKC pathway, but it is not clear which active ingredient plays a role in it and is worth further exploration. Besides, this research on FSE is limited to the cellular level; hence the hypoglycemic effect at the animal level remains to be explored.

In conclusion, FSE promoted GLUT4 expression and translocation through the AMPK, Akt, and G protein-PLC-PKC pathways. FSE increased Ca^{2+} concentration by external Ca^{2+} influx and internal Ca^{2+} release of G protein-PLC-IP3-IP3R signals to assist GLUT4 traffic and PM fusion, ultimately leading to glucose uptake (Figure 9). Therefore, FSE is expected to become an effective drug for the treatment of insulin resistance.

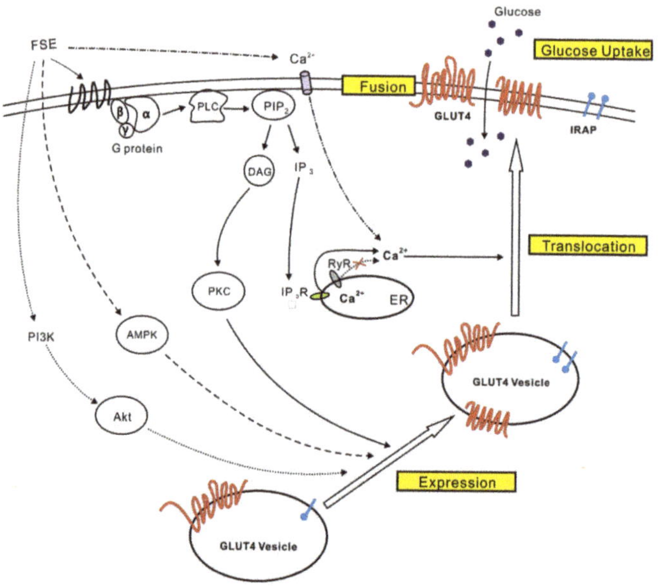

Figure 9. Proposed mechanism of FSE for the enhancement of glucose uptake in L6 cells. FSE promotes GLUT4 expression and translocation via the activation the AMPK, IP3K/Akt, and G protein-PLC-PKC pathways. Moreover, the increase in cytosolic Ca^{2+} induced by the G-protein-PLC-IP3-IP3R-Ca^{2+} pathway or/and by extracellular Ca^{2+} influx assists GLUT4 trafficking and fusion to PM, ultimately triggering glucose uptake.

4. Materials and methods

4.1. Reagents and Solutions

Alpha-MEM (α-MEM) and penicillin streptomycin solution were purchased from Gibco (Gran Island, NY, USA). Fetal bovine serum (FBS) was purchased from Hyclone (Logan, UT, USA). The glucose assay kit was purchased from Cayman Chemical Company (Ann Arbor, MI, USA). Fluo-4 AM was obtained from Invitrogen (Camarillo, CA, USA). Compound C was purchased from Selleckchem (Houston, TX, USA). Wortmannin, BAPTA-AM, U73122, Ryanodine, and 2-APB were purchased from Sigma (St. Louis, MO, USA). Gallein and PTX were purchased from Tocris Bioscience (Bristol, UK). Gö6983 was from EMD Millipore (Billerica, MA, USA). GLUT4 antibody, β-actin antibody, phospho-AMPKα (Thr172) antibody, AMPK antibody, phospho-Akt (Ser473) antibody, Anti-Akt antibody, and phospho-PKC pan (Thr410) antibody were from Cell Signaling Technology (Beverly, MA, USA). HRP goat anti-mouse and goat anti-rabbit IgG antibody were from CWBIO (Beijing, China), anti-c-myc mouse monoclonal antibody and FITC antibody were purchased from TransGen Biotech (Beijing, China), Phorbol 12-myristate 13-acetate (PMA) was purchased from Ascent Scientific (Cambridge, MA), metformin and insulin were obtained from Yuanye biological (shanghai, China). 2 mM Ca^{2+} (pss): 135 NaCl, 5 KCl, 1 $MgCl_2$, 2 $CaCl_2$, 10 HEPES, and 10 glucose (pH 7.4). 0 mM Ca^{2+}-EGTA: 135 NaCl, 5 KCl, 1 $MgCl_2$, 0.5 EGTA, 10 HEPES, and 10 glucose (pH 7.4). PBS buffer: 137 NaCl, 2.7 KCl, 10 Na_2HPO_4, 2 KH_2PO_4, and the volume is adjusted to 1 L with ultrapure water (PH 7.4).

4.2. Plant Collection and Preparation

Dried plant material was ground into a fine powder using a commercial electric blender and stored in air-tight containers. Fifty grams of leaf material was soaked in 500 mL of 70% industrial ethanol for 30 h, and then refluxed in a 60 °C water bath. The extraction procedure was repeated three times in order to extract as much of the components as possible. The extract was filtered using Whatman no. 1 filter paper and dried under a stream of cold air. The ethanolic extract of Folium Sennae (FSE) was dissolved in 3% dimethylsulfoxide (DMSO) for biological detection.

4.3. L6 Cell Culture and Treatment

L6 myoblasts were grown in α-MEM containing 10% (*v*/*v*) FBS, 100 units/mL penicillin, and 100 μg/mL streptomycin in 5% CO_2 at 37 °C. L6 cells were harvested after about 80% confluent and used in all experiments. Prior to any treatment, the cells were serum-deprived for 2 h. After treatment, the cells were divided into different drug treatment groups.

4.4. Amount of Glucose Uptake into Cells

The glucose uptake stimulatory effect of FSE was determined in L6 cells by a previously reported method [60] with slight modifications [61,62]. Briefly, L6 cells were grown in 96-well culture plates at 37 °C under 5% CO_2 and cultured for 3–4 days until the cells were confluent. Next, cells were starved for 2 h with 100 μL serum-free α-MEM medium and then treated with 60 μg/mL FSE or 100 nM insulin or vehicle control dissolved in 100 μL serum-free α-MEM medium for 1 h. Insulin was used as positive control. The concentration of glucose remaining in the media was determined according to the glucose assay kit manufacturer's instructions using an Infinite M200 Pro microplate reader (Tecan, Croedig, Austria) with a 505 nm wavelength. Meanwhile, cell numbers from each group were analyzed using tetrazolium salt (3-(4,5-dimethylthiazol-2-yl)-2,5-diphenyltetrazolium) bromide (MTT). For analysis, 20 μL of MTT substrate was added to each well and the plates were incubated for an additional 4 h at 37 °C with 5% CO_2. The medium was removed, and the cells were solubilized in 150 μL DMSO. The colorimetric analysis was performed at a wavelength of 492 nm. The amount of glucose uptake in each group was calculated by using the amount of glucose uptake for the corresponding cell counts. Three independent experiments were conducted, comparing the control group (control), the insulin group (insulin), and the added drug group (FSE).

4.5. Western Blotting Analyses

L6 cells were serum-deprived for 2 h, then treated with FSE (60 μg/mL for 30 min), insulin (100 nM for 30 min), PMA (200 nM for 4 h) or metformin (100 μg/mL overnight), Wortmannin (100 nM for 30 min), Gö6983 (10 μM for 30 min), Compound C (10 μM for 30 min). Next, the cells were placed on ice, washed three times with cold PBS, and treated with a protease inhibitor cocktail (Roche, Basel, Switzerland) and phosphatase inhibitor cocktail (Selleckchem, Houston, TX, USA) at 4 °C. Cells were then lysed as described previously [60]. After cell debris was removed, supernatants containing proteins were collected. Equal amounts of protein were separated by 10% (*v*/*v*) SDS-PAGE and transferred to polyvinylidene difluoride (PVDF) membranes. Blots were incubated with 5% BSA blocking solution at 4 °C, overnight with a primary antibody (1:1000), and then incubated with corresponding horseradish peroxidase-conjugated secondary antibody (1:10,000) for 1 h at room temperature. The intensity of protein bands was quantitated using a ChemiDoc XRS system (Bio-Rad, Hercules, CA, USA).

4.6. RT-PCR

The L6 cells were subjected to the same western blotting operation described above and divided into control, insulin, and FSE groups. Total RNA was extracted using TRIzol reagent (Invitrogen) including chloroform extraction and isopropanol precipitation. The RNA initial extract of each sample was washed and dried with 75% ethanol and then dissolved in 50 μL DEPC water. The quality of each RNA extraction was confirmed by electrophoresis on a 1% agarose gel. Next, 2 μg of total RNA from each sample was reverse-transcribed using the RevertAid First Strand cDNA Synthesis Kit (Thermo Scientific, Wilmington, DE, USA) in a 20 μL reaction according to the manufacturer's protocol. The PCR conditions were set as follows: initial activation of Taq polymerase at 95 °C for 10 min, 35 cycles of PCR amplification at 95 °C for 15 s, and annealing/elongation at 60 °C for 1 min. cDNA products were diluted with RNAse-free water, and then real-time PCR was performed using the FastStart Universal SYBR Green PCR Master ROX (Roche) system on the 7500 Fast Real-Time PCR System instrument (Applied Biosystems, Foster City, CA, USA). Primer sequences were as follows: rat GAPDH (NCBI RefSeq NM_017008.4), F: 5′-TACAGCAACAGGGTGGTGGAC-3′, R: 5′-GGGATGGAATTGTGAGGGAGA-3′; rat GLUT4 (NCBI RefSeq NM_012751.1), F: 5′-CTTCCTTCTATTTGCCGTCCTC-3′, R: 5′-GCTGCTGTTTCCTTCATCCTG-3′; rat IRAP (NCBI Refseq NM_001113403.2), F: 5′-GTGGGGACTAAGGGCGAAAA- 3′ R:5′-CATACATCCGGACCTCCACG-3′. Relative quantification results obtained for the target genes were normalized using the $2^{-\Delta\Delta CT}$ method.

4.7. Fluorescence Microscopy for Detection of IRAP Translocation and Ca^{2+}

L6 cells were transfected with pIRAP-mOrange cDNAs (presented by Professor Xu Tao, Chinese Academy of Sciences) using Lipofectamine 2000 as per the manufacturer's protocol [2]. Stably expressing IRAP-mOrange of L6 cells (L6 IRAP-mOrange) were seeded into a glass slide and incubated overnight until differentiated and confluent over the slides. Cells were starved in serum-free α-MEM for 2 h. For loading the dye, cells were incubated in 2 μM fluo4-AM (Invitrogen, Carlsbad, CA, USA) for 20 min at 37 °C, followed by a wash with PSS, and then treated with 60 μg/mL FSE or other related signaling pathway protein inhibitors. Red fluorescence (555 nm) and green fluorescence (488 nm) images of cells were simultaneously taken with the LSM700 laser scanning confocal microscope (Carl Zeiss, Jena, Germany). The IRAP-mOrange translocation and intracellular Ca^{2+} levels were monitored as spatial and temporal changes in the fluorescence intensity of the indicator mOrange and dye Fluo4, respectively. In the absence of stimulation, GLUT4 and IRAP are present in intracellular GLUT storage vesicles (GSVs). Many studies have reported that GLUT4 and IRAP displayed a high co-localization relationship [63], thus, detecting the IRAP can indirectly reflect the localization of GLUT4. The images were captured with 555 nm or 488 nm excitation laser every 10 s in the first 5 min and then every 5 min over 25 min.

4.8. Immunofluorescence of GLUT4 Fusion with PM

L6 cells were transfected by lentivirus with GV348 plasmid DNA encoding myc, GLUT4, and mOrange constructs of the myc-GLUT4-mOrange fusion protein. GLUT4myc cDNA was constructed by inserting the human c-myc epitope (14 amino acids) into the first ectodomain of GLUT4, as described [64]. Live cell imaging was performed to measure membrane fusion and GLUT4 trafficking with myc and mOrange as molecular probes, respectively [42]. A single clone containing the highest fluorescence intensity was selected and used for the following experiments. The GV348-myc-GLUT4-mOrange of L6 cells were seeded onto the glass slide, incubated until they reached 80% confluence, and then serum-deprived for 2 h. In addition to the control group and the 100 nM insulin-positive control group of 2 mM Ca^{2+}, the cells were treated with 60 μg/mL FSE under the conditions of 2 mM Ca^{2+}, 0 mM Ca^{2+}, and 0 mM Ca^{2+}+BAPTA-AM, respectively. After 30 min of stimulation, the cells were fixed with 4% paraformaldehyde. Then, 50 mM glycine was used to remove impurities which would cause background signals. Then samples were blocked with PBS containing with 2% FBS for 1 h. Afterward, cells were labeled with anti-c-myc mouse monoclonal antibody (1:200) and goat anti-mouse IgG (H+L) FITC-conjugated secondary antibody (1:200). Cell images of green fluorescent protein (FITC) and mOrange fluorescence were measured by the LSM700 microscope (Carl Zeiss).

4.9. Statistical Analysis

Data are presented as the mean ± SEM of at least three independent experiments. All statistical analyses were performed using OriginPro 8 (OriginLab, Northampton, MA, USA). Multigroup comparisons were conducted by one-way analysis of variance and differences between two group means were compared by Student's *t*-test. p values < 0.05 were considered to represent statistical significance. The n values represent the number of cells.

5. Conclusions

The present study showed that FSE promoted GLUT4 expression and translocation in L6 cells via the AMPK, PI3K/Akt, and G protein-PLC-PKC signaling pathways. It also increased Ca^{2+} concentration in the form of external Ca^{2+} influx and Ca^{2+} pool release, assisting GLUT4-PM fusion to enhance glucose uptake. These results suggested the possibility of FSE being used as a novel hypoglycemic agent for the treatment of T2DM.

Supplementary Materials: Supplementary materials are available online. Figure S1: MTT test with different treatment groups. Figure S2: Comparative images with insulin treatment.

Author Contributions: P.Z. and Q.M. contributed equally to this study. P.Z. contributed to study design and guidance. Q.M. conducted the experiments and wrote the manuscript. J.Q. provided the raw materials for FSE. D.T. and J.L. participated in data interpretation. J.S., Q.-H.L., P.Z., and X.Y. supervised this study and edited the manuscript.

Funding: The present study was financially supported by the National Natural Science Foundation of China (grant nos. 31070744, 81573561, and 81774000), Fundamental Research Funds for the Central Universities, South-Central University for Nationalities (CZR18003, CZP17060, and CZP17048), and Wuhan Applied Basic Research Program of Science and Technology (2017060201010217).

Acknowledgments: Authors are thankful to Tao Xu for providing the IRAP-mOrange L6 cell lines. We are also deeply grateful to Pingsheng Liu for providing L6 cells.

Conflicts of Interest: The authors declare no conflict of interest.

References

1. Kang, O.H.; Shon, M.Y.; Kong, R.; Seo, Y.S.; Zhou, T.; Kim, D.Y.; Kim, Y.S.; Kwon, D.Y. Anti-diabetic effect of black ginseng extract by augmentation of AMPK protein activity and upregulation of GLUT2 and GLUT4 expression in db/db mice. *BMC Complement. Altern. Med.* **2017**, *17*, 341. [CrossRef] [PubMed]
2. Yang, J.; Zhao, P.; Wan, D.; Zhou, Q.; Wang, C.; Shu, G.; Mei, Z.; Yang, X. Antidiabetic Effect of Methanolic Extract from Berberis julianae Schneid. via Activation of AMP-Activated Protein Kinase in Type 2 Diabetic Mice. *Evid. Based Complement. Altern. Med.* **2014**, *2014*, 106206. [CrossRef] [PubMed]
3. Zhang, M.; Li, X.; Liang, H.; Cai, H.; Hu, X.; Bian, Y.; Dong, L.; Ding, L.; Wang, L.; Yu, B.; et al. Semen Cassiae Extract Improves Glucose Metabolism by Promoting GlUT4 Translocation in the Skeletal Muscle of Diabetic Rats. *Front. Pharmacol.* **2018**, *9*, 235. [CrossRef] [PubMed]
4. Huang, Y.; Hao, J.; Tian, D.; Wen, Y.; Zhao, P.; Chen, H.; Lv, Y.; Yang, X. Antidiabetic Activity of a Flavonoid-Rich Extract From Sophora davidii (Franch.) Skeels in KK-Ay Mice via Activation of AMP-Activated Protein Kinase. *Front. Pharmacol.* **2018**, *9*, 760. [CrossRef] [PubMed]
5. Cai, Y.; Wang, Y.; Zhi, F.; Xing, Q.C.; Chen, Y.Z. The Effect of Sanggua Drink Extract on Insulin Resistance through the PI3K/AKT Signaling Pathway. *Evid. Based Complement. Altern. Med.* **2018**, *2018*, 9407945.
6. Kamakura, R.; Son, M.J.; de Beer, D.; Joubert, E.; Miura, Y.; Yagasaki, K. Antidiabetic effect of green rooibos (Aspalathus linearis) extract in cultured cells and type 2 diabetic model KK-A(y) mice. *Cytotechnology* **2015**, *67*, 699–710. [CrossRef] [PubMed]
7. Choi, J.; Kim, K.J.; Koh, E.J.; Lee, B.Y. Gelidium elegans Extract Ameliorates Type 2 Diabetes via Regulation of MAPK and PI3K/Akt Signaling. *Nutrients* **2018**, *10*, 51. [CrossRef] [PubMed]
8. Kadan, S.; Sasson, Y.; Saad, B.; Zaid, H. Gundelia tournefortii Antidiabetic Efficacy: Chemical Composition and GLUT4 Translocation. *Evid. Based Complement. Altern. Med.* **2018**, *2018*, 8294320. [CrossRef] [PubMed]
9. Chanda, D.; Luiken, J.J.; Glatz, J.F. Signaling pathways involved in cardiac energy metabolism. *FEBS Lett.* **2016**, *590*, 2364–2374. [CrossRef] [PubMed]
10. Zaid, H.; Antonescu, C.N.; Randhawa, V.K.; Klip, A. Insulin action on glucose transporters through molecular switches, tracks and tethers. *Biochem. J.* **2008**, *413*, 201–215. [CrossRef] [PubMed]
11. Vlavcheski, F.; Baron, D.; Vlachogiannis, I.A.; MacPherson, R.E.K.; Tsiani, E. Carnosol Increases Skeletal Muscle Cell Glucose Uptake via AMPK-Dependent GLUT4 Glucose Transporter Translocation. *Int. J. Mol. Sci.* **2018**, *19*, 1321. [CrossRef] [PubMed]

12. Wright, D.C. Mechanisms of calcium-induced mitochondrial biogenesis and GLUT4 synthesis. *Appl. Physiol. Nutr. Metab.* **2007**, *32*, 840–845. [CrossRef] [PubMed]
13. Li, Q.; Zhu, X.; Ishikura, S.; Zhang, D.; Gao, J.; Sun, Y.; Contreras-Ferrat, A.; Foley, K.P.; Lavandero, S.; Yao, Z.; et al. Ca^{2+} signals promote GLUT4 exocytosis and reduce its endocytosis in muscle cells. *Am. J. Physiol. Endocrinol. Metab.* **2014**, *307*, E209–E224. [CrossRef] [PubMed]
14. Lanner, J.T.; Katz, A.; Tavi, P.; Sandstrom, M.E.; Zhang, S.J.; Wretman, C.; James, S.; Fauconnier, J.; Lannergren, J.; Bruton, J.D.; et al. The role of Ca^{2+} influx for insulin-mediated glucose uptake in skeletal muscle. *Diabetes* **2006**, *55*, 2077–2083. [CrossRef] [PubMed]
15. Contreras-Ferrat, A.E.; Toro, B.; Bravo, R.; Parra, V.; Vasquez, C.; Ibarra, C.; Mears, D.; Chiong, M.; Jaimovich, E.; Klip, A.; et al. An inositol 1,4,5-triphosphate (IP3)-IP3 receptor pathway is required for insulin-stimulated glucose transporter 4 translocation and glucose uptake in cardiomyocytes. *Endocrinology* **2010**, *151*, 4665–4677. [CrossRef] [PubMed]
16. Wijesekara, N.; Tung, A.; Thong, F.; Klip, A. Muscle cell depolarization induces a gain in surface GLUT4 via reduced endocytosis independently of AMPK. *Am. J. Physiol. Endocrinol. Metab.* **2006**, *290*, E1276–E1286. [CrossRef] [PubMed]
17. Waller, A.P.; Kalyanasundaram, A.; Hayes, S.; Periasamy, M.; Lacombe, V.A. Sarcoplasmic reticulum Ca^{2+} ATPase pump is a major regulator of glucose transport in the healthy and diabetic heart. *Biochim. Biophys. Acta* **2015**, *1852*, 873–881. [CrossRef] [PubMed]
18. Contreras-Ferrat, A.; Llanos, P.; Vasquez, C.; Espinosa, A.; Osorio-Fuentealba, C.; Arias-Calderon, M.; Lavandero, S.; Klip, A.; Hidalgo, C.; Jaimovich, E. Insulin elicits a ROS-activated and an IP(3)-dependent Ca(2)(+) release, which both impinge on GLUT4 translocation. *J. Cell Sci.* **2014**, *127*, 1911–1923. [CrossRef] [PubMed]
19. Deng, B.; Zhu, X.; Zhao, Y.; Zhang, D.; Pannu, A.; Chen, L.; Niu, W. PKC and Rab13 mediate Ca^{2+} signal-regulated GLUT4 traffic. *Biochem. Biophys. Res. Commun.* **2018**, *495*, 1956–1963. [CrossRef] [PubMed]
20. Singh, S.; Loke, Y.K.; Furberg, C.D. Long-term risk of cardiovascular events with rosiglitazone: A meta-analysis. *JAMA* **2007**, *298*, 1189–1195. [CrossRef] [PubMed]
21. Schuster, D.P.; Duvuuri, V. Diabetes mellitus. *Clin. Podiatr. Med. Surg.* **2002**, *19*, 79–107. [CrossRef]
22. Li, W.L.; Zheng, H.C.; Bukuru, J.; De Kimpe, N. Natural medicines used in the traditional Chinese medical system for therapy of diabetes mellitus. *J. Ethnopharmacol.* **2004**, *92*, 1–21. [CrossRef] [PubMed]
23. Chen, J.; Mangelinckx, S.; Adams, A.; Wang, Z.T.; Li, W.L.; De Kimpe, N. Natural flavonoids as potential herbal medication for the treatment of diabetes mellitus and its complications. *Nat. Prod. Commun.* **2015**, *10*, 187–200. [PubMed]
24. Zaid, H.; Mahdi, A.A.; Tamrakar, A.K. Natural Active Ingredients for Diabetes and Metabolism Disorders Treatment. *Evid. Based Complement. Altern. Med.* **2016**, *2016*, 2965214. [CrossRef] [PubMed]
25. Testa, R.; Bonfigli, A.R.; Genovese, S.; De Nigris, V.; Ceriello, A. The Possible Role of Flavonoids in the Prevention of Diabetic Complications. *Nutrients* **2016**, *8*, 310. [CrossRef] [PubMed]
26. Kundu, S.; Roy, S.; Nandi, S.; Ukil, B.; Lyndem, L.M. Senna alexandrina Mill. induced ultrastructural changes on Hymenolepis diminuta. *J. Parasit. Dis.* **2017**, *41*, 147–154. [CrossRef] [PubMed]
27. Rama Reddy, N.R.; Mehta, R.H.; Soni, P.H.; Makasana, J.; Gajbhiye, N.A.; Ponnuchamy, M.; Kumar, J. Next Generation Sequencing and Transcriptome Analysis Predicts Biosynthetic Pathway of Sennosides from Senna (*Cassia angustifolia* Vahl.), a Non-Model Plant with Potent Laxative Properties. *PLoS ONE* **2015**, *10*, e0129422. [CrossRef] [PubMed]
28. Muanda, F.N.; Bouayed, J.; Djilani, A.; Yao, C.; Soulimani, R.; Dicko, A. Chemical Composition and, Cellular Evaluation of the Antioxidant Activity of Desmodium adscendens Leaves. *Evid. Based Complement. Altern. Med.* **2011**, *2011*, 620862. [CrossRef] [PubMed]
29. Elansary, H.O.; Szopa, A.; Kubica, P.; Ekiert, H.; Ali, H.M. Bioactivities of Traditional Medicinal Plants in Alexandria. *Evid. Based Complement. Altern. Med.* **2018**, *2018*, 1463579. [CrossRef] [PubMed]
30. Susunaga-Notario Adel, C.; Perez-Gutierrez, S.; Zavala-Sanchez, M.A.; Almanza-Perez, J.C.; Gutierrez-Carrillo, A.; Arrieta-Baez, D.; Lopez-Lopez, A.L.; Roman-Ramos, R.; Flores-Saenz, J.L.; Alarcon-Aguilar, F.J. Bioassay-guided chemical study of the anti-inflammatory effect of Senna villosa (Miller) H.S. Irwin & Barneby (Leguminosae) in TPA-induced ear edema. *Molecules* **2014**, *19*, 10261–10278. [PubMed]

31. Pereira, R.M.; Ferreira-Silva, G.A.; Pivatto, M.; Santos Lde, A.; Bolzani Vda, S.; Chagas de Paula, D.A.; Oliveira, J.C.; Viegas Junior, C.; Ionta, M. Alkaloids derived from flowers of Senna spectabilis, (-)-cassine and (-)-spectaline, have antiproliferative activity on HepG2 cells for inducing cell cycle arrest in G1/S transition through ERK inactivation and downregulation of cyclin D1 expression. *Toxicol. In Vitro* **2016**, *31*, 86–92. [CrossRef] [PubMed]
32. Hishe, H.Z.; Ambech, T.A.; Hiben, M.G.; Fanta, B.S. Anti-nociceptive effect of methanol extract of leaves of Senna singueana in mice. *J. Ethnopharmacol.* **2018**, *217*, 49–53. [CrossRef] [PubMed]
33. Hiben, M.G.; Sibhat, G.G.; Fanta, B.S.; Gebrezgi, H.D.; Tesema, S.B. Evaluation of Senna singueana leaf extract as an alternative or adjuvant therapy for malaria. *J. Tradit. Complement. Med.* **2016**, *6*, 112–117. [CrossRef] [PubMed]
34. Thilagam, E.; Parimaladevi, B.; Kumarappan, C.; Mandal, S.C. Alpha-Glucosidase and alpha-amylase inhibitory activity of Senna surattensis. *J. Acupunct. Meridian. Stud.* **2013**, *6*, 24–30. [CrossRef] [PubMed]
35. Ayinla, T.M.; Owoyele, V.B.; Yakubu, T.M. Effect of Ethanolic Leaf Extract of Senna Fistula on some Haematological Parameters, Lipid Profile and Oxidative Stress in Alloxan-induced Diabetic Rats. *Niger. J. Physiol. Sci.* **2015**, *30*, 87–93. [PubMed]
36. Malematja, R.O.; Bagla, V.P. Potential Hypoglycaemic and Antiobesity Effects of Senna italica Leaf Acetone Extract. *Evid. Based Complement. Altern. Med.* **2018**, *2018*, 5101656. [CrossRef] [PubMed]
37. Ismail, M.A.; Mateos, L.; Maioli, S.; Merino-Serrais, P. 27-Hydroxycholesterol impairs neuronal glucose uptake through an IRAP/GLUT4 system dysregulation. *J. Exp. Med.* **2017**, *214*, 699–717. [CrossRef] [PubMed]
38. Li, Y.; Zheng, L.; Wang, D.; Zhang, X.; Li, J.; Ali, S.; Lu, J.; Zong, H.; Xu, X. Staurosporine as an agonist for induction of GLUT4 translocation, identified by a pH-sensitive fluorescent IRAP-mOrange2 probe. *Biochem. Biophys. Res. Commun.* **2016**, *480*, 534–538. [CrossRef] [PubMed]
39. Jiang, L.; Fan, J.; Bai, L.; Wang, Y.; Chen, Y.; Yang, L.; Chen, L.; Xu, T. Direct quantification of fusion rate reveals a distal role for AS160 in insulin-stimulated fusion of GLUT4 storage vesicles. *J. Biol. Chem.* **2008**, *283*, 8508–8516. [CrossRef] [PubMed]
40. Zeng, B.; Chen, G.L.; Daskoulidou, N.; Xu, S.Z. The ryanodine receptor agonist 4-chloro-3-ethylphenol blocks ORAI store-operated channels. *Br. J. Pharmacol.* **2014**, *171*, 1250–1259. [CrossRef] [PubMed]
41. Yu, H.; Rathore, S.S.; Davis, E.M.; Ouyang, Y.; Shen, J. Doc2b promotes GLUT4 exocytosis by activating the SNARE-mediated fusion reaction in a calcium- and membrane bending-dependent manner. *Mol. Biol. Cell* **2013**, *24*, 1176–1184. [CrossRef] [PubMed]
42. Xie, X.; Gong, Z.; Mansuy-Aubert, V.; Zhou, Q.L.; Tatulian, S.A.; Sehrt, D.; Gnad, F.; Brill, L.M.; Motamedchaboki, K.; Chen, Y.; et al. C2 domain-containing phosphoprotein CDP138 regulates GLUT4 insertion into the plasma membrane. *Cell Metab.* **2011**, *14*, 378–389. [CrossRef] [PubMed]
43. Xing, Q.; Chen, Y. Antidiabetic Effects of a Chinese Herbal Medicinal Compound Sangguayin Preparation via PI3K/Akt Signaling Pathway in db/db Mice. *Evid. Based Complement. Altern. Med.* **2018**, *2018*, 2010423. [CrossRef] [PubMed]
44. Tian, C.; Chang, H. Wushenziye Formula Improves Skeletal Muscle Insulin Resistance in Type 2 Diabetes Mellitus via PTP1B-IRS1-Akt-GLUT4 Signaling Pathway. *Evid. Based Complement. Altern. Med.* **2017**, *2017*, 4393529. [CrossRef] [PubMed]
45. Zhang, C.; Jiang, Y.; Liu, J.; Jin, M.; Qin, N.; Chen, Y.; Niu, W.; Duan, H. AMPK/AS160 mediates tiliroside derivatives-stimulated GLUT4 translocation in muscle cells. *Drug Des. Dev. Ther.* **2018**, *12*, 1581–1587. [CrossRef] [PubMed]
46. Beaton, N.; Rudigier, C.; Moest, H.; Muller, S.; Mrosek, N.; Roder, E.; Rudofsky, G.; Rulicke, T.; Ukropec, J.; Ukropcova, B.; et al. TUSC5 regulates insulin-mediated adipose tissue glucose uptake by modulation of GLUT4 recycling. *Mol. Metab.* **2015**, *4*, 795–810. [CrossRef] [PubMed]
47. Waller, A.P.; Burns, T.A.; Mudge, M.C.; Belknap, J.K.; Lacombe, V.A. Insulin resistance selectively alters cell-surface glucose transporters but not their total protein expression in equine skeletal muscle. *J. Vet. Intern. Med.* **2011**, *25*, 315–321. [CrossRef] [PubMed]
48. Werno, M.W.; Chamberlain, L.H. S-acylation of the Insulin-Responsive Aminopeptidase (IRAP): Quantitative analysis and Identification of Modified Cysteines. *Sci. Rep.* **2015**, *5*, 12413. [CrossRef] [PubMed]

49. Grigorash, B.B.; Suvorova, I.I.; Pospelov, V.A. AICAR-Dependent Activation of AMPK Kinase Is Not Accompanied by G1/S Block in Mouse Embryonic Stem Cells. *Mol. Biol. (Mosk)* **2018**, *52*, 489–500. [CrossRef] [PubMed]
50. Wang, C.; Deng, Y.; Yue, Y.; Chen, W.; Zhang, Y.; Shi, G.; Wu, Z. Glutamine Enhances the Hypoglycemic Effect of Insulin in L6 Cells via Phosphatidylinositol-3-Kinase (PI3K)/Protein Kinase B (AKT)/Glucose Transporter 4 (GLUT4) Signaling Pathway. *Med. Sci. Monit.* **2018**, *24*, 1241–1250. [CrossRef] [PubMed]
51. Nishizaki, T. Dioleoylphosphoethanolamine Retains Cell Surface GLUT4 by Inhibiting PKCalpha-Driven Internalization. *Cell. Physiol. Biochem.* **2018**, *46*, 1985–1998. [CrossRef] [PubMed]
52. Litosch, I. Regulating G protein activity by lipase-independent functions of phospholipase C. *Life Sci.* **2015**, *137*, 116–124. [CrossRef] [PubMed]
53. Whitehead, J.P.; Molero, J.C.; Clark, S.; Martin, S.; Meneilly, G.; James, D.E. The role of Ca^{2+} in insulin-stimulated glucose transport in 3T3-L1 cells. *J. Biol. Chem.* **2001**, *276*, 27816–27824. [CrossRef] [PubMed]
54. Klip, A. The many ways to regulate glucose transporter 4. *Appl. Physiol. Nutr. Metab.* **2009**, *34*, 481–487. [CrossRef] [PubMed]
55. Song, P.; Kim, J.H.; Ghim, J.; Yoon, J.H.; Lee, A.; Kwon, Y.; Hyun, H.; Moon, H.Y.; Choi, H.S.; Berggren, P.O.; et al. Emodin regulates glucose utilization by activating AMP-activated protein kinase. *J. Biol. Chem.* **2013**, *288*, 5732–5742. [CrossRef] [PubMed]
56. Jing, D.; Bai, H.; Yin, S. Renoprotective effects of emodin against diabetic nephropathy in rat models are mediated via PI3K/Akt/GSK-3beta and Bax/caspase-3 signaling pathways. *Exp. Ther. Med.* **2017**, *14*, 5163–5169. [PubMed]
57. Lee, M.S.; Sohn, C.B. Anti-diabetic properties of chrysophanol and its glucoside from rhubarb rhizome. *Biol. Pharm. Bull.* **2008**, *31*, 2154–2157. [CrossRef] [PubMed]
58. Anand, S.; Muthusamy, V.S.; Sujatha, S.; Sangeetha, K.N.; Bharathi Raja, R.; Sudhagar, S.; Poornima Devi, N.; Lakshmi, B.S. Aloe emodin glycosides stimulates glucose transport and glycogen storage through PI3K dependent mechanism in L6 myotubes and inhibits adipocyte differentiation in 3T3L1 adipocytes. *FEBS Lett.* **2010**, *584*, 3170–3178. [CrossRef] [PubMed]
59. Alkhalidy, H.; Moore, W.; Zhang, Y.; McMillan, R. Small Molecule Kaempferol Promotes Insulin Sensitivity and Preserved Pancreatic beta-Cell Mass in Middle-Aged Obese Diabetic Mice. *J. Diabetes Res.* **2015**, *2015*, 532984. [CrossRef] [PubMed]
60. Zhou, Q.; Yang, X.; Xiong, M.; Xu, X.; Zhen, L.; Chen, W.; Wang, Y.; Shen, J.; Zhao, P.; Liu, Q.H. Chloroquine Increases Glucose Uptake via Enhancing GLUT4 Translocation and Fusion with the Plasma Membrane in L6 Cells. *Cell. Physiol. Biochem.* **2016**, *38*, 2030–2040. [CrossRef] [PubMed]
61. Zhou, F.; Furuhashi, K.; Son, M.J.; Toyozaki, M.; Yoshizawa, F.; Miura, Y.; Yagasaki, K. Antidiabetic effect of enterolactone in cultured muscle cells and in type 2 diabetic model db/db mice. *Cytotechnology* **2017**, *69*, 493–502. [CrossRef] [PubMed]
62. Zhao, Y.; He, J.; Yang, L.; Luo, Q.; Liu, Z. Histone Deacetylase-3 Modification of MicroRNA-31 Promotes Cell Proliferation and Aerobic Glycolysis in Breast Cancer and Is Predictive of Poor Prognosis. *J. Breast Cancer* **2018**, *21*, 112–123. [CrossRef] [PubMed]
63. Huang, M.; Deng, S.; Han, Q.; Zhao, P.; Zhou, Q.; Zheng, S.; Ma, X.; Xu, C.; Yang, J.; Yang, X. Hypoglycemic Activity and the Potential Mechanism of the Flavonoid Rich Extract from Sophora tonkinensis Gagnep. in KK-Ay Mice. *Front. Pharmacol.* **2016**, *7*, 288. [CrossRef] [PubMed]
64. Wang, Q.; Khayat, Z.; Kishi, K.; Ebina, Y.; Klip, A. GLUT4 translocation by insulin in intact muscle cells: Detection by a fast and quantitative assay. *FEBS Lett.* **1998**, *427*, 193–197. [CrossRef]

Sample Availability: Samples of the compounds are available from the authors.

molecules

MDPI

Article

Phytochemical and Analytical Characterization of Novel Sulfated Coumarins in the Marine Green Macroalga *Dasycladus vermicularis* (Scopoli) Krasser

Anja Hartmann [1,*], Markus Ganzera [1], Ulf Karsten [2], Alexsander Skhirtladze [3] and Hermann Stuppner [1]

1 Institute of Pharmacy, Pharmacognosy, CMBI, University of Innsbruck, Innrain 80-82, 6020 Innsbruck, Austria; markus.ganzera@uibk.ac.at (M.G.); hermann.stuppner@uibk.ac.at (H.S.)
2 Institute of Biological Sciences, Applied Ecology & Phycology, University of Rostock, Albert-Einstein-Str. 3, 18059 Rostock, Germany; ulf.karsten@uni-rostock.de
3 Department of Phytochemistry, Iovel Kutateladze Institute of Pharmacochemistry, Tbilisi State Medical University, 0159 Tbilisi, Georgia; aleksandre.skhirtladze@yahoo.com
* Correspondence: Anja.Hartmann@uibk.ac.at; Tel.: +43-512-507-58430

Academic Editor: Pinarosa Avato
Received: 11 September 2018; Accepted: 17 October 2018; Published: 23 October 2018

Abstract: The siphonous green algae form a morphologically diverse group of marine macroalgae which include two sister orders (Bryopsidales and Dasycladales) which share a unique feature among other green algae as they are able to form large, differentiated thalli comprising of a single, giant tubular cell. Upon cell damage a cascade of protective mechanisms have evolved including the extrusion of sulfated metabolites which are involved in the formation of a rapid wound plug. In this study, we investigated the composition of sulfated metabolites in *Dasycladus vermicularis* (Dasycladales) which resulted in the isolation of two phenolic acids and four coumarins including two novel structures elucidated by nuclear magnetic resonance spectroscopy (NMR) as 5,8′-di-(6(6′),7(7′)-tetrahydroxy-3-sulfoxy-3′-sulfoxycoumarin), a novel coumarin called dasycladin A and 7-hydroxycoumarin-3,6-disulfate, which was named dasycladin B. In addition, an analytical assay for the chromatographic quantification of those compounds was developed and performed on a reversed phase C-18 column. Method validation confirmed that the new assay shows good linearity ($R^2 \geq 0.9986$), precision (intra-day R.S.D $\leq$ 3.71%, inter-day R.S.D $\leq$ 7.49%), and accuracy (recovery rates ranged from 104.06 to 97.45%). The analysis of several samples of *Dasycladus vermicularis* from different collection sites, water depths and seasons revealed differences in the coumarin contents, ranging between 0.26 to 1.61%.

Keywords: siphonous green algae; sulfated coumarins; *Dasycladus vermicularis*; isolation and quantification

1. Introduction

Dasycladus vermicularis (Scopoli) Krasser is an evolutionarily ancient, small siphonous green alga, which is widely distributed throughout tropical to temperate regions such as several Atlantic islands (Canary islands, Madeira, Antilles), many regions in the Mediterranean Sea, Central America (Belize), Caribbean islands, South America (Brazil), and Asia (Japan, South China Sea, Philippines) [1]. This chlorophyte inhabits well-illuminated shallow waters (0.3–20 m) with high light exposures in the upper littoral zone on rocky substrates and are often covered by a thin layer of sediment [2]. To thrive under enhanced doses of UV radiation, photo-protective mechanisms are needed. In 1983, Menzel et al. [3] isolated and identified 3,6,7-trihydroxycoumarin (thyc) as a UV absorbing compound from

D. vermicularis for the first time, which was also the first report of coumarins in algae. Subsequently, several studies have been carried out to investigate the relevance of thyc in *D. vermicularis*. They indicated an elevated excretion of thyc due to increasing UV exposure and temperatures suggesting that this compound is a natural sunscreen/UV protectant [4–6]. Another very remarkable characteristic of *D. vermicularis* is its morphology. *D. vermicularis* is a member of the so-called siphonous green macro algae comprising unique giant single cells without cross walls. These thalli can grow up to 10 cm long, gaining stability by surrounding themselves with a calcareous coating which supports the long unicellular algae with sufficient stability to grow upright. Siphonous algae typically contain a huge central vacuole and a thin layer of cytoplasm, the latter inhabiting multiple nuclei (Bryopsidales) or just one nucleus (Dasycladales) [7]. After cell damage, for example due to herbivory, a rapid wound closure is essential for the survival of such organisms. Therefore, immediately upon injury a cascade of biochemical reactions is induced to assimilate cellular contents into an insoluble wound plug initially formed by gelling, followed by a slower hardening process (1–2 h) [8,9]. This mechanism is indispensable to avoid cytoplasmic loss and limits the intrusion of extracellular components, herbivore attack or pathogenic invasion, which could otherwise result in high mortality rates [8,10]. A few years ago Welling et al. [8] investigated both the intact and wounded alga to monitor changes in chemical composition, which may be involved in the wound plug formation. This study surprisingly revealed the dominant secondary metabolite to be 6,7-dihydroxycoumarin-3-sulfate (dhycs) in the methanolic extracts of intact *D. vermicularis*, while the previously reported major compound 3,6,7-trihydroxycoumarin was only found in the methanolic extracts after wounding. Thus, the dhycs is supposed to act as a precursor and is transformed into the more active thyc in the presence of sulfatases. According to Welling et al. [9] thyc acts as an intermediate which is rapidly oxidized and serves as a protein cross-linker for the formation of a wound sealing co-polymer in combination with amino acid side chains from the alga. Such polymerization processes are known from other marine organisms, which are usually involved in bioadhesive processes that are needed for sessile marine organisms such as tubeworms and mussels to attach themselves to surfaces. For example, the common blue mussel *Mytilus edulis* uses a metal centered chelate that initiates the biopolymerisation process which includes secondary metabolites such as protein-bound-dopamine [11]. Sulfated secondary metabolites are widely distributed among marine species and are stored therein in a dormant state. They are then transformed enzymatically into more active metabolites, for example, psammaplin A sulfate from the sponge *Aplysinella rhax* or zosteric acid, an antifouling metabolite in the seagrass *Zostera marina*. Both metabolites are converted upon tissue disruption to their desulfated form thereby increasing activity as a defensive metabolite [12,13]. Kurth et al. [14] just recently revealed the presence of two sulfated phenolic acids in *D. vermicularis* namely 4-(sulfooxy)benzoic acid (SBA) and 4-(sulfooxy)phenylacetic acid (SPA), which are also proposed to exist in a dormant state prior to transformation to more active desulfated metabolites. However, these two sulfated phenolic acids are most likely not involved in the wound plug formation, but could be serving as biofilm inhibitor. In this study we investigated the phytochemical composition of *D. vermicularis* extracts of different polarities. The coumarin composition of this alga seems to be more complex than previously described, and hence we report on two novel coumarins from *D. vermicularis* and their analysis via HPLC-MS and NMR. Coumarins are natural benzopyrone derivatives with a variety of desirable pharmacological properties which are commonly found in higher plants [15], however sulfated molecules are rather uncommon and beyond that *D. vermicularis* is the first alga known to contain these secondary metabolites. Therefore, we report on the first validated HPLC assay for the separation and quantification of sulfated coumarins in algae which has been applied to samples from three different sampling sites across the Mediterranean Sea to compare their coumarin content.

2. Results

2.1. Isolation and Identification of the Coumarins

With the aim of isolating the major compounds present in *Dasycladus vermicularis* four coumarins and two phenolic acids were isolated from the methanol and the aqueous extract. A sample (2.5 g) of the aqueous extract was separated by means of repeated flash chromatography and semi-preparative HPLC, which resulted in the isolation of compounds **1**, **4** and **8**. Compounds **2**, **3** and **7** were obtained from 4.5 g of crude methanol extract by silica gel and Sephadex LH 20 column chromatography. ^{1}H- and ^{13}C-NMR shift values of all isolated coumarins are summarized in Table 1. The shift values for thyc were in good agreement with literature values [16]. Compounds **1** and **2** were identified as new natural products.

Table 1. NMR shift values of compounds isolated from the marine green alga *Dasycladus vermicularis*; spectra were recorded on a 600 MHz NMR instrument in deuterated water.

Position	Dasycladin A (1) in D_2O		HMBC C	Dasycladin B (2) in D_2O		HMBC C
	δ_H	δ_C, Type		δ_H	δ_C, Type	
2		163.3, C			161.0, C	
3		136.1, C			134.1, C	
4	7.40 (s)	134.4, CH	2, 3, 5, 9	7.94 (s)	133.3, CH	2, 3, 5, 9
5		118.3, C		7.64 (s)	122.4, CH	4, 6, 7, 9
6		144.1, C			137.6, C	
7		152.7, C			153.0, C	
8	7.10 (s)	106.8, CH	6, 7, 9, 10	7.05 (s)	105.1, CH	6, 7, 9, 10
9		150.2, C			151.1, C	
10		113.5, C			112.1, C	
2′		163.0, C				
3′		135.8, C				
4′	7.96 (s)	135.8, CH	2′, 3′, 5′, 9′			
5′	7.28 (s)	115.8, CH	4′, 6′, 7′, 9′			
6′		145.7, C				
7′		151.5, C				
8′		111.2, C				
9′		147.7, C				
10′		113.9, C				

Compound **1** was isolated as a yellowish amorphous powder. Its molecular formula was established as $C_{18}H_{10}O_{16}S_2$ by HR-ESI–MS (m/z 544.934, calcd. for $[C_{18}H_{10}O_{16}S_2\text{-H}]^-$, 544.936) indicating the presence of a sulfated dicoumarin. Fragments at m/z 464.9 $[\text{M-H-80}]^-$ and 385.0 $[\text{M-H-80-80}]^-$ could be attributed to the loss of sulfate groups, respectively. The melting point was measured to as 278–280 °C The IR spectra shows a strong and characteristic S=O stretching vibration at about 1038 cm^{-1} for the R-OSO_3H groups, 1689 and 1629 cm^{-1} for (C=O), 3059 and 3203 cm^{-1} (OH). In the ^{1}H-NMR (Table 1) spectrum, four singlet aromatic proton resonances at δ_H 7.96 (1H, s, H-4′), 7.40 (1H, s, H-4), 7.28 (1H, s, H-5′), 7.10 (1H, s, H-8) were observed. The ^{13}C-NMR (Table 1) spectrum showed eighteen carbon signals, which were assigned by DEPT experiments to four aromatic methines and fourteen quaternary carbons, two of which (δ_C 163. 3 and 163.0) could be attributed to intramolecular ester groups. The spectroscopic data suggested that **1** is composed of two identical coumarin moieties substituted in positions C-3(C-3′), C-6(C-6′), and C-7 (C-7′). The absence of corresponding signals in the ^{1}H-NMR spectrum and the low field-shifted C-5 and C-8′ signals in the ^{13}C-NMR spectrum indicated that the two symmetric coumarin moieties were connected at 5–8′ through a C-C bond. Localization of the two sulfate groups was established based on the low field-shifted signals of C-3 and C-3′ as well as by comparison of NMR data with those of thyc (**4**) [16] and compound **3**. HSQC and HMBC experiments of **1** were useful to assign all signals in the ^{1}H and ^{13}C spectra. C-4 (δ 134.4) and C-8 (δ 106.8) were used to assign the H-4 (7.40, s) and H-8 (7.10, s) as well as C-4′ (δ 135.8) and C-5′ (δ 115.8) which were assigned to H-4′ (7.96, s) and H-5′ (7.28, s) by ^{1}H-^{13}C HSQC.

The HMBC spectrum showed key correlation peaks between the proton signal at δ_H 7.93 (1H, s, H-4′) and carbon resonances at δ_C 163.0 (C-2′), 147.7 (C-9′), 135.8 (C-3′), 115.8 (C-5′); and between the proton signal at δ_H 7.38 (1H, s, H-4) and carbon resonances at δ_C 163.3 (C-2), 150.3 (C-9), 136.1 (C-3), 118.3 (C-5). Thus, compound **1** was identified as 5,8′-di-(6(6′),7(7′)-tetrahydroxy-3-sulfoxy-3′-sulfoxycoumarin), a new coumarin for which we propose the trivial name "dasycladin A".

Compound **2** was also isolated as a yellowish amorphous powder. The molecular formula of $C_9H_6O_{11}S_2$ was determined by HR-ESI–MS (negative mode) with a mass peak at m/z 352.928 (calcd. for $[C_9H_6O_{11}S_2\text{-H}]^-$, 352.926). The mass spectrum showed a fragment at m/z 272.8 $[\text{M-H-80}]^-$ corresponding to the loss of a sulfate moiety. The melting point was measured as 233–238 °C. The IR spectra shows a strong and characteristic S=O stretching vibration at about 1038 cm^{-1} for the R-OSO$_3$H groups, 1697 cm^{-1} for (C=O), 3217 cm^{-1} (OH). The ^{1}H-NMR spectrum (Table 1) of **2** showed signals for three aromatic protons at δ_H 7.94 (1H, s, H-4), 7.64 (1H, s, H-5), 7.05 (1H, s, H-8). In the ^{13}C-NMR (Table 1) spectrum nine carbon signals, including three aromatic methines and six quaternary carbons were observed. HSQC and HMBC experiments of Compound **2** were useful to assign all signals in the ^{1}H- and ^{13}C-NMR spectra. C-4 (δ 133.3), C-5 (δ 122.4) and C-8 (δ 105.2) were used to assign the protons H-4 (7.94, s), H-5 (7.64, s) and H-8 (7.05, s) by ^{1}H-^{13}C HSQC. The HMBC spectrum showed correlation peaks between the proton signal at δ_H 7.94 (1H, s, H-4) and carbon resonances at δ_C 161.1 (C-2), 151.1 (C-9), 134.2 (C-3), 122.4 (C-5); between the proton signal at δ_H 7.64 (1H, s, H-5) and carbon resonances at δ_C 152.9 (C-7), 151.1 (C-9), 137.7 (C-6), 133.3 (C-4); and between the proton signal at δ_H 7.04 (1H, s, H-8) and carbon resonances at δ_C 152.9 (C-7), 151.1 (C-9), 137.7 (C-6), 112.3 (C-10). These spectroscopic data suggested that compound **2** is 3,6,7-trisubstituted coumarin. The low field-shifted signal of C-3 and the up field-shifted of C-6 indicated that the sulfate groups were attached at these carbons. The structure of **2** was deduced as 7-hydroxycoumarin-3,6-disulfate. Compound **2** represents a new coumarin for which we propose the trivial name "dasycladin B".

NMR spectra and HR-ESI–MS data for the novel sulfated coumarins **1** and **2** are shown in Figures S1A–E and S2A–E in the Supplementary Material.

2.2. HPLC-Method Development

A HPLC method was developed for quantification of the coumarins. Four coumarins were isolated as described above and used as standards in addition to the two synthetized sulfated phenolic acids and their educts (see Figure 1). Several different stationary phases were screened for the separation of the coumarins and phenolic acids in *D. vermicularis*, such as Zorbax SB-C18 3.5 µm, Hyperclone ODS 3 µm, YMC-triart C-18, 3.5 µm and Kinetex C-18 2.6 µm. However, the best separation was achieved on the Gemini C 18 110 Å, 3 µm (150 mm × 4.6 mm). The latter column yielded the best results concerning separation efficiency and peak shape, resulting in an optimum separation within less than 25 min (Figure 2).

5,8′-Di-(6(6′),7(7′)-tetrahydroxy-3-sulfoxy-3′-sulfoxycoumarin) (**1**) eluted first (13.12 min), followed by 7-hydroxycoumarin-3,6-disulfate (**2**; 16.58 min), the sulfated phenolic acids 4-(sulfooxy)benzoic acid and 4-(sulfooxy)phenylacetic acid (**5**; 17.73 min, **6**; 18.3 min), then 6,7-dihydroxycoumarin-3-sulfate (**3**; 18.81 min), 3,6,7-trihydroxycoumarin (**4**; 20.63 min), 4-(hydroxyl)phenylacetic acid (**7**; 21.62 min), and finally 4-(hydroxyl)-benzoic acid (**8**; 22.07 min).

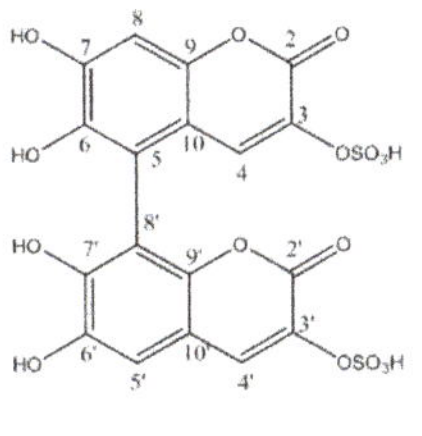

5,8′-di-(6(6′),7(7′)-tetrahydroxy-3-sulfoxy-3′-sulfoxycoumarin (**1**)

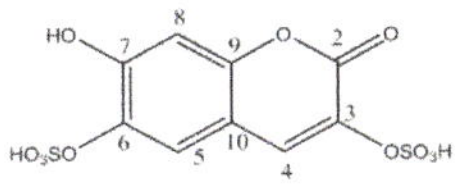

7-hydroxycoumarin-3,6-disulfate (**2**)

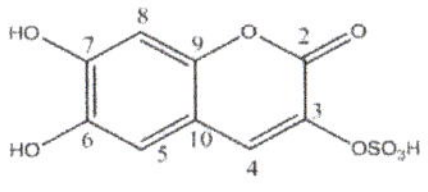

6,7-dihydroxycoumarin-3-sulfate (**3**)

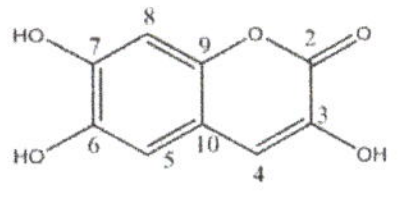

3,6,7-trihydroxycoumarin (**4**)

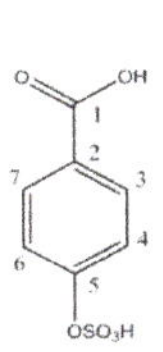

4-(sulfooxy)benzoic acid (**5**)

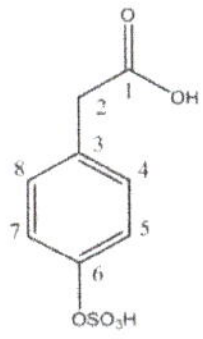

4-(sulfooxy)phenylacetic acid (**6**)

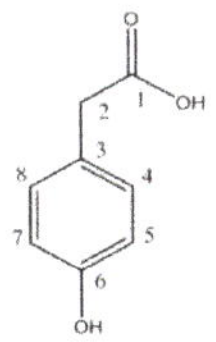

4-(hydroxy)phenylacetic acid (**7**)

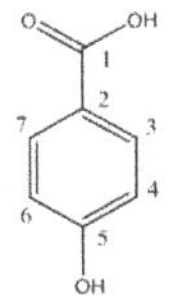

4-(hydroxy)benzoic acid (**8**)

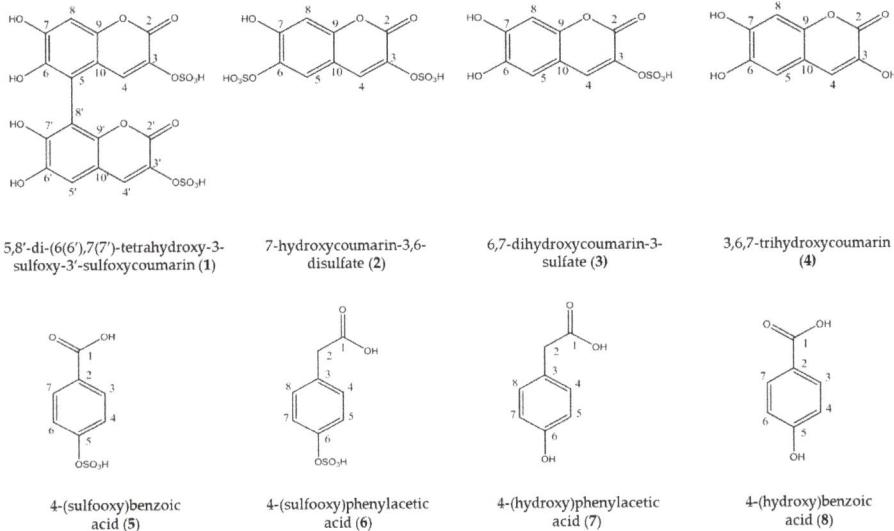

Figure 1. Chemical structure of the isolated coumarins from the marine green alga *Dasycladus vermicularis*, the sulfated phenolic acids and their educts.

2.3. Method Validation

The new analytical method was validated according to the ICH guidelines [17] by establishing calibration curves of the two coumarin standards **1** and **4**, as well as the phenolic acids 4-hydroxy-benzoic acid and 4-hydroxyphenylacetic acid and their sulfated products 4-(sulfooxy)benzoic acid (SBA) and 4-(sulfooxy)phenylacetic acid (SPA) **5**–**8**. Sufficient material was not available for **2** and **3**. Excellent determination coefficients ($R^2 \geq 0.9986$) were obtained within a concentration range of 0.859–1154 μg/mL. Individual calibration levels were obtained by serial dilution, and each solution was analyzed under optimum HPLC conditions in triplicate. Limit of detection (LOD) and limit of quantification (LOQ) were calculated using defined concentration equivalents to S/N ratios of 3 (LOD) and 10 (LOQ). LOD and LOQ values ranged from 0.014–1.939 μg/mL, and from 0.044–5.876 μg/mL, respectively (Table 2). Selectivity of the method was assured by no visible co-elution (shoulders) in the relevant signals, LC-MS data, and by very consistent UV-spectra (as confirmed by the peak purity option in the operating software). The methods precision was confirmed by its repeatability, as well as inter- and intra-day variation which were determined in *D. vermicularis* sample (DV-2). For this purpose five individual samples at 250 mg/25 mL were extracted and analyzed on each of three consecutive days (Table 3). Intra-day (RSD $\leq$ 5.99%) and inter-day precision (RSD $\leq$ 7.49%) were within accepted limits. Accuracy was assured by spiking accurately weighed samples of DV-2 with three different concentrations of the standard substances. For all compounds the observed recovery rates were acceptable and ranged from 95.6 to 104.6%. Only for 3,6,7-trihydroxcoumarin the value for the low spike was at 91.3% (Table 3). This compound appeared to be stable in solution for at least several h, however when added to the extract it degrades rapidly and therefore the recovery rates are poor, especially at the lower concentrations.

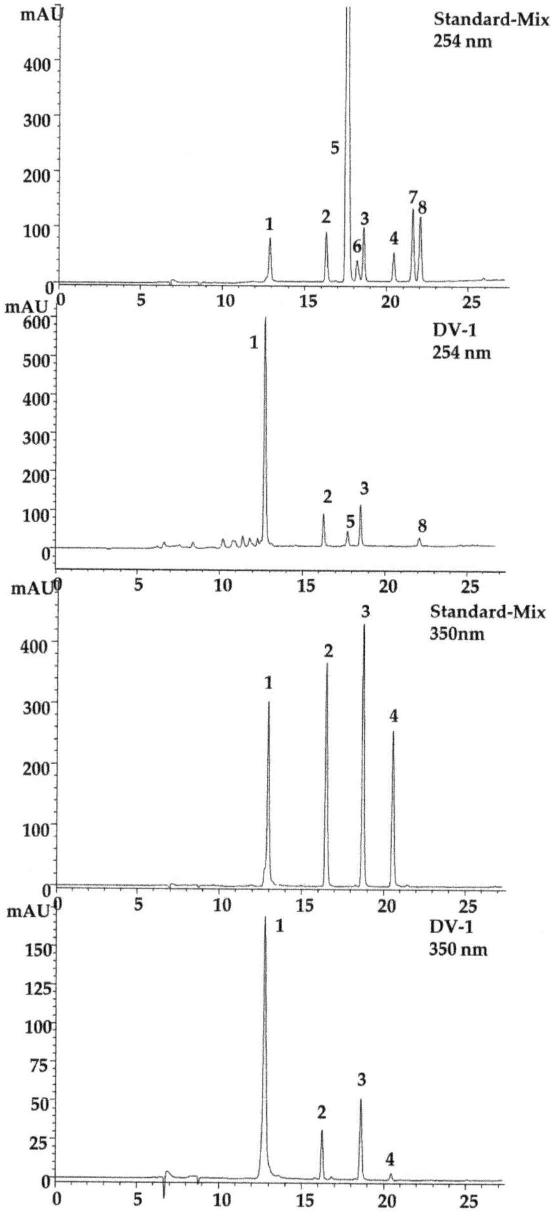

Figure 2. HPLC separation of all standards **1** to **8** at 254 nm and all coumarins **1** to **4** isolated from the marine green alga *Dasycladus vermicularis* at 350 nm, and the sample DV-1 from the marine green alga *Dasycladus vermicularis* at 254 nm and 350 nm under optimized conditions (column: Gemini C18, 110 Å column (150 × 4.6 mm, 3 µm); mobile phase (A) aqueous 20 mM ammonium acetate solution with 1.5% acetic acid and (B) methanol/water (9:1) with 20 mM ammonium acetate and 1.5% acetic acid. Gradient: 2% B to 15% B from 0 to 5 min and 15% B to 60% B from 5–20 min and 60% B to 98% B from 20–25 min; detection at 254 nm and 350 nm, flow rate 0.3 mL/min, injection volume 5 µL and 40 °C oven temperature. Peak assignment is according to Figure 1.

Table 2. Calibration data for the coumarins isolated from the marine green alga *Dasycladus vermicularis* and the respective phenolic acids.

Parameter	1 (Dasycladin A)	4 (thyc)	5 (SBA)	6 (SPA)	7 (4-OH-PAA)	8 (4-OH-BA)
Regr. Equation	Y = 22.953x − 7.904	Y = 67.354x − 296.52	Y = 19.684x + 22.158	Y = 0.652x − 1.475	Y = 97.057x + 14.771	Y = 2.110x + 2.757
σ rel of the slope	0.09	0.683	0.116	0.175	0.049	0.339
R	0.9999	0.9986	0.9999	1.000	1.000	1.000
Range (μg/mL)	440–0.859	445–6.953	629–1.229	1154–18.031	124.75–0.975	483–3.770
LOD [1]	0.192	0.589	0.039	1.939	0.014	1.045
LOQ [2]	0.581	1.784	0.117	5.876	0.044	3.168

[1] LOD: limit of detection determined with purified standards (in μg/mL). [2] LOQ: limit of quantification determined with purified standards (in μg/mL).

Table 3. Accuracy and precision of the new coumarin assay.

Substance	Accuracy [1]			Precision [2]			
	High Spike	Medium Spike	Low Spike	Day 1	Day 2	Day 3	Intra-Day
1	99.49	95.63	101.89	7.49	1.57	1.38	1.86
2	-	-	-	2.22	4.43	6.65	3.71
3	-	-	-	6.39	4.37	2.81	5.99
4	97.49	97.87	91.34	-	-	-	-
5	102.62	99.58	99.40	-	-	-	-
6	98.70	103.23	100.72	-	-	-	-
7	97.45	104.06	103.77	-	-	-	-
8	102.10	99.50	98.85	-	-	-	-

[1] Expressed as recovery rates in percent (sample DV-2 Alonissos). [2] maximum relative standard deviation (peak area) within one and three consecutive days (n = 5; sample: DV-2).

2.4. Analysis of Samples

Four different samples of *D. vermicularis*, all originating from the Mediterranean Sea, were analyzed for their coumarin content. For further details on collection sites, seasons and water depths see Supplementary Material Table S1. As expected, the total amount of coumarins in sample DV-2 (1.60–1.80 m depth) was much lower (3.66 mg/g DW) compared to sample DV-3 (0.30–0.80 m depth; 10.17 mg/g DW). The quantity of the monomeric sulfated coumarins **2** and **3** was the same, while the content of the dimeric compound **1** was about three times higher in the sample that was collected from shallow waters. The two samples that were collected from the same spot in Volos, Greece (DV-3 and DV-4) indicated that there might be seasonal changes in the coumarin content of *D. vermicularis* as well. In November (sample DV-4; 4.27 mg/g DW), the total coumarin content was only half the amount as in August (sample DV-3; 10.17 mg/g DW). The sample that was harvested from Malaga, Spain (DV-1) showed the highest amount of coumarins with 16.09 mg/g DW. The dimeric coumarin **1** was the most abundant compound in all samples, followed by **3**, the 6,7-dihydroxycoumarin-3-sulfate, and 7-hydroxycoumarin-3,6-disulfate (**2**). Thyc, which is reported to be the sole metabolite of compound **3**, only occurred in traces in the highest concentrated samples DV-1 and DV-3. Phenolic acids were also present in all samples, however, in much lower content. All samples contained 4-hydroxybenzoic acid and at a higher concentration its sulfated precursor 4-(sulfooxy)benzoic acid. All quantitative results are summarized in Figure 3. 4-(Sulfooxy)phenylacetic acid which was reported to be present in *D. vermicularis* in a previous publication by Kurth et al. [14] could not be detected in the samples by DAD; however, LC-MS revealed the presence of this compound in all samples. In addition to the standard compounds, three other signals were tentatively identified as coumarins based on the typical UV and MS-spectra; they are marked with a star (Figure 4). The compounds a* and b* both have UV absorption maxima of 346 nm and m/z of 465 [M-H$^-$]. These two compounds may be monosulfated dicoumarins. The assignment of other signals was easily possible by comparison to standards. For example, the determination of coumarins in sample DV-1 is shown in Figure S5 in the Supplementary Material. Chromatograms were recorded at 254 nm and 350 nm, the other traces show the identification of individual compounds by LC-MS in EIC mode.

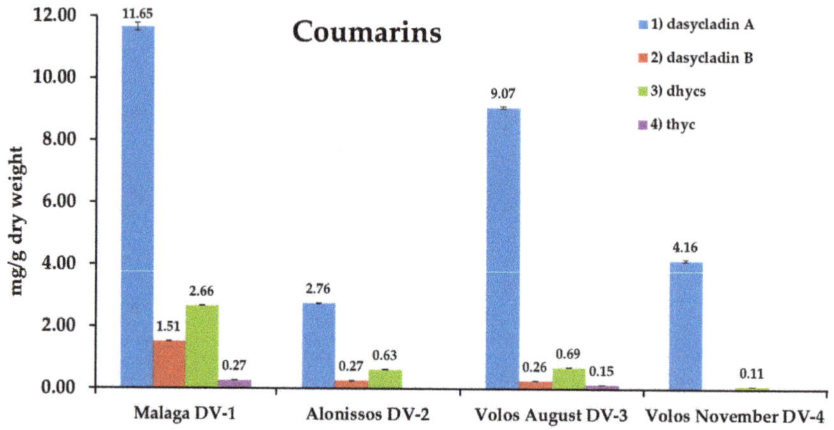

(A)

Figure 3. *Cont.*

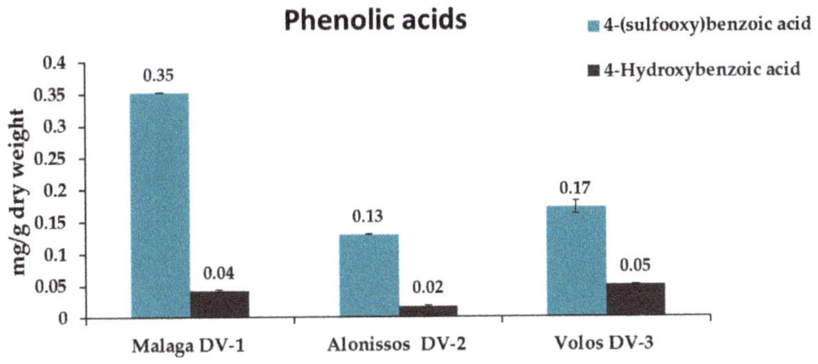

(B)

Figure 3. Quantification of the coumarins (**1**) dasycladin A, (**2**) dasycladin B, (extbf3) 6,7-dihydroxycoumarin-3-sulfate, (**4**) 3,6,7-trihydroxycoumarin. Concentrations are given as mg coumarins/g dry weight (**A**) and as mg/g phenolic acids as dry weight (**B**) (n = 3) in the green alga *Dasycladus vermicularis* collected at different sampling sites and dates in the Mediterranean Sea.

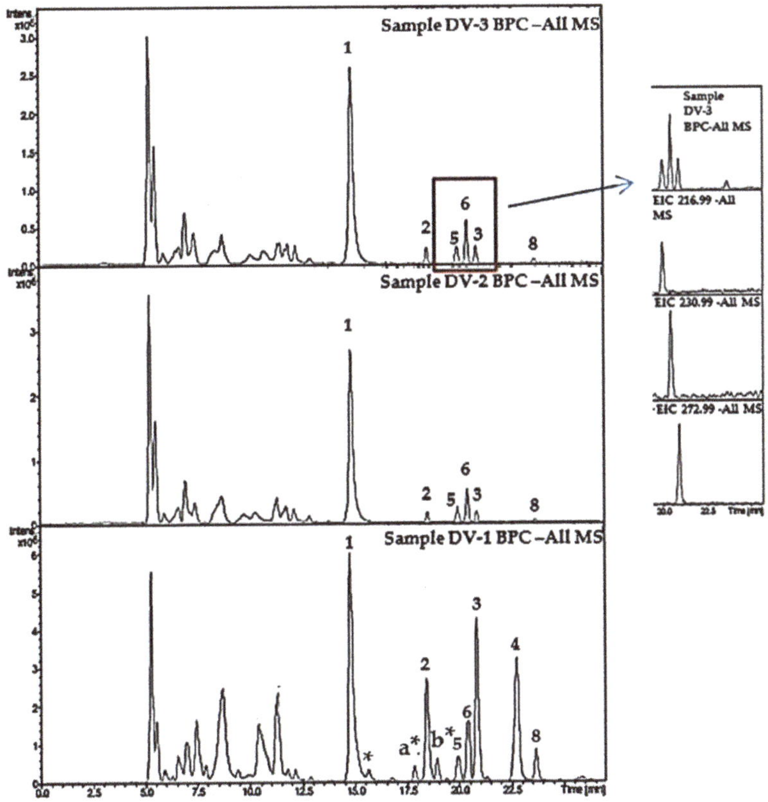

Figure 4. Base peak chromatograms of all extracts DV1-DV3 prepared from the marine green alga *Dasycladus vermicularis*. The red area is enlarged and shows the extracted ion chromatograms (EIC) for the sulfated phenolic acids SBA (**5**) and SPA (**6**). Tentatively identified minor coumarins are marked with a star (similar UV spectra) and with **a*** and **b*** (similar UV spectra and molecular weight).

3. Discussion

The chemical composition of coumarins and phenolic acids in the marine green alga *D. vermicularis* was investigated in detail in this study, revealing that the coumarin composition is more complex than previously reported [8]. Dasycladin A is the major compound, which probably degrades to the previously reported 6,7 dihydroxycoumarin-3 sulfate. Similarly, it can be speculated that dasycladin B is metabolized to the corresponding monosulfated coumarin first and afterwards to the more active metabolite 3,6,7-trihydroxycoumarin, since the sulfated compounds have been reported as dormant forms which are enzymatically transferred into active metabolites through sulfatases [9]. The sulfated phenolic acids SPA and SBA were both present in the extract, however at very low concentrations. These findings are highlighted with red in Figure 4 and are in good agreement with the LC-MS data published by Kurth et al. [14]. Coumarins in general show a wide range of different pharmacological activities, including anti-HIV, anti-tumor, anti-hypertensive, anti-coagulant, anti-inflammatory just to name a few. They have become important lead compounds in drug research due to their high bioavailability, low molecular weight, and low toxicity [15,18]. For simple coumarins anti-oxidative activity has been reported especially for compounds with free hydroxyl groups. Likewise, the C-7 free hydroxyl group is important for anti-bacterial activity and is also important for an anti-inflammatory activity [19]. The C-6 free hydroxyl group is important for both anti-bacterial and anti-fungal activity. A free hydroxyl group in position 3 (e.g., Compound **4** in this study) is especially important for a strongly enhanced inhibition of 5-Lipoxygenase and α-D-glucosidase [20]. Sulfated coumarins are rather uncommon but due to their negative charge they could bind to heparin receptors or inhibit platelet aggregation [21].

Besides recently developed HPLC-DAD, LC-MS and SFC methods for the separation of furo-pyrano- and monocoumarins on reversed phase columns [22–24], this study presents the first method for the separation of the definitive more polar sulfated coumarins. Their content was found to be quite variable in the different samples suggesting that water depth and seasonal changes including fluctuations in the visible and ultraviolet part of solar radiation might have a strong influence. *D. vermicularis* has been reported to excrete UV-absorbing brown-green substances under in-situ conditions staining the nearby seawater and thus being beneficial as photo-protective compounds for other macroalgae living in the vicinity [6]. The responsible compounds were later identified as coumarins and since they are accumulated in the outer parts of the siphonous cell walls, particularly after UV exposure, they are considered to act as UV-sunscreens [6]. 3,6,7-trihydroxycoumarin (thyc) was found to be preferentially localized in the apical part of the *D. vermicularis* thallus, which usually experiences highest natural insolation, particularly in the internal part of the cell wall and around the tonoplast. The percentage of UVR absorbed by both thyc layers could be measured from the in-vitro total thallus concentration of thyc and histological measurements of these layers. While the cell wall thyc layer absorbed 88% of the incident UVR irradiance, the one close to the vacuole membrane absorbed a similar fraction with 87.5% [6]. These data strongly support the hypothesis of coumarins/phenolics as natural sunscreen compounds reducing biologically harmful UVR from reaching sensitive biomolecules in the cell such as DNA and proteins. Phenolic compounds also play an important role in the interaction of macroalgae with their environment. They are relevant for different supporting or protective tissues, for example in cell wall formation, they can be involved in defense mechanisms, for example in anti-herbivory or having antibacterial effects, and signaling properties, for example in allelopathy [25].

The conspicuous decrease of coumarin content in November could make *D. vermicularis* more susceptible to abiotic and biotic stressors, but UVR and biotic interactions are less strong in late autumn compared to summer in the Mediterranean Sea. However, a larger number of samples from different origins, seasons and water depths is definitely needed to examine the qualitative and quantitative metabolic composition of *D. vermicularis* and its chemical reaction after wounding or other stress situations.

4. Materials and Methods

4.1. Reagents and Chemicals

All solvents used for isolation, synthesis and analytical studies were of analytical grade and purchased from Merck (Darmstadt, Germany). HPLC grade water was produced by a Sartorius arium 611 UV water purification system (Sartorius Göttingen, Germany). Reagents for the synthesis of 4-(sulfooxy)benzoic acid and 4-(sulfooxy)phenylacetic acid (4-hydroxybenzoic acid, sulphur trioxide pyridine complex (Pyr*SO_3), and 4-hydroxyphenylacetic acid) were purchased from Sigma Aldrich (Taufkirchen, Germany). Deuterated water for NMR experiments was obtained from Euriso-top (Saint-Aubin Cedex, France).

4.2. Algal Material

Four samples of *Dasycladus vermicularis* were analyzed. DV-1(330 g dry weight) was collected in September 1998 from the upper part of the infralittoral zone (0.5 m depth) in the Cabo de Gata-Nijar Natural Park (36° 52′ N, 2° 12′ W, Almerıa, Southern Spain) and identified by Prof. Felix Figueroa (University of Malaga), freeze-dried and sent to Ulf Karsten, who stored the material under cool, dry and dark conditions prior to further processing in Innsbruck. Sample DV-2 was harvested in August 2017 in Alonissos, Greece (39°08′23.8″ N, 23°50′43.3″ E) at 1.80 m depth; Sample DV-3 and DV-4 were both harvested in Volos, Greece (39°1900.0″ N, 23°01′11.5″ E), DV-3 in August 2017 and DV-4 in November 2017 at 30–80 cm depth. All samples from Greece were collected and identified by the author (A. Hartmann). All samples were air-dried and voucher specimen of all samples are stored at the Institute of Pharmacy, Pharmacognosy, University of Innsbruck.

4.3. Instrumentation

NMR experiments were conducted on an Avance II 600 spectrometer (Bruker, Karlsruhe, Germany) operating at 600.19 (^{1}H) and 150.91 MHz (^{13}C). Spectra of the respective compounds were recorded in deuterated solvents from Euriso-Top adding 3-(trimethylsilyl)-propionic acid sodium salt (TMSP) as an internal standard. Infrared (IR) spectra were recorded on an ALPHA Fourier transform (FT)-IR apparatus (Bruker, Billerica, MA, USA) equipped with a platinum attenuated total reflection module. Analytical HPLC experiments were carried out on an Agilent 1100 system (Agilent, Waldbronn, Germany) equipped with a binary pump, autosampler, diode array detector and column oven. For the purification of the compounds a semi-preparative HPLC from Dionex (ThermoFisher, Waltham, MA, USA), comprising of a HPG-3200 pump, a VWD-3100 detector, column oven and a fraction collector was utilized. Additionally, the exact mass of the novel compounds **1** and **2** were determined in negative ESI mode on a micrOTOF-Q II MS (Bruker, Bremen, Germany). The settings were: nebulizer gas: 4.4 psi, dry gas: 4 L/min, dry temperature: 180 °C, capillary voltage: 2.5 kV, set capillary V 3500, set endplate offset V-500.

4.4. Isolation and Structural Analysis of Coumarins

Dried algal material of *Dasycladus vermicularis* (300 g, DV-1, Malaga), were finely ground to powder and subsequently extracted five times with 100% dichloromethane (p.a.) for 15 min in an ultrasonic bath. After centrifugation at 1537× *g*, the combined solutions were evaporated to dryness at 40 °C under reduced pressure to yield 1.13 g of crude dichloromethane extract (DV-1D). The plant material was subsequently extracted with 100% methanol (p.a.) using the same procedure to yield 4.71 g of crude methanol extract (DV-1M). The algal residue was extracted for a third time using the same procedure with a 1:1 mixture of water and methanol to yield 7.9 g crude aqueous extract. The crude methanol extract (4.5 g) was separated into 10 fractions (DV-M-S1-10) on silica gel (40–63 μm particle size) using a dichloromethane/ethyl acetate/methanol/water gradient. Fraction DasyM-S7 was further purified using size-exclusion chromatography on Sephadex LH-20 material with methanol:water (1:1) as eluent to obtain 16 subfractions (DV-M 7.1-16). This resulted in the isolation of compounds **2** (5.24 mg) and **3**

(4.04 mg). A portion (2.5 g) of the crude aqueous extract was first separated using flash chromatography (on RP-18 material (80 g Reveleris cartridge, 40 µm) and a water/methanol gradient, containing 0.25% formic acid in each solvent. 20 subfractions were obtained (DV-W-R1-20). Fraction 18 resulted in the pure compound **4**. DV-W-R6 (39.56 mg) was purified by semi-preparative HPLC on a Lichrosorb RP-18 (250 × 10 mm, 7 µm) column with a gradient of 2–50 % methanol in water within 25 min at a flow of 1 mL/min. The oven temperature was set to 20 °C and the UV-detector signal to 350 nm, resulting in 7.91 mg of compound **1**. Fraction DV-W-R14 (123 mg) was re-chromatographed on a smaller C18 column using flash chromatography which resulted in 2.6 mg of compound **8**. The samples were dissolved in deuterated water with sodium trimethylsilyl propionate (TSP) as internal standard and in case of 3,6,7-trihydroxycoumarin deuterated methanol was used. NMR data of the isolated coumarins are summarized in Table 1. The shift values for thyc were in good agreement to literature values [16]. NMR spectra for the novel sulfated coumarins **1** and **2** are shown in Figure 1A–D and Figure 2A–D in the Supplementary Material. Compounds **3** and **4** are known natural products. Their structures were identified by comparison of their reported spectroscopic data, including ESI-MS and NMR data:

6,7-Dihydroxycoumarin-3-sulfate (**3**, Figure 1): UV_{max} 268, 346 nm. It was assigned with a molecular formula $C_9H_5O_8S$ of ESI-MS, m/z 272.98 $[M-H]^-$. ^{1}H-NMR (600 MHz, D_2O + 0.05% TSP) δ(ppm): 7.87 (s, 1H), 7.10 (s, 1H), 6.95 (s, 1H) ^{13}C NMR δ(ppm): 163.6 (C-2), 135.9 (C-3), 135.8 (C-4), 115.7 (C-5), 145.1 (C-6), 151.8 (C-7), 106.0 (C-8), 149.7 (C-9), 114.2 (C-10) [9].

3,6,7-Trihydroxycoumarin (**4**, Figure 1): UV_{max} 268, 346 nm. It was assigned with a molecular formula $C_9H_6O_5$ of ESI-MS, m/z 193.14 $[M-H]^-$. ^{1}H-NMR (600 MHz, D_2O + 0.05% TSP) δ(ppm): 6.94 (s, 1H), 6.79 (s, 1H), 6.73 (s, 1H) ^{13}C-NMR δ (ppm): 161.7 (C-2), 140.3 (C-3), 117.6 (C-4), 111.6 (C-5), 144.5 (C-6), 148.0 (C-7), 103.5 (C-8), 145.3 (C-9), 113.9 (C-10) [16].

4.5. Sample Preparation

The powdered dried alga (200 mg) was extracted three times with 8 mL of water: methanol (1:1) each by 15 min of sonication (Sonorex 35 KHz, Bandelin, Berlin, Germany). After centrifugation (1000× *g* for 3 min), the supernatants were combined in a 25 mL volumetric flask. Samples were measured immediately after extraction.

4.6. Analytical Conditions

Experiments were performed on an Agilent 1100 HPLC system using a Gemini C18, 110 Å column (150 × 4.6 mm, 3 µm) from Phenomenex (Aschaffenburg, Germany). The mobile phase (A) contained water with 20 mM ammonium acetate and 1.5% acetic acid and (B) methanol/water (9:1) with 20 mM ammonium acetate and 1.5% acetic acid. Elution was performed in gradient mode starting with 2% B to 15% B from 0 to 5 min, 15% B to 60% B from 5–20 min and 60% B to 98% B from 20–25 min, followed by 10 min of re-equilibration with 98% A. The DAD was set to 254 nm and 350 nm, and flow rate, sample volume and column temperature were adjusted to 0.3 L/min, 5 µL and 40 °C, respectively. HPLC-MS experiments were carried out on an Agilent 1260 HPLC system coupled to an amaZon iontrap mass spectrometer (Bruker, Bremen, Germany). The chromatographic conditions were as described before; MS-spectra were recorded in negative ESI mode, with a drying gas temperature of 220 °C, the nebulizer gas (nitrogen) set to 23 psi, and a nebulizer flow (nitrogen) of 6 L/min. The scanned mass range was between m/z 70–1500, at a capillary voltage of 4.5 kV.

4.7. Synthesis of 4-(sulfooxy)benzoic Acid and Synthesis of 4-(sulfooxy)phenylacetic Acid

The synthesis of the two sulfated phenolic acids **5** and **6** was carried out as described recently by Kurth et al. [14], however using smaller quantities. 4-Hydroxybenzoic acid (1.5 g), sulfur trioxide pyridine complex (Pyr*SO_3, 1.72 g) were dissolved in water free pyridine (25 mL) and stirred in a 250 mL round bottomed flask at 25 °C for 48 h. For the synthesis of SPA, 4-hydroxyphenylacetic acid (0.75 g) and sulfur trioxide pyridine complex (Pyr*SO_3, 0.83 g) were used. Subsequently, the pyridine was removed by evaporation at 40 °C under reduced pressure. The remaining yellow-brown oil was dissolved in water (20 mL, HPLC grade) and the solution adjusted to pH 6–7 (pH-Meter, Mettler Toledo, Greifensee, Switzerland) using 25% potassium hydroxide. The aqueous solution was washed three times in a separatory funnel. A white precipitate was formed and filtered off after phase separation. Subsequently, the clear aqueous solution was evaporated at 45 °C under reduced pressure to give a white residue, which was re-dissolved in water and adjusted to pH 10 again using 25% KOH. To cleave the anhydride side products this solution was stirred at 60 °C for 1 h and subsequently neutralized using diluted sulfuric acid and afterwards evaporated again. The yellow-white residue was suspended in 10 mL water at 40 °C (5 mL for the synthesis of SPA). A white precipitate was formed by adding 20 mL (10 mL) of methanol, which was filtered off and subsequently washed with 10 mL (5 mL) of methanol. The methanol fractions were combined and left at 4 °C for 24 h in the fridge, so that a crystalline precipitate was formed; it was filtered off and the solution evaporated to dryness. The so obtained raw product was suspended in the ultrasonic bath using 2 mL (1 mL) methanol (HPLC-grade), which resulted in a white powder in a yellow solution. This step was repeated twice. Finally the product was washed with acetone and dried at 70 °C to give 660.93 mg (44% yield) SBA and 253.86 mg SPA (33.8% yield).

SBA: ^{1}H-NMR (600 MHz, D_2O + 0.05% TSP) δ(ppm): 7.91 (d, 2H; J = 8.4 Hz); 7.36 (d, 2H; J = 8.4 Hz), ^{13}C-NMR δ(ppm): 177.7(C, C-1), 123.9 (C, C-2), 136.8 (CH,C-3,C-7), 133.3 (CH, C-4,C-6), 156.4 (C, C-5) HPLC–MS m/z [M − H]$^-$: 216.99

SPA: ^{1}H-NMR (600 MHz, D_2O + 0.05% TSP) δ(ppm): 3.55 (s, 2H; J = 8.4 Hz), 7.26 (d, 2H; J = 8.5 Hz), 7.32 (d, 2H), ^{13}C-NMR δ(ppm): 183.5 (C, C-1), 46.5 (CH_2, C-2), 124.2 (C, C-3), 133.1 (CH,C5; CH, C7), 138.1 (CH,C4; CH,C8), 152.3 (C, C-6), HPLC–MS m/z [M − H]$^-$: 231.00.

4.8. Synthesis of 3,6,7-trihydroxycoumarin

The synthesis of thyc was performed as previously published by Cotelle et al. [26] Briefly, 2,4,5 trihydroxybenzaldehyde (2.31 g), acetylglycine (2.10 g) and sodium acetate (1.59 g) were weighted into a round bottomed flask (100 mL), acetic anhydride (7.5 g) was added and the mixture was heated under reflux for 4 h (130 °C). The solution was cooled to room temperature and ice water (10 mL) was added. The precipitate was filtered, washed with ethanol/water (50:50) and dried to give 3-acetamido-6,7-diacetoxycoumarin. A solution of this intermediate (1.59 g) in 3 M HCl (50 mL) plus acetic acid (2 mL) was refluxed for 1 h and subsequently cooled to room temperature. The obtained precipitate was washed again with water to give pure 3,6,7-trihydroxycoumarin (667.2 mg).

Supplementary Materials: The following are available online. Table S1: Origin of analyzed samples, Figure S2A–E: NMR spectra and HR-ESI-MS spectra of Compound **1**, Figure S3A–E: NMR spectra and HR-ESI-MS spectra of Compound **2,** Figure S4: UV spectra of the 4 Coumarins recorded on line by DAD, Figure S5: Determination of coumarins (**1**: dasycladin A, **2**: dasycladin B, **3**: 6,7-dihydroxycoumarin-3sulfate, **4**: 3,6,7-trihydroxycoumarin) in the marine green alga *Dasycladus vermicularis*.

Author Contributions: A.H. did all analytical work, isolated/elucidated the coumarins and wrote the manuscript; M.G. aided in analytical questions and corrected the manuscript; U.K. supplied and identified the algae and edited the first draft. A.S. aided in the structure elucidation of the novel coumarins.

Funding: This work was financially supported by the Austrian Science Fund (FWF), project P296710 and EMBO (ASTF 448-2016).

Acknowledgments: We thank Barbara Matuszczak for measuring the IR spectra.

Conflicts of Interest: The authors declare no conflict of interest.

References

1. Guiry, M.D.; Guiry, M.D.; Guiry, G.M. *AlgaeBase*; World-Wide Electronic Publication, National University of Ireland: Galway, Ireland. Available online: http://www.algaebase.org (accessed on 18 October 2018).
2. Carrillo, J.M.A. Algunas observaciones sobre la distribucion vertical de las algas en la Isla del Hierro (canarias). *Vieraea. Fol. Sci. Biol. Canar.* **1980**, *10*, 3–16.
3. Menzel, D.; Kazlauskas, R.; Reichelt, J. Coumarins in the Siphonalean Green Algal Family Dasycladaceae Kutzing (Chlorophyceae). *Bot. Mar.* **1983**, *26*, 23–29. [CrossRef]
4. Gomez, I.; Pérez-Rodríguez, E.; Viñegla, B.; Figueroa, F.L.; Karsten, U. Effects of solar radiation on photosynthesis, UV-absorbing compounds and enzyme activities of the green alga *Dasycladus vermicularis* from southern Spain. *J. Photochem. Photobiol. B* **1998**, *47*, 46–57. [CrossRef]
5. Perez-Rodriguez, E.; Aguilera, J.; Gomez, I.; Figueroa, F.L. Excretion of coumarins by the Mediterranean green alga *Dasycladus vermicularis* in response to environmental stress. *Mar. Biol.* **2001**, *139*, 633–639. [CrossRef]
6. Perez-Rodriguez, E.; Aguilera, J.; Figueroa, F.L. Tissular localization of coumarins in the green alga *Dasycladus vermicularis* (Scopoli) Krasser: A photoprotective role? *J. Exp. Bot.* **2003**, *54*, 1093–1100. [CrossRef] [PubMed]
7. Coneva, V.; Chitwood, D.H. Plant architecture without multicellularity: Quandaries over patterning and the soma-germline divide in siphonous algae. *Front. Plant. Sci.* **2015**, *6*, 287. [CrossRef] [PubMed]
8. Welling, M.; Pohnert, G.; Küppert, F.C.; Ross, C. Rapid Biopolymerisation During Wound Plug Formation in Green Algae. *J. Adhes.* **2009**, *85*, 825–838. [CrossRef]
9. Welling, M.; Ross, C.; Pohnert, G.A. Desulfatation-Oxidation Cascade Activates Coumarin-Based Cross-Linkers in the Wound Reaction of the Giant Unicellular Alga *Dasycladus vermicularis*. *Angew. Chem.-Int. E* **2011**, *50*, 7691–7694. [CrossRef] [PubMed]
10. Ross, C.; Vreeland, V.; Waite, J.H.; Jacobs, R.S. Rapid assembly of a wound plug: Stage one of a two-stage wound repair mechanism in the giant unicellular chlorophyte *Dasycladus vermicularis* (Chlorophyceae). *J. Phycol.* **2005**, *41*, 46–54. [CrossRef]
11. Sever, M.J.; Weisser, J.T.; Monahan, J.; Srinivasan, S.; Wilker, J.J. Metal-mediated cross-linking in the generation of a marine-mussel adhesive. *Angew. Chem.-Int. E.* **2004**, *43*, 448–450. [CrossRef] [PubMed]
12. Thoms, C.; Schupp, P.J. Activated chemical defense in marine sponges—A case study on *Aplysinella rhax*. *J. Chem. Ecol.* **2008**, *34*, 1242–1252. [CrossRef] [PubMed]
13. Kurth, C.; Cavas, L.; Pohnert, G. Sulfation mediates activity of zosteric acid against biofilm formation. *Biofouling* **2015**, *31*, 253–263. [CrossRef] [PubMed]
14. Kurth, C.; Welling, M.; Pohnert, G. Sulfated phenolic acids from Dasycladales siphonous green algae. *Phytochemtry* **2015**, *117*, 417–423. [CrossRef] [PubMed]
15. Haensel, R.; Sticher, O. *Pharmakognosie Phytopharmazie*, 9th ed.; Springer Medizin Verlag GmbH: Heidelberg, Germany, 2010; pp. 419–420.
16. Bailly, F.; Maurin, C.; Teissier, E.; Vezin, H.; Cotelle, P. Antioxidant properties of 3-hydroxycoumarin derivatives. *Bioorg. Med. Chem.* **2004**, *12*, 5611–5618. [CrossRef] [PubMed]
17. ICH Harmonization for Better Health. Available online: http://www.ich.org/products/guidelines.html (accessed on 6 August 2018).
18. Zhu, J.J.; Jiang, J.G. Pharmacological and Nutritional Effects of Natural Coumarins and Their Structure-Activity Relationships. *Mol. Nutr. Food Res.* **2018**, *62*, 1701073. [CrossRef] [PubMed]
19. Kayser, O.; Kolodziej, H. Antibacterial Activity of Simple Coumarins: Structural Requirements for Biological Activity. *Naturforschung C* **1999**, *54*, 169. [CrossRef]
20. Aihara, K.; Higuchi, T.; Hirobe, M. 3-Hydroxycoumarins: First direct preparation from coumarins using a $Cu^{2(+)}$-ascorbic acid-O_2 system, and their potent bioactivities. *Biochem. Biophys. Res. Commun.* **1990**, *168*, 169–175. [CrossRef]
21. Verespy, S.; Metha, A.Y.; Afosah, D.; Al-Horani, R.A.; Desai, U.R. Allosteric partial Inhibition of Monomeric Proteases. Sulfated Coumarins Induce Regulation, not just Inhibition of Thrombin. *Sci. Rep.* **2016**, *6*, 24043. [CrossRef] [PubMed]

22. Li, B.; Zhang, X.; Wang, J.; Zhang, Z.; Gao, B.; Shi, S.; Wang, X.; Li, J.; Tu, P. Simultaneous characterization of fifty coumarins from the roots of *Angelica dahurica* by off-line two-dimensional high-performance liquid chromatography coupled with electrospray ionization tandem mass spectrometry. *Phytochem. Anal.* **2014**, *25*, 229–240. [CrossRef] [PubMed]
23. Wu, Y.; Wang, F.; Ai, Y.; Ma, W.; Bian, Q.; Lee, D.; Dai, R. Simultaneous determination of seven coumarins by UPLC-MS/MS: Application to a comparative pharmacokinetic study in normal and arthritic rats after administration of Huo Luo Xiao Ling Dan or single herb. *J. Chromatogr. B* **2015**, *991*, 108–117. [CrossRef] [PubMed]
24. Li, G.J.; Wu, H.J.; Wang, Y.; Hung, W.L.; Rouseff, R.L. Determination of citrus juice coumarins, furanocoumarins and methoxylated flavones using solid phase extraction and HPLC with photodiode array and fluorescence detection. *Food Chem.* **2019**, *15*, 29–38. [CrossRef] [PubMed]
25. Schoenwaelder, M.E.A. The Biology of Phenolic Containing Vesicles. *Algae* **2008**, *23*, 163–175. [CrossRef]
26. Cotelle, P.; Vezin, H. EPR of free radicals formed from 3-hydroxyesculetin and related derivatives. *Res. Chem. Intermed.* **2003**, *29*, 365–377. [CrossRef]

Sample Availability: Samples of the compounds/fractions are available from the authors upon request.

molecules

MDPI

Article

Antinociceptive Effects of Cardamonin in Mice: Possible Involvement of $TRPV_1$, Glutamate, and Opioid Receptors

Chung Pui Ping [1], Tengku Azam Shah Tengku Mohamad [1], Muhammad Nadeem Akhtar [2], Enoch Kumar Perimal [1], Ahmad Akira [1], Daud Ahmad Israf Ali [1,3] and Mohd Roslan Sulaiman [1,3,*]

1 Department of Biomedical Sciences, Faculty of Medicine and Health Sciences, Universiti Putra Malaysia Selangor, Serdang 43400, Malaysia; puiping.chung@gmail.com (C.P.P.); azamshah@upm.edu.my (T.A.S.T.M.); enoch@upm.edu.my (E.K.P.); ahmadakira@upm.edu.my (A.A.); daudaia@upm.edu.my (D.A.I.A.)
2 Laboratory of Natural Products, Institute of Bioscience, Universiti Putra Malaysia, Selangor, Serdang 43400, Malaysia; nadeemupm@gmail.com
3 Faculty of Industrial Sciences & Technology, University Malaysia Pahang, Pahang, Gambang 26300, Malaysia
* Correspondence: mrs@upm.edu.my; Tel.: +60-38-947-2346

Received: 3 July 2018; Accepted: 30 July 2018; Published: 3 September 2018

Abstract: Pain is one of the most common cause for hospital visits. It plays an important role in inflammation and serves as a warning sign to avoid further injury. Analgesics are used to manage pain and provide comfort to patients. However, prolonged usage of pain treatments like opioids and NSAIDs are accompanied with undesirable side effects. Therefore, research to identify novel compounds that produce analgesia with lesser side effects are necessary. The present study investigated the antinociceptive potentials of a natural compound, cardamonin, isolated from *Boesenbergia rotunda* (L) Mansf. using chemical and thermal models of nociception. Our findings showed that intraperitoneal and oral administration of cardamonin (0.3, 1, 3, and 10 mg/kg) produced significant and dose-dependent inhibition of pain in abdominal writhing responses induced by acetic acid. The present study also demonstrated that cardamonin produced significant analgesia in formalin-, capsaicin-, and glutamate-induced paw licking tests. In the thermal-induced nociception model, cardamonin exhibited significant increase in response latency time of animals subjected to hot-plate thermal stimuli. The rota-rod assessment confirmed that the antinociceptive activities elicited by cardamonin was not related to muscle relaxant or sedative effects of the compound. In conclusion, the present findings showed that cardamonin exerted significant peripheral and central antinociception through chemical- and thermal-induced nociception in mice through the involvement of $TRPV_1$, glutamate, and opioid receptors.

Keywords: cardamonin; antinociceptive; $TRPV_1$; glutamate; opioid

1. Introduction

Cardamonin or 2′,4′-dihydroxy-6′-methoxychalcone ($C_{16}H_{14}O_4$) is a naturally occurring chalcone. Cardamonin was firstly isolated from the seeds of *Amomum subulatum* [1] and later from other plant species, such as *Boesenbergia pandurata*, *Alpinia rafflesiana*, *Alpinia katsumadai*, *Alpinia henryi*, and *Campomanesia adamantium*. Previous report showed that cardamonin exerted antiproliferative activity and induced apoptosis in PC-3 [2], myeloma [3], and A549 cell lines [4]. In addition, cardamonin was capable to protect lipopolysaccharide (LPS)-induced septic mice against acute lung injury [5] and showed nephroprotective effect against cisplatin-induced renal injury [6]. Furthermore, cardamonin could exert inhibition of platelet aggregation [7], vasorelaxant effect [8], improvement in insulin resistance and vascular complication in a high fructose-fed rat model [9], suppression of lipid accumulation in vitro [10], inhibition of pigmentation in human normal melanocytes [11], and anti-pruritic activity [12].

In vitro study showed that cardamonin inhibits the release of pro-inflammatory mediators [13] and it was supported by the findings on inhibitory action of cardamonin upon the expression of NO and PGE_2 via interruption of the NF-κB pathway [14,15]. This mechanism of action is common to phenolic compounds showing protective effects [16,17]. In vivo study also presented the capability of cardamonin in suppressing NO generation in LPS-challenged ICR mice [18]. NO has been reported to be involved in generation of pain perception through a series of pathway [19]. Since cardamonin reduces generation of NO, we believe that cardamonin may show antinociceptive activityies.

Recently, the antinociceptive profile of cardamonin has been reported through PBQ-induced writhing and carrageenan-induced hyperalgesia test [20], but there is still no report on the possible mechanism of antinociceptive action of cardamonin. Thus, the present study was aimed to examine the antinociceptive effect of cardamonin in chemical- and thermal-induced nociception using mice models.

2. Results

2.1. *Evaluation of the Antinociceptive Activity*

2.1.1. Acetic Acid–Induced Abdominal Writhing Test

The effect of cardamonin in acetic acid-induced abdominal writhing response in mice is depicted in Figure 1. Cardamonin produced significant reduction in the number of writhing in both routes of administration, intraperitoneally (Panel a) and orally (Panel b) at $p < 0.001$. Cardamonin administered intraperitoneally (i.p.) showed 45, 56, 80, and 100% of inhibition against acetic acid-induced pain as compared to control at doses of 0.3, 1, 3, and 10 mg/kg respectively, with calculated ED_{50} (and its respective confidence interval) of 2.1 (1.9–2.5) mg/kg. Oral administration (p.o.) of cardamonin exhibited 39%, 40%, 63% and 77% of inhibition as compared to control at doses of 0.3, 1, 3, and 10 mg/kg, respectively, with calculated ED_{50} (and its respective confidence interval) of 2.5 (2.0–3.3) mg/kg. Indomethacin, produced significant inhibition in acetic acid-induced abdominal pain with 80% (i.p.) and 60% (p.o.) of inhibition respectively, as compared to control at $p < 0.001$.

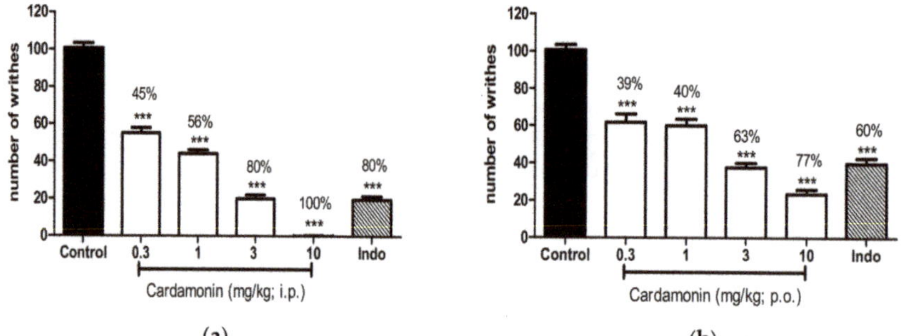

Figure 1. (**a**) Effect of cardamonin (0.3, 1, 3, 10 mg/kg, i.p.) administered intraperitoneally against acetic acid-induced nociception. (**b**) Effect of cardamonin (0.3, 1, 3, 10 mg/kg, i.p.) administered orally against acetic acid-induced nociception. Each column represents the mean ± S.E.M. of 6 mice. Control group received only the vehicle (ethanol: Tween 20: distilled water in 5:5:90, *v*/*v*/*v*) used to dilute the compound. Indomethacin (Indo, 10 mg/kg) was used as positive control. The asterisks denote the significance levels compared with the control group (one-way ANOVA, followed by Dunnett's post hoc test); *** $p < 0.001$. Values in parentheses were percentage of inhibition.

2.1.2. Formalin-Induced Paw Licking Test

Cardamonin treated animals showed significant analgesic effect on both early neurogenic phase (0–5 min) and late inflammatory phase (15–35 min) in the formalin-induced paw licking test as shown in Figure 2 (Panel a and b respectively). Cardamonin inhibited the inflammatory pain better in comparison with the neurogenic pain at all dosage use, especially at 1 mg/kg (98%) and 3 mg/kg (99%) against inflammatory pain. Morphine (5 mg/kg; s.c.) produced significant inhibition ($p < 0.001$) against formalin-induced pain at both the early neurogenic phase (96%) and late inflammatory phase (99%). In contrast, indomethacin significantly inhibits formalin-induced pain better at the late inflammatory phase (70% of inhibition) than the early neurogenic phase (31% of inhibition).

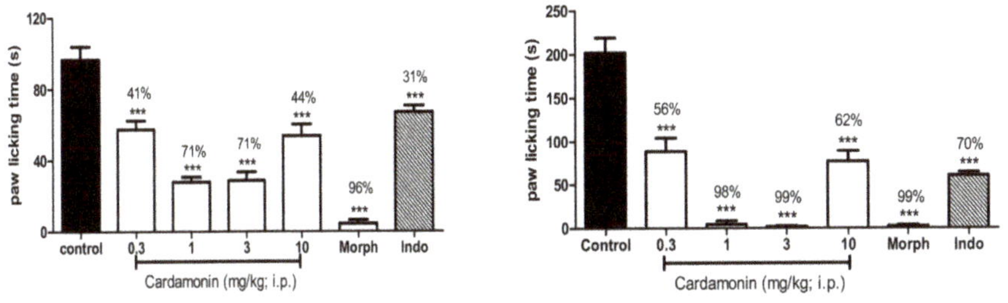

(**a**) (**b**)

Figure 2. (**a**) Effect of cardamonin (0.3, 1, 3, 10 mg/kg, i.p.) in formalin-induced paw licking test (early phase) in mice. (**b**) Effect of cardamonin (0.3, 1, 3, 10 mg/kg, i.p.) in formalin-induced paw licking test (late phase) in mice. Each column represents the mean ± S.E.M. of 6 mice. Control group received only the vehicle used to dilute the compound. Morphine (Morph, 5 mg/kg, s.c.) and indomethacin (Indo, 10 mg/kg, i.p.) were used as positive control. The asterisks denote the significance levels compared with the control group (one-way ANOVA, followed by Dunnett's post hoc test); *** $p < 0.001$. Values in parentheses were percentage of inhibition.

2.1.3. Hot Plate Test

i.p. administration of cardamonin and morphine significantly increased the latency time of nociceptive responses in the hot plate test at the temperature of 52 ± 0.2 °C compared with vehicle-treated animals (Table 1).

Table 1. Effect of cardamonin on the hot plate test in mice. Results were expressed in mean ± S.E.M of latency time (s) of 6 mice. Statistical significance was determined by two-way ANOVA followed by Bonferroni post hoc test.

Treatment	Dose	Latency Time (s)							
	(mg/kg)	0 min	30 min	60 min	90 min	120 min	150 min	180 min	210 min
Control		6.17 ± 0.17	6.83 ± 0.31	6.67 ± 0.33	6.67 ± 0.21	6.83 ± 0.31	6.67 ± 0.21	6.83 ± 0.31	6.33 ± 0.21
Cardamonin (i.p.)	0.3	6.34 ± 0.16	6.99 ± 0.52	7.01 ± 0.27	8.26 ± 0.33	8.28 ± 0.56	9.08 ± 1.09 *	8.36 ± 0.59	6.83 ± 0.55
	1	7.05 ± 0.22	6.84 ± 0.56	7.03 ± 0.16	7.11 ± 0.28	8.04 ± 0.67	8.97 ± 0.44 *	8.50 ± 0.37	7.22 ± 0.26
	3	6.95 ± 0.25	6.83 ± 0.25	7.59 ± 0.25	7.65 ± 0.16	8.37 ± 0.41	8.92 ± 0.24 *	7.52 ± 0.51	6.71 ± 0.36
	10	6.63 ± 0.20	7.45 ± 0.46	8.08 ± 0.46	9.14 ± 0.72 *	10.09 ± 0.89 ***	9.21 ± 0.83 **	8.07 ± 0.33	7.48 ± 0.15
Naloxone (i.p.) + Cardamonin (i.p.)	1 + 5	7.30 ± 0.24	8.70 ± 0.28	8.54 ± 0.32	8.60 ± 0.25	11.33 ± 0.59 ###	11.62 ± 0.50 ##	9.40 ± 0.58	8.45 ± 0.66
Morphine (s.c.)	5	7.50 ± 0.34	18.33 ± 0.67 ***	17.00 ± 0.82 ***	16.33 ± 0.42 ***	16.33 ± 0.99 ***	15.33 ± 0.62 ***	15.17 ± 0.40 ***	14.83 ± 0.40 ***
Naloxone (i.p.) + Morphine (s.c.)	5 + 5	7.30 ± 0.29	8.93 ± 0.82 ###	11.18 ± 0.74 ###	10.76 ± 0.61 ###	10.10 ± 0.84 ###	9.01 ± 0.83 ###	7.64 ± 0.30 ###	6.92 ± 0.30 ###

* $p < 0.05$ as compared to control; ** $p < 0.01$ as compared to control; *** $p < 0.001$ as compared to control; ## $p < 0.01$ as compared to the group receiving appropriate drug/compound at the same dose without naloxone; ### $p < 0.001$ as compared to the group receiving appropriate drug/compound at the same dose without naloxone.

2.2. *Investigation of the Mechanisms of Action*

2.2.1. Involvement of the $TRPV_1$ Receptor

Cardamonin showed significant inhibition against capsaicin-induced nociception at 1, 3 and 10 mg/kg with $p < 0.001$ in Figure 3. The maximum inhibition was produced by cardamonin at the dose of 3 mg/kg with 66% inhibition compared to control. Likewise, capsazepine and indomethacin significantly exhibited 89% and 74% inhibition, respectively.

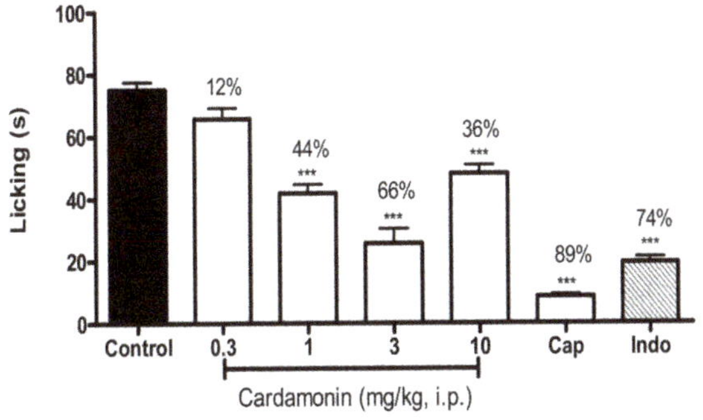

Figure 3. Effect of cardamonin (0.3, 1, 3, 10 mg/kg, i.p.) against capsaicin-induced nociception. Each column represents the mean ± S.E.M. of 6 mice. Control group receives only the vehicle used to dilute the compound. Capsazepine (Cap, 0.17 mmol/kg, i.p.) was used as the positive control for capsaicin-induced nociception. Indomethacin (Indo, 10 mg/kg, i.p.) was used as positive control. The asterisks denote the significance levels compared with the control group (one-way ANOVA, followed by Dunnett's post hoc test); *** $p < 0.001$. Values in parentheses are percentage of inhibition.

2.2.2. Involvement of the Glutamate Receptor

Using the glutamate-induced nociception study, it was observed that cardamonin produced significant antinociceptive activities at all dosage (Figure 4). The percentage of inhibition for were 46%, 44%, 66%, and 84% for 0.3, 1, 3, and 10 mg/kg of cardamonin, respectively, as in comparison with control. Indomethacin showed 69% of significant inhibition against glutamate-induced nociception at $p < 0.001$.

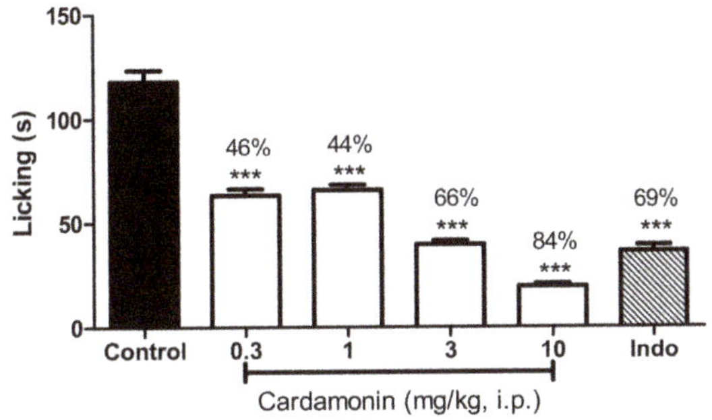

Figure 4. Effect of cardamonin (0.3, 1, 3, 10 mg/kg, i.p.) against glutamate-induced nociception. Each column represents the mean ± S.E.M. of 6 mice. Control group receives only the vehicle used to dilute the compound. Indomethacin (Indo, 10 mg/kg, i.p.) was used as positive control. The asterisks denote the significance levels compared with the control group (one-way ANOVA, followed by Dunnett's post hoc test), *** $p < 0.001$. Values in parentheses are percentage of inhibition.

2.2.3. Involvement of the Opioid Receptors

Pre-treatment of mice with the non-specific opioid receptor antagonist, naloxone (5 mg/kg; i.p.) significantly reversed the antinociceptive effect of cardamonin (1 mg/kg; i.p.) at $p < 0.001$ only in the early neurogenic phase, but not the late inflammatory phase (Figure 5). The effect of morphine (5 mg/kg; s.c.) was significantly reversed by naloxone in both the early neurogenic phase as well as late inflammatory phase. This suggested that opioid system might be involved in the centrally activated antinociceptive activity by cardamonin.

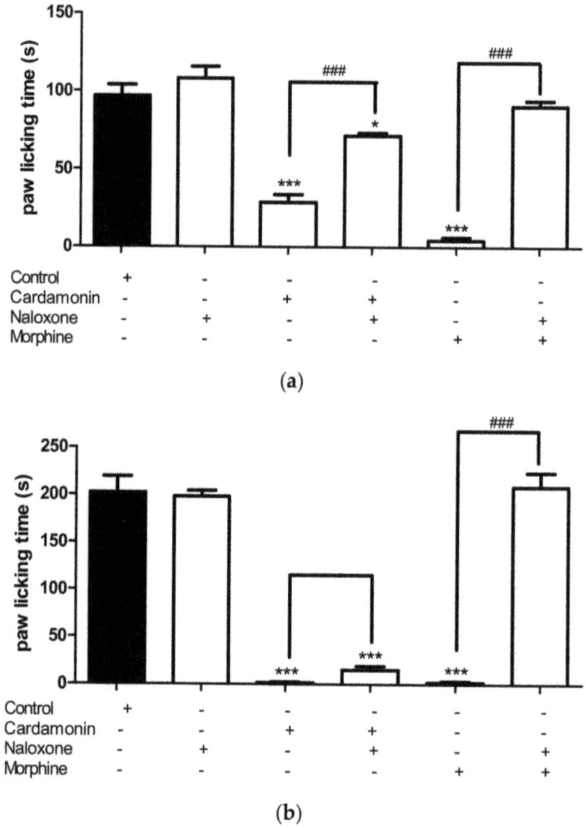

Figure 5. (**a**) Effect of naloxone (5 mg/kg, i.p.) on antinociception caused by cardamonin (1 mg/kg, i.p.) in the early phase in formalin-induced paw licking test. (**b**) Effect of naloxone (5 mg/kg, i.p.) on antinociception caused by cardamonin (1 mg/kg, i.p.) in the and the late phase in formalin-induced paw licking test. The asterisks and hash denote the significance levels (one-way ANOVA, followed by Tukey's post hoc test), * $p < 0.05$, *** $p < 0.001$, ### $p < 0.001$.

2.3. *Toxicity Assessment*

After seven days of observation, no mortality was reported at all doses of cardamonin used. During the observation period, the animals did not show any signs of abnormal behavior and locomotor activity. The observations were done qualitatively.

2.4. Motor Coordination Evaluation

Animals subjected to rota rod task after administration of cardamonin (10 mg/kg; i.p.) did not show any disturbance in motor coordination. The mean ± S.E.M. in the rota rod test for control, cardamonin (10 mg/kg) and diazepam (4 mg/kg) were 114.7 ± 5.33 s, 120.0 ± 0.00 s, and 38.83 ± 4.38 s, respectively.

3. Discussion

According to the Third National Health and Morbidity Survey 2006, 7% of the Malaysian population were suffering from chronic persistent pain [21]. Chronic pain has become a prevalent health problem among the older generation in Malaysia [22]. This has led to higher hospitalization rates among the elderly and severely interferes with the quality of life.

Non-steroidal anti-inflammatory drugs (NSAIDs), opioids, and analgesic adjuvants are the major classes of pharmacological therapies for pain relief currently available in modern medicine [23]. In spite of pain relieving effects, prolonged usage of these drugs leads to undesirable side effects such as gastrointestinal bleeding, renal toxicity, hypotension and respiratory depression [24,25]. These adverse effects have limited the usage of well-known effective pain relieving medicines. Research has been continuously carried out to seek for alternative pharmacologically potent analgesic treatment with fewer or milder side effects.

Previous studies have demonstrated an increase in NOS and TNF-α gene expression in the injected paw of animals after intraplantar administration of CFA [26]. It was postulated that NO capable of inducing peripheral hyperalgesia by regulating the expression of cyclooxygenase (COX) which then results in an increase of prostaglandin release [27]. Thus, with the reports of the inhibitory effect of cardamonin upon the release of pro-inflammatory mediators and also inhibition of both the NO and PGE_2 [13–15], we suggest that cardamonin possess antinociceptive effect in both chemical- and thermal-induced nociception models in mice.

The present study demonstrated the antinociceptive effects of cardamonin, either through intraperitoneal or oral administration, at doses that did not produce impairment of motor coordination. It showed a dose-dependent inhibition in acetic acid-induced abdominal writhing test in mice. This result support the finding on antinociceptive activity of cardamonin in PBQ-induced writhing test [20]. The acetic acid–induced abdominal writhing model has been utilized as a screening tool for the assessment of antinociceptive and also anti-inflammatory properties of potential analgesic agents [28]. Following acetic acid administration into the peritoneal cavity of the animals, chemical mediators released directly or indirectly at the free nerve endings of sensory polymodal neurons. They also reported on the increase level of prostaglandins, especially PGE_2 in the peritoneal fluid following acetic acid injection [29]. In line with the in vitro finding where cardamonin exerted inhibitory action of PGE_2 secretion and down regulation of COX-2 gene expression, we suggest that the antinociceptive mechanism of cardamonin may be linked partly to the disruption of the LOX and/or COX in the peripheral tissues, leading to decrease in PGE_2 synthesis, which then interferes with the mechanism of signal transduction in primary afferent nociceptors. It has also been previously reported that cardamonin inhibits inflammatory cytokines like TNF-α, IL-1β and IL-6 and interferes with the NF-κB signaling pathway [15] that may additionally explain the antinociceptive effects of cardamonin.

The commonly used analgesic agent NSAIDs inhibits the synthesis of prostaglandin, and in the present study, indomethacin exerted a significant inhibition in the acetic acid–induced pain model. As shown in Figure 2, cardamonin at the dose of 3 mg/kg has similar analgesic effect as indomethacin at dose 10 mg/kg. However, acetic acid–induced nociceptive model has good sensitivity but poor specificity. This is due to the suppressing effect of abdominal writhes by muscle relaxants or other types of drugs to misinterpretation of the results [30,31]. Thus, formalin-induced paw licking and hot plate test were carried out in the present study to avoid this problem.

The responses of formalin-induced paw licking is biphasic [32]. The first phase reflects the neurogenic pain whereby formalin-injected into the paw directly sensitize the C-fiber primary afferent nociceptors. The second phase is the result of inflammatory response caused by the action of inflammatory mediators, or to some extent, the central sensitization of the dorsal horn neurons [32,33]. Substance P and bradykinin was reported release during the neurogenic phase, whereas histamine, serotonin, prostaglandins and also bradykinin were involved in the inflammatory phase [34]. Centrally acting analgesics such as morphine inhibit nociception in both phases equally; in contrast, peripherally acting analgesics such as indomethacin only inhibit the second phase [33,34]. The present study indicates that cardamonin at all doses reduce paw lickings induced by formalin in both phases. Thus it was suggested that cardamonin works both centrally and peripherally, which also implies that cardamonin not only possess antinociceptive response but also anti-inflammatory activity.

In line with its centrally acting properties, cardamonin exert significant prolongation in response latency time to thermal stimuli as in the hot plate assessment. Hot plate test is a sensitive and specific thermal model for the evaluation of the involvement of central analgesic activity, or in other words supra-spinal activity [35,36]. Thus, the present study provides strong evidence that cardamonin exert centrally mediated antinociceptive activity as it decreases nociception in the first phase of formalin test and increased nociceptive threshold in the hot plate test. In addition, pre-treatment with non-selective opioid antagonist, naloxone has significantly antagonized the antinociceptive effect of cardamonin and morphine in both the formalin-induced paw licking and hot plate test. These finding suggest that the central antinociceptive mechanism of cardamonin could involve the activation of opioid receptors or modulation of the effect of endogeneous opioid peptides.

In order to further understand the antinociceptive action of cardamonin, capsaicin-induced neurogenic paw licking test was carried out. Capsaicin, the pungent ingredient of hot chili peppers, upon administered, it directly stimulates the transient receptor potential cation channel V1 ($TRPV_1$) which found on the sensory C-fibers. Capsaicin also mediates the release of excitatory amino acids (glutamate and aspartate), nitric oxide and pro-inflammatory mediators and thus transmitting the nociceptive impulses to the central spinal system [37]. In this study, cardamonin also exhibit significant reduction in nociceptive responses in capsaicin-induced paw licking assessment.

Another interesting finding of this study reveals that cardamonin exhibit significant inhibitory nociceptive response against intraplantar injection of glutamate into mouse hind paw. Glutamate-induced nociceptive responses appears to involve peripheral, spinal and supra-spinal sites of action and is mediated by both of the activation of *N*-methyl-*D*-aspartate (NMDA) and α-amino-3-hydroxyl-5-methyl-isoxazolepropionate (non-NMDA) receptors, as well as by nitric oxide release or by some NO-derived substances. The release of nitric oxide eventually increased the synthesis or release of pro-inflammatory mediators such as cytokine, reactive oxygen species (ROS) as well as prostanoids followed by enhanced inflammatory reaction [38]. The present study strongly suggests that antinociceptive activity induced by cardamonin in the glutamate test, at least in part, could be due to its interaction with the glutamatergic system or its ability to inhibit NO production.

Finally, the present study provides convincing evidence that systemic administration of cardamonin was largely devoid of significant effect on motor coordination of animals in the rota rod assessment. Therefore, the possibility of non-specific muscle relaxation and sedative effects of cardamonin-induced antinociception could be eliminated. The result of preliminary acute toxicity investigation showed that no occurrence of animal mortality over the period of observation. The study conducted qualitatively by observing signs of toxicity indicated that cardamonin have a reasonably low toxicity profile and should be regarded as safe while detailed quantitative assessments to be carried out in the future.

4. Materials and Methods

4.1. Plant Material

Five kilograms of *Boesenbergia rotunda* were purchased from the local market in Serdang, Malaysia and was authenticated by a resident botanist at the Institute of Bioscience, Universiti Putra Malaysia (IBS, UPM), Malaysia. A voucher specimen (SK1780/10) was deposited at the Herbarium,

Laboratory of Natural Products, IBS, UPM and small part of the rhizomes were cultivated at the Medicinal Plant Garden, IBS, UPM for future reference.

4.2. Extraction and Isolation

The fresh rhizomes of *B. rotunda* were sliced into small flat pieces and dried under shadow for one weak. The dried rhizomes were ground into fine powder by using domestic food processor. The dried powder 2.5 kg was dissolved in distilled methanol for two-three days. The methanolic extract was filtrate and concentrate on rotary evaporator to obtained 255 gm crude extract. The methanolic extract was subjected to solvent extraction. The crude methanolic extract was dissolved in 250 mL distilled water and transferred into separating funnel. About 150 mL hexane was added into aqueous layer and subsequently extracted with chloroform, ethyl acetate, and butanol. The chloroform layer finally passed over sodium sulfate anhydrous to remove the moisture. The chloroform extract was subjected to flash column chromatography by using ethyl acetate and hexane as eluents. Finally, the compound (Figure 6) was purified from chloroform extract and identify as cardamonin (CARD) after performing the detailed NMR spectroscopic and chromatographic methods, respectively. The purity of the compound was 98.0%.

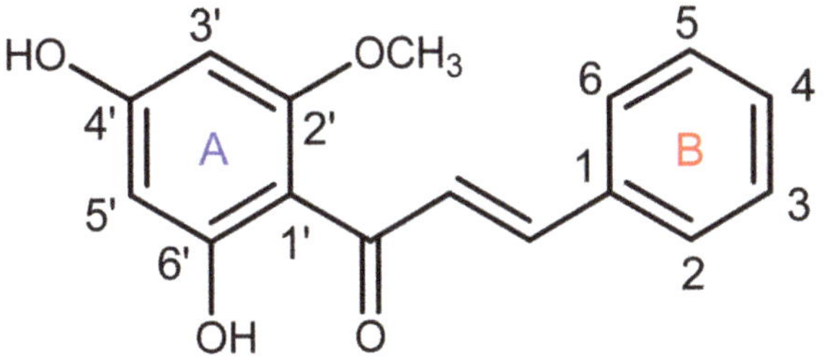

Figure 6. The chemical Structure of cardamonin.

(Cardamonin): (E)-1-(4′,6′dihydroxy-2′-methoxyphenyl)-3-phenylprop-2-en-1-one. (*E*)-1-(4′,6′-dihydroxy-2′-methoxyphenyl)-3-phenylprop-2-en-1-one: yellow needles crystals: m.p. 192–194 °C, EI-MS *m*/*z* 270.23, (molecular formula $C_{16}H_{16}O_4$). IR max (cm^{-1}, KBr disc): 3256 (OH), 1632 (C=O), 1544, 1490, 1288, 1326, 1228 cm^{-1}. ^{1}HNMR ($CDCl_3$, 500 MHz): δ 7.92 (d, 1H, J = 15.5 Hz, Hβ), 7.80 (d, 1H, J = 15.5 Hz, Hα), 7.62 (br, d, 2H, H-2,6), 7.46 (m, 3H, H-3,4,5), 6.12 (br, s, 1H, H-3′), 5.98 (br, s, 1H, H-5′), 3.85 (s, 3H, OMe, C-2′). int.): *m*/*z* 270 ([M^+], 269 (54), 253 (5), 193 (100), 131 (35, 103 (39), 77 (32).

4.3. Experimental Animals

All animal care and the antinociceptive experimental procedures performed were in accordance with the ethical guidelines for investigations of experimental pain in conscious animals (Zimmermann, 1983) and approved by the Animal Care Unit Committee (ACUC), Faculty of Medicine and Health Sciences, Universiti Putra Malaysia (UPM/FPSK/PADS/BR-UUH/00425). The antinociceptive experiments were carried out using male ICR mice (20–30 g). They were housed in groups of 10 per cage and maintained on a 12/12-h light/dark cycle (lights were switched on at 06:00 h), at the animal house facility, Faculty of Medicine and Health Sciences, Universiti Putra Malaysia. Food and water were available ad libitum, except during the experimental procedure. The animals were habituated to the condition of the laboratory at least 2 h before testing and were used only once throughout the experiments. The number of animals and intensities of noxious stimuli used were the minimum necessary to demonstrate consistent effects of drug treatments. All efforts were made to minimize animal suffering. At the end of the experiments, the animals were anesthetized and euthanized by cervical dislocation. In all experiments, data were collected by a blinded, randomized, and controlled design.

4.4. Drugs and Chemicals

Tween 20, absolute ethanol, acetic acid, formalin, morphine hydrochloride, naloxone, indomethacin, diazepam, capsaicin, capsazepine, and glutamate were purchased from Sigma Chemical Co. (St. Louis, MO, USA). All drugs used were dissolved in physiological saline (0.9% NaCl). Cardamonin and indomethacin were dissolved in ethanol, Tween 20 and distilled water in 5:5:90 (*v*/*v*/*v*) fractions. Respective controls received only solvent vehicle, whereby it had no effect per se on nociceptive responses. All drugs, chemicals, and CARD solutions were freshly prepared and administered intraperitoneally (i.p.) in a volume of 10 mL/kg, unless otherwise stated in the method.

4.5. Evaluation of the Antinociceptive Activity

4.5.1. Acetic Acid–Induced Abdominal Writhing Test

The acetic acid–induced abdominal writhing test was conducted as previously described [39]. Mice were pre-treated with CARD (0.3, 1, 3 and 10 mg/kg; i.p.), 30 min prior to injection of 0.6% acetic acid (10 mL/kg; i.p.). Indomethacin (10 mg/kg) was used as reference drug and was administered by i.p. route, 30 min before the nociceptive agent. Following the injection of acetic acid, the animals were immediately placed into a perspex chamber, and the number of writhing was recorded for 30 min, starting from 5 min post-injection. Antinociceptive activity of CARD was expressed as a reduction in the mean number of abdominal writhes in the group pre-treated with CARD compared with the control group.

4.5.2. Formalin-Induced Paw Licking Test

The formalin-induced paw licking test was carried out as previously described [40]. Mice used were individually adapted in an observation chamber made of transparent acrylic. CARD (0.3, 1, 3, and 10 mg/kg; i.p.) or vehicle (10 mL/kg; i.p.) was administered 30 min before the formalin injection. Indomethacin (10 mg/kg; i.p.) and morphine (5 mg/kg; s.c.) were used as positive control drug and were administered 30 min and 1 h before the test. After 30 min, 20 μL of 2.5% of formalin solution (*v*/*v* in distilled water) was injected subcutaneously into the ventral surface of the right hind paw of the mice. The amount of time (in seconds) spent on licking and biting the injected paw was recorded up to 35 min after formalin injection as an indicator of nociceptive behavior. The initial nociceptive scores normally peaked at 0–5 min (early phase) and 15–35 min (late phase) after formalin injection, representing the neurogenic and inflammatory pain responses, respectively.

4.5.3. Hot Plate Test

The antinociceptive property of cardamonin for thermal noxious stimuli was evaluated according to the method described previously [41]. The metal surface of the hot plate (Model 7280, Ugo Basile, VA, Italy) was set and maintained at temperature of 52 $\pm$ 0.2 °C. Mice were then placed into the Plexiglas cylinder on the heated metal surface individually and the time elapsed between placement and licking the forepaws, or jumping were recorded as response latency time. The reaction time was recorded before and at 30, 60, 90, 120, 180 and 210 min after administration of cardamonin (0.3, 1, 3, and 10 mg/kg; i.p.) or vehicle (10 mL/kg; i.p.). Morphine (5 mg/kg; s.c.) was used as a reference drug. A cut-off time of 20 s was defined as complete analgesia and to avoid tissue damage.

4.6. Investigation of the Mechanisms of Action

4.6.1. Involvement of the $TRPV_1$ Receptor

The involvement of $TRPV_1$ in antinociceptive activity by CARD was investigated by using capsaicin-induced paw licking model. The procedure implemented was similar to that described previously [42]. Mice were pre-treated with CARD (0.3, 1, 3, and 10 mg/kg; i.p.), capsazepine (0.17 mmol/kg; i.p.), indomethacin (10 mg/kg; i.p.) or vehicle (10 mL/kg; i.p.) prior to injection of

20 μL of capsaicin (1.6 μg/paw) intraplantarly (i.pl) into the ventral surface of the right hind paw of the mice. The animals were observed individually for 5 min after capsaicin injection. The amount of time spent licking the injected paw was recorded and was considered as an indication of pain behavior.

4.6.2. Involvement of the Glutamate Receptor

The participation of glutamate receptor in antinociceptive activity by cardamonin was investigated through glutamate-induced paw licking model. The experiment was carried out as previously described [38]. Mice were pre-treated with CARD (0.3, 1, 3, and 10 mg/kg; i.p.), indomethacin (10 mg/kg; i.p.) or vehicle (10 mL/kg; i.p.). After 30 min, 20 μL of glutamate (10 μmol/paw; i.pl.) was injected into the ventral surface of right hind paw of the mice. The mice were then observed individually for 15 min after glutamate injection. The amount of time spent licking the glutamate-injected paw was recorded and was considered as an indication of pain behavior.

4.6.3. Involvement of the Opioid Receptors

To investigate the possible involvement of the opioid system in the antinociceptive activity of cardamonin, separate groups of mice were pre-treated with the non-selective opioid receptor antagonist, naloxone (5 mg/kg; i.p.) 15 min prior to the administration of cardamonin (1 mg/kg; i.p.), morphine (5 mg/kg; s.c.) or vehicle (10 mL/kg; i.p.). After 30 min (for i.p. administration) and 60 min (for s.c. administration), the mice were subjected to the formalin-induced paw licking test and hot plate test [42].

4.7. Toxicity Assessment

The acute toxicity study was conducted to assess the toxicity of cardamonin as described previously [41]. Animals were fasted overnight prior to the test with free access to water ad libitum. Mice were divided into groups and were administered with experimental doses of cardamonin (0.3, 1, 3 and 10 mg/kg) orally (p.o.) and intraperitoneally (i.p.). The control group received the vehicle (10 mL/kg). After administration of cardamonin, the animals were observed for 4 h for any abnormal behaviors, respiratory distress, motor impairment, sedation, and hyper-excitability qualitatively. In addition, any incidence of mortality was recorded up to 24 h after administration of cardamonin. Animals were given free access to standard pellet and water throughout the study.

4.8. Motor Coordination Test

Rota-rod test was conducted to investigate the possible sedative and motor-coordination effect of cardamonin. The method employed was similar to that described previously with slight modification [43]. Mice that successfully remain on the revolving bar of the rota rod apparatus (Model 7600, Ugo Basile) revolving at a speed of 20 rounds per min for two consecutive periods of 60 s were selected 24 h prior to the test. The selected mice were administered with cardamonin (10 mg/kg; i.p.), vehicle (10 mL/kg; i.p.) or diazepam (4 mg/kg; i.p.) 30 min prior to the experiment. Motor performance was evaluated as the latency of permanence(s) on the revolving bar up to 120 s at the time of 30, 60, and 90 s after the treatment. The average time of the animals remain on the revolving bar was recorded.

4.9. Statistical Analysis

The data collected was expressed as mean ± S.E.M. obtained from 6 animals per group and analyzed using one-way ANOVA followed by Dunnett's post hoc test, unless otherwise stated. The differences between means were considered as statistically significant at $p < 0.05$. The experimental ED_{50} (effective dose producing a 50% reduction in abdominal writhes) and its 95% confidence intervals (CI) were determined by linear regression using GraphPad Prism (Version 5, GraphPad Software,

La Jolla, CA, USA). The percentages of inhibition were calculated by comparing the results of treatment group with control group.

5. Conclusions

In conclusion, the present study demonstrated that systemic administration of cardamonin at a dose which does not cause any toxic effects and interference of motor co-ordination exerted significant peripheral and central antinociception when assessed in the chemical- and thermal-induced nociception test models in mice through the involvement of $TRPV_1$, glutamate, and opioid receptors. The precise mechanism underlying the antinociceptive activity of cardamonin remains to be investigated. Currently, a study to determine the possible mechanism(s) of action responsible for cardamonin-induced antinociceptive activity is in progress.

Author Contributions: Conceptualization, M.R.S., E.K.P., A.A., D.A.I.A. and C.P.P.; Methodology, C.P.P.; Software, C.P.P.; Validation, T.A.S.T.M., M.N.A., E.K.P., and A.A.; Formal Analysis, C.P.P.; Investigation, C.P.P.; Resources, T.A.S.T.M., M.N.A., E.K.P., A.A., D.A.I.A. and M.R.S.; Data Curation, All authors; Writing-Original Draft Preparation, All authors; Writing-Review & Editing, All authors; Visualization, All authors; Supervision, T.A.S.T.M., M.N.A., E.K.P., A.A., D.A.I.A. and M.R.S.; Project Administration, M.R.S.; Funding Acquisition, M.R.S.

Funding: This research was funded by Universiti Putra Malaysia Research Grant (GP-IBT/2013/9409600).

Acknowledgments: The authors would like to thank the Faculty of Medicine and Health Sciences and Institute of Bioscience, Universiti Putra Malaysia, for providing the necessary support for this study.

Conflicts of Interest: The authors declare no conflict of interest.

References

1. Bheemasankara, R.C.; Namosiva, R.T.; Suryaprakasam, S. Cardamonin and alpinetin from the seeds of *Amomum subulatum*. *Planta Medica* **1976**, *29*, 391–392.
2. Pascoal, A.C.; Ehrenfried, C.A.; Lopez, B.G.; de Araujo, T.M.; Pascoal, V.D.; Gilioli, R.; Anhe, G.F.; Ruiz, A.L.; Carvalho, J.E.; Stefanello, M.E. Antiproliferative Activity and Induction of Apoptosis in PC-3 Cells by the Chalcone Cardamonin from *Campomanesia adamantium* (Myrtaceae) in a Bioactivity-Guided Study. *Molecules* **2014**, *19*, 1843. [CrossRef] [PubMed]
3. Qin, Y.; Sun, C.-Y.; Lu, F.-R.; Shu, X.-R.; Yang, D.; Chen, L.; She, X.-M.; Gregg, N.M.; Guo, T.; Hu, Y. Cardamonin exerts potent activity against multiple myeloma through blockade of NF-κB pathway in vitro. *Leuk. Res.* **2012**, *36*, 514–520. [CrossRef] [PubMed]
4. Tang, Y.; Fang, Q.; Shi, D.; Niu, P.; Chen, Y.; Deng, J. mTOR inhibition of cardamonin on antiproliferation of A549 cells is involved in a FKBP12 independent fashion. *Life Sci.* **2014**, *99*, 44–51. [CrossRef] [PubMed]
5. Wei, Z.; Yang, J.; Xia, Y.F.; Huang, W.Z.; Wang, Z.T.; Dai, Y. Cardamonin protects septic mice from acute lung injury by preventing endothelial barrier dysfunction. *J. Biochem. Mol. Toxicol.* **2012**, *26*, 282–290. [CrossRef] [PubMed]
6. El-Naga, R.N. Pre-treatment with cardamonin protects against cisplatin-induced nephrotoxicity in rats: Impact on NOX-1, inflammation and apoptosis. *Toxicol. Appl. Pharmacol.* **2014**, *274*, 87–95. [CrossRef] [PubMed]
7. Jantan, I.; Raweh, S.M.; Sirat, H.M.; Jamil, S.; Mohd Yasin, Y.H.; Jalil, J.; Jamal, J.A. Inhibitory effect of compounds from Zingiberaceae species on human platelet aggregation. *Phytomedicine* **2008**, *15*, 306–309. [CrossRef] [PubMed]
8. Wang, Z.-T.; Lau, C.-W.; Chan, F.L.; Yao, X.; Chen, Z.-Y.; He, Z.-D.; Huang, Y. Vasorelaxant effects of cardamonin and alpinetin from *Alpinia henryi* K. Schum. *J. Cardiovasc. Pharmacol.* **2001**, *37*, 596–606. [CrossRef] [PubMed]
9. Liao, Q.; Shi, D.-H.; Zheng, W.; Xu, X.-J.; Yu, Y.-H. Antiproliferation of cardamonin is involved in mTOR on aortic smooth muscle cells in high fructose-induced insulin resistance rats. *Eur. J. Pharmacol.* **2010**, *641*, 179–186. [CrossRef] [PubMed]
10. Zhang, T.; Yamamoto, N.; Yamashita, Y.; Ashida, H. The chalcones cardamonin and flavokawain B inhibit the differentiation of preadipocytes to adipocytes by activating ERK. *Arch. Biochem. Biophys.* **2014**, *554*, 44–54. [CrossRef] [PubMed]

11. Cho, M.; Ryu, M.; Jeong, Y.; Chung, Y.-H.; Kim, D.-E.; Cho, H.-S.; Kang, S.; Han, J.-S.; Chang, M.-Y.; Lee, C.-K.; et al. Cardamonin suppresses melanogenesis by inhibition of Wnt/β-catenin signaling. *Biochem. Biophys. Res. Commun.* **2009**, *390*, 500–505. [CrossRef] [PubMed]
12. Park, M.K.; Choi, J.K.; Kim, H.J.; Nakahata, N.; Lim, K.M.; Kim, S.Y.; Lee, C.H. Novel inhibitory effects of cardamonin on thromboxane A_2-induced scratching response: Blocking of Gh/transglutaminase-2 binding to thromboxane A_2 receptor. *Pharmacol. Biochem. Behav.* **2014**, *126*, 131–135. [CrossRef] [PubMed]
13. Ahmad, S.; Israf, D.A.; Lajis, N.H.; Shaari, K.; Mohamed, H.; Wahab, A.A.; Ariffin, K.T.; Hoo, W.Y.; Aziz, N.A.; Kadir, A.A.; et al. Cardamonin, inhibits pro-inflammatory mediators in activated RAW 264.7 cells and whole blood. *Eur. J. Pharmacol.* **2006**, *538*, 188–194. [CrossRef] [PubMed]
14. Israf, D.A.; Khaizurin, T.A.; Syahida, A.; Lajis, N.H.; Khozirah, S. Cardamonin inhibits COX and iNOS expression via inhibition of p65NF-κB nuclear translocation and κ-B phosphorylation in RAW 264.7 macrophage cells. *Mol. Immunol.* **2007**, *44*, 673–679. [CrossRef] [PubMed]
15. Chow, Y.-L.; Lee, K.-H.; Vidyadaran, S.; Lajis, N.H.; Akhtar, M.N.; Israf, D.A.; Syahida, A. Cardamonin from *Alpinia rafflesiana* inhibits inflammatory responses in IFN-γ/LPS-stimulated BV2 microglia via NF-κB signalling pathway. *Int. Immunopharmacol.* **2012**, *12*, 657–665. [CrossRef] [PubMed]
16. Menghini, L.; Ferrante, C.; Leporini, L.; Recinella, L.; Chiavaroli, A.; Leone, S.; Pintore, G.; Vacca, M.; Orlando, G.; Brunetti, L. An hydroalcoholic chamomile extract modulates inflammatory and immune response in HT29 cells and isolated rat colon. *Phytother. Res.* **2016**, *30*, 1513–1518. [CrossRef] [PubMed]
17. Locatelli, M.; Macchione, N.; Ferrante, C.; Chiavaroli, A.; Recinella, L.; Carradori, S.; Zengin, G.; Cesa, S.; Leporini, L.; Leone, S. Graminex Pollen: Phenolic Pattern, Colorimetric Analysis and Protective Effects in Immortalized Prostate Cells (PC3) and Rat Prostate Challenged with LPS. *Molecules* **2018**, *23*, e1145. [CrossRef] [PubMed]
18. Takahashi, A.; Yamamoto, N.; Murakami, A. Cardamonin suppresses nitric oxide production via blocking the IFN-γ/STAT pathway in endotoxin-challenged peritoneal macrophages of ICR mice. *Life Sci.* **2011**, *89*, 337–342. [CrossRef] [PubMed]
19. Schmidtko, A.; Tegeder, I.; Geisslinger, G. No NO, no pain? The role of nitric oxide and cGMP in spinal pain processing. *Trends Neurosci.* **2009**, *32*, 339–346. [CrossRef] [PubMed]
20. Park, M.K.; Lee, H.J.; Choi, J.K.; Kim, H.J.; Kang, J.H.; Lee, E.J.; Kim, Y.R.; Kang, J.H.; Yoo, J.K.; Cho, H.Y.; et al. Novel anti-nociceptive effects of cardamonin via blocking expression of cyclooxygenase-2 and transglutaminase-2. *Pharmacol. Biochem. Behav.* **2014**, *118*, 10–15. [CrossRef] [PubMed]
21. Cardosa, M.; Osman, Z.J.; Nicholas, M.; Tonkin, L.; Williams, A.; Aziz, K.A.; Ali, R.M.; Dahari, N.M. Self-management of chronic pain in Malaysian patients: Effectiveness trial with 1-year follow-up. *Transl. Behav. Med.* **2012**, *2*, 30–37. [CrossRef] [PubMed]
22. Zaki, L.R.M.; Hairi, N.N. Chronic pain and pattern of health care utilization among Malaysian elderly population: National Health and Morbidity Survey III (NHMS III, 2006). *Maturitas* **2014**, *79*, 435–441. [CrossRef] [PubMed]
23. Williams, M.; Kowaluk, E.A.; Arneric, S.P. Emerging molecular approaches to pain therapy. *J. Med. Chem.* **1999**, *42*, 1481. [CrossRef] [PubMed]
24. Smith, M.D.; Wang, Y.; Cudnik, M.; Smith, D.A.; Pakiela, J.; Emerman, C.L. The Effectiveness and Adverse Events of Morphine versus Fentanyl on a Physician-staffed Helicopter. *J. Emerg. Med.* **2012**, *43*, 69–75. [CrossRef] [PubMed]
25. Sostres, C.; Gargallo, C.J.; Arroyo, M.T.; Lanas, A. Adverse effects of non-steroidal anti-inflammatory drugs (NSAIDs, aspirin and coxibs) on upper gastrointestinal tract. *Best Pract. Res. Clin. Gastroenterol.* **2010**, *24*, 121–132. [CrossRef] [PubMed]
26. Chen, Y.; Boettger, M.K.; Reif, A.; Schmitt, A.; Uceyler, N.; Sommer, C. Nitric oxide synthase modulates CFA-induced thermal hyperalgesia through cytokine regulation in mice. *Mol. Pain* **2010**, *6*, 1–11. [CrossRef] [PubMed]
27. Cury, Y.; Picolo, G.; Gutierrez, V.P.; Ferreira, S.H. Pain and analgesia: The dual effect of nitric oxide in the nociceptive system. *Nitric Oxide* **2011**, *25*, 243–254. [CrossRef] [PubMed]
28. De Souza, M.M.; Pereira, M.A.; Ardenghi, J.V.; Mora, T.C.; Bresciani, L.F.; Yunes, R.A.; Monache, F.D.; Cechinel Filho, V. Filicene obtained from *Adiantumcuneatum* interacts with the cholinergic, dopaminergic, glutamatergic, GABAergic, and tachykinergic systems to exert antinociceptive effect in mice. *Pharmacol. Biochem. Behav.* **2009**, *93*, 40–46. [CrossRef] [PubMed]

29. Deraedt, R.; Jouquey, S.; Delevallee, F.; Flahaut, M. Release of prostaglandins E and F in an algogenic reaction and its inhibition. *Eur. J. Pharmacol.* **1980**, *61*, 17–24. [CrossRef]
30. Ikeda, Y.; Ueno, A.; Naraba, H.; Oh-ishi, S. Involvement of vanilloid receptor VR1 and prostanoids in the acid-induced writhing responses of mice. *Life Sci.* **2001**, *69*, 2911–2919. [CrossRef]
31. Le Bars, D.; Gozariu, M.; Cadden, S.W. Animal models of nociception. *Pharmacol. Rev.* **2001**, *53*, 597–652. [PubMed]
32. Omote, K.; Kawamata, T.; Kawamata, M.; Namiki, A. Formalin-induced release of excitatory amino acids in the skin of the rat hindpaw. *Brain Res.* **1998**, *787*, 161–164. [CrossRef]
33. Hunskaar, S.; Hole, K. The formalin test in mice: Dissociation between inflammatory and non-inflammatory pain. *Pain* **1987**, *30*, 103–114. [CrossRef]
34. Shibata, M.; Ohkubo, T.; Takahashi, H.; Inoki, R. Modified formalin test: Characteristic biphasic pain response. *Pain* **1989**, *38*, 347–352. [CrossRef]
35. Abbott, F.V.; Melzack, R. Brainstem lesions dissociate neural mechanisms of morphine analgesia in different kinds of pain. *Brain Res.* **1982**, *251*, 149–155. [CrossRef]
36. Nemirovsky, A.; Chen, L.; Zelman, V.; Jurna, I. The antinociceptive effect of the combination of spinal morphine with systemic morphine or buprenorphine. *Anesthesia Analg.* **2001**, *93*, 197–203. [CrossRef]
37. Sakurada, T.; Matsumura, T.; Moriyama, T.; Sakurada, C.; Ueno, S.; Sakurada, S. Differential effects of intraplantar capsazepine and ruthenium red on capsaicin-induced desensitization in mice. *Pharmacol. Biochem. Behav.* **2003**, *75*, 115–121. [CrossRef]
38. Beirith, A.; Santos, A.R.S.; Calixto, J.B. Mechanisms underlying the nociception and paw oedema caused by injection of glutamate into the mouse paw. *Brain Res.* **2002**, *924*, 219–228. [CrossRef]
39. Sulaiman, M.R.; Tengku Mohamad, T.A.; Shaik Mossadeq, W.M.; Moin, S.; Yusof, M.; Mokhtar, A.F.; Zakaria, Z.A.; Israf, D.A.; Lajis, N. Antinociceptive activity of the essential oil of *Zingiber zerumbet*. *Planta Medica* **2010**, *76*, 107. [CrossRef] [PubMed]
40. Mohamad, A.S.; Akhtar, M.N.; Zakaria, Z.A.; Perimal, E.K.; Khalid, S.; Mohd, P.A.; Khalid, M.H.; Israf, D.A.; Lajis, N.H.; Sulaiman, M.R. Antinociceptive activity of a synthetic chalcone, flavokawin B on chemical and thermal models of nociception in mice. *Eur. J. Pharmacol.* **2010**, *647*, 103–109. [CrossRef] [PubMed]
41. Ong, H.M.; Mohamad, A.S.; Makhtar, N.; Khalid, M.H.; Khalid, S.; Perimal, E.K.; Mastuki, S.N.; Zakaria, Z.A.; Lajis, N.; Israf, D.A. Antinociceptive activity of methanolic extract of *Acmella uliginosa* (Sw.) Cass. *J. Ethnopharmacol.* **2011**, *133*, 227–233. [CrossRef] [PubMed]
42. Ming-Tatt, L.; Khalivulla, S.I.; Akhtar, M.N.; Mohamad, A.S.; Perimal, E.K.; Khalid, M.H.; Akira, A.; Lajis, N.; Israf, D.A.; Sulaiman, M.R. Antinociceptive activity of a synthetic curcuminoid analogue, 2, 6-bis-(4-hydroxy-3-methoxybenzylidene) cyclohexanone, on nociception-induced models in mice. *Basic Clin. Pharmacol. Toxicol.* **2012**, *110*, 275–282. [CrossRef] [PubMed]
43. Perimal, E.K.; Akhtar, M.N.; Mohamad, A.S.; Khalid, M.H.; Ming, O.H.; Khalid, S.; Tatt, L.M.; Kamaldin, M.N.; Zakaria, Z.A.; Israf, D.A. Zerumbone-induced antinociception: Involvement of the L-arginine-nitric oxide-cGMP-PKC-K^+ ATP channel pathways. *Basic Clin. Pharmacol. Toxicol.* **2011**, *108*, 155–162. [CrossRef] [PubMed]

Sample Availability: Samples of the compounds are available from the authors.

molecules

MDPI

Article

Identification and Growth Inhibitory Activity of the Chemical Constituents from *Imperata Cylindrica* Aerial Part Ethyl Acetate Extract

Yan Wang, James Zheng Shen, Yuk Wah Chan and Wing Shing Ho *

School of Life Sciences, Chinese University of Hong Kong, Shatin, Hong Kong, China; 1155070144@link.cuhk.edu.hk (Y.W.); james_shen_zheng@alumni.cuhk.net (J.Z.S.); anthony.chan@link.cuhk.edu.hk (Y.W.C.)

* Correspondence: ws203ho@cuhk.edu.hk; Tel.: +852-9313-3054

Received: 27 June 2018; Accepted: 16 July 2018; Published: 21 July 2018

Abstract: *Imperata cylindrica* (L.) Raeusch. (IMP) aerial part ethyl acetate extract has anti-proliferative, pro-apoptotic, and pro-oxidative effects towards colorectal cancer in vitro. The chemical constituents of IMP aerial part ethyl acetate extract were isolated using high-performance liquid chromatography (HPLC) and identified with tandem mass spectrometry (ESI-MS/MS) in combination with ultraviolet-visible spectrophotometry and 400 MHz NMR. The growth inhibitory effects of each identified component on BT-549 (breast) and HT-29 (colon) cancer cell lines were evaluated after 48/72 h treatment by MTT assay. Four isolated compounds were identified as trans-p-Coumaric acid (**1**); 2-Methoxyestrone (**2**); 11, 16-Dihydroxypregn-4-ene-3, 20-dione (**3**); and Tricin (**4**). Compounds (**2**), (**3**), and (**4**) exhibited considerable growth inhibitory activities against BT-549 and HT-29 cancer cell lines. Compounds (**2**), (**3**), and (**4**) are potential candidates for novel anti-cancer agents against breast and colorectal cancers.

Keywords: *Imperata cylindrica*; HPLC; ESI-MS/MS; growth inhibitory activity; cancer

1. Introduction

Imperata cylindrica (L.) Raeusch. (IMP) is widely used for the treatment of hemorrhage, improvement of urination, and enhancement of the immune system [1]. Amounts of bio-active compounds isolated from IMP rhizomes and leaves were identified including benzoic acid and its derivatives [2], lignans [3], phenolic compounds [4], steroids [5], methoxylated flavonoids [6], and chromones [7].

Cancer is one of the leading causes of death worldwide. Herbal medicines are commonly used as both complementary ingredients and alternative therapies in cancer treatments. Potential bio-active components from herbal medicines can be isolated and purified using a high-performance liquid chromatography (HPLC) system. A tandem MS/MS detection system providing fragmentation information of the targets is one of the best choices adopted in chemical structural characterization and drug discovery [8,9].

Our previous study demonstrated that IMP aerial part ethyl acetate extract had growth-inhibiting, pro-apoptotic, and pro-oxidative effects on a colorectal cancer cell line HT-29 in vitro [10]. The present study aims to isolate the chemical constituents from IMP aerial part ethyl acetate extract and identify the bio-active compounds with considerable growth inhibitory activity against cancers.

2. Results

2.1. *Isolation, Identification, and Quantification of Compounds* (1)–(4)

Chemical structures of four compounds isolated from IMP aerial part ethyl acetate extract are shown in Figure 1.

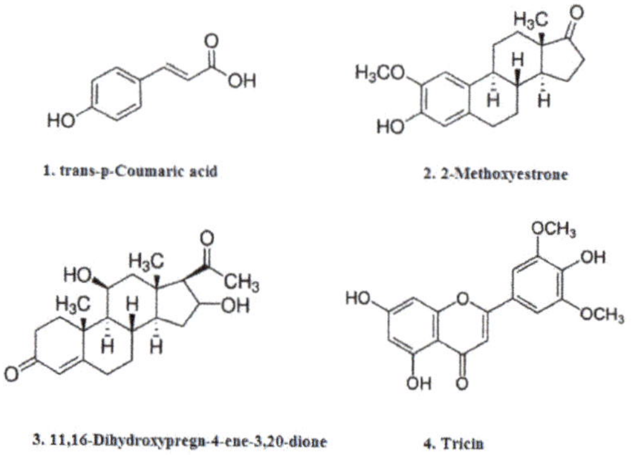

Figure 1. Chemical structures of compounds (**1**)–(**4**) isolated from IMP aerial part ethyl acetate extract. These are trans-p-Coumaric acid (**1**); 2-Methoxyestrone (**2**); 11, 16-Dihydroxypregn-4-ene-3, 20-dione (**3**); and Tricin (**4**).

2.1.1. Compound (1): Trans-p-Coumaric Acid

The molecular formula of compound (**1**), $C_9H_8O_3$, was identified by comparing the liquid chromatographic retention time, UV absorption spectrum, and ESI-MS/MS spectrum with the trans-p-Coumaric acid standard (Sigma Aldrich, St. Louis, MO, USA). The HPLC chromatogram of compound (**1**) and trans-p-Coumaric acid standard (in methanol) possessed the same identical retention time (Figure 2A,B).

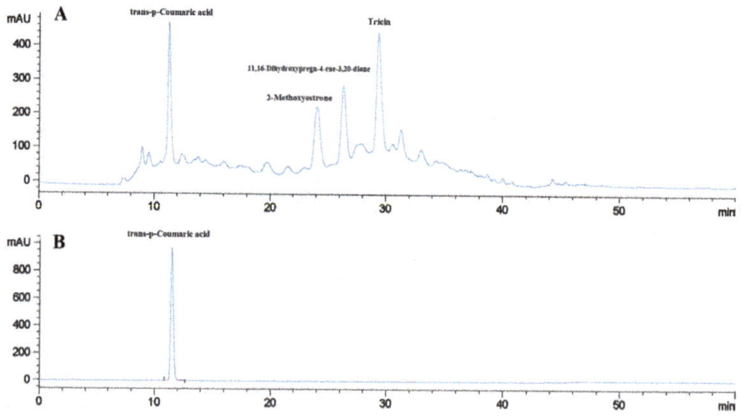

Figure 2. HPLC-DAD chromatogram of IMP aerial part ethyl acetate extract at 323 nm. IMP aerial part ethyl acetate extract solution (10 mg/mL in methanol, 20 μL) was analyzed in the 60 min HPLC gradient program. (**A**) The retention time of the trans-p-Coumaric acid standard (0.125 mg/mL in methanol, 20 μL) purchased from Sigma (**B**) was consistent with compound (**1**) in IMP aerial part ethyl acetate extract fingerprint.

The MS/MS fragmentation pattern of compound (**1**) accurately matched with the MS^2 spectrum from the NIST14 mass spectral database and the trans-p-Coumaric standard (Figure 3).

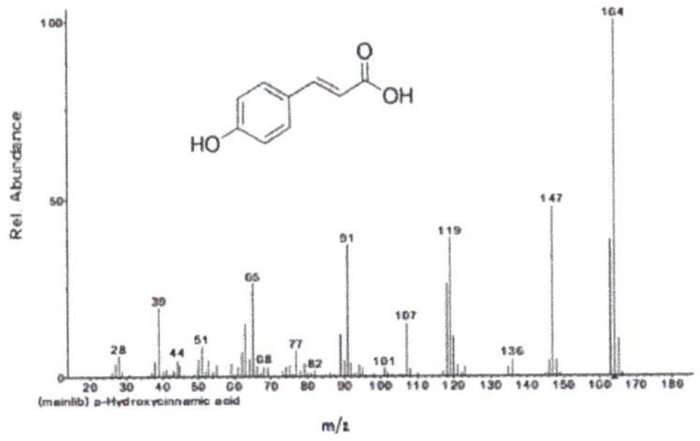

(A)

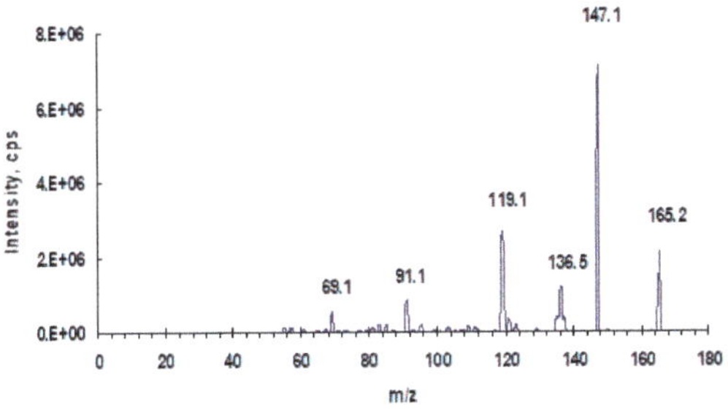

(B)

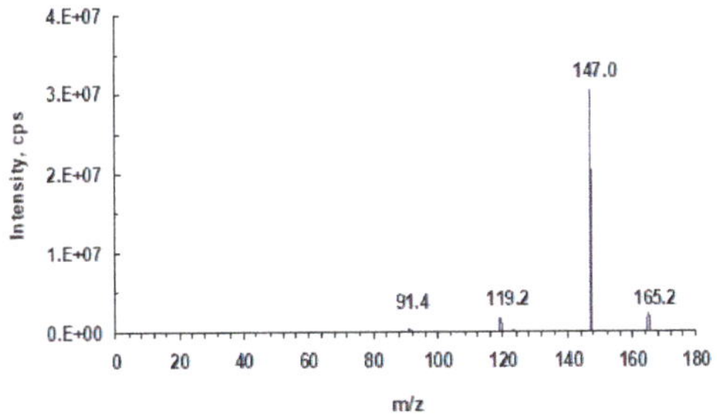

(C)

Figure 3. Relevant tandem mass (MS/MS) spectra. (**A**) trans-p-Coumaric acid spectrum (from NIST 14 mass spectral library); (**B**) isolated and purified compound (**1**); (**C**) trans-p-Coumaric acid standard (Sigma).

2.1.2. Compound (2): 2-Methoxyestrone

The molecular formula of compound (**2**), $C_{19}H_{24}O_3$, was identified with the MS/MS spectrum by searching the NIST14 mass spectral database (Figure 4).

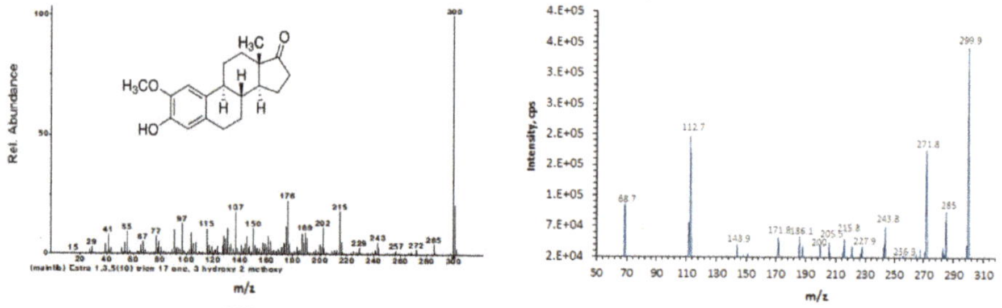

(A) (B)

Figure 4. Relevant tandem mass (MS/MS) spectra. (**A**) 2-Methoxyestrone (from NIST 14 mass spectral library); (**B**) isolated and purified compound (**2**).

2.1.3. Compound (3): 11, 16-Dihydroxypregn-4-ene-3, 20-dione

The molecular formula of compound (**3**): $C_{21}H_{30}O_4$, was identified with the MS/MS spectrum by searching the NIST14 mass spectral database (Figure 5).

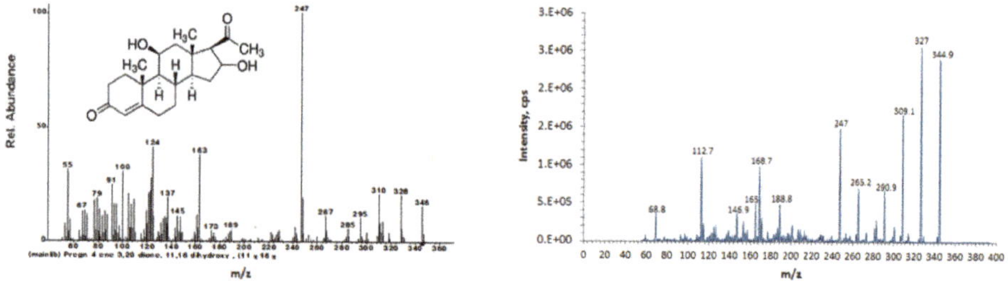

(A) (B)

Figure 5. Relevant tandem mass (MS/MS) spectra. (**A**) 11, 16-Dihydroxypregn-4-ene-3, 20-dione (from NIST 14 mass spectral library); (**B**) isolated and purified compound (**3**).

2.1.4. Compound (4): Tricin

The molecular formula of compound (**4**), $C_{17}H_{14}O_7$, was identified by comparing the MS/MS spectrum with the published literature [11] (Figure 6A,B). The UV spectrum (Figure 6C), obtained using λ_{max} at 351 nm, was consistent with the previous description [12].

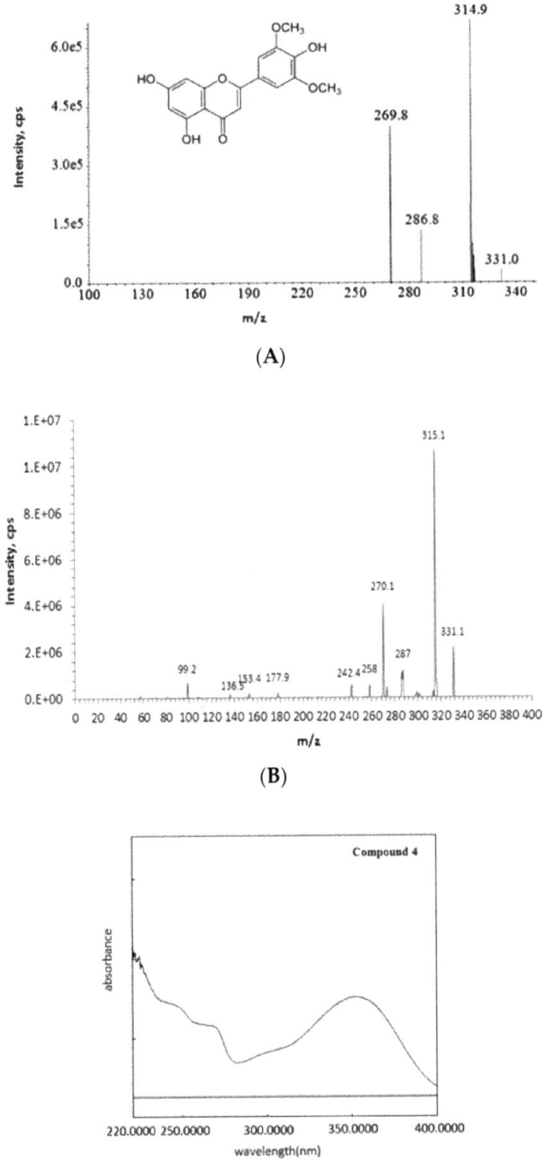

Figure 6. Relevant tandem mass (MS/MS) spectra. (**A**) Tricin (from literature [11]); (**B**) isolated and purified compound (**4**). (**C**) Compound (**4**) has absorption peaks (λ_{max}) at 351 nm. A control of 100% methanol was used and auto-zeroed automatically by the software.

1H-NMR (400 MHz, DMSO-d_6) δ (ppm): 12.964 (1H, s, 5-OH), 10.804 (s, 1H, 7-OH), 9.318 (s, 1H, 4-OH), 7.330 (2H, s, H-6′ and H-2′), 6.984 (1H, s, H-3), 6.564 (1H, d, *J* = 2.0 Hz, H-8), 6.209 (1H, d, *J* = 2.0 Hz, H-6), 3.887 (6H, s, 2OCH_3). 13C-NMR (100 MHz, DMSO-d_6) δ (ppm): 181.75 (C-4), 164.08 (C-2), 163.61 (C-7), 161.35 (C-5), 157.28 (C-9), 148.41 (C-3′ and C-5′), 139.81 (C-4′), 120.34 (C-1′), 104.35

(C-3), 103.68 (C-2′ and C-6′), 103.55 (C-10), 98.77 (C-6), 94.14 (C-8), 56.32 (2OCH_3). DEPT90-NMR (DMSO-d_6) δ (ppm): 94.12 (C-8), 98.75 (C-6), 103.53 (C-10), 104.31 (C-3). DEPT135-NMR (DMSO-d_6) δ (ppm): 56.31 (2OCH_3), 94.13 (C-8), 98.76 (C-6), 103.54 (C-10), 104.3 (C-3). DEPT spectra revealed that there were two primary carbons, five tertiary carbons, and ten quaternary carbons. A signal at δ3.887 (s, 6H) observed in the 1H-NMR spectrum and a signal at δ 56.32 observed in the 13C-NMR spectrum indicated that there were two equivalent methoxy groups. The NMR results (Figure 7) were consistent with the published data [13,14].

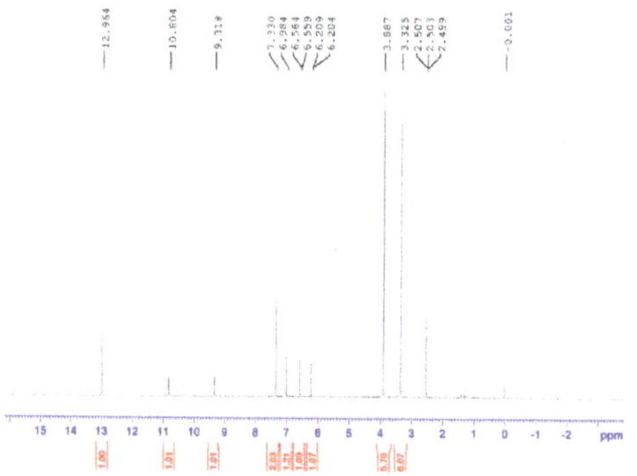

(A)

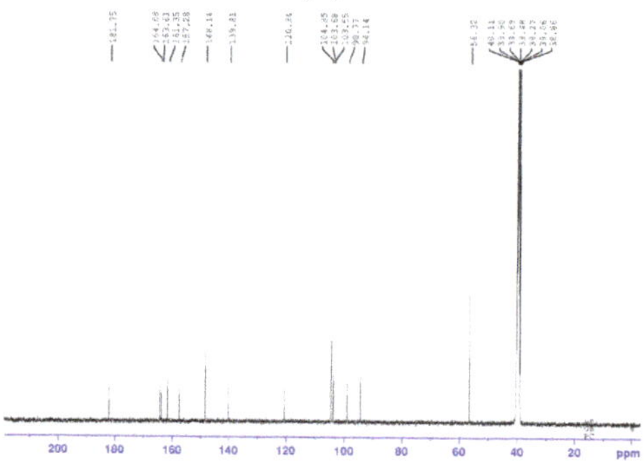

(B)

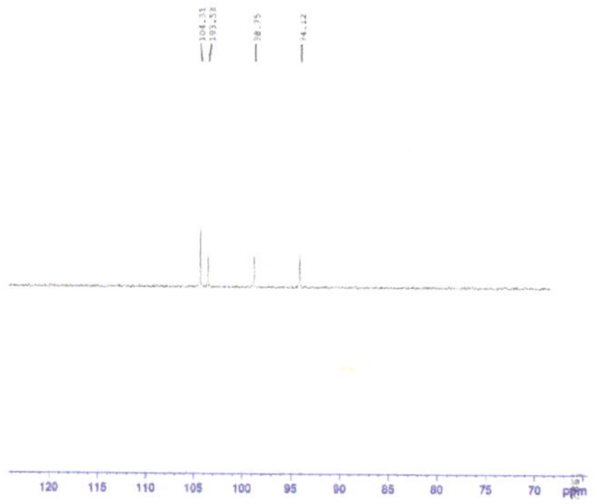

(C)

Figure 7. *Cont.*

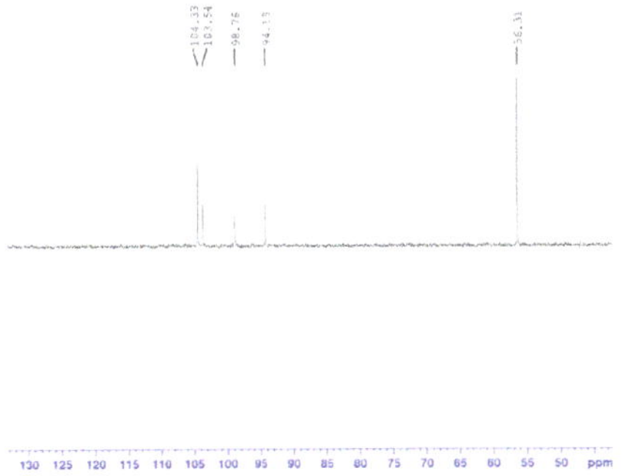

(D)

Figure 7. NMR spectra of Tricin. Purified Compound (**4**) in DMSO-d_6 solution was conducted NMR analysis. ^{1}H, ^{13}C, DEPT90, and DEPT135-NMR spectra are shown in (**A**–**D**), respectively.

Compounds (**1**)–(**4**) identified by tandem mass spectrometry (MS^2) are listed in Table 1.

Table 1. Characteristics of compound (**1**)–(**4**) identified by tandem mass spectrometry.

Analyte	Ion Mode	Molecular Formula	CAS No.	MS/MS Fragments (*m/z*)
trans-p-Coumaric acid	$[M+H]^+$	$C_9H_8O_3$	501-98-4	165.7, 147.4, 136.3, 118.9, 90.5
2-Methoxyestrone	$[M-H]^-$	$C_{19}H_{24}O_3$	362-08-3	299.9, 285.0, 271.8, 256.3, 243.8
11, 16-Dihydroxypregn-4-ene-3, 20-dione	$[M-H]^-$	$C_{21}H_{30}O_4$	55622-61-2	344.9, 327.0, 309.1, 290.9, 265.2, 247.0
Tricin	$[M+H]^+$	$C_{17}H_{14}O_7$	520-32-1	331.1, 315.0, 287.0, 270.1, 258.0, 242.4

2.1.5. Content of Analytes in IMP Aerial Part Ethyl Acetate Extract

Quantitative analysis of each isolated and purified compound in IMP aerial part ethyl acetate extract was determined by HPLC-DAD. The linearity of the calibration curve, limit of detection (LOD), and limit of quantification (LOQ) are listed in Table 2.

Table 2. Content of analytes in IMP aerial part ethyl acetate extract.

Analytes	Calibration Curves [a]	R^2 [b]	Linear Range (mg/mL)	LOD [c] (μg/mL)	LOQ [d] (μg/mL)	Contents of Analytes (mg/g Extract, *n* = 3)
trans-p-Coumaric acid	$y = 114751x - 31.91$	0.9999	0.0010–0.25	0.30	0.95	0.12 ± 0.010
2-Methoxyestrone	$y = 13217x + 195.65$	0.9992	0.031–1.00	7.28	24.84	0.86 ± 0.042
11,16-Dihydroxypregn-4-ene-3, 20-dione	$y = 15063x + 1173.70$	0.9995	0.12–2.50	6.71	22.91	0.65 ± 0.13
Tricin	$y = 35025x - 126.29$	0.9999	0.016–2.00	3.23	11.02	0.59 ± 0.041

[a] y, the value of peak area (by HPLC-DAD at 323 nm); x, the value of concentration (mg/mL); [b] R^2, correlation coefficient for six points on the calibration curves ($n = 3$); [c] LOD, limit of detection (S/N = 3); [d] LOQ, limit of quantification (S/N = 10).

2.2. *Growth Inhibitory Evaluation of Compounds* (**1**)–(**4**) *on Breast Cancer and Colorectal Cancer In Vitro*

The purified dried powder of each compound was dissolved in DMSO with a gradient of concentrations (μM). The growth inhibitory effects of compounds (**1**)–(**4**) on BT-549 (breast cancer cell line) were evaluated after 48/72 h treatment by MTT assay (Figure 8). Data are presented as mean values ±SD from three independent studies ($n = 3$).

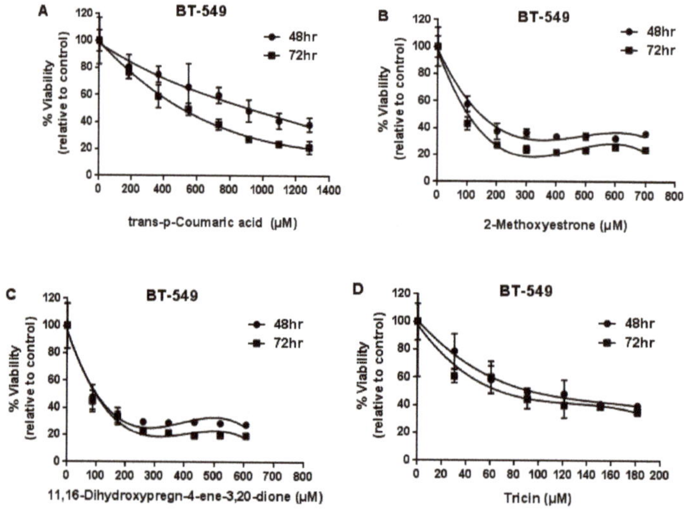

Figure 8. The growth inhibitory effects of compound (**1**)–(**4**) on BT-549 (breast cancer cell line) were evaluated after 48/72 h treatment by MTT assay.

The growth inhibitory effects of compounds (**1**)–(**4**) on HT-29 (colon cancer cell line) are shown in Figure 9.

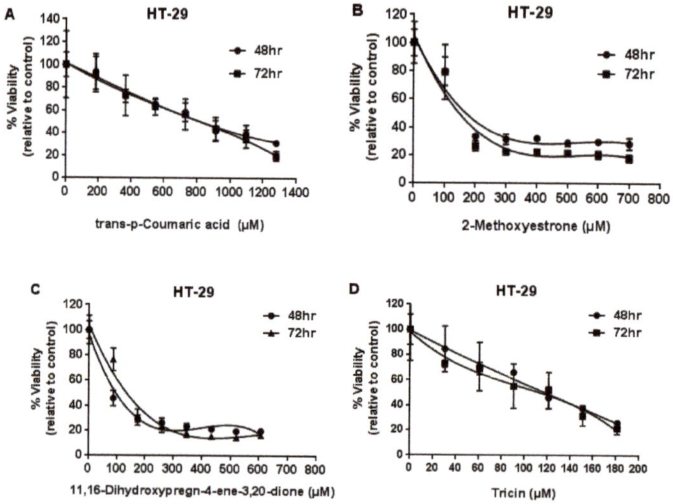

Figure 9. The growth inhibitory effects of compounds (**1**)–(**4**) on HT-29 (colon cancer cell line) were evaluated after 48/72 h treatment by MTT assay.

The half-maximal inhibitory concentration (IC50) of compounds (**2**), (**3**), and (**4**) on BT-549 breast cancer cell line (72 h) was 102, 97, and 68 μM, respectively. IC50 of compounds (**2**), (**3**), and (**4**) on a HT-29 colon cancer cell line (72 h) was 147, 134, and 114 μM, respectively. There were no statistically significant differences between 48 h and 72 h treatment groups ($p > 0.05$) (Table 3).

Table 3. IC50 of compounds (**1**)–(**4**) on BT-549 and HT-29 cancer cell lines.

Cancer Unit		Treatment Group (48/72 h)			
		Trans-p-Coumaric Acid	2-Methoxyestrone	11,16-Dihydroxypregn-4-ene-3, 20-dione	Tricin
BT-549	μg/mL	151/83	43/31	35/34	31/23
	μM	920/507	144/102 [a]	101/97 [a]	95/68 [a]
HT-29	μg/mL	135/135	51/44	33/46	39/38
	μM	821/821	169/147 [a]	96/134 [a]	118/114 [a]

[a] Numbers identified refer to the considerable growth inhibitory activity with half-maximal inhibitory concentration (IC50 < 150 μM).

3. Discussion

A previous study showed that the 50% growth inhibitory effect (GI50) of the IMP aerial part ethyl acetate extract against HT-29 was 14.5 μg/mL [10]. The three isolated compounds, including 2-Methoxyestrone (**2**), 11, 16-Dihydroxypregn-4-ene-3, 20-dione (**3**), and Tricin (**4**), have considerable growth inhibitory activities on BT-549 and HT-29 with the IC50 values among 23–51 μg/mL. Synergy and positive interactions between isolated constituents may contribute to the greater effect of the crude extract against cancers that can be further investigated.

Compound (**1**), trans-p-Coumaric acid, was able to induce apoptosis of HCT-15 colon cancer cells through a ROS-mitochondrial pathway with an IC 50 value of 1400 μM [15]. Natural trans-p-Coumaric acid exists in a wide variety of edible plants. The phenolic components from flaxseed oil was reported to have cytotoxic and pro-oxidant effects on MCF-7 human breast cancer cells [16]. The high gastric absorption efficiency of p-Coumaric acid was observed in rats, which makes it a potential bio-active compound in vivo [17]. Compound (**2**), 2-Methoxyestrone, is one kind of metabolite of estrone and estradiol. It is worth mentioning that 2-Methoxyestradiol was under a phase II clinical trial and expected to be a novel oral drug against multiple human melanoma, including breast cancer and ovarian cancer [18,19]. Metabolic inter-conversion between 2-Methoxyestrone and 2-Methoxyestradiol are based on the enzymatic catalyze reactions. Reductive activity promotes 2-Methoxyestrone conversion to 2-Methoxyestradiol. 2-Methoxyestrone can be formed by the enzymatic oxidation of 2-Methoxyestradiol [20]. Our study first reported the growth inhibitory activities of compound (**3**), 11, 16-Dihydroxypregn-4-ene-3, 20-dione, against BT-549 and HT-29 cancer cell lines. The structure of 11, 16-Dihydroxypregn-4-ene-3, 20-dione is similar to the well-known endogenous steroid (11α-Hydroxyprogesterone, $C_{21}H_{30}O_3$). Transformations of 11α-Hydroxyprogesterone generate a series of metabolites. Amounts of metabolites with different isoforms were identified as novel candidates of steroid drugs [21]. The molecular mechanisms of 11, 16-Dihydroxypregn-4-ene-3, 20-dione against cancers can be further investigated. Compound (**4**), Tricin, a well-studied bio-active flavonoid, is widely distributed in rice bran and bamboo leaves [22,23]. A previous study also isolated Tricin from the aerial part of *Imperata cylindrica* (L.) Beauv. [5]. Tricin was reported to have remarkable anti-cancer potential against SW-480 colon cancer cells and MDA-MB-468 breast cancer cells, and is safe for clinical development as a cancer preventive agent [24–28].

4. Materials and Methods

4.1. Cells, Chemicals and Reagents

BT-549 and HT-29 cell lines were obtained from ATCC (Manassas, VA, USA). BT-549 and HT-29 cells were cultured at 37 °C in a humidified atmosphere of 5% CO_2 in RPMI 1640 (Gibco, Carlsbad, CA, USA) supplemented with 10% fetal bovine serum (FBS) (Gibco, Carlsbad, CA, USA). Acetonitrile (ACN) (E. Merck, Darmstadt, Germany), Methanol (E. Merck, Darmstadt, Germany) and trifluoroacetic acid (TFA) (Sigma Aldrich, St. Louis, MO, USA) were of HPLC grade, and distilled and deionized water (ddH_2O) was prepared using a Millipore water purification system (Millipore, Milford, MA, USA). All other reagents used in this study were of analytical reagent grade or higher and purchased from Sigma Aldrich.

4.2. *Preparation of Powder Extract of IMP Aerial Part*

The extraction method was described previously [10].

4.3. *HPLC Analysis*

The HPLC fingerprint was analyzed on a HP1100 series system (Santa Clara, CA, USA) equipped with a diode-array detector. An extract solution of 50 mg/mL (dissolved in methanol) was filtered with a 0.22 μm polytetrafluoroethylene (PTFE) membrane. A 15 μL sample was injected to a semi-preparative HPLC column (ALLTIMA C18, 5 μm, 250 mm × 10 mm i.d. Hichrom, Searle, UK) and detected at 323 nm. The initial mobile phase composed of solvent A (0.1% TFA in ddH_2O) and solvent B (100% methanol). The gradient for the HPLC analysis was programmed as follows: 0–5 min, 65% B; 5–15 min, 70% B; at a flow rate of 1.5 mL/min; 15–25 min, 80% B, at a flow rate of 1.0 mL/min; 25–40 min, 85% B, at a flow rate of 0.8 mL/min; 40–50 min, 100% B, at a flow rate of 2.0 mL/min, and then was held for additional 5 min.

4.4. *Isolation and Purification of Compounds* (**1**)–(**4**) *by HPLC*

Fractions were collected manually by observing the elution profile of the chromatography workstation. The elution profile was programmed with the gradient mobile phase composed of solvent A (0.1% TFA in ddH_2O), solvent B (100% methanol), and solvent C (100% ACN). Fractions were isolated and purified with the semi-preparative HPLC column (ALLTIMA C18, 5 μm, 250 mm × 10 mm i.d. Hichrom, Searle, UK). The gradients used for collecting each fraction were set as follows: Fraction (1), 0–14 min, 60% C; 14–19 min, 100%; at a flow rate of 1.5 mL/min; Fractions (2) and (3), 0–15 min, 85% B; 15–18 min, 100% B; at a flow rate of 2.0 mL/min; Fraction (4), 0–15 min, 85% B; at a flow rate of 2.0 mL/min; and 15–17 min, 100% B; at a flow rate of 2.5 mL/min. The purity of each HPLC fraction was calculated based on the proportion of the target peak area. The purified HPLC eluent was lyophilized and stored at −20 °C for further use.

4.5. *Mass Spectrometry*

The identification of each purified component was performed on a tandem mass spectrometer equipped with an electrospray ionization source. Each purified compound was dissolved in methanol at an appropriate concentration and was infused into the QTRAP 5500 mass spectrometer system (AB SCIEX, Framingham, MA, USA) equipped with a Turbo VTM Spray ion source. Multiple reaction monitoring (MRM) in both positive and negative mode was used to enhance the selectivity of detection. The source-dependent parameters for the mass spectrometer (MS) were set as follows: ion spray voltage (IS) = ±5500 V; curtain gas (CUR) = 20 psi; collision gas (CAD) = 10 psi; nebulizer gas (GS1) = 12 psi, heater gas (GS2) = 0 psi, and source temperature (TEM) = 0 °C. The fraction-dependent parameters were set as follows: declustering potential (DP) = +120.0 V/−130.0 V; entrance potential (EP) = ±10.0 V; collision cell exit potential (CXP) = ±13.0 V. The MS/MS optimized collision energy applied to compounds (**1**)–(**4**) was given as follows: 25 V in positive mode, 25 V in negative mode, 25 V in negative mode, and 40 V in positive mode, respectively. For trans-p-Coumaric acid standard, the collision energy applied was 10 V in positive mode. Raw data and images of spectra were generated by Analyst® Software (Redwood, CA, USA) and modified using Excel® (Redmond, WA, USA).

4.6. *Ultraviolet-Visible Spectrophotometry*

The UV spectrum of compound (**4**) was measured using a Shimadzu UV-3600 spectrophotometer (Shimadzu Corporation, Kyoto, Japan). Each absorption spectrum was recorded from 200.00 nm to 400.00 nm. Profiles were generated by UVProbe 2.21 Software (Shimadzu Corporation, Kyoto, Japan). A control of 100% methanol was set and auto-zeroed automatically by software.

4.7. NMR Analysis

A 5 mg sample of purified compound (**4**) was dissolved in DMSO-d_6, and 1H NMR (400 MHz), 13C NMR (100 MHz), DEPT 90, DEPT 135 spectra were recorded using the Bruker Avance III 400 MHz NMR spectrometer spectroscopy (Bruker Corporation, Solna, Sweden). All chemical shifts were reported in δ (ppm) relative to tetramethylsilane (TMS).

4.8. Quantitative Analysis

The content of each identified compound in IMP aerial part ethyl acetate extract was determined using a HPLC-DAD system. The linearity and range was evaluated by constructing a calibration curve (peak area vs concentration). Quantification was performed upon six levels of external standards. The limit of detection (LOD) was determined as the concentration with a signal-to-noise ratio of three, and the limit of quantification (LOQ) was determined as the concentration with a signal-to-noise ratio of ten.

4.9. MTT Assay

The growth inhibitory effects of compounds (**1**)–(**4**) on HT-29 (colon) and BT-549 (breast) cancer cell lines were evaluated. Cells were seeded at 4×10^3 cells per 96-well and incubated for 24 h. The cells were then treated by 0.5% DMSO (as solvent control) or various concentrations of compounds (as treatment group) and incubated at 37 °C for 48 and 72 h. The MTT assay and data analysis were performed as previously described [29].

4.10. Data Analysis

All statistics were calculated with SPSS 17.0 software and data were expressed as mean ± standard deviation (SD) for each analyte. For MS/MS spectrometry analysis, each mass spectrum shown was the average spectra of each sample detected with ten repetitions in each analysis. Compounds were identified by comparing the tandem mass (MS/MS) fragmentation patterns with those in the literatures, NIST14 mass spectral database, and the MS Search Program v.2.2 (National Institute of Standards and Technology, Gaithersburg, MD, USA). For the viability assay, a nonlinear regression test was applied to obtain a fit curve ($R^2 > 0.98$). Analysis of the differences between the 48/72 h treatment groups was carried out by one-way ANOVA (coupled with a post-test, Dunnett's test) with * $p < 0.05$.

5. Conclusions

In this study, it is the first time that trans-p-Coumaric acid (**1**); 2-Methoxyestrone (**2**); 11, 16-Dihydroxypregn-4-ene-3, 20-dione (**3**), and Tricin (**4**) were isolated and identified from IMP aerial part ethyl acetate extract. 2-Methoxyestrone, 11, 16-Dihydroxypregn-4-ene-3, 20-dione and Tricin possess considerable growth inhibitory activities against BT-549 breast and HT-29 colon cancer cell lines. The data provided important information about the bio-active components from IMP aerial part ethyl acetate extract. *Imperata cylindrica* (L.) Raeusch., one kind of traditional herbal medicine, has rational medical application potentials with respect to breast and colorectal cancer prevention.

Author Contributions: Y.W. and W.S.H. designed the experiments and wrote the paper; Y.W. and J.Z.S. purified each compound by HPLC system; Y.W.C. conducted the tandem MS analysis and analyzed the data; Y.W. identified each compound; J.Z.S. performed the MTT assay and evaluated the growth inhibitory activities of each purified compound against breast cancer and colon cancer cell lines. All authors approved the final manuscript.

Funding: This research was funded by Keenway Industries Ltd. (grant number 6903088).

Acknowledgments: We are grateful to the Biomedical Technology Support Center of Hong Kong Science and Technology Parks Corporation for their help with the mass spectrometry analysis and the generous support from Keenway Industries Ltd. (grant No. 6903088) to W.S.H.

Conflicts of Interest: The authors declare no conflict of interest.

Abbreviations

HPLC-DAD, high-performance liquid chromatography–diode array detector (HPLC-DAD); ESI-MS/MS, electrospray ionization tandem mass spectrometry; NMR, nuclear magnetic resonance; IMP, Imperata cylindrica; MTT, 3-(4,5-Dimethylthiazol-2-yl)-2,5-Diphenyltetrazolium Bromide; ACN, acetonitrile; TFA, trifluoroacetic acid; λmax, wavelength of maximum absorption; LOD, limit of detection; LOQ, limit of quantification; IC50, half-maximal inhibitory concentration; TMS, tetramethylsilane; SD, standard deviation.

References

1. Pinilla, V.; Luu, B. Isolation and partial characterization of immunostimulating polysaccharides from *Imperata cylindrica*. *Planta Med.* **1999**, *65*, 549–552. [CrossRef] [PubMed]
2. Eussen, J.H.H.; Niemann, G.J. Growth inhibiting substances from leaves of *Imperata cylindrica* (L.) Beauv. *Z. Pflanzenphysiol.* **1981**, *102*, 263–266. [CrossRef]
3. Matsunaga, K.; Shibuya, M.; Ohizumi, Y. Graminone B, a novel lignan with vasodilative activity from *Imperata cylindrica*. *J. Nat. Prod.* **1994**, *57*, 1734–1736. [CrossRef] [PubMed]
4. Matsunaga, K.; Shibuya, M.; Ohizumi, Y. Imperanene, a novel phenolic compound with platelet aggregation inhibitory activity from *Imperata cylindrica*. *J. Nat. Prod.* **1995**, *58*, 138–139. [CrossRef] [PubMed]
5. Mohamed, G.A.; Abdel-Lateff, A.; Fouad, M.A.; Ibrahim, S.R.; Elkhayat, E.S.; Okino, T. Chemical composition and hepato-protective activity of *Imperata cylindrica* Beauv. *Pharmacogn. Mag.* **2009**, *5*, 28–36.
6. Liu, R.H.; Chen, S.S.; Ren, G.; Shao, F.; Huang, H.L. Phenolic compounds from roots of *Imperata cylindrica* var. major. *Chin. Herb. Med.* **2013**, *5*, 240–243. [CrossRef]
7. An, H.J.; Nugroho, A.; Song, B.M.; Park, H.J. Isoeugenin, a novel nitric oxide synthase inhibitor isolated from the rhizomes of *Imperata cylindrica*. *Molecules* **2015**, *20*, 21336–21345. [CrossRef] [PubMed]
8. Tine, Y.; Renucci, F.; Costa, J.; Wélé, A.; Paolini, J. A Method for LC-MS/MS profiling of coumarins in *Zanthoxylum zanthoxyloides* (Lam.) B. Zepernich and Timler extracts and essential oils. *Molecules* **2017**, *22*, 174. [CrossRef] [PubMed]
9. Chen, G.; Pramanik, B.N.; Liu, Y.H.; Mirza, U.A. Applications of LC/MS in structure identifications of small molecules and proteins in drug discovery. *J. Mass Spectrom.* **2007**, *42*, 279–287. [CrossRef] [PubMed]
10. Kwok, A.H.Y.; Wang, Y.; Ho, W.S. Cytotoxic and pro-oxidative effects of *Imperata cylindrica* aerial part ethyl acetate extract in colorectal cancer in vitro. *Phytomedicine* **2016**, *23*, 558–565. [CrossRef] [PubMed]
11. Lam, P.Y.; Zhu, F.Y.; Chan, W.L.; Liu, H.; Lo, C. Cytochrome P450 93G1 is a flavone synthase II that channels flavanones to the biosynthesis of Tricin O-linked conjugates in rice. *Plant Physiol.* **2014**, *165*, 1315–1327. [CrossRef] [PubMed]
12. Li, M.; Pu, Y.; Yoo, C.G.; Ragauskas, A.J. The occurrence of Tricin and its derivatives in plants. *Green Chem.* **2016**, *18*, 1439–1454. [CrossRef]
13. Kwon, Y.S.; Kim, C.M. Antioxidant constituents from the stem of Sorghum bicolor. *Arch. Pharm. Res.* **2003**, *26*, 535–539. [CrossRef] [PubMed]
14. Kong, C.; Xu, X.; Zhou, B.; Hu, F.; Zhang, C.; Zhang, M. Two compounds from allelopathic rice accession and their inhibitory activity on weeds and fungal pathogens. *Phytochemistry* **2004**, *65*, 1123–1128. [CrossRef] [PubMed]
15. Jaganathan, S.K.; Supriyanto, E.; Mandal, M. Events associated with apoptotic effect of p-Coumaric acid in HCT-15 colon cancer cells. *World J. Gastroenterol.* **2013**, *19*, 7726–7734. [CrossRef] [PubMed]
16. Sorice, A.; Guerriero, E.; Volpe, M.G.; Capone, F.; La Cara, F.; Ciliberto, G.; Colonna, G.; Costantini, S. Differential response of two human breast cancer cell lines to the phenolic extract from flaxseed oil. *Molecules* **2016**, *21*, 319. [CrossRef] [PubMed]
17. Konishi, Y.; Zhao, Z.; Shimizu, M. Phenolic acids are absorbed from the rat stomach with different absorption rates. *J. Agric. Food Chem.* **2006**, *54*, 7539–7543. [CrossRef] [PubMed]
18. Dobos, J.; Tímár, J.; Bocsi, J.; Burián, Z.; Nagy, K.; Barna, G.; Peták, I.; Ladányi, A. In vitro and in vivo anti-tumor effect of 2-methoxyestradiol on human melanoma. *Int. J. Cancer* **2004**, *112*, 771–776. [CrossRef] [PubMed]
19. Lakhani, N.J.; Sparreboom, A.; Xu, X. Characterization of in vitro and in vivo metabolic pathways of the investigational anticancer agent, 2-methoxyestradiol. *J. Pharm. Sci.* **2007**, *96*, 1821–1831. [CrossRef] [PubMed]
20. Zhu, B.T.; Conney, A.H. Is 2-Methoxyestradiol an endogenous estrogen metabolite that inhibitsmammary carcinogenesis? *Cancer. Res.* **1998**, *58*, 2269–2277. [PubMed]

21. Choudhary, M.I.; Nasir, M.; Khan, S.N.; Atif, M.; Ali, R.A.; Khalil, S.M.; Rahman, A. Microbial hydroxylation of hydroxyprogesterones and α-glucosidase inhibition activity of their metabolites. *Z. Naturforsch.* **2007**, *62*, 593–599. [CrossRef]
22. Lee, D.E.; Lee, S.; Jang, E.S.; Shin, H.W.; Moon, B.S.; Lee, C.H. Metabolomic profiles of Aspergillus oryzae and Bacillus amyloliquefaciens during rice koji fermentation. *Molecules* **2016**, *21*, 773. [CrossRef] [PubMed]
23. Jiao, J.J.; Zhang, Y.; Liu, C.M.; Liu, J.E.; Wu, X.Q.; Zhang, Y. Separation and purification of Tricin from an antioxidant product derived from bamboo leaves. *J. Agric. Food Chem.* **2007**, *55*, 10086–10092. [CrossRef] [PubMed]
24. Hudson, E.A.; Dinh, P.A.; Kokubun, T.; Simmonds, M.S.; Gescher, A. Characterization of potentially chemopreventive phenols in extracts of brown rice that inhibit the growth of human breast and colon cancer cells. *Cancer Epidemiol. Biomarkers. Prev.* **2000**, *9*, 1163–1170. [PubMed]
25. Cai, H.; Hudson, E.A.; Mann, P.; Verschoyle, R.D.; Greaves, P.; Manson, M.M.; Steward, W.P.; Gescher, A.J. Growth-inhibitory and cell cycle-arresting properties of the rice bran constituent Tricin in human-derived breast cancer cells in vitro and in nude mice in vivo. *Br. J. Cancer* **2004**, *91*, 1364–1371. [CrossRef] [PubMed]
26. Verschoyle, R.D.; Greaves, P.; Cai, H.; Borkhardt, A.; Broggini, M.; D'Incalci, M.; Riccio, E.; Doppalapudi, R.; Kapetanovic, I.M.; Steward, W.P.; et al. Preliminary safety evaluation of the putative cancer chemopreventive agent Tricin, a naturally occurring flavone. *Cancer Chemother. Pharmacol.* **2006**, *57*, 1–6. [CrossRef] [PubMed]
27. Zhou, J.M.; Ibrahim, R.K. Tricin-a potential multifunctional nutraceutical. *Phytochem. Rev.* **2010**, *9*, 413–424. [CrossRef]
28. Jang, M.H.; Ho, J.K.; Hye, J.J. Tricin, 4′,5′,7′-trihydroxy-3′,5′-dimethoxyflavone, exhibits potent antiangiogenic activity in vitro. *Int. J. Oncol.* **2016**, *49*, 1497–1504. [CrossRef]
29. Zheng, Y.M.; Shen, J.Z.; Wang, Y.; Lu, A.X.; Ho, W.S. Anti-oxidant and anti-cancer activities of Angelica dahurica extract via induction of apoptosis in colon cancer cells. *Phytomedicine* **2016**, *15*, 1267–1274. [CrossRef] [PubMed]

Sample Availability: Samples of the compounds are not available from the authors.

molecules

MDPI

Article

Cytotoxicity-Guided Isolation of Two New Phenolic Derivatives from *Dryopteris fragrans* (L.) Schott

Tong Zhang [1], Li Wang [2], De-Hua Duan [1], Yi-Hao Zhang [1], Sheng-Xiong Huang [2,*] and Ying Chang [1,*]

1 College of Life Science, Northeast Agricultural University, Harbin 150030, China; shmzhyzt@163.com (T.Z.); myrddh@163.com (D.-H.D.); yhzneau@163.com (Y.-H.Z.)

2 State Key Laboratory of Phytochemistry and Plant Resources in West China, Kunming Institute of Botany, Chinese Academy of Sciences, Kunming 650201, China; jasminewangli@126.com

* Correspondence: sxhuang@mail.kib.ac.cn (S.-X.H.); changying@neau.edu.cn (Y.C.); Tel.: +86-871-6521-5112 (S.-X.H.); +86-451-5519-0410 (Y.C.)

Academic Editor: Pinarosa Avato
Received: 29 May 2018; Accepted: 1 July 2018; Published: 6 July 2018

Abstract: *Dryopteris fragrans* is a valuable medicinal plant resource with extensive biological activities including anti-cancer, anti-oxidation, and anti-inflammation activities. This work aims to study further the cytotoxic constituents from *Dryopteris fragrans*. In this work, two new phenolic derivatives known as dryofragone (**1**) and dryofracoumarin B (**2**) with six known compounds (**3–8**) were isolated from the petroleum ether fraction of the methanol extract of the aerial parts of *Dryopteris fragrans* (L.) Schott by two round cytotoxicity-guided tracking with the 3-(4,5-dimethyl-2-thiazolyl)-2,5-diphenyl-2-*H*-tetrazolium bromide (MTT) assay and cell counting kit-8 (CCK-8) assay. Their structures were elucidated by the extensive spectroscopic analysis (^{1}H-NMR, ^{13}C-NMR, and two dimensions NMR), chemical derivatization, and comparison with data reported in the literature. All the isolates were evaluated for their cytotoxicity against nine cancer cell lines as well as their in vitro immunomodulatory activity. The results showed that compounds have a modest cytotoxicity toward human HeLa cell line with IC_{50} value below 30 μM and compounds **4** and **5** may modulate immunity to affect the growth of tumor cells.

Keywords: cytotoxicity-guided; phenolic derivatives; *Dryopteris fragrans*; chemical derivatization; immuno-regulation activity

1. Introduction

Dryopteris fragrans (L.) Schott (Figure 1) belonging to the genus Dryopteris is a perennial herb with aroma widely distributed throughout the world and is mostly distributed in the alpine and volcanic regions of Northeast China [1,2]. *D. fragrans* has been used as folk medicine for treating arthritis and skin diseases such as psoriasis, dermatophytosis, and more [3]. Previous phytochemical investigations on this plant have led to the identification of terpenoids [4], phloroglucinols [5], glucosides [6], and other phenolic derivatives such as coumarin [3]. The earlier biological studies have shown that *D. fragrans* was a valuable medicinal plant resource with extensive biological activities including anti-cancer, anti-oxidation, insect repellent, anti-microbial, and anti-inflammation activities [3–7].

Of its various biological effects, the mechanism of anti-cancer effects has been studied most. Dryofragin, which is a derivative of phloroglucinol, was found to activate the endogenous pathway of apoptosis by affecting the changes of ROS in mitochondria and inducing changes in mitochondria in breast cancer cell MCF-7 and to cause tumor cell apoptosis by the apoptosis-related protein Bcl-2, Bax, Caspase-9, Caspase-3, and PARP [8]. It has also been reported to be an inhibitor of migration and invasion of the human osteosarcoma cell line U2OS through the PI3K/Akt and MAPK energy pathway involving MMP-2/9 and TIMP-1/2 proteins [9]. Aspidin PB, which is another phloroglucinol derivative from *D. fragrans*, has been recorded as a tumor cell-inhibiting agent for its impact on cyclin p53/p21 and mitochondrial changes in human osteosarcoma cells Saos-2, U2OS, and HOS [10]. In addition, there have been many other reports on compounds from *D. fragrans* with cytotoxicity [11–13]. To further study cytotoxic constituents from *D. fragrans*, a cytotoxicity-guided isolation of the extract of *D. fragrans* was designed. The isolation of two new phenolic derivatives and six known compounds by cytotoxicity-guided tracking as well as their cytotoxicity and immunomodulatory activity detection is described in this paper.

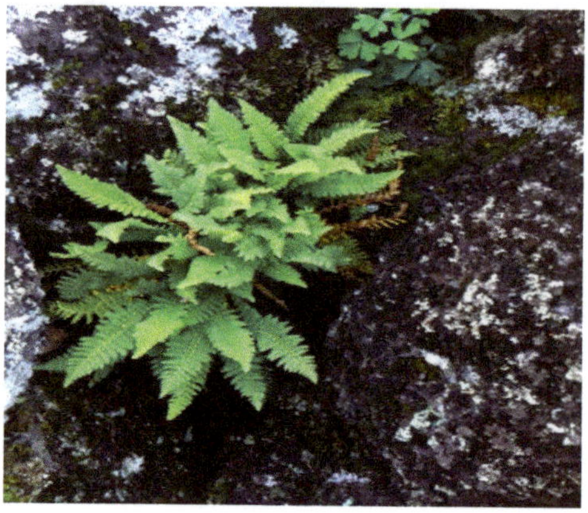

Figure 1. *Dryopteris fragrans* plant.

2. Results and Discussion

2.1. Determination of Isolated Compounds

After two round cytotoxicity screening by MTT [14] and CCK-8 [15] assay, Fractions SG1-SG7 from the petroleum ether-soluble part with prominent cytotoxic activities were selected as the bioactive sites (Figures S1 and S2). Two new phenolic derivatives known as dryofragone (**1**) and dryofracoumarin B (**2**) (Figure 2) along with six known compounds (**3–8**) (Figure 2), were isolated from the above seven bioactive fractions by using extensive chromatographic methods like silica gel, MCI gel, Sephadex LH-20, and HPLC. The known compounds were identified as dryofracoumarin A (**3**) [3], vitamin E quinone (**4**) [16], albicanol (**5**) [5], 2′,4′-dihydroxy-6′-methoxy-3′,5′-dimethylchalcone (**6**) [17], norflavesone (**7**) [18], and aspidinol (**8**) [19] by comparing their ^{1}H- and ^{13}C-NMR data with that reported in the literature.

Compound **1** was obtained as yellow powder from $CHCl_3$. The HR-ESI-MS data (*m/z* 239.0926 $[M - H]^-$, calcd for 239.0925) of **1** showed the molecular formula $C_{12}H_{16}O_5$, which correspond to five degrees of unsaturation. The IR spectrum of **1** displayed hydroxyls (3321 cm^{-1}), carbonyl groups (1714 cm^{-1}), and double bonds (1607 cm^{-1}) absorptions. The red shifted hydroxyl signal (3321 cm^{-1}) also showed that some hydroxyls in **1** were involved in the hydrogen bonding interaction. The ^{1}H-NMR spectrum of **1** (Table 1) showed one 3H-singlet at δ_H 1.54 for a tertiary methyl group, one 3H-singlet at δ_H 3.91 for a methoxy group, one 3H-triplet at δ_H 1.01 for a primary methyl group, and an olefinic proton at δ_H 5.37. The ^{13}C-NMR spectrum of **1** revealed 12 resonance signals including two ketone carbons at δ_C 196.3 (conjugated) and 203.7, two pair of olefinic carbons (δ_C 189.4, 176.0, 104.5 and 94.5) with two oxygenated sites (δ_C 189.4 and 176.0), an oxygenated tertiary carbon (δ_C 75.4), a methoxy carbon (δ_C 57.4), two aliphatic methylene carbon (δ_C 41.0 and 18.7), and two methyl carbons (δ_C 30.2 and 14.1). The above evidence indicated that compound **1** presumably possessed an oxygenated phloroglucinol core [20]. This inference was further confirmed by the 2D-NMR spectra

(Figure 3). The long-range HMBC couplings—H-4/C-2, C-3, C-5, and C-6 as well as Me-11/C-1, C-2, and C-3 demonstrated the presence of a cyclohexadiene moiety with two oxygen-bearing carbon at C-2 and C-5. The HMBC correlation from a methoxy at δ_H 3.91 (Me-12) to a quaternary olefinic carbon at δ_C 176.0 (C-3) revealed that a methoxy was located at C-3. Furthermore, a butyryl was linked to C-6, which was supported by the HMBC correlations from protons at C-8 (δ_H 2.99 and 2.92) to carbons at δ_C 104.5 (C-6), 203.7 (C-7), 18.7 (C-9), and 14.1 (C-10), respectively. The CD experiment towards compound **1** was performed. However, the CD spectrum (Figure S9) of **1** showed no characteristic cotton effect. Compound **1** was considered to be a pair of enantiomers.

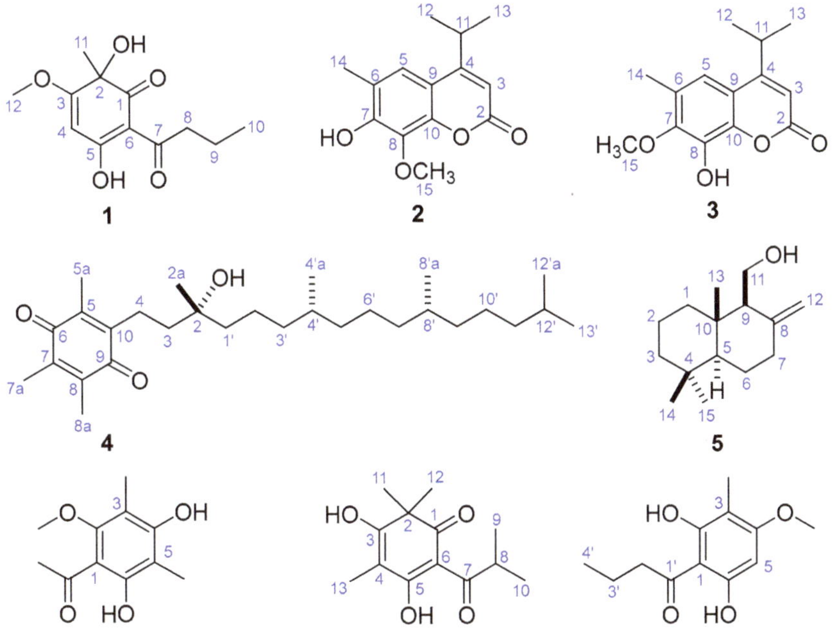

Figure 2. Structures of compounds **1–8**.

Table 1. NMR data for Compound **1** (TMS as the internal standard, δ in ppm, J in Hz) [a].

No.	δ_H	δ_C	No.	δ_H	δ_C
1		196.32 (C)	8a	2.99 (1H, m)	41.04 (CH_2)
2		75.37 (C)	8b	2.92 (1H, m)	
3		176.04 (C)	9	1.69 (2H, m)	18.71 (CH_2)
4	5.37 (1H, s)	94.49 (CH)	10	1.01 (3H, t, J = 7.4)	14.07 (CH_3)
5		189.34 (C)	11	1.54 (3H, s)	30.20 (CH_3)
6		104.49 (C)	12	3.91 (3H, s)	57.35 (CH_3)
7		203.65 (C)			

[a] ^{1}H-NMR and ^{13}C-NMR data were recorded in $CDCl_3$ at 600 MHz and 150 MHz, respectively.

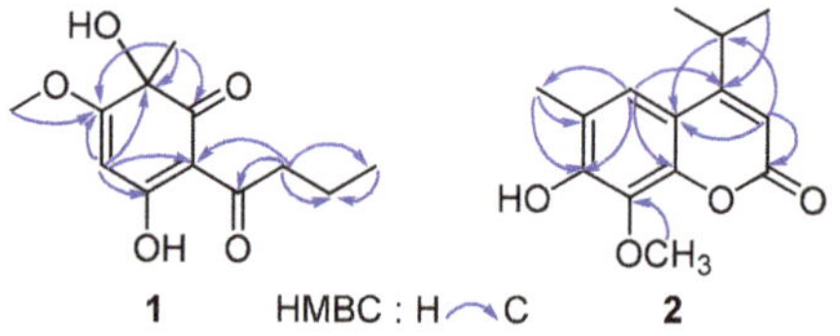

Figure 3. Key HMBC correlations of **1** and **2**.

Therefore, the structure of **1** was concluded to be a new acylphloroglucinol, 6-isobutyryl-2, 5-dihydroxy-2-methyl-3-methoxy-cyclohexa-3,5-dien-1-one, and was named dryofragone.

Compound **2** was obtained as a mixture with compound **3** initially. The ^{13}C-NMR spectrum of the mixture revealed 28 resonance signals (Figure S12) in which half were consistent with the data reported for a coumarin and dryofracoumarin A (**3**) [3]. However, the ESI-MS data (*m*/*z* 249[M + H]$^+$, 271[M + Na]$^+$, 287[M + K]$^+$) of the mixture showed only one molecular weight (248 Da), which aligned with that of **3**. Consequently, the other half of carbon resonance signals in the ^{13}C-NMR for the mixture, which were highly similar with that of **3**, were supposed to be of an isomer of **3** featuring exchanged positions of hydroxyl and methoxy groups in the coumarin core. Based on the large space size of tert-butyl dimethyl silicyl group, which can strike the balance of molecular polarity for compounds **2** and **3** and the high yield of the desilication step, a silicon etherification-desilication procedure was designed for the isolation of the mixture (See Section 3.5 and Figure 4). NMR data of compounds **2** and **3** are shown in Table 2. After the chemical derivatization, compound **2** was afforded as a simplex. The IR spectrum of **2** exhibited a signal of hydroxyl with no hydrogen bonds (3548 cm^{-1}), a strong band at 1668 cm^{-1} for the lactone subunit in coumarin core, and absorptions (1636, 1602, 1572 cm^{-1}) of benzene ring moiety in coumarin. The HR-ESI-MS data (*m*/*z* 247.0975 [M − H]$^-$, calcd for 247.0976) indicated a molecular formula $C_{14}H_{16}O_4$ with seven degrees of unsaturation for **2**. The HMBC correlations (Figure 3) from Me-12 and -13 (δ_H 1.30 × 2) to C-4 (δ_C 163.0) as well as the correlations from H-11(δ_H 3.25) to C-3 (δ_C 107.8), C-4 (δ_C 163.0), and C-9 (δ_C 112.2), which suggests that an isopropyl was fused to C-4. Another HMBC correlation Me-15/C-8 verified that a methoxyl group was linked to C-8. In addition, the HMBC correlations from an isolated methyl (δ_H 2.31) to C-5 (δ_C 120.0), C-6 (δ_C 121.1), and C-7 (δ_C 150.0) inferred a methyl at C-6 in **2**. The above analyses disclosed our former hypothesis. As a result, the structure of **2** was determined to be 7-hydroxy-6-methyl-8-methoxy-4-isopropyl-2H-chromen-2-one, which was given the trivial name of dryofracoumarin B.

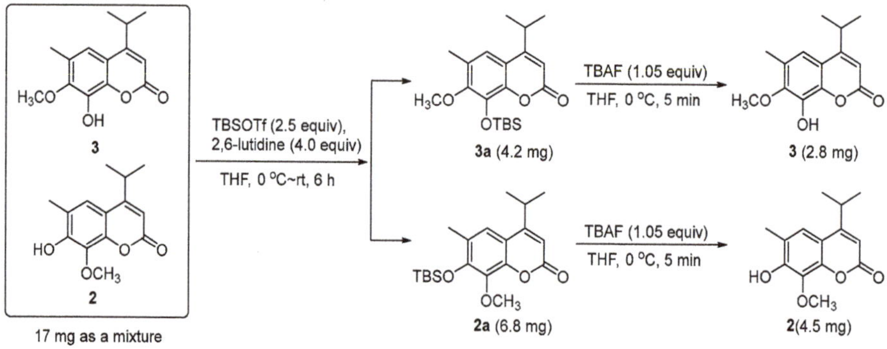

Figure 4. Silicon etherification involved the isolation of **2** and **3**.

Table 2. NMR data for compound **2** and **3** (TMS as the internal standard, δ in ppm, J in Hz) [a].

No.	2		3	
	δ_H	δ_C	δ_H	δ_C
1				
2		161.5 (C)		161.1 (C)
3	6.16 (1H, s)	107.8 (CH)	6.22 (1H, s)	109.2 (CH)
4		163.0 (C)		163.0 (C)
5	7.17 (1H, s)	120.0 (CH)	7.01 (1H, s)	115.5 (CH)
6		121.1 (C)		127.5 (C)
7		150.0 (C)		147.8 (C)
8		133.6 (C)		136.7 (C)
9		112.2 (C)		114.5 (C)
10		145.5 (C)		141.3 (C)
11	3.25 (1H, m)	28.7 (CH)	3.25 (1H, m)	28.7 (CH)
12	1.30 (3H, d, J = 6.8)	22.1 (CH_3)	1.31 (3H, d, J = 6.8)	21.9 (CH_3)
13	1.30 (3H, d, J = 6.8)	22.1 (CH_3)	1.31 (3H, d, J = 6.8)	21.9 (CH_3)
14	2.31 (3H, s)	15.9 (CH_3)	2.32 (3H, s)	16.3 (CH_3)
15	4.08 (3H, s)	61.9 (OCH_3)	3.95 (3H, s)	60.5 (OCH_3)

[a] ^{1}H-NMR and ^{13}C-NMR data were recorded in $CDCl_3$ at 600 MHz and 150 MHz, respectively.

2.2. In Vitro Cytotoxicity and Immunomodulatory Activity Detection

For all the isolates, their cytotoxicities against nine human cancer cell lines known as HepG2, A549, HeLa, U251, HOS, MG63, U2OS, MB231, and SKBR-3 as well as their immuno-regulation activities were evaluated. The cytotoxicities were screened using the CCK-8 assay [15]. The IC_{50} values of cytotoxicities for the eight compounds are shown in Table 3. For compounds isolated by cytotoxicity-guided tracking, they exhibited moderate activities to the HeLa cell line and weak activities to glioma, liver cancer, and lung cancer cell lines. However, they were not very sensitive to osteosarcoma and breast cancer cell lines when compared to the crude extract. For their immuno-regulation activities, LPS stimulated THP-1 cells were used as the in vitro model for the detection [21]. Fenofibrate (Feno) pre-treatment (20 μM) was used as a positive control [21]. The results for immuno-regulation activities are shown in Figure 5. Only compounds **4** and **5** could enhance the secretion of the factors *TNF-α* and *IL-1β*. The results showed that compounds **4** and **5** may activate the LPS signaling pathway, which may modulate immunity to affect the growth of tumor cells.

Table 3. IC_{50} values (μM) of cytotoxicity for eight compounds against nine human cancer cell lines.

Compound	HepG2	A549	HeLa	U251	HOS	MG63	U2OS	MB231	SKBR-3
1	-	45.86 ± 1.64	25.37 ± 2.62	46.13 ± 1.90	-	-	-	-	-
2	45.52 ± 3.21	47.70 ± 2.43	15.12 ± 4.01	46.14 ± 2.40	-	-	-	25.59 ± 2.30	-
3	48.39 ± 2.15	38.01 ± 3.56	-	-	-	-	-	38.09 ± 2.40	-
4	38.13 ± 1.03	37.41 ± 1.24	1.24 ± 0.08	-	-	-	47.56 ± 2.23	41.95 ± 2.35	-
5	-	49.74 ± 3.35	-	-	-	-	-	-	-
6	-	47.42 ± 2.25	-	-	-		-	-	-
7	-	40.03 ± 0.98	-	-	-	-	-	-	
8	18.02 ± 0.89	-	17.76 ± 3.43	41.21 ± 1.35	43.67 ± 2.52	22.76 ± 2.65	36.36 ± 1.32	39.61 ± 1.50	33.40 ± 1.50
Taxol [a]	5.32 ± 0.12	3.46 ± 0.23	0.17 ± 0.02	5.02 ± 0.21	3.71 ± 0.33	5.86 ± 0.24	1.01 ± 0.03	6.23 ± 0.36	3.12 ± 0.25

Note: IC_{50} values represented the means ± SD of six independent experiments and "-" means the IC_{50} value is above 50 μM. [a] Taxol was used as a positive control.

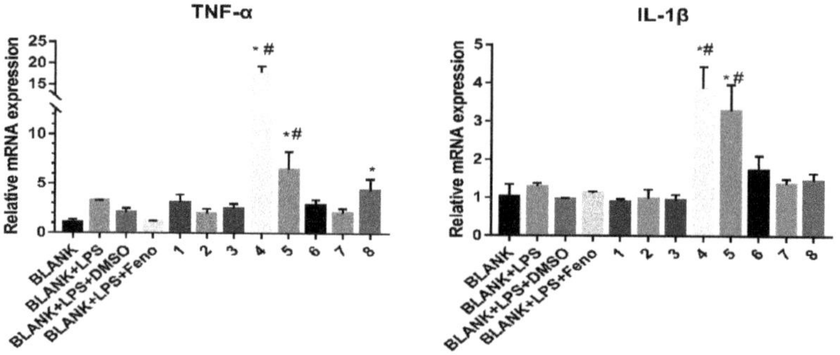

(A) (B)

Figure 5. The influence of eight compounds on immuno-regulation factors over a period of 24 h. (**A**) for the factor *TNF-α* and (**B**) for the factor *IL-1β*. The "*" indicates that there were significant differences ($p < 0.05$) between other compounds and the BLANK group amd the "#" indicates that there were significant differences ($p < 0.05$) between other compounds and the BLANK + LPS group. Each value represented the means ± SD of three independent experiments.

3. Materials and Methods

3.1. General Experimental Procedures

Optical rotations were recorded in MeOH using a JASCO P-1020 Polarimeter (Jasco Corp., Tokyo, Japan). UV spectra were acquired in MeOH with a Shimadzu UV-2401PC UV-VIS spectrophotometer (Shimadzu Corp., Kyoto, Japan). IR spectra were measured on a Bruker Tensor 27 FTIR Spectrometer with KBr disks (Bruker Corp., Karlsruhe, Germany). ^{1}H-NMR, ^{13}C-NMR, and 2D NMR spectra were recorded in $CDCl_3$ using a Bruker AVANCE III-600 spectrometer or a Bruker DRX-400 spectrometer (Bruker Corp., St. Gallen, Switzerland). TMS was used as the internal standard. ESI-MS spectra were recorded using a Waters Xevo TQ-S Ultra High Pressure Liquid Chromatography Triple Quadrupole Mass Spectrometer (Waters Corp., Manchester, UK). HR-ESI-MS data were obtained using an Agilent G6230 Q-TOF mass instrument (Agilent Corp., Santa Clara, CA, USA). Column chromatography (CC) was performed using a silica gel (200–300 mesh, Qingdao Marine Chemical Inc., Qingdao, China), MCI gel CHP 20P (75–150 μm, Mitsubishi Corp., Tokyo, Japan), and Sephadex LH-20 (25–100 mm, Pharmacia Biotech Ltd., Uppsala, Sweden). Thin-layer chromatography (TLC) was performed using pre-coated silica gel GF254 plates (0.25 mm in thickness for analysis and 0.60 mm thickness for preparation, Qingdao Marine Chemical Inc., Qingdao, China) with various solvent systems. Spots were visualized under UV light (254 nm) and colored by iodine and by spraying silica gel plates with 10% H_2SO_4 in MeOH followed by heating. Preparative HPLC separations were performed on a CXTH system equipped with a UV3000 detector (Beijing Chuangxintongheng Instruments Co. Ltd., Beijing, China), and a Kromasil C_{18} column (250 mm × 20 mm i.d., 5 mm, EKA Chemicals Corp., Bohus, Sweden) using a flow rate of 8.0 mL/min at a column temperature of 25 °C. Semi-preparative HPLC was conducted on a HITACHI Chromaster system (Hitachi Ltd., Tokyo, Japan) equipped with an Agilent ZORBAXSB-C_{18} column (150 mm × 9.4 mm i.d., 5 mm, Agilent Corp., Santa Clara, CA, USA) using a flow rate of 3.0 mL/min at a column temperature of 25 °C. The detection was performed with a DAD detector.

3.2. Plant Material

The aerial parts of *Dryopteris fragrans* (L.) Schott were collected in June 2016 from the Wudalianchi scenic area, Heihe City, Helongjiang Province, China and identified by Prof. Baodong Liu from the

Harbin Normal University. A voucher specimen (No. df-20070702-9) was deposited in the Plant Herbarium of Northeast Agricultural University in Harbin, China.

3.3. Determination of Anti-Tumor Fraction of *Dryopteris fragrans*

After methanol extraction, the crude extract was then partitioned with petroleum ether (rt), dichloromethane (DCM) (rt), EtOAc (rt), and n-BuOH (rt) in sequence. The crude extract was divided into six parts (the whole extracts, petroleum ether layer, DCM layer, EtOAc layer, n-BuOH layer, and water phase). Each fraction was dissolved in DMSO and the final concentration of DMSO in the cell culture medium was no more than 0.1%. The osteosarcoma cell lines HOS and MG63 were used as the first round screening target in MTT [14] for the above six parts of the crude extracts. As shown in Figure S1, petroleum ether fraction of crude extracts had the most obvious cytotoxic effects at the point of 48 h. The petroleum ether fraction was then divided into 14 sub-fractions (Fr SG1-SG14) by using silica gel column chromatography. The above 14 fractions were then subjected to MTT or CCK-8 assay [15] against HepG2, MB231, and MG63 cell lines, respectively. As shown in Figure S2, Fractions SG1–SG7 from the petroleum ether-soluble part exhibited prominent cytotoxic activities.

3.4. Extraction and Isolation

The air-dried aerial parts of *Dryopteris fragrans* (L.) Schott powder (2 kg) were extracted with 100% methanol (20 L × 2 d × 3) and ultrasonized (40 Hz) for 4 h at each time. After filtration, the filtrate was concentrated to yield the crude extract. The crude extract was then suspended in water (1.5 L) and partitioned with petroleum ether (3 × 1.5 L), DCM (3 × 1.5 L), EtOAc (3 × 1.5 L), and n-BuOH (3 × 1.5 L) sequentially. Guided by the first round cytotoxicity screening, the petroleum ether fraction (54 g) was chosen for further isolation. The petroleum ether-soluble part was then subjected to silica gel CC and eluted with petroleum ether–EtOAc (1:0–0:1) to create 14 fractions (SG1–SG14). According to the second round cytotoxicity screening, Fractions SG1–SG7 were selected as the isolation targets for the next step. Fractions SG1 and SG2 were not actually involved in the next step because their low polarities made an effective separation on column chromatography difficult.

Fraction SG3 (5.93 g) was submitted to the silica gel CC (petroleum ether–EtOAc 1:0–0:1) and Sephadex LH-20 CC (MeOH–$CHCl_3$ 1:1) and followed by preparative TLC (petroleum ether–EtOAc 11:2, Rf = 0.53) to afford compound **4** (14.4 mg). Compound **5** (103.2 mg) was isolated from Fraction SG4 (5.01 g) by undergoing a protocol of repeated silica gel CC (petroleum ether–EtOAc 1:0–10:1), Sephadex LH-20 CC (MeOH–CHCl3 1:1), and preparative TLC (petroleum ether–EtOAc 8:1, Rf = 0.40). Fraction SG6 (3.54 g) was chromatographed on MCI CC (MeOH–H_2O 40:60 to 100:0) to yield 16 sub-fractions (Fr M1–M16). Further purification of Fr. M6 by semi-preparative HPLC (MeOH: H_2O 53:47) resulted in the isolation of compounds **6** (15.8 mg) and **7** (10.0 mg). Fraction SG7 (2.49 g) was further separated by MCI CC (MeOH–H_2O 20:80 to 100:0) to yield 11 fractions (Fr. M_21–M_211). Compound **1** (4.5 mg) was purified from Fraction M_24 using semi-preparative HPLC (MeOH:H_2O 58:42). In the same way, compound **8** (2.0 mg) was obtained from Fraction M_27. Compounds **2** and **3** were obtained as a mixture (17.0 mg) from Fraction M_26 by semi-preparative HPLC (MeOH:H_2O 77:23). They were separated by a silicon etherification-desilication procedure (See Section 3.5).

Dryofragone (**1**): yellow powder ($CHCl_3$). $[\alpha]_D^{23.7}$ −20.3 (*c* 0.10, MeOH); UV (MeOH) λ_{max} (log ε): 198 (3.17) nm, 241 (3.38) nm, 276 (3.20) nm, 320 (3.14) nm, IR (KBr) ν_{max} IR (KBr) ν_{max} 3321, 2929, 1714, 1607, 1533, 1442, 1231, 1104; ^{1}H-NMR (600 MHz, $CDCl_3$): δ_H 5.37 (1H, s, H-4), 3.91 (3H, s, Me-12), 2.99 (1H, m, H-8a), 2.92 (1H ,m, H-8b), 1.69 (2H, m, H-9), 1.54 (3H, s, Me-11), 1.01 (3H, t, *J* = 7.4 Hz, Me-10); 203.7 (C-7), 196.3 (C-1), 189.4 (C-5), 176.0 (C-3), 104.5 (C-6), 94.5 (C-4), 75.4 (C-2), 57.4 (C-12), 41.0 (C-8), 30.2 (C-11), 18.7 (C-9),14.1 (C-10), ESI-MS *m/z* 239 $[M-H]^-$, and HR-ESI-MS *m/z* 239.0926 $[M-H]^-$ (calcd for $C_{12}H_{15}O_5$, 239.0925).

3.5. Silicon Etherification Involved Isolation of 2 and 3

3.5.1. Silicon Etherification of the Mixture of Compounds 2 and 3

With regard to the solution of the mixture of Compounds **2** and **3** (17 mg, 0.068 mmol) in dry DCM (0.5 mL), 2,6-luditine (30 μL, 0.27 mmol, 4.0 equiv) was added at 0 °C, which is followed by the addition of TBSOTf (35 μL, 0.17 mmol, 2.5 equiv). The resulting mixture was warmed to room temperature (rt) naturally, stirred for 6 h, and then quenched with water (2.0 mL). The mixture was then stirred for 10 min, followed by an extraction with EtOAc (10.0 mL) three times, and the EtOAc layer was dried over anhydrous Na_2SO_4 and subsequently concentrated. The residue was further purified by semi-preparative HPLC (85% MeOH in H_2O, 3 mL/min, a HITACHI Chromaster system equipped with a DAD detector, an Agilent ZORBAX SB-C_{18} column, 150 mm × 9.4 mm i.d., 5 μm) to yield compound **2a** (6.8 mg, t_R = 19.8 min) and **3a** (4.2 mg, t_R = 15.8 min) as white solids. Compound **2a**: ^{1}H-NMR (400 MHz, $CDCl_3$): δ_H 7.17 (1H, s, H-5), 6.18 (1H, s, H-3), 3.91 (3H, s, Me-15), 3.24 (1H, m, H-11), 2.29 (3H, s, Me-14), 1.30 (6H, d, J = 6.8 Hz, Me-12, 13), 1.03 (9H, s, Me-19, 20, 21), 0.24 (6H, s, Me-16, 17), ^{13}C-NMR (100 MHz, $CDCl_3$): δ_C 162.5 (C-4), 161.7 (C-2), 150.1 (C-7), 146.9 (C-10), 138.3 (C-8), 126.5 (C-6), 119.5 (C-5), 113.4 (C-9), 108.5 (C-3), 61.1 (C-15), 28.7 (C-11), 26.1 × 3 (C-19, 20, 21), 22.1 × 2 (C-12, 13), 19.0 (C-18), 17.7 (C-14), −4.0 × 2 (C-16, 17). Compound **3a**: ^{1}H-NMR (400 MHz, $CDCl_3$): δ_H 7.07 (1H, s, H-5), 6.21 (1H, s, H-3), 3.82 (3H, s, Me-15), 3.24 (1H, m, H-11), 2.32 (3H, s, Me-14), 1.30 (6H, d, J = 6.8 Hz, Me-12, 13), 1.08 (9H, s, Me-19, 20, 21), 0.25 (6H, s, Me-16, 17), ^{13}C-NMR (100 MHz, $CDCl_3$): δ_C 162.2 (C-4), 161.4 (C-2), 152.5 (C-7), 145.3 (C-10), 137.2 (C-8), 127.8 (C-6), 117.0 (C-5), 115.4 (C-9), 109.8 (C-3), 60.2 (C-15), 28.7 (C-11), 25.9 × 3 (C-19, 20, 21), 22.1 × 2 (C-12, 13), 18.8 (C-18), 16.4 (C-14), −4.2 × 2 (C-16, 17).

3.5.2. Desilication of Compound 2a

To a solution of compound **2a** (6.8 mg, 0.0188 mmol) in dry THF (0.1 mL), TBAF (1 M in THF, 19 μL, 0.0197 mmol, 1.05 equiv) was added at 0 °C. The resulting mixture was stirred at 0 °C for 5 min and then quenched by adding 1.0 mL of the saturated ammonium chloride aqueous solution. The resulting mixture was then extracted by EtOAc (5.0 mL) three times and the combined organic extracts were dried over anhydrous Na_2SO_4 and were then concentrated. The residue was purified by using flash column chromatography on the silica gel (200–300 mush, 1.0 × 3.0 cm, petroleum ether/EtOAc 4:1), which yielded compound **2** (4.5 mg, 96.6% yield) as a white solid. Compound **2**: UV (MeOH) λ_{max} (log ε): 206 (3.81) nm, 218 (3.52) nm, 250 (2.78) nm, 330 (3.29) nm; IR (KBr) ν_{max} 3548, 3466, 3169, 2942, 1668, 1602, 1460, 1404, 1229, 1094, 1024, 925, 856; ^{1}H-NMR (600 MHz, $CDCl_3$): δ_H 7.17 (1H, s, H-5), 6.16 (1H, s, H-3), 4.08 (3H, s, Me-15), 3.25 (1H, m, H-11), 2.31 (3H, s, Me-14), 1.30 (3H, d, J = 6.8 Hz, Me-12), 1.30 (3H, d, J = 6.8 Hz, Me-13); ^{13}C-NMR (150 MHz, $CDCl_3$): δ_C 163.0 (C-4), 161.5 (C-2), 150.0 (C-7), 145.5 (C-10), 133.6 (C-8), 121.1 (C-6), 120.0 (C-5), 112.2 (C-9), 107.8 (C-3), 61.9 (C-15), 28.7 (C-11), 22.1 (C-12), 22.1 (C-13), 15.9 (C-14), HR-ESI-MS: m/z 247.0975[M − H]$^-$, calcd. 247.0976 for $C_{14}H_{15}O_4$.

3.5.3. Desilication of Compound 3a

To a solution of compound **3a** (4.2 mg, 0.0116 mmol) in dry THF (0.1 mL), TBAF (1 M in THF, 12 μL, 0.0121 mmol, 1.05 equiv) was added at 0 °C. The resulting mixture was stirred at 0 °C for 5 min and then quenched by adding 1.0 mL of saturated ammonium chloride aqueous solution. The resulting mixture was then extracted by EtOAc (5.0 mL) three times and the combined organic extracts were dried over anhydrous Na_2SO_4 and concentrated. The residue was purified by flash column chromatography on the silica gel (200–300 mush, 1.0 × 3.0 cm, petroleum ether/EtOAc 4:1), which yielded compound **3** (2.8 mg, 97.4% yield) as a white solid. Compound **3**: ^{1}H-NMR (600 MHz, $CDCl_3$): δ_H 7.01 (1H, s, H-5), 6.22 (1H, s, H-3), 3.95 (3H, s, Me-15), 3.25 (1H, m, H-11), 2.32 (3H, s, Me-14), 1.31 (6H, d, J = 6.8 Hz, Me-12, 13); ^{13}C-NMR (150 MHz, $CDCl_3$): δ_C 163.0 (C-4), 161.1 (C-2),

147.8 (C-7), 141.3 (C-10), 136.7 (C-8), 127.5 (C-6), 115.5 (C-5), 114.5 (C-9), 109.2 (C-3), 60.5 (C-15), 28.7 (C-11), 21.9 (C-12 & C-13), and 16.3 (C-14).

3.6. MTT and CCK-8 Assay

Human HepG2, HeLa, U251, HOS, MG63, U2OS, MB231, and SKBR-3 cells were obtained from the Cell Library of Committee on Type Culture Collection of Chinese Academy of Sciences (Shanghai, China). Cells were cultured at 37 °C, 5% CO_2 in the Dulbecco's Modified Eagle's medium (DMEM), Minimum Eagle's medium (MEM), or the Roswell Park Memorial Institute (RPMI) medium containing 10% FBS, 100 U/mL penicillin, and 100 U/mL streptomycin.

Compounds **1–8** were dissolved in DMSO and diluted with DMEM medium (containing 1% FBS and 100 U/mL penicillin/streptomycin) for certain concentrations (1.5625 μM, 3.125 μM, 6.25 μM, 12.5 μM, 25 μM, 50 μM, and 100 μM). The concentration of DMSO in the final solutions was no more than 0.1%. Human HepG2, HeLa, U251, HOS, MG63, U2OS, MB231, and SKBR-3 cells were seeded in 96-well micro-titer plates (100 μL, 1×10^4 cells/well). When the cells grew to certain concentrations (70%–80% of the well), the medium was removed and the diluted compounds (200 μL) were added to each well. Blank (only medium) and control (cells with DMEM medium) group were set to calculate the cell viability and Taxol was used as a positive control. After 48 h, the 96-well micro-titer plates were taken out from the incubator and the medium was removed. When using the MTT assay, DMEM medium (200 μL) should be first added into the well and then followed by MTT (20 μL, 5 mg/mL dissolved in PBS). After culturing for 4 h, the 96-well micro-titer plates were taken out from the incubator and the medium was removed and then 150 μL of DMSO was added into the well. The absorbance was measured by a microplate reader (Bio-Rad, America) at 560 nm. When using CCK-8 assay, DMEM medium (100 μL) should be first added into the well and then CCK-8 (Dojindo, Kumamoto, Japan) followed. After culturing for 2.5 h, the 96-well micro-titer plates were taken out from the incubator and the absorbance was measured by a microplate reader at 450 nm. The cell viability = (Lab group − Blank group)/(Control group − Blank group) and the IC_{50} value was calculated by the software GraphPad Prism 7.0 with the cell viability value.

3.7. Immunoregulation Activity

THP-1 cells were obtained from the Harbin medical university and was cultured in RPMI medium. The cell was seeded in 6-well plate (2 mL, 2×10^6 cell/well) and starved for 12 h. Lipopolysaccharide (LPS, Sigma, St. Louis, MI, USA) (2 mg/mL in PBS) was then added in the well to stimulate the cell. One hour later, each compound was dissolved in DMSO at a concentration of 20 μM. It was added in the well and cultivated for 24 h. The cell was then collected. Following the manufacturer's instructions, the Trizol reagent (Invitrogen, Carlsbad, CA, USA) was used to isolate the total RNA of THP-1 cell. The extracted total RNA was dissolved in RNA enzyme-free water and added into a 100 μL reaction mixture for reverse transcription into complementary DNA (cDNA). The extracted RNA solution contained 8 μg, 8 μL of 50 pmol/μL Oligo d(T)18 and the volume was brought up to 46 μL with RNA enzyme-free water, incubated at 70 °C for 5 min, and then 4 °C for 5 min. Afterward, 20 μL of 2.5 μmol/mL dNTP, 20 μL of 5× RT buffer, 8 μL of dTT, 2 μL of RNA inhibitor, and 4 μL of M-MLV were added and the mixture was incubated at 42 °C for 3 h. The 100 μL mixture was stored at −20 °C for qualitative PCR (qPCR). Detected via qPCR, the gene expression levels were identified with a LightCycler® 480 System (Roche, Basel, Switzerland) using the TransStart® Tip Green qPCR SuperMix (TRANSGEN BIOTECH, Beijing, China). The cDNA was added into a 20 μL reaction mixture: 10 μL of 2× TransStart® Tip Green qPCR SuperMix, 2 μL of cDNA Template (100–200 pg), 0.8 μL of primer mixture (10 μM), 0.4 μL of Passive Reference Dye (50×), and 6.8 μL of ddH_2O. The PCR procedure includes a temperature of 94 °C and a time period of 30 s followed by 40 cycles at 94 °C for 5 s, 57 °C for 15 s, and 72 °C for 10 s. The β-actin gene was used a control to quantify other genes. The results were calculated using $2^{-\Delta\Delta Ct}$ where ΔΔCt = (Ct Target − Ct β-actin)Lab − (Ct Target − Ct β-actin) Control. Primers of the target gene TNF-α, IL-1β, and β-actin were designed by Primer 5.0 software following the published gene sequence in GenBank: TNF-α Forward: CAGCAAGGGACAGCAGAGG, Reverse: AGTATGTGAGAGGAAGAGAACC; IL-1β Forward: TGATGGCTTATTACAGTGGCAATG, Reverse: TGATGGCTTATTACAGTGGCAATG; β-actin Forward: ATCGGCAATGAGCGGTTCC, Reverse: ATCGGCAATGAGCGGTTCC.

4. Conclusions

In this work, two new phenolic derivatives dryofragone (**1**) and dryofracoumarin B (**2**) were isolated from *Dryopteris fragrans* by cytotoxicity-guided tracking. Two coumarin isomers dryofracoumarin B (**2**) and dryofracoumarin A (**3**) were separated by a silicon etherification-desilication procedure. Compounds (**4**) and (**6**) were first reported in this plant. The cytotoxicity and immuno-regulation activity were examined among the eight compounds and the relationship between cytotoxicity and immuno-regulation activity revealed that compounds may activate the LPS signaling to regulate the growth of tumor cells through immuno-regulation. This relation needs further study.

Supplementary Materials: The following are available online. Supplementary materials included Figures S1 and S2: Two round screening of cytotoxicity with MTT or CCK-8 assay, Figures S3–S27: Spectrum and Spectroscopy data of compounds **1–3**, **2a** and **3a**, and NMR spectral data of compounds **4–8**.

Author Contributions: S.-X.H. and Y.C. handled the conceptualization. T.Z. managed the data curation. T.Z. performed a formal analysis. S.-X.H. and Y.C. handled the funding acquisition. T.Z., L.W., D.-H.D., and Y.-H.Z. were responsible for the methodology. L.W. handled the software. S.-X.H. and Y.C. supervised the project. T.Z. wrote the original draft. Writing—review & editing, L.W. took part in reviewing and editing the manuscript.

Acknowledgments: This work received no external funding and was financially supported by the National Natural Science Foundation of China (No. 81522044 to S.-X.H.), the Applied Basic Research Foundation of Yunnan Province (No. 2013HA022 to S.-X.H.), Foundation from Chinese Academy of Sciences (QYZDB-SSW-SMC051 to S.-X.H.), and the National Natural Science Foundation of China (No. 31570189 to Y.C.). We appreciate the help of Yunzhou Wu and Wenfei Wang in this work.

Conflicts of Interest: The authors declare no conflict of interest.

References

1. Kuang, H.; Zhang, Y.; Li, G.; Zeng, W.; Wang, H.; Song, Q. A new phenolic glycoside from the aerial parts of *Dryopteris fragrans*. *Fitoterapia* **2008**, *79*, 319–320. [CrossRef] [PubMed]
2. Patama, T.T.; Widen, C.J. Phloroglucinol derivatives from *Dryopteris fuscoatra* and *D. hawaiiensis*. *Phytochemistry* **1991**, *30*, 3305–3310. [CrossRef]
3. Zhao, D.D.; Zhao, Q.S.; Liu, L.; Chen, Z.Q.; Zeng, W.M.; Lei, H.; Zhang, Y.L. Compounds from *Dryopteris fragrans* (L.) Schott with cytotoxic activity. *Molecules* **2014**, *19*, 3345–3355. [CrossRef] [PubMed]
4. Huang, Y.H.; Zeng, W.M.; Li, G.Y.; Liu, G.Q.; Zhao, D.D.; Wang, J.; Zhang, Y.L. Characterization of a new sesquiterpene and antifungal activities of chemical constituents from *Dryopteris fragrans* (L.) Schott. *Molecules* **2013**, *19*, 507–513. [CrossRef] [PubMed]
5. Ito, H.; Muranaka, T.; Mori, K.; Jin, Z.X.; Tokuda, H.; Nishino, H.; Yoshida, T. Ichthyotoxic phloroglucinol derivatives from *Dryopteris fragrans* and their anti-tumor promoting activity. *Chem. Pharm. Bull.* **2000**, *31*, 1190–1195. [CrossRef]
6. Peng, B.; Bai, R.F.; Li, P.; Han, X.Y.; Wang, H.; Zhu, C.C.; Zeng, Z.P.; Chai, X.Y. Two new glycosides from *Dryopteris fragrans* with anti-inflammatory activities. *J. Asian Nat. Prod. Res.* **2016**, *18*, 59–64. [CrossRef] [PubMed]
7. Li, X.J.; Wang, W.; Luo, M.; Li, C.Y.; Zu, Y.G.; Mu, P.S.; Fu, Y.J. Solvent-free microwave extraction of essential oil from *Dryopteris fragrans* and evaluation of antioxidant activity. *Food Chem.* **2012**, *133*, 437–444. [CrossRef] [PubMed]
8. Zhang, Y.; Luo, M.; Zu, Y.; Fu, Y.; Gu, C.; Wang, W.; Yao, L.; Efferth, T. Dryofragin, a phloroglucinol derivative, induces apoptosis in human breast cancer MCF-7 cells through ROS-mediated mitochondrial pathway. *Chem. Biol. Interact.* **2012**, *199*, 129–136. [CrossRef] [PubMed]
9. Wan, D.; Jiang, C.; Hua, X.; Wang, T.; Chai, Y. Cell cycle arrest and apoptosis induced by aspidin PB through the p53/p21 and mitochondria-dependent pathways in human osteosarcoma cells. *Anti Cancer Drugs* **2015**, *26*, 931–941. [CrossRef] [PubMed]

10. Su, Y.; Wan, D.; Song, W. Dryofragin inhibits the migration and invasion of human osteosarcoma U2OS cells by suppressing MMP-2/9 and elevating TIMP-1/2 through PI3K/AKT and p38 MAPK signaling pathways. *Anti Cancer Drugs* **2016**, *27*, 660–668. [CrossRef] [PubMed]
11. Sun, Y.; Gao, C.; Luo, M.; Wang, W.; Gu, C.; Zu, Y.; Li, J.; Efferth, T.; Fu, Y. Aspidin PB, a phloroglucinol derivative, induces apoptosis in human hepatocarcinoma HepG2 cells by modulating PI3K/Akt/GSK3β pathway. *Chem. Biol. Interact.* **2013**, *201*, 1–8. [CrossRef] [PubMed]
12. Sun, Y.; Mu, F.; Li, C.; Wang, W.; Luo, M.; Fu, Y.; Zu, Y. Aspidin BB, a phloroglucinol derivative, induces cell cycle arrest and apoptosis in human ovarian HO-8910 cells. *Chem. Biol. Interact.* **2013**, *204*, 88–97. [CrossRef] [PubMed]
13. Zhong, Z.C.; Zhao, D.D.; Liu, Z.D.; Jiang, S.; Zhang, Y.L. A new human cancer cell proliferation inhibition sesquiterpene, dryofraterpene A, from medicinal plant *Dryopteris fragrans* (L.) Schott. *Molecules* **2017**, *22*, 180. [CrossRef] [PubMed]
14. Elisia, I.; Popovich, D.G.; Hu, C.; Kitts, D.D. Evaluation of viability assays for anthocyanins in cultured cells. *Phytochem. Anal.* **2008**, *19*, 479–486. [CrossRef] [PubMed]
15. Kang, D.; Gong, Y.; Zhu, Y.; Li, A.; Dong, N.; Piao, Y.; Yuan, Y. The biological activity of *H. pylori* SlyD in vitro. *Helicobacter* **2013**, *18*, 347–355. [CrossRef] [PubMed]
16. Cho, J.G.; Lee, D.Y.; Lee, J.W.; Lee, D.G.; Lee, Y.H.; Kim, S.Y.; Kim, S.H. Acyclic diterpenoids from the leaves of *Capsicum annuum*. *J. Korean Soc. Appl. Biol. Chem.* **2009**, *52*, 128–132. [CrossRef]
17. Amzad, H.M. Synthesis of 2′,4′-dihydroxy-6′-methoxy-3′,5′-dimethylchalcone. *Bangladesh J. Sci. Ind. Res.* **2001**, *36*, 50–54.
18. Ayräs, P.; Lötjönen, S.; Widén, C.J. NMR spectroscopy of naturally occurring phloroglucinol derivatives. *Planta Med.* **1981**, *42*, 187–194. [CrossRef] [PubMed]
19. Lobo-Echeverri, T.; Rivero-Cruz, J.F.; Su, B.N.; Chai, H.B.; Cordell, G.A.; Pezzuto, J.M.; Swanson, S.M.; Soejarto, D.D.; Kinghorn, A.D. Constituents of the leaves and twigs of *Calyptranthes pallens* collected from an experimental plot in Southern Florida. *J. Nat. Prod.* **2005**, *68*, 577–580. [CrossRef] [PubMed]
20. Ito, T.; Nisa, K.; Rakainsa, S.K.; Lallo, S.; Morita, H. New phloroglucinol derivatives from Indonesian *Baeckea frutescens*. *Tetrahedron* **2017**, *73*, 1177–1181. [CrossRef]
21. Yang, L.; Guo, H.; Li, Y.; Meng, X.; Yan, L.; Dan, Z.; Wu, S.; Zhou, H.; Peng, L.; Xie, Q.; et al. Oleoylethanolamide exerts anti-inflammatory effects on LPS-induced THP-1 cells by enhancing PPARα signaling and inhibiting the NF-κB and ERK1/2/AP-1/STAT3 pathways. *Sci. Rep.* **2016**, *6*, 34611. [CrossRef] [PubMed]

Sample Availability: Samples of the compounds **1–8** are available from the authors.

molecules

MDPI

Review

Terpene Derivatives as a Potential Agent against Antimicrobial Resistance (AMR) Pathogens

Nik Amirah Mahizan [1], Shun-Kai Yang [1], Chew-Li Moo [1], Adelene Ai-Lian Song [2], Chou-Min Chong [3], Chun-Wie Chong [4], Aisha Abushelaibi [5], Swee-Hua Erin Lim [5] and Kok-Song Lai [1,5,*]

1. Department of Cell and Molecular Biology, Faculty of Biotechnology and Biomolecular Sciences, Universiti Putra Malaysia, 43400 Serdang, Selangor, Malaysia
2. Department of Microbiology, Faculty of Biotechnology and Biomolecular Sciences, Universiti Putra Malaysia, 43400 Serdang, Selangor, Malaysia
3. Department of Aquaculture, Faculty of Agriculture, Universiti Putra Malaysia, 43400 Serdang, Selangor, Malaysia
4. School of Pharmacy, Monash University Malaysia, Jalan Lagoon Selatan, Bandar Sunway 47500, Selangor, Malaysia
5. Health Sciences Division, Abu Dhabi Women's College, Higher Colleges of Technology, 41012 Abu Dhabi, UAE

* Correspondence: laikoksong@upm.edu.my; Tel.: +60-389468021

Academic Editor: Pinarosa Avato
Received: 24 April 2019; Accepted: 3 June 2019; Published: 19 July 2019

Abstract: The evolution of antimicrobial resistance (AMR) in pathogens has prompted extensive research to find alternative therapeutics. Plants rich with natural secondary metabolites are one of the go-to reservoirs for discovery of potential resources to alleviate this problem. Terpenes and their derivatives comprising of hydrocarbons, are usually found in essential oils (EOs). They have been reported to have potent antimicrobial activity, exhibiting bacteriostatic and bactericidal effects against tested pathogens. This brief review discusses the activity of terpenes and derivatives against pathogenic bacteria, describing the potential of the activity against AMR followed by the possible mechanism exerted by each terpene class. Finally, ongoing research and possible improvisation to the usage of terpenes and terpenoids in therapeutic practice against AMR are discussed.

Keywords: terpenes; terpenoids; antimicrobial resistance; synergy

1. Introduction

The increase of antimicrobial resistance (AMR) in microbiological pathogens has spurred a global mandate to identify potentially effective alternatives [1]. AMR is defined as inefficacious infection-associated treatment with an antimicrobial agent that used to be effective [2]. The rise of AMR is contributed by both intrinsic and extrinsic factors. For instance, evolution of intrinsic factors in microbes include development of structural attributes [3] such as microbial biofilm production [4], and insertion of transposons [5]. On the other hand, extrinsic contributing factors include excessive antibiotic usage resulting from non-judicious prescribing practices, fueled by increased competition in the production and marketing of antimicrobials within the pharmaceutical industry [6]. As a whole there is also inadequate public education, in tandem with a lack of consistent regulatory systems in place. Both of these, coupled with improper infection control in healthcare, poor sanitation, and water hygiene in low-middle income countries (LMIC), are expanding the AMR challenge [1,7].

Laxminarayan et al. [7] reported that the antibiotic usage in growth and disease prevention on veterinary, agriculture, aquaculture, and horticulture are the main contributors in the non-clinical setting. In the clinical settings however, lack of antibiotic stewardship and uncertain diagnoses by physicians add to emerging pathogen resistance. In fact, as far back as in 1959, the potentially adverse consequences related to antibiotic misuse resulting in selection pressure to the development of resistance were observed. Recent genetic mutations in pathogens which were aided by chromosomal genes and inter species gene transmission has resulted in the rise of resistant microbes such as methicillin resistant *Staphylococcus aureus* (MRSA), *Escherichia coli* ST131 and *Klebsiella* ST258; this further contributes to the dissemination of resistant genes such as *Klebsiella pneumoniae* carbapenemase (KPC), NDM-1, and Enterobacteriaceae-producing extended-spectrum β-lactamases (ESBL) [7].

The continuous dissemination of AMR not only contributes to new resistance mechanisms; it will also have a detrimental impact whereby the efficacy of current antibiotics are drastically reduced, leading to therapeutic failure [8]. It is worrisome to note that in 2010, there were almost 1000 resistant cases worldwide associated with β-lactamases, a 10-fold increase since 1990 [9]. Correlation between antibiotic misuse and AMR is clearly evidenced when quinolone misuse caused the revival of MRSA 30 years after it was first introduced in 1962, while carbapenem misconduct via overuse causing resistance in Enterobacteriaceae has significantly increased over the past decade [7]. In addition, loss of function of ampicillin and gentamicin under the World Health Organisation (WHO) recommended dosage in neonatal infection-related pathogens such as *Klebsiella* spp. and *E. coli* was common in the hospitals of developing countries [10]. This was attributed to the high mortality rates of sepsis cases caused by carbapenem-resistant *Enterobacteriaceae* and *Acinetobacter* spp. in neonatal nurseries. It was also noted by Saleem [11] that in Pakistan, common oral antibiotics such as cefixime and ciprofloxacin have become inefficient in Gram-negative pathogens such as *E. coli*, bacteria commonly associated with urinary infection. Barbieri [2] stated in his review that dissemination of AMR inadvertently affected health systems in the community in LMICs due to the escalating cost of accessing necessary therapies and the prolonged duration of illness caused by AMR which increases treatment time.

Bacterial resistance is commonly mediated by transfer of resistance genes [12]. Overall, there are four main ways in which resistance is acquired, firstly, via inactivation of the drug (Figure 1) as reported by Shen [13]. The modification of the antibiotics which occurred based on their target location (bacterial cell wall, cytoplasm, and genome) rendered ineffective to that antibiotic [14]. The second method is the specific modification (Figure 1) at the target such as penicillin-binding protein (PBPs) in MRSA [15]. Similar modifications may arise from mutational or post-translational modifications [3]. Furthermore, porin mutation causes reduction in the number of porins, preventing antibiotic entry and thus increased resistance to antibiotics [16]. Mutations can either be acquired from existing genes (vertical transfer) or new genes can be acquired from other cells (horizontal gene transfer) [17]. Third is the ability of the bacteria to obtain genes for metabolic pathways, these genes then prevent antimicrobial agents from binding to their target. For instance, mobile genes in resistant *Enterococcus* spp. can be disseminated to susceptible strains via horizontal transfer mediated by conjugative plasmids [18]. Finally, the fourth method of bacterial resistance is the reduction of antimicrobial agent intracellularly due to the presence of a bacterial efflux pump. In fact, some resistant bacteria increase impermeability in the cell membrane or increase active efflux, both of which result in reduced drug concentration (Figure 1) in the bacterial cell [19]. The up-regulation in expression of efflux pump has been found to be a major resistance mechanism in many bacteria [20].

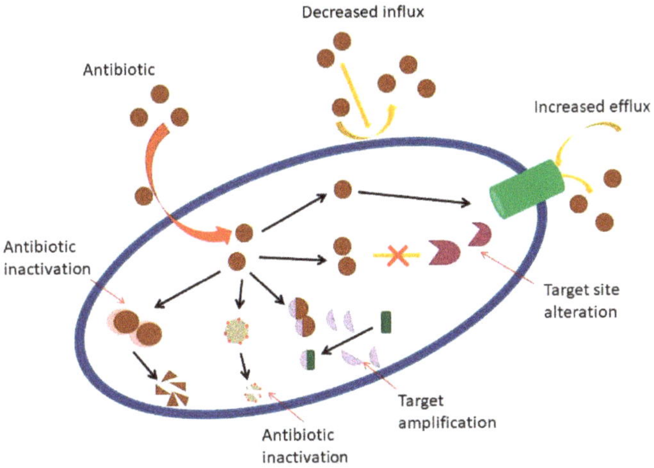

Figure 1. Overall mechanisms of antibiotic resistance in bacteria. Picture adapted from [17].

Strategies to curb the ongoing emergence of AMR require the involvement from various parties. They include policy makers to develop antibiotic regulations, pharmacists and physicians to practice proper antibiotic stewardship, the pharmaceutical industry to invest in new antibiotic discovery, as well as academics to provide adequate public education [7]. Some strategies for control and containment of AMR included extensive surveillance of antimicrobials, especially for antibiotic prescriptions amongst health care providers, avoiding unnecessary use of antimicrobials in the agricultural sectors, limiting drugs advertising, improvising on sanitation, in tandem with continuous research of novel drugs and invention of nanotechnology; these were some of the measures to be implemented [7]. A shift in focus towards alternative therapies targeting AMR mechanisms would also be an important aspect and these include incorporation of antimicrobial peptides (AMPs), phage therapy, metalloantibiotics, lipopolysaccharides, efflux pump inhibitors, and phytochemicals [1].

Antimicrobial agents may comprise of naturally-occurring compounds such as phytochemicals and essential oils (EOs) [21]. They can also be either semi-synthetic or synthetic [22] in nature. Natural secondary metabolites which have a molecular weight ≤500 g/mol may have the ability to act as adjuvants for antimicrobials and exhibit synergy effects [2,23]. Exploration of new antimicrobial agents via biotransformation such as through microbial modification may present an important alternative [24]. Combination therapy of an antimicrobial agent with a low molecular weight natural product, such as terpene derivatives have shown promising effects, with the ability to eliminate fungal and bacterial biofilm production [4]. Terpenes and their derivatives are secondary metabolites which are commonly found in EOs and have been shown to have antimicrobial activities against susceptible and resistant pathogens [25]. Combination therapy between natural compounds and drugs may be able to recover the loss of function for existing antimicrobial agents [26], potentiating the action of drugs. Wagner and Merzenich [27] reported that the potentiation of antimicrobial agents was accomplished via several mechanisms in combinatorial therapy; these provide a multi-targeted pharmacokinetic effect, allowing simultaneous destruction of existing resistance mechanisms in a specific pathogen.

EOs are naturally produced from aromatic plants such as herbs as their secondary metabolites. Usually EOs exist in liquid form, are volatile and exhibit good solubility in lipids and inorganic compounds that are less dense compared to water. They can be extracted from various parts of the plant organ such as flowers, buds, leave, bark, twigs, stem, wood, seed, or root [28] by various methods which include solvent extraction (solvent, supercritical CO_2, subcritical water), distillation (steam, hydrodistillation, hydrodiffusion), solvent-free (microwave) and combination method (solvent + steam) [29]. Generally, plants store their EOs in specific cellular compartments such as in the secretory cells, cavities, or glandular trichomes. EOs primarily function as protection against plant pests and infections [30]. In particular, EOs have been reported to be a prominent antimicrobial, antioxidant, and insecticidal agent, significantly inhibiting microbial biofilm production and the growth of bacteria, yeasts, and molds [31]. Previously our group has also focused on the bacterial membranous disruption effect when subjected to treatment with EOs [32]. A list of reports summarized in Table 1 indicate various antimicrobial activities possessed by EOs. In 2018, our research group demonstrated synergistic activity when peppermint (*Mentha x piperita* L. Carl) essential oil was added to meropenem against resistant *E. coli* [33]. Recently, our research group established a mode of action of EO from cinnamon bark against KPC-KP via oxidative stress [34]. There are challenges involved in working with EOs. They are laborious to handle as they need to be extracted and purified before being tested and manipulated. Furthermore, despite EOs being used for testing, it is difficult to ascertain as to which bioactive component in EOs is contributing to the antimicrobial activity. Acquisition of EOs will also require higher cost as compared to synthetic additives because they need to be processed prior to screening for their activity. One method to resolve the cost issue involves downscaling the volume via extraction of the antimicrobial compounds. This review in particular will focus on one such compound commonly found in EOs, namely the terpenes and their antimicrobial potential and their possible mechanisms of action.

Table 1. Essential oils extracted from plant against tested pathogens.

Plants spp.	Common Name	Pathogens Tested	MIC/Sensitivity/ Inhibition Zone	Citation
Eugenia caryophyllata	Clove	*Burkholderia cepacia* complex	ES	[35]
Origanum vulgare	Oregano	*B. cepacia* complex	ES	[35]
Thymus vulgaris	Thyme	*B. cepacia* complex	ES	[35]
Eucalyptus camadulensis	Eucalyptus	*Streptococcus pyogenes*	1 mg mL^{-1}	[36]
		Fusarium oxysporum f. sp. *lycopersici*	15.93% to 72.5%	[37]
Mentha spicata	Spearmint	*S. pyogenes*	2 mg mL^{-1}	[36]
		E. coli	21 mm at 150 μL	[38]
		Salmonella thyphi	13 mm at 150 μL	
		S. aureus	12 mm at 150 μL	
Cymbopogon citratus	Lemongrass	*Acinetobacter baumannii*	0.65% (v/v)	[39]
		F. oxysporum f. sp. *lycopersici*	250 ppm	[37]
Syzygium aromaticum	Clove	*Candida albicans*	360 μg mL^{-1}	[40]
		F. oxysporum f. sp. *lycopersici*	125 ppm	[37]
Pelargonium graveolens	Geranium	*B. cepacia* complex	0.4% (v/v)	[41]
		Prototheca zopfii	3.5 to 4.0 μL mL^{-1}	[42]
Laurus nobilis	Bay laurel	*S. typhimurium*	3 % (v/v)	[43]
		E. coli	1 % (v/v)	[44]
		Candida spp.	250 to 500 μg mL^{-1}	
Melaleuca alternifolia	Tea tree	*Campylobacter* spp.	0.00%	[45]
Leptospermum petersonii	Manuka	*Campylobacter* spp.	0.01%	[45]
Backhousia citriodora	Lemon myrtle	*Campylobacter* spp.	0.01%	[45]
Lavandula angustifolia	Lavender	*S. aureus*	2 mg mL^{-1}	[46]
		Pseudomonas aeruginosa	2 mg mL^{-1}	
		C. albicans	3 mg mL^{-1}	
Mentha x piperita	Peppermint	*Clostridium perfringens*	10 mg mL^{-1}	[47]
		Fusarium oxysporum f. sp. *lycopersici*	500 ppm	[37]
Chamaemelum nobile	Roman chamomile	*Porphyromonas gingivalis*	20.5 ± 0.5 mm	[48]
Origanum majorana	Marjoram	*Micrococcus luteus*	0.097 mg mL^{-1}	[49]
		Vibrio alginolyticus	0.39 mg mL^{-1}	
Foeniculum vulgare	Fennel	*Candida* spp.	1.56 to 12.48 mg mL^{-1}	[50]
Pinus sylvestris	Pine	*Pseudomonas* spp.	4.33 ± 0.58 mm	[51]
Cedrus atlantica	Cedarwoood	*E. coli*	0.4 μL mL^{-1}	[52]
		Bacillus subtilis	0.2 μL mL^{-1}	
		Bacillus cereus	0.4 μL mL^{-1}	
Aniba rosaeodora	Rosewood	*Trichophyton mentagrophytes*	0.002 M	[53]

ES: extremely sensitive.

2. Terpenes and Their Derivatives

Terpenes are large hydrocarbon groups that consist of 5-carbon isoprene (C5H8) units as their basic building block. They are synthesized via two pathways which are the non-mevalonate pathway; the Methylerythritol Phosphate (MEP) and the mevalonate pathway from Acetyl CoA precursor. Their backbones can be reorganized into cyclic structure by cyclases. The commonly found terpenes which differ in numbers of isoprene units are the monoterpenes and sesquiterpenes; however longer chains such as diterpenes and triterpenes also exist [47,54]. P-Cymene, limonene, sabinene, terpinene, carene, and pinene are examples belonging to the terpene groups. Most terpenes possess reduced antimicrobial activities [54]. Terpenoids are derivatives of terpenes which takes place when modification of terpenes occur, such as with the addition/removal of functional groups [2]. Therefore, the antimicrobial activity of terpenoids are determined from their functional group [55]. For instance, the shifting or removal of a methyl group and addition of oxygen by a specific enzyme result in derivation of terpenes. The hydroxyl group of the phenolic terpenoids and delocalized electrons are amongst the antimicrobial determining factors. Linalool, menthol, carvacrol, thymol, linalyl acetrate, piperitone, geraniol, and citronella are amongst the best studied terpenoids.

2.1. *Bioactive Terpenes and Terpenoids*

Terpenoids represent a large group of phytochemicals with promising antimicrobial activity [2]. The chemical diversity of terpenoids have led to discovery of over 40,000 structural varieties, with a few classes serving as pharmaceutical agents, some of which include terpenoid derived indole alkaloids [56]. There are a total of eight different classes of terpenoids (hemiterpenoids, monoterpenoids, sesquiterpenoids, diterpenoids, sesterpenoids, triterpenoids, tetrapenoids, and polyterpenoids) which differ in the number of isoprene (C5H8) units. Recently in 2017, it was reported that 67% of potentiators belong to monoterpenes and sesquiterpenes [4]. Meanwhile, specifically among the discovered potentiators of antibacterial drugs, 75% were terpenes; these include classes of mono-, di-, and tri-terpenes [4].

Although the antibacterial mode of action of terpenes remains largely unknown, Griffin et al. [55] reported in his study that most terpenoids are able to inhibit two crucial processes which are essential to microbial survival, this includes oxygen uptake and oxidative phosphorylation. Aerobic microbes require oxygen in order to yield energy for their growth. Previously, it was proven that low oxygen concentrations caused limitation in bacterial respiration rates [57]. Meanwhile, oxidative phosphorylation is a crucial biochemical process responsible for cellular respiration that takes place in the cytoplasmic membrane. Thus, terpene interaction leads to alteration in cellular respiration which later causes uncoupling of oxidative phosphorylation in the microbe [58]. Additionally, carbonylation of terpenoids was believed to increase bacteriostatic activity but not necessarily the bactericidal activity. A bacteriostatic agent is an agent that stops or inhibits microbial growth, while a bactericidal is responsible for killing the microbe. Terpenoids have also been found to exhibit antiseptic potential according to their solubility in water. Lipophilicity and/or hydrophobicity and presence of hydroxyl groups in the terpenes are amongst the determining elements of their antibacterial action [58]. In skin barrier-associated treatment, terpenes have also been reported to affect the lipid membrane activity by interacting with lipophilic tails of intermembrane lipid and polar head groups which, at the end, affects the lipodial intermembrane and polar transmembrane pathways [59].

2.1.1. Monoterpenes and Monoterpenoids

Monoterpenes comprise of two isoprene units and exist in many plants. It has been reported by Griffin et al. [55] that monotepenes possess antimicrobial activity. For instance, carvacrol, thymol, menthol, and geraniol were able to work against Gram-positive and Gram-negative bacteria. Geraniol was also later claimed to efficiently increase the susceptibility of the Gram-negative multi-drug resistant (MDR) *Enterobacter aerogenes* by becoming a potent efflux pump inhibitor [60]. Trombetta et al. [61]

claimed in his study that three monoterpenes linalyl acetate, (+) menthol and thymol showed positive responses against *S. aureus* and *E. coli*. Other compounds such as carvacrol, trans-cinnamaldehyde and (+)-carvone were reported to possess potent inhibitory activity against *E. coli* and *S. typhimurium* [30]. In addition, other types of monoterpenes such as halogenated monoterpenes recorded good cytotoxic, antimalarial, and antialgal effects while monocyclic monoterpenes had been reported to exhibit potent insecticidal, as well as antifungal effects [62].

In fact, in as early as 1979, Kurita et al. [63] had listed a total of 13 monoterpenes ((+)-terpinen-4-ol, γ-terpinene, α-terpinene, terpinolene, α-pinene 1,8-cineole, ρ-cymene, (+)-limonene, β-myrcene, (+)-β-pinene, (±)-linalool, α-phellandrene, α-terpinoel) which exhibited antifungal properties against 14 fungal strains. The phenolic monoterpenes such as carvacrol, eugenol and thymol were found to be highly active against bacteria [64]. There were twenty one monoterpenes (borneol, d-3-carene, carvacrol, carvacrol methyl ester, *cis/trans* citral, eugenol, geraniol, Geranyl acetate, *cis*-hex-3-en-1-ol, R(+)limonene, (2)-linalool, menthone, nerol, α-pinene, β-pinene, (+)sabinene, α-terpinene, terpinen-4-ol, α-terpineole, (−)-thujone, thymol) which were previously reported regarding their antimicrobial activity against 25 bacterial strains [65]. Phenol monoterpenes, such as carvacrol were also reported to inhibit biofilm development of *S.aureus* and *S. typhimurium* [66]. Recently, our research group found one monoterpene compound, linalool, extracted from lavender essential oil which exhibited strong antimicrobial activity against resistant *K. pneumoniae* [34]. The proposed mechanism of action for the compound was membrane disruption [34].

Monoterpene ketones were also found to exhibit antimicrobial properties [67]. In comparison, alcoholic monoterpenes are more bactericidal agents rather than bacteriostatic agents. In line with this, Bhatti et al. [67] reported that monoterpenes alcohol of terpinen-4-ol, α-terpineol, 1, 8-cineole and linalool exhibited good antifungal activity and suggested alcohol moieties as determinants of antifungal activity. In addition, myrcene, one of the acyclic monoterpene alcohols showed a negative response against fungal specimens; this infers that the cyclic structure of monoterpenes may also be the structure responsible for this activity [68]. Monoterpenes consisting of aldehydes, however, possessed a potent antimicrobial activity which can be explained through its carbon double bond arrangements; this creates high electronegativity. The observations of nine monoterpenes (α-terpinene, γ-terpinene, α-pinene, ρ-cymene, terpinen-4-ol, α-terpineol, thymol, citral and 1, 8-cineole) against *Herpes simplex virus* type 1 (HSV-1) were made by Thompson in 1989. Later in 2010, Dunkic et al. [69] listed a few more monoterpenes having considerable activity against HSV-1 which are borneol, bornyl acetate, and isoborneol, 1, 8-cineole, thujone, and camphor. Thymol and carvacrol were also noted to be powerful agents against the *Tobacco mosaic virus* (TMV) and *Cucumber mosaic virus* (CMV) [70].

2.1.2. Sesquiterpenes and Sesquiterpenoids

It has been long recognized that sesquiterpenes possess antimicrobial activites [55]. Back in 2011, Torres-Romero et al. [71] identified one of dihydro-β agarofuran sesquiterpenes, namely 1α-acetoxy-6β, 9β-dibenzoyloxy-dihydro-β-agarofuran inhibits the growth of *Bacillus* spp. [71]. Farnesol, which is an isoprenoid natural acyclic sesquiterpene alcohol showed moderate effects against *Streptococcus mutans* and *Streptococcus sobrinus* biofilm formation [72]. Farnesol also showed antibacterial activity against *S. aureus* and *S. epidermidis* whereby it inhibited the biofilm development [73]. Two studies conducted by Masako [74] evidenced that combinations of farnesol with xylitol have positive effects against atopic dermatitis caused by *S. aureus* without altering the microbial flora and successfully inhibited the biofilm production of *S. aureus*. Sesquiterpenes were also incorporated in the combination therapy using existing drugs.

A recent study conducted by Castelo-Branco et al. [75] showed potentiation effects of a combination therapy of farnesol with amoxicillin, doxycycline, ceftazidime, and sulfamethoxazole-trimethoprim against *B. pseudomallei*. A phenol sesquiterpene, xanthorrhizol was found to reduce 60% of *Staphylococcus mutans* cell adherence ability [76], and inhibited the growth of *Mycobacterium smegmatis* [77]. Recently, it was discovered that sesquiterpenes have potent antibiotic enhancement against MRSA and also

Gram-negative bacteria [4]. In 2011, Gonçalves et al. [78] reported a significantly larger inhibition zone when sesquiterpenes were incorporated into antibiotic discs. The experiment was conducted against MDR strains of *S. aureus* with a combination of sets of available antibiotics such as tetracycline, erythromycin, penicillin, and vancomycin.

2.1.3. Diterpenes and Diterpenoids

Diterpene is a class of terpene with broad biological activities [79]. Previously, 60 terpenoids have been tested for their minimum inhibitory concentration (MIC) against *P. aeruginosa, E. coli, S. aureus,* and *C. albicans* [55]. They were then classified into five groups to determine their activity patterns. Hydrogen bond was found to be the factor that determines the positive antimicrobial activity. On the other hand, low water solubility was discovered to be the factor of antimicrobial inactivity. Griffin [55] suggested that inhibition of microbial oxygen uptake and oxidative phosphorylation are likely mechanisms of action responsible for the antimicrobial properties of the diterpene class. Separately, diterpene derivatives such as ent-kaurane and ent-pimarane are able to inhibit growth of the dental caries pathogens. The MIC value of 2–10 mg/mL confirmed the antibacterial potential of the compounds [80]. Additionally, the diterpenoid salvipisone prevented cell adherence and biofilm developments of *S. aureus* and *S. epidermidis* [81].

Besides sesquiterpenes, diterpenes also function as a good antibiotic enhancer against MRSA. Moreover, diterpenes have been widely used in combination therapy with antibiotics [82]. For instance, clerodane diterpenoid 16αhydroxycleroda-3, 13 (14)-Z-dien-15, 16-olide (CD) extracted from leaves of *Polyathia longifolia* enhanced the efficacy of oxacillin, tetracycline, daptomycin, and linezolid against clinical isolates of MRSA. All MICs of the antibiotic dropped significantly between 10–80, 4–16, 2–8 and 2–4-folds respectively when combined with CD. Gupta et al. [82] then proposed the in vivo mechanism of CD in reversing the resistance of clinical isolates of MRSA. The same clinical MRSA isolates were tested with CD combined with norfloxacin, ciprofloxacin, and ofloxacin. qRT-PCR analysis showed that the expression of genes coding for efflux pumps were significantly modulated in cells treated with CD alone and in combination with antimicrobial drugs. In fact, the results of time-kill assay showed the MIC in combination of CD with norfloxacin was half of the MIC of CD and norfloxacin alone, undoubtedly decreasing the viability of bacterial cells. Unfortunately, despite the promising effects offered by CD, sourcing to obtain CD became the bottleneck for further testing [4].

Salvipisone and aethiopinone are diterpenoids isolated from roots of *Salvia sclarea* [81]. They were shown to express antibacterial and antibiofilm activities against *S. aureus, Enterococcus faecalis* and *S. epidermidis*. Both salvipisone and aethiopinone were also tested for their synergistic activity when combined with antimicrobial drugs alongside oxacillin, vancomycin, and linezolid against MRSA and Methicillin resistant *Staphylococcus epidermidis* (MRSE). It was discovered that they were either bactericidal or bacteriostatic against planktonic cultures of tested MRSA and MRSE [83]. Remarkably, the MIC was achieved with 50% reduction in the dose of antibiotic when diterpenoids were used in combination.

2.1.4. Triterpenes and Triterpenoids

Triterpenes comprises of six isoprene units. It was reported that *Pandanaceae* containing triterpenes in the form of 24, 24-dimethyl-5β-tirucall-9 [11], 25-dien-3-one showed promising activities against tubercular strains. Another triterpene, Oleanic acid (OA) is potent against pathogens such as *Mycobacterium tuberculosis*. OA also had promising synergy against MDR when combined with rifampicin, isoniazide, and ethambutol with significant MIC reduction of 128–16 fold, 32–4 fold, and from 128 to 16 fold, respectively [2].

Besides OA, bonianic acid A and B are two triterpenoids that were extracted from *Radermachera boniana*. Both compounds were found to be active against *M. tuberculosis*. There are at least six known molecules which include OA, ergosterol peroxide, and ursolic acid (UA). In fact, the combination of both ergosterol peroxide and UA showed synergistic activity against *M. tuberculosis* [84]. The reports conducted by Cunha et al. [85] depicted that OA and UA that were isolated from *Miconia ligustroides*, resulted in significant antibacterial activity when tested on selected bacteria (*B. cereus, Vibrio cholerae, S. choleraesuis, K. pneumoniae and S. pneumoniae*). When UA was used against *B. cereus*, the MIC value was 20 μg/mL and OA showed MIC value of 80 μg/mL against *B. cereus* and *S. pneumoniae*. In 2013, a study conducted by Zhou et al. [86] showed that UA and OA were active against planktonic cariogenic microorganism and their biofilm. Later in 2015, Liu et al. [31] expanded the research and reported the combinatory effects of UA and xylitol against biofilm produced by *S. mutans and S. sobrinus*. Moreover, OA and UA were reported to enhance antimicrobial activity against *Listeria monocytogenes* without affecting toxin secretion; this influenced the virulence factors of *L. monocytogenes* and inhibited the capacity of biofilm production from these bacteria [45].

OA also exhibited strong interactions alongside aminoglycoside (gentamicin and kanamycin) against *A. baumanii*, but not with other classes of which ampicillin, norfloxacin, chloramphenicol, tetracycline, and rifampicin are examples [4]. Based on time-kill assay, the bactericidal effects of gentamicin were significantly greater when combined with OA compared to gentamicin alone [4]. Three triterpenoids, amyrin, betulinic acid, and betulinaldehyde were extracted from the bark of *Callicarpa farinose* Roxb (Verbenaceae) and were shown to exhibit potent antimicrobial activity against clinical methicillin-resistant (MRSA) and methicillin-susceptible (MSSA) with MICs ranging from 2 to 512 μg/mL [87].

While there is no firm report specifically on modes of action by terpenoids, the mechanisms of action of phytochemicals found in nature have been proposed. Typically, phytochemicals aim either for disruption of the bacterial cell membranes, modulation of bacterial efflux pump, suppression of bacterial biofilm development or inhibition of some virulence factors which include enzymes and toxins [2]. For instance, carvacrol was found to be responsible for sub-lethal injury to bacterial cells due to alteration of fatty acid compositions, while other reports state that carvacrol and thymol caused disintegration of the outer membrane and disruption of the cytoplasmic membrane of Gram-negative bacteria [30]. Antimicrobial activity effects of some terpenoids are summarized in Table 2 while the postulated mode of action of terpenes on antibiotic resistance pathogens and as combination therapies are depicted in Figure 2.

Table 2. Summary of antimicrobial activity effects of some terpenoid class.

Terpenoids Class	Chemical Compounds	Tested Microorganism	Antimicrobial Effect	Reference
Monoterpenes and monoterpenoids	Carvacrol Thymol Geraniol	Resistant *Enterobacter aerogenes*	Efflux pump inhibition	[60]
	Linalyl acetate (+)- Menthol Thymol	*S. aureus* *E. coli*	Growth inhibition	[61]
	Carvacrol Trans-cinnamaldehyde (+)-Carvone	*E. coli* *S. typhimurium*	Growth inhibition	[30]
	(+)-Terpinen-4-ol γ-Terpinene α-Terpinene Terpinolene α-Pinene 1,8-Cineole ρ-Cymene (+)-Limonene β-Myrcene (+)-β-Pinene (±)-Linalool α-Phellandrene α-Terpinoel	*T. mentagrophytes* *Trichophyton violaceum* *Microsporium gypseum* *Histoplasma capsulatum* *Blastomyces dermatitidis* … etc.	Growth inhibition	[63]

Table 2. *Cont.*

Terpenoids Class	Chemical Compounds	Tested Microorganism	Antimicrobial Effect	Reference
	Carvacrol Eugenol Thymol	*Acinetobacter calcoacetica* *Aeromonas hydrophila* *B. subtilis*	Growth inhibition	[64]
	Borneol d-3-Carene Carvacrol Carvacrol methyl ester *cis/trans* Citral Eugenol Geraniol Geranyl acetate *cis*-hex-3-en-1-ol R(+)Limonene (2)-Linalool Menthone Nerol α-Pinene β-Pinene (+)sabinene α-Terpinene Terpinen-4-ol α-terpineole (−)-Thujone Thymol	*S. aureus* *E. coli* *Salmonella typhia* *S. typhimurium* *Salmonella enteritidis* *A. hydrophila* *Yersinia* sp. *Vibrio anguillarum* *Shigella* sp. *Vibrio parahaemolyticus C. albicans* *Penicillium expansum* *Aspergillus niger* … etc.	Growth inhibition	[65]
	Carvacrol	*S.aureus* *S. typhimurium*	Biofilm inhibition	[66]
	Linalool	Resistant *K. pneumoniae carbapenemase* (KPC)	Cell membrane disruption	[34]
	Terpinen-4-ol α-Terpineol 1, 8-Cineole Linalool	*A. niger* *Botrytis cinerea*	Growth inhibition	[67]
	α-Terpinene γ-Terpinene α-Pinene ρ-Cymene Terpinen-4-ol α-Terpineol Thymol Citral 1, 8-Cineole Borneol Bornyl acetate Isoborneol 1, 8-Cineole Thujone Camphor	*Herpes simplex virus* type 1 (HSV-1)	Growth inhibition	[69]

Table 2. *Cont.*

Terpenoids Class	Chemical Compounds	Tested Microorganism	Antimicrobial Effect	Reference
	Thymol Carvacrol	*Tobacco mosaic virus* (TMV) *Cucumber mosaic virus* (CMV)	Growth inhibition	[70]
Sesquiterpenes and Sesquiterpenoids	1α-Acetoxy-6β, 9β-dibenzoyloxy-dihydro-β-agarofuran	*Bacillus* spp.	Growth inhibition	[71]
	Farnesol	*Streptococcus mutans* *Streptococcus sobrinus*	Biofilm formation inhibition	[72]
		S. aureus *S. epidermidis*		[73] [74]
		B. pseudomallei	Potentiation effect—combination therapy	[75]
	Xanthorrhizol	*Staphylococcus mutans*	Reduction of cell adherence ability	[76]
		Mycobacterium smegmatis	Growth inhibition	[77]
Diterpenes and diterpenoids	(-)-Carvone Thymol Dihydrocarveol (-)-Perilla alcohol Carvacrol (-)-Carveol … etc.	*P. aeruginosa* *E. coli* *S. aureus* *C. albicans*	Growth inhibition	[55]
	Ent-kaurane Ent-pimarane	Dental carries pathogens	Growth inhibition	[80]
	Salvipisone	*S. aureus* *S. epidermidis*	Bacterial cell adherence prevention Biofilm development inhibition	[81]
	16αHydroxycleroda-3, 13 (14)-Z-dien-15, 16-olide (CD)	MRSA	Antibiotic potentiation Efflux pump modulation	[82]
	Salvipisone Aethiopinone	*S. aureus* *Enterococcus faecalis* *S. epidermidis*	Biofilm production inhibition	[81]
		MRSA MRSE	Synergistic activity alongside antibiotic	[83]

Table 2. *Cont.*

Terpenoids Class	Chemical Compounds	Tested Microorganism	Antimicrobial Effect	Reference
Triterpenes and triterpenoids	24, 24-Dimethyl-5β-tirucall-9	Tubercular strains	Growth inhibition	[11]
	25-Dien-3-one Oleanic acid (OA) Bonianic acid A Bonianic acid B	*Mycobacterium tuberculosis*	Synergistic activity alongside antibiotic	[2]
	OA Ergosterol peroxide Ursolic acid (UA)		Synergistic activity—combination therapy	
	OA UA	*B. cereus* *Vibrio cholerae* *S. choleraesuis* *K. pneumoniae* *S. pneumoniae*	Growth inhibition	[85]
		Planktonic cariogenic microorganism *S. mutans* *S. sobrinus*	Biofilm inhibition	[86] [31]
		Listeria monocytogenes		[45]
	OA	*A. baumanii*	Antibiotic potentiation	[4]
	Amyrin Betulinic acid Betulinaldehyde	MRSA MMSA	Growth inhibition	[87]

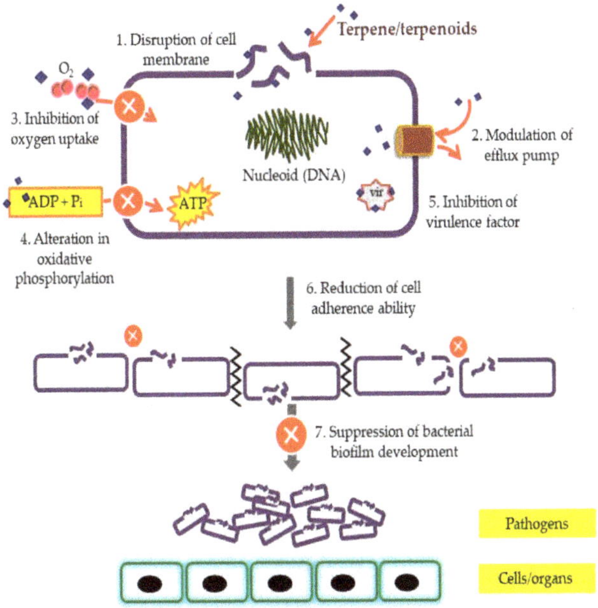

Figure 2. Postulated mode of action of terpene/terpenoids on antibiotic resistance pathogens and as combination therapies.

2.2. Therapeutic Implementation

2.2.1. Drugs and Antibiotics

Combination therapy with terpenes have been widely seen in current therapeutic practice especially in antifungal drugs [26]. It was shown that fluconazole which had once lost its efficacy, had been potentiated by monoterpenes, thymol, and carvacrol when subjected against 38 fluconazole-sensitive *C. albicans, C. tropicalis,* and *C. glabrata* and 11 fluconazole-resistant *C. albicans, C. krusei, C. glabrata, C. tropicalis,* and *C. parapsilopsis*. The combination analysis showed that of the strains tested, 32 out of 38 strains and eight out of 10 strains have obtained a Fractional Inhibitory Concentration (FIC) index of less than 0.5 [88]. FIC is a term used to express the degree of synergy interaction between antibacterial drugs whereby FIC < 0.5 shows positive synergism while FIC > 0.5 shows negative synergism [89]. The sequiterpene, farnesol, also showed potentiation activity with fluconazole against candidiasis [88]. Previously, it was reported that three diterpene compounds, ent-clerodanes (bacchotricuneatin, bacrispine and hawtriwaic acid) which were isolated from *Baccharis* extract synergistically reduced the dose of the anti-fungal drug Terbinafine against *Trichophyton rubrum* [90]. Another triterpene, retigeric acid, found in the lichenized fungi family, Lobariaceae exhibited strong potentiation when combined with either fluconazole, itraconazole or ketoconazole against azole-resistant *C. albicans* strains [91]. It was proposed that facilitation of azole uptake or membranous repair associated with azoles were the modes of action of retigeric acid.

Prior to the development of novel drugs, in vitro and in vivo testing are usually performed to ascertain the safety and efficacy of the compound to better understand the physiological effects. Despite a number of published in vitro reports pertaining to terpenes antimicrobial testing, incorporation of various terpenes in clinical trials focusing on antimicrobial activity is still lacking due to insufficient data on the in vivo system. Most in vivo testing for terpenes and its derivatives has been conducted for human health associated with anti-inflammatory, anti-tumorigenic, anti-cancer, transdermal delivery medium and neuroprotective [92] aspects. However, incorporation of terpenes into household products and cosmetics due to antibacterial properties showed increasing assurance in vivo, inhibiting multiple species of bacteria [93]. In 2006, Mondello et al. [94] demonstrated in vivo activity of the monoterpene terpinen-4-ol which is the main bioactive constituent of *Malaleuca alternifolia* Cheel (tea tree) oil against azole-susceptible and resistant human pathogenic candida species. In this demonstration, terpinen-4-ol was able to clear a well-established model of rat vaginal candidiasis. Terpenes which were found in *Cassia occidentalis* and *Phyllanthus niruri* showed antimalarial activity in vivo using mice against *Plasmodium berghei* [95]. In addition, β-sitosterol was tested in the treatment of culture proven pulmonary tuberculosis (PTB) patients using blinded randomized placebo-controlled trials. Two groups of patients consisting of a sitosterol group and a placebo group were set up upon the treatment. Patients were hospitalized for the duration of treatment and checked monthly with regards to sputum culture positivity, chest radiography, weight gain, hematology, liver function, and Mantoux test response. At the end of trials, it was reported that the sitosterol group marked a greater weight gain, lymphocyte and eosinophils count compared to the other group [96].

2.2.2. Terpenes Bioavailability

In order to ensure greater therapeutic effect from drugs, terpene bioavailability should be determined. It was reported that while natural volatile terpenes from 1,8-cineole of uncrushed capsule from the plasma yielded relatively 100% of bioavailability, limomene and α-pinene were only detectable for a few subjects [97]. In 2017, research conducted by Papada et al. [98] demonstrated positive bioavailability of major terpenes from Mastiha powder after 30 min of ingestion with the highest peak between 2–4 h post ingestion. The plasma analysis was done using ultra-high-pressure liquid chromatography high-resolution MS (UHPLC-HRMS/MS). The bioavailability bottleneck of medicinal herbs including terpenes, however, had been improved ever since phytosome technology arrival. It was reported that the bioavailability of *Ginkgo biloba* extract (GBE) which constitutes of the terpene, lactone, was improved significantly with 2–4 times greater plasma concentration compared to a non-phytosome delivery method [99].

2.2.3. Evaluation of Compounds Interaction in Combination Therapies

Combination therapies using natural products such as the terpenoids may synergistically, additively, or antagonistically affect the treatments. Zacchino et al. [4] reported in a review that the nature of interaction between phytochemical and antimicrobial drugs can be determined using the median-effect method of Chou [89] which permits the calculation of combination index (CI). As for combination therapy, both agents at a fixed ratio will result in IC_{50} respectively; these are mixed with two-fold dilutions of both agents with a fixed ratio. The CI will resolve synergistic (CI < 1), additive (CI = 1) and antagonistic effects (CI > 1). In addition, another method that contributed significantly in synergistic activity was to calculate the Dose Reduction Index (DRI), also known as the reversal enhancement ratio, that measures how many folds the dose of antimicrobial drugs may be cut down when used in combination rather than alone. One of the measures that can be used to evaluate synergism is through checkerboard assay.

In our previous study, through this method, peppermint essential oil was proven to synergistically react with meropenem. MIC of individual peppermint oil and meropenem were 8% and 4 µg/mL respectively. Meanwhile when used in combination, the MIC of peppermint oil and meropenem were reduced to 1% and 0.5 µg/mL respectively. The CI value of 0.26 obtained in checkerboard assay had portrayed a high synergism. Last year, our group carried out extensive analysis to investigate the additive interaction of cinnamon bark oil and meropenem. The shift of attention towards synergism between compounds and antibiotics have caused researchers to overlook the additive effects, thus we conducted the study to understand additive interaction which focused on the effect on the bacterial membrane [100].

2.2.4. Methods for Antimicrobial Evaluation

Both in vitro and in vivo experimental systems can be used to evaluate the antimicrobial activity of either synthetic compounds or naturally-acquired compounds. Nevertheless, in vitro approaches have been more commonly used due to their feasibility. In vivo studies, however, are seldom applied due to limitations in detecting the actual mechanism of action. Susceptibility testing which determines the MIC of a compound against bacteria is routinely done using variations in the methods of MIC assay such as rapid *p*-Iodonitrotetrazolium chloride (INT) colorimetric assay, micro- or macro-dilution and disc diffusion methods. However, Griffin et al. [55] stated in his study that the disc diffusion method is prone to problems as the method was highly dependent on water solubility and suitability of the test agent to be diffused through the agar. In combination therapy, however, the effects are assessed through the checkerboard assay which investigated the interaction between agents. The checkerboard antibiofilm microsomal triglyceride transfer protein (MTP) assay through which the checkerboard microdilution was seeded with biofilm have also been used in an experiment associated with biofilm producing bacteria [88]. By performing the checkerboard assay, an important index called the FIC will reveal the potential of an individual compound [4]. The Dose Reduction Index (DRI) [89] can also be conducted in a compound combination analysis in order to find out the dosage reductions ruled out by individual compounds that affected the MIC of the second compound. A greater DRI disclosed better adjuvant capabilities for a given effect level [89]. More extensively, further analysis usually includes isobolograms and time-kill studies.

3. Perspectives

3.1. Ongoing Research

Effective management and treatment of microbial resistance are among the main priorities in healthcare. Terpene derivatives are an important and promising source of novel antibiotics. Indeed, ent-kaurenoids (ent-kaur-15-en-18, 20-diol and ent-kaur-15-en-18-ol) extracted from *Senegalia nigrescens* are among the novel terpene derivatives discovered recently. Both in vitro and in silico anti-quorum sensing evaluation have demonstrated potential anti-quorum sensing against *Chromobacterium violaceum* [101]. In addition, it was reported that antiquorum sensing does not contribute towards evolution of MDR pathogens as there is no enforcement of selection pressure [32]. Additionally, terpenoids found in microbial volatile compounds (MVCs) have exhibited the ability to combat and modulate antibiotic resistance in human and animal pathogens [102].

With the success of terpenoids in the treatment of microbial resistance, the hunt for new terpenoids has been an important quest amongst the scientific community as a potential application. For instance, screening for terpenoids was conducted on semi-arid plants such as *Caesalpinia pulcherrima, Lawsonia inermis, Pithecellobium dulce, Euphorbia tithymaloides, Punica granatum, Plumeria obtusa, Carica papaya, Cassia fistula, Cordia dichotoma, Euphorbia prostrate, Nerium oleander*, and *Cyanthillium cinereum* [103]. A separate study conducted in 2018 identified three terpenoid derivatives (α-pinene—45.44%, 3-carene—38.34%, and terpinolene—5.36%) of *Cupressus torulosa* essential oil. The compounds are effective against pathogens including *B.subtilis, Pseudomonas alcaligenes, M. luteus*, and *B. cereus* [104]. This can mitigate AMR problems by manipulating combinatory therapeutics of existing antimicrobial agents with terpenoid derivatives. *Ganoderma lucidum* (Reishi) which is a medicinal mushroom, contains several triterpenoid substances such as ganoderic acid and lucidenic acid. The compounds were then evaluated for their therapeutic effects whereby they exhibited anti-human immunodeficiency virus (HIV) activity by inhibiting the effects of HIV progression [105].

3.2. *Application of Terpenoids in Clinical Settings: Challenges*

As mentioned previously, terpenes and terpenoids had been known to exert antimicrobial activity against a wide variety of bacteria, both Gram-positive and Gram-negative. Clinical trials regarding highlighting the application of terpenes had been performed in several studies. In addition, β-sitosterol had also demonstrated immune enhancing ability in tuberculosis patients, demonstrating significant weight gain and higher white blood cell counts which resulted in faster recovery [106]. However, the application of terpenes as antimicrobials in the clinical phase is yet to be explored. This can be attributed to several factors, as the mode of actions of terpenes is not fully understood and the amount of time and resources required for clinical trials are limited and not always rewarding [107]. Terpenes consist of a diverse group of lipophilic organic compounds, resulting in different structures which affect their mode of action. β-caryophyllene showed poor antimicrobial activity against a panel of bacteria [108]. In the event whereby terpenes with efficient antimicrobial activities have been discovered, the safety of the terpenes would often be the next obstacle prior to clinical trials. Certain terpenes are reported to be toxic at low dosage and thus not preferred [109]. For instance, even at 1% dose of eugenol, it was reported to effectively inhibit growth of *Dermanyssus gallinae* at 20% of the pathogen population. Eugenol, geraniol, and citral found in plant essential oils were able to administer 100% mortality when used undiluted. This shows that some undiluted terpenes are highly toxic upon direct usage [110]. Generally, the unfavorable toxicity of terpenes towards whole cells takes place due to disturbance; primarily disrupting cell membrane integrity which eventually leads to cell lysis [111]. Due to the lipophilic nature of terpenes, upon ingestion, they are easily absorbed by epidermal cells before reaching the site of infection. Thus, delicate drug delivery systems are required for their application into clinical trials.

3.3. *Future Prospects*

The evidenced antimicrobial activity of terpenes and their derivatives need to be further expounded with the aid of automation and advancement in technology. Experimental analyses will need to be more streamlined to become more precise, resulting in less ambiguity so that the results obtained can be ensured and are consistent. This will reduce the time taken for experimental work and more time can be spent for extended analyses. Researchers may then study the modification effects of natural products with a special focus on terpenoids. Structural modifications of natural compounds produced either synthetically or via biotransformation may offer a new facet in finding novel AMR solutions as it explores new antimicrobial agents. In addition, delivery methods involving existing treatments against AMR should be improved and new inventions can be investigated. Combination therapeutics may be enhanced by exploring more antimicrobial adjuvants which will synergistically affect treatment outcomes with greater efficiency and less side effects. Natural terpenes and terpenoids which are available at very low prices such as carvacrol, thymol, and geraniol [4], should be optimally used for development of good antibacterial combination drugs. However, application at the pharmaceutical level remains challenging as the in vivo after effect is, currently, still very much unexplored. Extended analysis involving well-designed clinical trials should be improved in order to manipulate potent compounds of terpenoids to the best of their functional potential.

4. Conclusions

From this review, it has been evidenced that some terpenes and their derivatives were proven to be potent antimicrobial agents against drug resistant pathogens which mainly include bacteria and fungi. Specific mechanisms of each class of terpenes have also been highlighted and as a whole, terpenes provide a possible mitigation route for AMR and navigating the dead end of the diminishing antibiotic pipeline, hence, an appropriate match between terpenoids and existing antimicrobial agents may provide ultimate therapeutic options for AMR-associated infections.

Author Contributions: Authors would also like to thank all the members of Floral Biotechnology Laboratory, UPM. K.-S.L. designed the manuscript. N.A.M. drafted the manuscript. S.-H.E.L. significantly refined the manuscript whereas K.-S.L., S.-K.Y., C.-L.M., A.A.-L.S., C.-M.C. and C.-W.C. edited the draft. All authors read and approved the final manuscript.

Funding: This research was funded by the HCT Research Grant (113123) from the Higher Colleges of Technology, UAE.

Acknowledgments: Special thanks are given to the HCT Research Grant for financial support of the research.

Conflicts of Interest: All authors declare no conflicts of interest.

References

1. Mandal, S.M.; Roy, A.; Ghosh, A.K.; Hazra, T.K.; Basak, A.; Franco, O.L. Challenges and future prospects of antibiotic therapy: From peptides to phages utilization. *Front. Pharmacol.* **2014**, *5*, 105. [CrossRef] [PubMed]
2. Barbieri, R.; Coppo, E.; Marchese, A.; Daglia, M.; Sobarzo-Sánchez, E.; Nabavi, S.F. Phytochemicals for human disease: An update on plant-derived compounds antibacterial activity. *Microbiol. Res.* **2017**, *196*, 44–68. [CrossRef] [PubMed]
3. Blair, J.M.; Webber, M.A.; Baylay, A.J.; Ogbolu, D.O.; Piddock, L.J. Molecular mechanisms of antibiotic resistance. *Nat. Rev. Microbiol.* **2015**, *1*, 42. [CrossRef] [PubMed]
4. Zacchino, S.A.; Butassi, E.; Cordisco, E.; Svetaz, L.A. Hybrid combinations containing natural products and antimicrobial drugs that interfere with bacterial and fungal biofilms. *Phytomedicine* **2017**, *37*, 14–26. [CrossRef] [PubMed]
5. Rajagopal, M.; Martin, M.J.; Santiago, M.; Lee, W.; Kos, V.N.; Meredith, T.; Gilmore, M.S.; Walker, S. Multidrug intrinsic resistance factors in *Staphylococcus aureus* identified by profiling fitness within high-diversity transposon libraries. *MBio* **2016**, *7*, 4. [CrossRef]
6. Lewis, K. Persister cells, dormancy and infectious disease. *Nat. Rev. Microbiol.* **2007**, *5*, 48–56. [CrossRef]
7. Laxminarayan, R.; Duse, A.; Wattal, C.; Zaidi, A.K.M.; Wertheim, H.F.L.; Sumpradit, N.; Vlieghe, E.; Hara, G.L.; Gould, I.M.; Goossens, H.; et al. Antibiotic resistance-the need for global solutions. *Lancet Infect. Dis.* **2013**, *13*, 1057–1098. [CrossRef]
8. Touani, F.K.; Seukep, A.J.; Djeussi, D.E.; Fankam, A.G.; Noumedem, J.A.K.; Kuete, V. Antibiotic-potentiation activities of four Cameroonian dietary plants against multidrug-resistant Gram-negative bacteria expressing efflux pumps. *BMC Complement. Altern. Med.* **2014**, *1*, 258. [CrossRef]

9. Davies, J.; Davies, D. Origins and Evolution of Antibiotic Resistance. *Microbiol. Mol. Biol. Rev.* **2010**, *3*, 417–433. [CrossRef]
10. Zaidi, A.K.M.; Huskins, W.C.; Thaver, D.; Bhutta, Z.A.; Abbas, Z.; Goldmann, D.A. Hospital-acquired neonatal infections in developing countries. *Lancet* **2005**, *365*, 1175–1188. [CrossRef]
11. Saleem, A.F.; Ahmed, I.; Mir, F.; Ali, S.R.; Zaidi, A.K.M. Pan-resistant Acinetobacter infection in neonates in Karachi, Pakistan. *J. Infect. Dev. Ctries.* **2010**, *4*, 30–37. [CrossRef]
12. Bush, K.; Courvalin, P.; Dantas, G.; Davies, J.; Eisenstein, B.; Huovinen, P.; Jacoby, G.A.; Kishony, R.; Kreiswirth, B.N.; Kutter, E.; et al. Tackling antibiotic resistance. *Nat. Rev. Microbiol.* **2011**, *9*, 894–896. [CrossRef]
13. Shen, J.; Davis, L.E.; Wallace, J.M.; Cai, Y.; Lawson, L.D. Enhanced diallyl trisulfide has in vitro synergy with amphotericin B against *Cryptococcus neoformans*. *Planta Med.* **1996**, *62*, 415–418. [CrossRef]
14. Yang, S.K.; Low, L.Y.; Yap, P.S.X.; Yusoff, K.; Mai, C.W.; Lai, K.S.; Lim, S.H. Plant-derived antimicrobials: Insights into mitigation of antimicrobial resistance. *Rec. Nat. Prod.* **2018**, *12*, 295–316. [CrossRef]
15. Spratt, B.G. Resistance to antibiotics mediated by target alterations. *Science* **1994**, *264*, 388–393. [CrossRef]
16. Baroud, M.; Dandache, I.; Araj, G.F.; Wakim, R.; Kanj, S.; Kanafani, Z.; Khairallah, M.; Sabra, A.; Shehab, M.; Dbaibo, G.; et al. Underlying mechanisms of carbapenem resistance in extended-spectrum β-lactamase-producing *Klebsiella pneumoniae* and *Escherichia coli* isolates at a tertiary care centre in Lebanon: Role of OXA-48 and NDM-1 carbapenemases. *Int. J. Antimicrob. Agents* **2013**, *41*, 75–79. [CrossRef]
17. Schmieder, R.; Edwards, R. Insights into antibiotic resistance through metagenomic approaches. *Future Microbiol.* **2012**, *7*, 73–89. [CrossRef]
18. Palmer, K.L.; Kos, V.N.; Gilmore, M.S. Horizontal gene transfer and the genomics of enterococcal antibiotic resistance. *Curr. Opin. Microbiol.* **2010**, *13*, 632–639. [CrossRef]
19. Nikaido, H. Prevention of drug access to bacterial targets: Permeability barriers and active efflux. *Science* **1994**, *264*, 382–388. [CrossRef]
20. Hancock, R.E.W. Mechanisms of action of newer antibiotics for Gram-positive pathogens. *Lancet Infect. Dis.* **2005**, *5*, 209–218. [CrossRef]
21. Moo, C.L.; Yang, S.K.; Yusoff, K.; Ajat, M.; Thomas, W.; Abushelaibi, A.; Lim, S.H.; Lai, K.S. Mechanisms of antimicrobial resistance (AMR) and alternative approaches to overcome AMR. *Curr. Drug Discov. Technol.* **2019**, *16*. [CrossRef]
22. Rudramurthy, G.R.; Swamy, M.K.; Sinniah, U.R.; Ghasemzadeh, A. Nanoparticles: Alternatives against drug-resistant pathogenic microbes. *Molecules* **2016**, *21*, 836. [CrossRef]
23. Langeveld, W.T.; Veldhuizen, E.J.A.; Burt, S.A. Synergy between essential oil components and antibiotics: A review. *Crit. Rev. Microbiol.* **2014**, *40*, 76–94. [CrossRef]
24. Yu, H.; Zhang, L.; Li, L.; Zheng, C.; Guo, L.; Li, W.; Sun, P.; Qin, L. Recent developments and future prospects of antimicrobial metabolites produced by endophytes. *Microbiol. Res.* **2010**, *165*, 437–449. [CrossRef]
25. Thapa, D.; Louis, P.; Losa, R.; Zweifel, B.; Wallace, R.J. Essential oils have different effects on human pathogenic and commensal bacteria in mixed faecal fermentations compared with pure cultures. *Microbiology* **2015**, *161*, 441–449. [CrossRef]
26. Lewis, R.E.; Kontoyiannis, D.P. Rationale for combination antifungal therapy. *Pharmacotherapy* **2001**, *21*, 149S–164S. [CrossRef]
27. Wagner, H.; Ulrich-Merzenich, G. Synergy research: Approaching a new generation of phytopharmaceuticals. *Phytomedicine* **2009**, *16*, 97–110. [CrossRef]
28. Oussalah, M.; Caillet, S.; Saucier, L.; Lacroix, M. Inhibitory effects of selected plant essential oils on the growth of four pathogenic bacteria: *E. coli* O157:H7, *Salmonella Typhimurium*, *Staphylococcus aureus* and *Listeria monocytogenes*. *Food Control* **2007**, *18*, 414–420. [CrossRef]
29. Tongnuanchan, P.; Benjakul, S. Essential oils: Extraction, bioactivities, and their uses for food preservation. *J. Food Sci.* **2014**, *7*. [CrossRef]
30. Helander, I.M.; Alakomi, H.L.; Latva-Kala, K.; Mattila-Sandholm, T.; Pol, I.; Smid, E.J.; Gorris, L.G.; Wright, A. Characterization of the action of selected essential oil components on Gram-negative bacteria. *Agric. Food Chem.* **1998**, *46*, 590–595. [CrossRef]
31. Liu, Q.; Niu, H.; Zhang, W.; Mu, H.; Sun, C.; Duan, J. Synergy among thymol, eugenol, berberine, cinnamaldehyde and streptomycin against planktonic and biofilm-associated food-borne pathogens. *Lett. Appl. Microbiol.* **2015**, *60*, 21–30. [CrossRef]

32. Yap, P.S.X.; Yang, S.K.; Lai, K.S.; Lim, S.H. Essential oils: The ultimate solution to antimicrobial resistance in *Escherichia coli*? In *Escherichia coli-Recent Advances on Physiology, Pathogenesis and Biotechnological Applications*; Samie, A., Ed.; Intech Open: Rijeka, Croatia, 2017; pp. 299–313.
33. Yang, S.K.; Yap, P.S.X.; Krishnan, T.; Yusoff, K.; Chan, K.G.; Yap, W.S.; Lai, K.S.; . Lim, S.H. Mode of action: Synergistic interaction of peppermint (*Mentha x piperita* L. Carl) essential oil and meropenem against plasmid-mediated resistant *E. coli*. *Rec. Nat. Prod.* **2018**, *12*, 582–594. [CrossRef]
34. Yang, S.K.; Yusoff, K.; Ajat, M.; Thomas, W.; Abushelaibi, A.; Akseer, R.; Lim, S.E.; Lai, K.S. Disruption of KPC-producing *Klebsiella pneumoniae* membrane via induction of oxidative stress by cinnamon bark (*Cinnamomum verum* J. Presl) essential oil. *PLoS ONE* **2019**, 1–20. [CrossRef]
35. Maida, I.; Lo Nostro, A.; Pesavento, G.; Barnabei, M.; Calonico, C.; Perrin, E.; Chiellini, C.; Fondi, M.; Mengoni, A.; Maggini, V.; et al. Exploring the anti- *Burkholderia cepacia* complex activity of essential oils: A preliminary analysis. *Evidence-Based Complement. Altern. Med.* **2014**, *2014*. [CrossRef]
36. Rasooli, I.; Shayegh, S.; Astaneh, S.D.A. The effect of *Mentha spicata* and *Eucalyptus camaldulensis* essential oils on dental biofilm. *Int. J. Dent. Hyg.* **2009**, *7*, 196–203. [CrossRef]
37. Sharma, A.; Rajendran, S.; Srivastava, A.; Sharma, S.; Kundu, B. Antifungal activities of selected essential oils against *Fusarium oxysporum* f. sp. lycopersici 1322, with emphasis on *Syzygium aromaticum* essential oil. *J. Biosci. Bioeng.* **2017**, *123*, 308–313. [CrossRef]
38. Shrigod, N.M.; Swami Hulle, N.R.; Prasad, R.V. Supercritical fluid extraction of essential oil from mint leaves (*Mentha spicata*): Process optimization and its quality evaluation. *J. Food Process Eng.* **2017**, *40*, 12488. [CrossRef]
39. Adukwu, E.C.; Bowles, M.; Edwards-Jones, V.; Bone, H. Antimicrobial activity, cytotoxicity and chemical analysis of lemongrass essential oil (*Cymbopogon flexuosus*) and pure citral. *Appl. Microbiol. Biotechnol.* **2016**, *100*, 9619–9627. [CrossRef]
40. De Andrade, F.B.; Midena, R.Z.; Koga-Ito, C.Y.; Duarte, M.A. Conventional and natural products against oral infections. Microbial pathogens and strategies for combating them: Science, technology and education. In *Pathogens and Strategies for Combating Them: Science, Technology and Education*; Méndez-Vilas, A., Ed.; FORMATEX Research Center: Badajoz, Spain, 2013; pp. 1574–1583.
41. Vasireddy, L.; Bingle, L.E.H.; Davies, M.S. Antimicrobial activity of essential oils against multidrug-resistant clinical isolates of the *Burkholderia cepacia* complex. *PLoS ONE* **2018**, *13*. [CrossRef]
42. Grzesiak, B.; Głowacka, A.; Krukowski, H.; Lisowski, A.; Lassa, H.; Sienkiewicz, M. The in vitro efficacy of essential oils and antifungal drugs against *Prototheca zopfii*. *Mycopathologia* **2016**, *181*, 609–615. [CrossRef]
43. Rafiq, R.; Hayek, S.; Anyanwu, U.; Hardy, B.; Giddings, V.; Ibrahim, S.; Tahergorabi, R.; Kang, H. Antibacterial and antioxidant activities of essential oils from *Artemisia herba-alba* Asso., *Pelargonium capitatum* radens and *Laurus nobilis* L. *Foods* **2016**, *5*, 28. [CrossRef]
44. Peixoto, L.R.; Rosalen, P.L.; Ferreira, G.L.S.; Freires, I.A.; de Carvalho, F.G.; Castellano, L.R.; Castro, R.D. Antifungal activity, mode of action and anti-biofilm effects of *Laurus nobilis Linnaeus* essential oil against *Candida* spp. *Arch. Oral Biol.* **2017**, *73*, 179–185. [CrossRef]
45. Kurekci, C.; Padmanabha, J.; Bishop-Hurley, S.L.; Hassan, E.; Al Jassim, R.A.M.; McSweeney, C.S. Antimicrobial activity of essential oils and five terpenoid compounds against *Campylobacter jejuni* in pure and mixed culture experiments. *Int. J. Food Microbiol.* **2013**, *166*, 450–457. [CrossRef]
46. De Rapper, S.; Viljoen, A.; Van Vuuren, S. The in vitro antimicrobial effects of *Lavandula angustifolia* essential oil in combination with conventional antimicrobial agents. *Evidence-Based Complement. Altern. Med.* **2016**. [CrossRef]
47. Swamy, M.K.; Akhtar, M.S.; Sinniah, U.R. Antimicrobial properties of plant essential oils against human pathogens and their mode of action: An updated review. *Evid.-Based Complement. Altern. Med.* **2016**. [CrossRef]
48. Al-Snafi, A.E. Medical importance of *Anthemis nobilis*—A review. *As. J. Pharm. Sci. Technol.* **2016**, *6*, 89–95.
49. Hajlaoui, H.; Mighri, H.; Aouni, M.; Gharsallah, N.; Kadri, A. Chemical composition and in vitro evaluation of antioxidant, antimicrobial, cytotoxicity and anti-acetylcholinesterase properties of Tunisian *Origanum majorana* L. essential oil. *Microb. Pathog.* **2016**, *95*, 86–94. [CrossRef]
50. Garzoli, S.; Božović, M.; Baldisserotto, A.; Sabatino, M.; Cesa, S.; Pepi, F.; Vicentini, C.B.; Manfredini, S.; Ragno, R. Essential oil extraction, chemical analysis and anti-Candida activity of *Foeniculum vulgare* Miller–new approaches. *Nat. Prod. Res.* **2018**, *32*, 1254–1259. [CrossRef]

51. Kačániová, M.; Terentjeva, M.; Vukovic, N.; Puchalski, C.; Roychoudhury, S.; Kunová, S.; Klūga, A.; Tokár, M.; Kluz, M.; Ivanišová, E. The antioxidant and antimicrobial activity of essential oils against Pseudomonas spp. isolated from fish. *Saudi Pharm. J.* **2017**, *25*, 1108–1116. [CrossRef]
52. Zrira, S.; Ghanmi, M. Chemical composition and antibacterial activity of the essential of *Cedrus atlantica* (Cedarwood oil). *J. Essent. Oil-Bearing Plants.* **2016**, *19*, 1267–1272. [CrossRef]
53. El Omari, K.; Hamze, M.; Alwan, S.; Jama, C.; Chihib, N.E. Antifungal activity of the essential oil of *Micromeria barbata* an endemic lebanese micromeria species collected at North Lebanon. *J. Mater. Environ. Sci.* **2016**, *7*, 4158–4167.
54. Nazzaro, F.; Fratianni, F.; De Martino, L.; Coppola, R.; De Feo, V. Effect of essential oils on pathogenic bacteria. *Pharmaceuticals* **2013**, *6*, 1451–1474. [CrossRef]
55. Griffin, S.G.; Wyllie, S.G.; Markham, J.L.; Leach, D.N. The role of structure and molecular properties of terpenoids in determining their antimicrobial activity. *Flavour Fragr. J.* **1999**, *14*, 322–332. [CrossRef]
56. Roberts, S.C. Production and engineering of terpenoids in plant cell culture. *Nat. Chem. Biol.* **2007**, *3*, 387–395. [CrossRef]
57. Shaw, M.K.; Ingraham, J.L. Synthesis of macromolecules by *Escherichia coli* near the minimal temperature for growth. *J. Bacteriol.* **1967**, *1*, 157–164.
58. Zengin, H.; Baysal, A. Antibacterial and antioxidant activity of essential oil terpenes against pathogenic and spoilage-forming bacteria and cell structure-activity relationships evaluated by SEM microscopy. *Molecules* **2014**, *11*, 17773–17798. [CrossRef]
59. Chen, J.; Jiang, Q.D.; Chai, Y.P.; Zhang, H.; Peng, P.; Yang, X.X. Natural terpenes as penetration enhancers for transdermal drug delivery. *Molecules* **2016**, *12*, 1709. [CrossRef]
60. Lorenzi, V.; Muselli, A.; Bernardini, A.F.; Berti, L.; Pagès, J.M.; Amaral, L.; Bolla, J.L. Geraniol restores antibiotic activities against multidrug-resistant isolates from Gram-negative species. *Antimicrob. Agents Chemother.* **2009**, *53*, 2209–2211. [CrossRef]
61. Trombetta, D.; Castelli, F.; Sarpietro, M.G.; Venuti, V.; Cristani, M.; Daniele, C.; Saija, A.; Mazzanti, G.; Bisignano, G. Mechanisms of antibacterial action of three monoterpenes. *Antimicrob. Agents Chemother.* **2005**, *49*, 2474–2478. [CrossRef]
62. De Inés, C.; Argandoña, V.H.; Rovirosa, J.; San-Martín, A.; Díaz-Marrero, A.R.; Cueto, M.; González-Coloma, A. Cytotoxic activity of halogenated monoterpenes from *Plocamium cartilagineum. Zeitschrift fur Naturforsch-Sect. C J. Biosci.* **2004**, *59*, 339–344. [CrossRef]
63. Kurita, N.; Miyaji, M.; Kuraney, R.; Takahara, Y.; Ichimura, K. Antifungal activity and molecular orbital energies of aldehyde compounds from oils of higher plants. *Agric. Biol. Chem.* **1979**, *43*, 2365–2371.
64. Dorman, H.J.D.; Deans, S.G. Antimicrobial agents from plants: Antibacterial activity of plant volatile oils. *J. Appl. Microbiol.* **2000**, *88*, 308–316. [CrossRef]
65. Liu, X.; Dong, M.; Chen, X.; Jiang, M.; Lv, X.; Zhou, J. Antimicrobial activity of an endophytic Xylaria sp. YX-28 and identification of its antimicrobial compound 7-amino-4-methylcoumarin. *Appl. Microbiol. Biotechnol.* **2008**, *78*, 241–247. [CrossRef]
66. Knowles, J.R.; Roller, S.; Murray, D.B.; Naidu, A.S. Antimicrobial action of carvacrol at different stages of dual-species biofilm development by *Staphylococcus aureus* and *Salmonella enterica* serovar typhimurium. *Appl. Environ. Microbiol.* **2005**, *71*, 797–803. [CrossRef]
67. Bhatti, H.N.; Khan, S.S.; Khan, A.; Rani, M.; Ahmad, V.U.; Choudhary, M.I. Biotransformation of monoterpenoids and their antimicrobial activities. *Phytomedicine.* **2014**, *21*, 1597–1626. [CrossRef]
68. Smid, E.J.; de Witte, Y.; Gorris, L.G.M. Secondary plant metabolites as control agents of postharvest Penicillium rot on tulip bulbs. *Postharvest Biol. Technol.* **1995**, *6*, 303–312. [CrossRef]
69. Dunkic, V.; Bezic, N.; Vuko, E.; Cukrov, D. Antiphytoviral activity of *Satureja montana* L. ssp. variegata (host) P. W. Ball essential oil and phenol compounds on CMV and TMV. *Molecules* **2010**, *15*, 6713–6721. [CrossRef]
70. Astani, A.; Reichling, J.; Schnitzler, P. Comparative study on the antiviral activity of selected monoterpenes derived from essential oils. *Phytother. Res.* **2010**, *24*, 673–679. [CrossRef]
71. Torres-Romero, D.; Jiménez, I.A.; Rojas, R.; Gilman, R.H.; López, M.; Bazzocchi, I.L. Dihydro-β-agarofuran sesquiterpenes isolated from *Celastrus vulcanicola* as potential anti-*Mycobacterium tuberculosis* multidrug-resistant agents. *Bioorganic Med. Chem.* **2011**, *19*, 2182–2189. [CrossRef]

72. Koo, H.; Pearson, S.K.; Scott-Anne, K.; Abranches, J.; Cury, J.A.; Rosalen, P.L.; Park, Y.; Marquis, R.E.; Bowen, W.H. Effects of apigenin and tt-farnesol on glucosyltransferase activity, biofilm viability and caries development in rats. *Oral Microbiol. Immunol.* **2002**, *17*, 337–343. [CrossRef]
73. Gomes, F.I.A.; Teixeira, P.; Azeredo, J.; Oliveira, R. Effect of farnesol on planktonic and biofilm cells of *Staphylococcus epidermidis*. *Curr. Microbiol.* **2009**, *59*, 118–122. [CrossRef]
74. Masako, K.; Yusuke, K.; Hideyuki, I.; Atsuko, M.; Yoshiki, M.; Kayoko, M.; Makoto, K. Corrigendum to "A novel method to control the balance of skin microflora. Part 2. A study to assess the effect of a cream containing farnesol and xylitol on atopic dry skin". *J. Dermatol. Sci.* **2005**, *39*, 197. [CrossRef]
75. Castelo-Branco, D.S.C.M.; Riello, G.B.; Vasconcelos, D.C.; Guedes, G.M.M.; Serpa, R.; Bandeira, T.J.P.G.; Monteiro, A.J.; Cordeiro, R.A.; Rocha, M.F.; Sidrim, J.J.; et al. Farnesol increases the susceptibility of *Burkholderia pseudomallei* biofilm to antimicrobials used to treat melioidosis. *J. Appl. Microbiol.* **2016**, *120*, 600–606. [CrossRef]
76. Rukayadi, Y.; Hwang, J.K. Effect of coating the wells of a polystyrene microtiter plate with xanthorrhizol on the biofilm formation of *Streptococcus mutans*. *J. Basic Microbiol.* **2006**, *46*, 410–415. [CrossRef]
77. Jin, J.; Guo, N.; Zhang, J.; Ding, Y.; Tang, X.; Liang, J.; Li, L.; Deng, X.; Yu, L. The synergy of honokiol and fluconazole against clinical isolates of azole-resistant *Candida albicans*. *Lett. Appl. Microbiol.* **2010**, *51*, 351–357. [CrossRef]
78. Gonçalves, O.; Pereira, R.; Gonçalves, F.; Mendo, S.; Coimbra, M.A.; Rocha, S.M. Evaluation of the mutagenicity of sesquiterpenic compounds and their influence on the susceptibility towards antibiotics of two clinically relevant bacterial strains. *Mutat. Res. -Genet. Toxicol. Environ. Mutagen.* **2011**, *723*, 18–25. [CrossRef]
79. Ambrosio, S.R.; Tirapelli, C.R.; da Costa, F.B.; de Oliveira, A.M. Kaurane and pimarane-type diterpenes from the Viguiera species inhibit vascular smooth muscle contractility. *Life Sci.* **2006**, *79*, 925–933. [CrossRef]
80. Souza, A.B.; Martins, C.H.G.; Souza, M.G.M.; Furtado, N.A.J.C.; Heleno, V.C.G.; De Sousa, J.P.B.; Rocha, E.M.; Bastos, J.K.; Cunha, W.R.; Veneziani, R.C.; et al. Antimicrobial activity of terpenoids from *Copaifera langsdorffii* Desf. against cariogenic bacteria. *Phythother. Res.* **2011**, *25*, 215–220. [CrossRef]
81. Różalski, M.; Walencka, E.; Różalska, B.; Wysokińska, H. Antimicrobial activity of diterpenoids from hairy roots of *Salvia sclarea* L.: Salvipisone as a potential anti-biofilm agent active against antibiotic resistant Staphylococci. *Phytomedicine.* **2007**, *14*, 31–35.
82. Gupta, V.K.; Tiwari, N.; Gupta, P.; Verma, S.; Pal, A.; Srivastava, S.K.; Darokar, M.P. A clerodane diterpene from *Polyalthia longifolia* as a modifying agent of the resistance of methicillin resistant *Staphylococcus aureus*. *Phytomedicine.* **2016**, *23*, 654–661. [CrossRef]
83. Walencka, E.; Rozalska, S.; Wysokinska, H.; Rozalski, M.; Kuzma, L.; Rozalska, B. Salvipisone and aethiopinone from *Salvia sclarea* hairy roots modulate staphylococcal antibiotic resistance and express anti-biofilm activity. *Planta Med.* **2007**, *73*, 545–551. [CrossRef]
84. Jiménez-Arellanes, A.; Luna-Herrera, J.; Cornejo-Garrido, J.; López-García, S.; Castro-Mussot, M.E.; Meckes-Fischer, M.; Mata-Espinosa, D.; Marquina, B.; Torres, J.; Hernández-Pando, R. Ursolic and oleanolic acids as antimicrobial and immunomodulatory compounds for tuberculosis treatment. *BMC Complement. Altern. Med.* **2013**, *13*, 258. [CrossRef]
85. Cunha, W.R.; De Matos, G.X.; Souza, M.G.M.; Tozatti, M.G.; Andrade, E.; Silva, M.L.; Martins, C.H.G.; Silva, R.D.; Da Silva Filho, A.A. Evaluation of the antibacterial activity of the methylene chloride extract of *Miconia ligustroides*, isolated triterpene acids, and ursolic acid derivatives. *Pharm. Biol.* **2010**, *48*, 166–169. [CrossRef]
86. Zhou, L.; Ding, Y.; Chen, W.; Zhang, P.; Chen, Y.; Lv, X. The in vitro study of ursolic acid and oleanolic acid inhibiting cariogenic microorganisms as well as biofilm. *Oral Dis.* **2013**, *19*, 494–500. [CrossRef]
87. Chung, P.Y.; Chung, L.Y.; Navaratnam, P. Potential targets by pentacyclic triterpenoids from *Callicarpa farinosa* against methicillin-resistant and sensitive *Staphylococcus aureus*. *Fitoterapia.* **2014**, *94*, 48–54. [CrossRef]
88. Lewis, R.E.; Diekema, D.J.; Messer, S.A.; Pfaller, M.A.; Klepser, M.E. Comparison of Etest, chequerboard dilution and time – kill studies for the detection of synergy or antagonism between antifungal agents tested against Candida species. *J. Antimicrob. Chemother.* **2002**, *49*, 345–351. [CrossRef]
89. Chou, T.C. Theoretical basis, experimental design, and computerized simulation of synergism and antagonism in drug combination studies. *Pharmacol. Rev.* **2006**, *58*, 621–681. [CrossRef]

90. Rodriguez, M.V.; Sortino, M.A.; Ivancovich, J.J.; Pellegrino, J.M.; Favier, L.S.; Raimondi, M.P.; Gattuso, M.A.; Zacchino, S.A. Detection of synergistic combinations of Baccharis extracts with Terbinafine against *Trichophyton rubrum* with high throughput screening synergy assay (HTSS) followed by 3D graphs. Behavior of some of their components. *Phytomedicine* **2013**, *13*, 1230–1239. [CrossRef]
91. Zacchino, S.A.; Butassi, E.; Di Liberto, M.; Raimondi, M.; Postigo, A.; Sortino, M. Plant phenolics and terpenoids as adjuvants of antibacterial and antifungal drugs. *Phytomedicine* **2017**, *37*, 27–48. [CrossRef]
92. Cho, K.S.; Lim, Y.R.; Lee, K.; Lee, J.; Lee, J.H.; Lee, I.S. Terpenes from forests and human health. *Toxicol. Res.* **2017**, *2*, 97. [CrossRef]
93. Schwab, W.; Fuchs, C.; Huang, F.C. Transformation of terpenes into fine chemicals. *Eur. J. Lipid Sci. Tech.* **2013**, *1*, 3–8. [CrossRef]
94. Mondello, F.; De Bernardis, F.; Girolamo, A.; Cassone, A.; Salvatore, G. In vivo activity of terpinen-4-ol, the main bioactive component of *Melaleuca alternifolia* Cheel (tea tree) oil against azole-susceptible and-resistant human pathogenic Candida species. *BMC infectious diseases* **2006**, *1*, 158. [CrossRef]
95. Tona, L.; Mesia, K.; Ngimbi, N.P.; Chrimwami, B.; Okond'Ahoka; Cimanga, K.; Bruyne, T.D.; Apers, S.; Hermans, N.; Totte, J.; et al. In-vivo antimalarial activity of *Cassia Occidentalism, Morinda morindoides* and *Phyllanthus niruri. Ann. Trop. Med. Parasitol.* **2001**, *1*, 47–57. [CrossRef]
96. Donald, P.R.; Lamprecht, J.H.; Freestone, M.; Albrecht, C.F.; Bouic, P.J.; Kotze, D.; Van Jaarsveld, P.P. A randomised placebo-controlled trial of the efficacy of beta-sitosterol and its glucoside as adjuvants in the treatment of pulmonary tuberculosis. *Int. J. Tuberc. Lung Dis.* **1997**, *6*, 518–522.
97. Kohlert, C.; Van Rensen, I.; März, R.; Schindler, G.; Graefe, E.U.; Veit, M. Bioavailability and pharmacokinetics of natural volatile terpenes in animals and humans. *Planta Med.* **2000**, *6*, 495–505. [CrossRef]
98. Papada, E.; Gioxari, A.; Brieudes, V.; Amerikanou, C.; Halabalaki, M.; Skaltsounis, A.L.; Smyrnioudis, I.; Kaliora, A.C. Bioavailability of terpenes and postprandial effect on human antioxidant potential. An open-label study in healthy subjects. *Mol. Nutr. Food Res.* **2018**, *3*, 1700751. [CrossRef]
99. Amin, T.; Bhat, S.V. A review on phytosome technology as a novel approach to improve the bioavailability of nutraceuticals. *Int. J. Adv. Res. Technol.* **2012**, *3*, 1–5.
100. Yang, S.K.; Yusoff, K.; Mai, C.W.; Lim, W.M.; Yap, W.S.; Lim, S.H.E.; Lai, K.S. Additivity vs. synergism: Investigation of the additive interaction of cinnamon bark oil and meropenem in combinatory therapy. *Molecules* **2017**, *22*, 1733. [CrossRef]
101. Bodede, O.; Shaik, S.; Chenia, H.; Singh, P.; Moodley, R. Quorum sensing inhibitory potential and in silico molecular docking of flavonoids and novel terpenoids from *Senegalia nigrescens. J. Ethnopharmacol.* **2018**, *216*, 134–146. [CrossRef]
102. Avalos, M.; van Wezel, G.P.; Raaijmakers, J.M.; Garbeva, P. Healthy scents: Microbial volatiles as new frontier in antibiotic research? *Curr. Opin. Microbiol.* **2018**, *45*, 84–91. [CrossRef]
103. Chudasama, R.G.; Dhanani, N.J.; Amrutiya, R.M.; Chandni, R.; Jayanthi, G.; Karthikeyan, K. Screening of selected plants from semi-arid region for its phytochemical constituents and antimicrobial activity. *J. Pharmacog. Phytochem.* **2018**, *7*, 2983–2988.
104. Gupta, S.; Bhagat, M.; Sudan, R.; Rajput, S.; Rajput, K. Analysis of chemical composition of *Cupressus torulosa* (D.Don) essential oil and bioautography guided evaluation of its antimicrobial fraction. *Indian J. Exp. Biol.* **2018**, *56*, 252–257.
105. Cör, D.; Knez, Ž.; Hrnčič, M.K. Antitumour, antimicrobial, antioxidant and antiacetylcholinesterase effect of *Ganoderma Lucidum* terpenoids and polysaccharides: A review. *Molecules* **2018**, *23*, 649. [CrossRef]
106. Bin Sayeed, M.; Karim, S.; Sharmin, T.; Morshed, M. Critical analysis on characterization, systemic effect, and therapeutic potential of beta-sitosterol: A plant-derived orphan phytosterol. *Medicines* **2016**, *3*, 29. [CrossRef]
107. Silver, L.L. Challenges of antibacterial discovery. *Clin. Microbiol. Rev.* **2011**, *24*, 71–109. [CrossRef]
108. Fidyt, K.; Fiedorowicz, A.; Strządała, L.; Szumny, A. β-caryophyllene and β-caryophyllene oxide—Natural compounds of anticancer and analgesic properties. *Cancer Medicine* **2016**, *5*, 3007–3017. [CrossRef]
109. De Moraes, M.M.; da Camara, C.A.G.; Da Silva, M.M.C. Comparative toxicity of essential oil and blends of selected terpenes of Ocotea species from Pernambuco, Brazil, against *Tetranychus urticae* Koch. *An. Acad. Bras. Cienc.* **2017**, *89*, 1417–1429. [CrossRef]

110. Sparagano, O.; Khallaayoune, K.; Duvallet, G.; Nayak, S.; George, D. Comparing terpenes from plant essential oils as pesticides for the poultry red mite (*Dermanyssus gallinae*). *Transbound. Emerg. Dis.* **2013**, *60*, 150–153. [CrossRef]
111. Van der Werf, M.J.; de Bont, J.A.; Leak, D.J. Opportunities in microbial biotransformation of monoterpenes. In *Biotechnology of Aroma Compounds*; Springer: Berlin/Heidelberg, Germany, 1997; pp. 147–177.

molecules

MDPI

Review

Marine Organisms as Potential Sources of Bioactive Peptides that Inhibit the Activity of Angiotensin I-Converting Enzyme: A Review

Dwi Yuli Pujiastuti [1,*], Muhamad Nur Ghoyatul Amin [1], Mochammad Amin Alamsjah [1,*] and Jue-Liang Hsu [2,3]

1 Department of Marine, Faculty of Fisheries and Marine, Universitas Airlangga, Surabaya 60115, Indonesia
2 Department of Biological Science and Technology, National Pingtung University of Science and Technology, Pingtung 91201, Taiwan
3 Research Center for Austronesian Medicine and Agriculture, National Pingtung University of Science and Technology, Pingtung 91201, Taiwan
* Correspondence: dwiyp@fpk.unair.ac.id (D.Y.P.); alamsjah@fpk.unair.ac.id (M.A.A.); Tel.: +62-31-5911451 (ext. 5197) (D.Y.P.); Fax: +62-31-5965741 (D.Y.P.)

Received: 11 June 2019; Accepted: 9 July 2019; Published: 12 July 2019

Abstract: Angiotensin I-converting enzyme (ACE) is a paramount therapeutic target to treat hypertension. ACE inhibitory peptides derived from food protein sources are regarded as safer alternatives to synthetic antihypertensive drugs for treating hypertension. Recently, marine organisms have started being pursued as sources of potential ACE inhibitory peptides. Marine organisms such as fish, shellfish, seaweed, microalgae, molluscs, crustaceans, and cephalopods are rich sources of bioactive compounds because of their high-value metabolites with specific activities and promising health benefits. This review aims to summarize the studies on peptides from different marine organisms and focus on the potential ability of these peptides to inhibit ACE activity.

Keywords: ACE inhibitory peptide; antihypertensive; bioactive peptides; hypertension; marine resources

1. Introduction

Hypertension or high blood pressure is generally caused by behavioral risk factors, ageing, and population growth. It emerged in upper-middle income countries among adults aged >25 years. Hypertension causes 9.4 million deaths each year worldwide [1]. Currently, hypertension is one of the leading causes of morbidity and mortality globally, followed by metabolic disorder [2]. It is a key risk factor for cardiovascular disease, heart attack, stroke, and arteriosclerosis. The common examination used to diagnose hypertension is the measurement of blood pressure; a systolic blood pressure (SBP) and diastolic blood pressure (DBP) higher than 140 mm Hg and 90 mm Hg, respectively, indicates hypertension. To mitigate the aberrations in blood pressure and restore normal physiological function, functional molecules derived from food have been widely pursued.

The renin angiotensin aldosterone system (RAAS) plays a significant role in the maintenance of arterial blood pressure and fluid balance and is regarded as the major target to combat hypertension [3]. In RAAS, angiotensinogen is cleaved by renin, producing angiotensin I. Angiotensin I is then converted to angiotensin II, a strong vasoconstrictor, by angiotensin I-converting enzyme (ACE). In addition, ACE inactivates the vasodilator bradykinin, which acts as a mediator of inflammation, a natriuretic peptide, and a potent stimulator of vasodilator prostaglandins, and is involved in nitric oxide synthesis [4]. Because the production of angiotensin II increases blood pressure [5,6], the inhibition of ACE is a reliable strategy to control hypertension [7]. ACE inhibitors decrease ACE activity and indirectly reduce the angiotensin II level, thereby exerting a vasorelaxation effect on blood vessels [8]. Captopril, enalapril, lisinopril, and benazepril are commonly used as effective synthetic ACE inhibitors and have been developed for treating hypertension. However, synthetic drugs usually cause undesirable side effects [9,10]. To reduce these side effects, food-derived ACE inhibitory peptides are preferred over synthetic drugs to combat hypertension. ACE inhibitory peptides are considered as potent antihypertensive drugs, and they do not have any undesirable side effects. ACE inhibitors are more effective than other hypertensive drugs in retarding the progression of renal damage and reducing proteinuria. Two health organization, namely the international society of hypertension-world health organization (ISHWHO) and the Canadian society of hypertension recommend ACE inhibitors as the first line of treatment for hypertension [11].

Proteins are an important macronutrient as they provide the necessary energy and amino acids essential for growth and the maintenance of normal bodily functions. Many physiological and functional properties of proteins are attributed to bioactive peptides [8]. Bioactive peptides derived from food protein have been growing attractive because of awareness of their health-boosting properties. Bioactive peptides from several natural and processed foods have now been isolated and characterized. They function as potential physiological modulators in the process of metabolism during intestinal digestion and are liberated depending on their structure, composition, and amino acid sequence. Some bioactive peptides have been identified to possess nutraceutical potential and promote overall human health [12], with the potential of being used as candidates for treating conditions, such as hypertension [13].

Bioactive peptides are usually isolated from milk and cheese. They are also isolated from other animal sources, such as meat, gelatin, eggs, and various fish species (salmon, sardine, tuna, and herring), and plant sources, such as mushroom, wheat, pumpkin, and sorghum [14]. For example, ACE inhibitory peptides derived from fish have been shown to have a favorable effect on blood pressure [7,15,16]. Unlike many synthetic ACE inhibitors, which cause dry cough and angioedema, natural peptide-inhibitors have no side effects and are considered to be safer and healthier [17]. In recent years, ACE inhibitors have been derived from food proteins, such as milk [18,19], corn [20,21], ovalbumin [22], legume [23,24], Chinese soft-shelled turtle eggs [25,26], bitter melon seeds [27], cheese [28,29], chicken eggs [30–33], casein [34–36], fish [37–39], and algae [40,41].

Oceans cover >70% of the earth's surface and are a rich resource for humans. There is increasing interest in marine organisms as new sources of natural products. Several compounds with unique biological activities have been isolated from marine organisms. The marine environment is rich in biological as well as chemical diversity; compounds isolated from marine organisms have been used as pharmaceuticals, nutraceuticals, cosmeceuticals, molecular probes, fine chemicals, and agrochemicals. Macro-and microorganisms in marine habitats possess a wide array of secondary metabolites, including terpenes, steroids, polyketides, peptides, alkaloids, polysaccharides, proteins, and porphyrins. Because the environment surrounding marine organisms is extreme, aggressive, and competitive, these organisms produce several secondary metabolites with a promising potential for use as drugs, nutritional supplements, and therapeutic agents [42–44]. Marine organisms, such as fish, shellfish, seaweed, microalgae, molluscs, crustaceans, and cephalopods, are rich sources of several functional compounds, such as bioactive peptides, enzymes, polyunsaturated fatty acids, vitamins, minerals, phenolic phlorotannins, and polysaccharides. Moreover, as some marine organisms, especially fish, are particularly rich sources of protein, they are ideal for generating protein-derived bioactive peptides [45,46]. Marine bioactive peptides have gained significant attention for their health promoting effects, such as antihypertensive, antioxidant, anticoagulant, antimicrobial, antithrombotic, and hypocholesterolemic properties [47]. Furthermore, compounds isolated from marine organisms have been commercially distributed in health markets [48]. In this review, we discuss the ACE inhibitory peptides derived from marine resources and provide information on their production, characterization, and potential health benefits. We also review the future prospects of ACE inhibitory peptides derived from marine organisms as therapeutic drugs to combat hypertension.

2. ACE Inhibitory Peptides Derived from Marine Organisms

Zinc ion (Zn^{2+})-dependent dipeptidyl carboxypeptidase, also known as ACE (EC 3.4.15.1), plays a pivotal role in the regulation of blood pressure because of its action in RAAS [49]. ACE is present in biological fluids, such as plasma and semen, and in many tissues, such as testis, intestinal epithelial cells, proximal renal tubular cells, brain, lungs, stimulated macrophages, vascular endothelium, and the medial and adventitial layers of blood vessel walls [4]. In humans, ACE exists in two isoforms: somatic ACE (sACE) and germinal ACE (gACE). sACE is distributed in many types of endothelial and epithelial cells, whereas gACE occurs in germinal cells in the testis, and is therefore also known as testicular ACE [6]. In RAAS, ACE cleaves the decapeptide angiotensin I (Asp-Arg-Val-Tyr-Ile-His-Pro-Phe-His-Leu) into the octapeptide angiotensin II (Asp-Arg-Val-Tyr-Ile-His-Pro-Phe) by removing the C-terminal dipeptide His-Leu. Angiotensin II stimulates the release of aldosterone and antidiuretic hormone or vasopressin, consequently increasing the retention of sodium and water; it also acts as a potent vasoconstrictor (Figure 1). These phenomena act in concert to directly increase the blood pressure [6]. Substrates of ACE include not only angiotensin I in RAAS and bradykinin in the kinin–kallikrein system, but also the haemoregulatory peptide *N*-acetyl-Ser-Asp-Lys-Pro, which is a putative bone marrow suppressor. It contributes to haemopoietic cell differentiation, regulating tissue and blood levels of the vasoactive hormones angiotensin II and bradykinin [50]. In addition, ACE shows endopeptidase activity against a wide range of substrates, such as cholecystokinin, substance P, and luliberin. The inhibition of ACE enzymatic activity on angiotensin I is one of the major challenges to combat hypertension-related disorders [51].

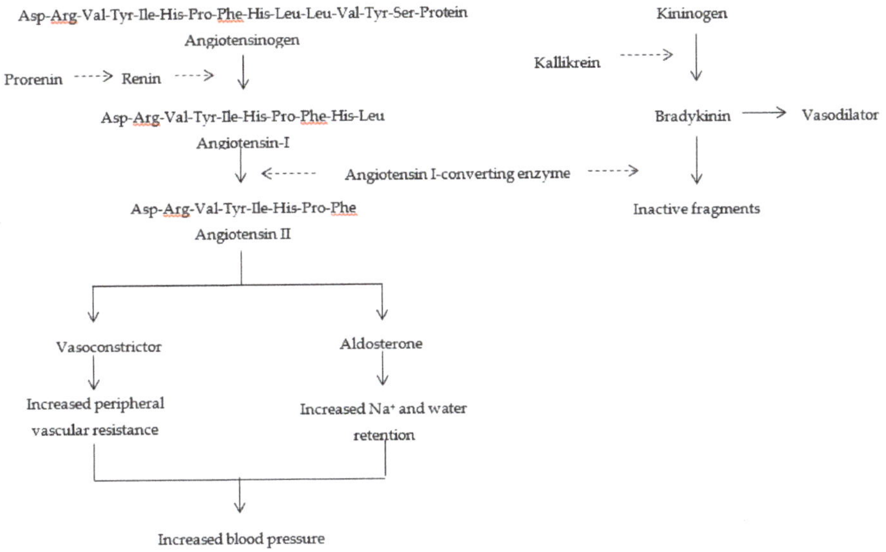

Figure 1. Role of angiotensin I-converting enzyme in the renin angiotensin aldosterone system and the kinin–kallikrein system [15].

Recently, natural marine products have been investigated as alternative synthetic drugs; they have been the topic of interest for many researchers due to their numerous beneficial effects, and some novel ACE-inhibitory compounds have been isolated from algae [52,53]. Marine proteins, such as Heshiko, a fermented mackerel product [38], sardine muscle [9], shark meat [54], Alaska pollock skin [55], marine shrimp [56], and chum salmon [57], exhibit ACE inhibitory activity. ACE inhibitory peptides usually contains 2–12 amino acid residues [10,58,59]. However, some studies have identified up to 27 amino acid residues in ACE inhibitory peptides [60,61]. Proteases, such as pepsin, chymotrypsin, alcalase, and trypsin, are frequently used in hydrolysis for generating ACE inhibitory peptides [9,10,55]. List of identified peptides derived from marine resources; origin, sequence peptides, and IC_{50} value, can be seen in Table 1.

Table 1. List of identified peptides derived from marine resources; origin, sequence peptides, and IC_{50} value.

Origin	Enzyme	Sequence Peptide	IC_{50} (μM)	Reference
	Fish			
Sea bream	Alkaline Protease	GY VY GF VIY	265 16 708 7.5	[62]
Lizard fish	Neutral Protease	MKCAF RVCLP	45.7 175	[63] [64]
Alaska pollock (*Theragra chalcogramma*)	Alcalase, Pronase E and Collagenase	GPL GPM	2.6 17.3	[55]
Grass carp	Alcalase	VAP	19.9	[10]
Atlantic salmon (*Salmo salar* L.)	Alcalase and Papain	AP VR	356.9 1301.1	[65]
Skipjack (*Katsuwonus pelamis*)	Alcalase	DLDLRKDLYAN MCYPAST MLVFAV	67.4 58.7 3.07	[66]
Yellowfin sole (*Limanda aspera*)	Chymotrypsin	MIFPGAGGPEL	268.3	[67]
Pacific cod	Pepsin	GASSGMPG LAYA	6.9 14.5	[68]
Paralichthys alivaceus	Pepsin	MEVFVP VSQLTR	79 105	[69]
Channa striatus	Thermolysin	VPAAPPK NGTWFEPP	0.45 0.63	[70]
	Microalgae			
Chlorella vulgaris	Pepsin	IVVE FAL AEL VVPPA AFL	315 26.3 57.1 79.5 63.8	[40]
Chlorella ellipsoidea	Alcalase	VEGY	128.4	[71]
Spirulina platensis	Pepsin	IAE IAPG VAF	34.7 11.4 35.8	[40]
	Molluscs			
Sea cucumber (*Acaudina molpadioidea*)	Bromelain and Alcalase	MEGAQEAQGD	15.9	[72]
Cuttlefish (*Sepia officinalis*)	Cuttlefish hepatopancreas	VYAP VIIF MAW	6.1 8.7 16.32	[73]
		GIHETTY EKSYELP VELYP	25.66 14.41 5.22	[74]
Squid (*Dosidicus gigas*) skin collagen	Esperase	GRGSVPAPGP	47.78	[75]
Corbicula fluminea	Protamex + Flavourzyme	VKP	3.7	[76]
		VKK	1045	

The potency of peptides derived from marine organisms is expressed as the half maximal inhibitory concentration (IC_{50}), which indicates the ACE inhibitor concentration that leads to 50% inhibition of ACE activity. Moreover, Lineweaver–Burk plots are usually used to determine the inhibition mode of

ACE inhibitory peptides. Most of the reported peptides act as competitive inhibitors of ACE. In the competitive inhibition mode, the inhibitor competes with the substrate and binds to the active site of ACE. In the non-competitive inhibition mode, the inhibitor binds to a site other than the active site. The binding of inhibitor to ACE alters the conformation of ACE, which prevents the substrate from binding to the active site of ACE. The enzyme, substrate, and inhibitor cannot form a complex; thus, the enzyme–substrate complex or enzyme–inhibitor complex is formed. In the uncompetitive inhibition mode, the inhibitor binds to only the substrate–enzyme complex. The C-terminal end of the inhibitory peptide associates with the active site pockets of ACE. ACE harbors three sub-sites: antepenultimate position (S1), penultimate position (S1′), and ultimate position (S2′). In the substrate, the amino acids Pro, Ala, Val, and Leu are the most favorable for S1; Ile is the most favorable for S1′; and Pro and Leu are the most favorable for S2′ [77]. The S1 sub-site includes Ala354, Glu384, and Tyr523 residues; S1′ pocket contains Glu162; and S2′ pocket includes Gln281, His353, His513, Lys511, and Tyr520 [78,79]. Many studies have shown that peptides with high ACE inhibitory activity contain Trp, Phe, Tyr, or Pro at the C-terminus and branched aliphatic amino acids at the N-terminus [49].

In China, soft-shelled turtle eggs have been used as a tonic food for a long time. Low-molecular weight peptides (<3 kDa) have been isolated from soft-shelled turtle egg by ultrafiltration and fractionated by reversed-phase high-performance liquid chromatography (RP-HPLC). In vitro screening of the resulting fractions for ACE inhibitory activity has revealed an IC_{50} value of 4.39 μM for the peptide IVRDPNGMGAW isolated from soft-shelled turtle egg white. This peptide has been identified as a competitive inhibitor of ACE [26]. The peptide AKLPSW, isolated from soft-shelled turtle egg yolk, has also been shown to exhibit potent ACE inhibitory activity, with an IC_{50} value of 15.3 μM, and inhibition kinetics has indicated that this peptide is a non-competitive inhibitor of ACE. The AKLPSW peptide significantly reduces the systolic blood pressure by approximately 13 mm Hg after 6 h of oral administration, thus confirming its antihypertensive effect [25]. In another study, Sardinella protein hydrolysates (SPHs) were obtained from fermentation with *Bacillus subtilis* (SPH-A26) and *Bacillus amyloliquefaciens* (SPH-An6). Approximately 800 peptides have been identified in SPH-A26 and SPH-An6 using nano electrospray ionization liquid chromatography tandem mass spectrometry. Of these 800 peptides, eight isolated from SPH-A26 and seven from SPH-An6 have been selected based on homologies with previously characterized peptides (Biopep data bank), as well as peptide length. Among the synthesized peptides, NVPVYEGY and ITALAPSTM show ACE inhibitory activity with IC_{50} values of 210 and 229 μM, respectively. Fermented SPHs have a potential for use as hypotensive nutraceutical ingredients [80]. The popular freshwater tilapia also reported the potential antihypertensive peptides from hydrolysate by using papain, bromelain, and pepsin. In order to enhance the activity, the hydrolysate was fractionated into four fractions (<1 kDa, 1–3 kDa, 3–5 kDa, and 5–10 kDa). The pepsin-hydrolyzed FPH (FPHPe) with the highest DH (23%) possessed the strongest ACE-inhibitory activity (IC_{50} of 0.57 mg/mL). Its <1 kDa ultrafiltration fraction (FPHPe1) suppressed both ACE (IC_{50} of 0.41 mg/mL). In addition, FPHPe1 significantly reduced SBP (maximum −33 mmHg), DBP (maximum −24 mmHg), mean arterial pressure (MAP) (maximum −28 mmHg), and hearth rates (HR) (maximum −58 beats) in SHRs [81].

The production of peptides with ACE inhibitory activity must consider the amino acid composition and molecular weight of hydrolysates. Purification is carried out to obtain a single peptide with a specific amino acid residues which is in accordance with characterized sequence of bioactive peptide inhibiting ACE. The pure peptide could be easily observed its activity and stability, as well as the dosage of peptide administration in the patients with hypertension symptom would be validly determined. Total hydrolysates with high molecular weight revealed lower activity for inhibiting the ACE rather than single peptide. The shorter amino acid residues is more visible to reach the target site when through the digestive tract and they can be absorbed easily. Then, lower-molecular weight peptides also have a higher probability of passing through the intestinal barrier and exerting biological function [65]. The C-terminal residue in tripeptides or dipeptides plays an important role in binding to sub-sites S1, S1′, and S2′ sub-sites within the active site of ACE [82]. Aromatic or hydrophobic amino acid residues, such as Trp, Phe, Tyr, and Pro, are more active if present at positions in the C-terminal end that bind to each of the three sub-sites of ACE. In addition, tripeptides or dipeptides with a branched aliphatic amino acid at the N-terminus show potent ACE inhibition. Basic amino acid residues, such as Lys and Arg, at the C-terminus also contribute to potent inhibition against ACE [83]. Many studies have shown that the C-terminal residue of potent ACE inhibitory peptides is usually a hydrophobic amino acid [39,70,74,84,85].

There is no correlation between competitive inhibitor with high ACE inhibitory activity. Several non-competitive inhibitors show high ACE inhibitory activity. The peptide Ala-Lys-Leu-Pro-Ser-Trp derived from soft-shelled turtle egg yolk exhibits a low IC_{50} value of 13.7 μM [25], whereas the peptide Val-Glu-Leu-Tyr-Pro isolated from cuttlefish muscle protein exhibits an even lower IC_{50} value of 5.22 μM [74]; both these peptides are considered non-competitive inhibitors. Moreover, some peptides inhibit ACE activity by the uncompetitive mode of inhibition. For example, the peptides Ile-Trp and Phe-Tyr have been ientified as uncompetitive inhibitors [86]; similarly, the peptides Tyr-Ley-Tyr-Glu-Ile-Ala and Tyr-Leu-Tyr-Glu-Ile-Ala-Arg-Arg have been identified as uncompetitive inhibitors [87]. Depending on the results of pre-incubation of the peptide with ACE, the ACE inhibitory peptides are divided into three categories: true inhibitors, prodrugs, and real substrates. A true inhibitor shows no significant difference in the IC_{50} value before and after pre-incubation with ACE, whereas a prodrug shows dramatic reduction in the IC_{50} value after pre-incubation with ACE. On the other hand, a real substrate shows an increase in the IC_{50} value after pre-incubation with ACE, suggesting a reduction in its inhibitory activity against ACE. Generally, the prodrug- and true inhibitor-type peptides are expected to exhibit long-lasting antihypertensive activity in spontaneously hypertensive rats used as a model to study hypertension in humans [88,89].

3. Generation of Bioactive Peptides

Protein hydrolysates have an excellent amino acid balance, are readily digestible, show rapid uptake, and contain bioactive peptides [90]. Bioactive peptides act as therapeutic agents and are characterized by high biological specificity, low toxicity, high structural diversity, high and wide spectrum of activity, and small size, which implies that they have a low likelihood of triggering undesirable immune responses [91]. Bioactive peptides are defined as protein fragments with beneficial effects on bodily functions and human health. Peptides isolated from food sources are structurally similar to endogenous peptides and therefore interact with the same receptors and play a prominent role as immune regulators, growth factors, and modifiers of food intake [92]. Depending on the sequence of amino acids, these peptides can exhibit diverse activities, including antimicrobial [93], antioxidant [94], antithrombotic [95], and antihypertensive [25].

Bioactive peptides are generally produced via enzymatic hydrolysis using digestive enzymes, fermentation using proteolytic starter cultures, or proteolysis using microorganism-or plant-derived enzymes. To generate short-chain functional peptides, enzymatic hydrolysis is used in combination with fermentation or proteolysis [96]. During growth, microorganisms release the protease enzyme into the extracellular medium, leading to proteolysis and peptide generation. Microorganisms are typically used for fermentation for several hours to several days, depending on the desired peptide and the type of fermentation [97]. During fermentation, microorganisms break down complex compounds into smaller molecules with various physiological functions [98]. Fermented marine food products are rich sources of bioactive compounds, including amino acids and peptides [99]. Digestive enzymes, such as trypsin, chymotrypsin, and pepsin, release the bioactive peptides for gastrointestinal digestion in vivo. To stimulate gastrointestinal digestion, several proteolytic enzymes, such as alcalase and thermolysin, engage with trypsin and pepsin. In addition, recombinant DNA technology and chemical synthesis have been used to produce bioactive peptides [92]. The physicochemical properties, such as molecular weight, isoelectric point, and hydrophilic or hydrophobic indices of the resulting peptides, change after enzymatic hydrolysis. Prominent amino acids, such as Pro and Val, play key roles in most antihypertensive peptides [91].

In the digestive system, bioactive peptides are absorbed through the intestine and enter the blood stream to exert systemic effects or local effects in the gastrointestinal tract. Dipeptides and tripeptides are easily absorbed in the intestine. To exert antihypertensive effects, bioactive peptides must reach the target cells after absorption through the intestine. Common bioactive peptides with antihypertensive effects include Val-Pro-Pro (VPP) and Ile-Pro-Pro (IPP); they are produced via fermentation using *Lactobacillus helveticus* and *Saccharomyces cerevisiae*. These two peptides have been detected in the aortal tissue using HPLC, and their effect on ACE activity was lower in the aorta in the study group than in the control group (saline) [14].

4. Screening Approach

The search for peptides capable of inhibiting ACE activity has been intensified. The pursue of ACE inhibitory peptides from marine, as well as other sources, has been substantiated. A reliable assay to determine the ability of peptides to inhibit ACE activity is of paramount concern. In vitro determination of ACE inhibitory peptides is preceded by enzymatic digestion or microbial fermentation, followed by the analysis of structure and chemical synthesis of active peptides. Most assays evaluating the ACE inhibitory activity of peptides have been performed as described previously [100]. The technique used to evaluate the ACE inhibitory activity of peptides must be simple, sensitive, and reliable. Several such methods have been developed, such as spectrophotometry, HPLC, fluorometric capillary electrophoresis, and radiochemistry. Among these, spectrophotometry is the most commonly used method to measure ACE inhibitory activity. This method involves the hydrolysis of hippuryl-histidyl-leucine (HHL) by ACE to hippuric acid (HA). The amount of HA produced from HHL is directly correlated with ACE activity [101]. The amount of HA formed is determined by measuring the absorbance at 228 nm (absorption maximum of HA) [102]. Although the spectrophotometry is useful, it is time consuming, complicated, and is unable to detect trace amounts of the sample.

In practice, results of different assays may vary because of the use of different substrates, such as the synthetic peptides HHL and furanacryloyl-L-phenylalanylglycyl-glycine (FAPGG), which are the most commonly used substrates, and the fluorescent molecule o-aminobenzoylglycyl-p-nitrophenylalanylproline for specific detection and quantification [103]. Results may also vary within the same assay because of the use of different test conditions or the use of ACE from different origins. Thus, ACE activity levels must be carefully controlled to obtain comparable and reproducible results [83,104].

HPLC is a common method to determine ACE inhibitory activity of peptides as it generates reproducible results. Although HPLC has been used for decades, it requires the extraction of the product from the reaction mixture using an organic solvent, which limits the number of samples that can be analyzed per day and is also a source of error [105]. Moreover, HPLC analysis shows peculiar results from samples with added inhibitor, which exhibit high HA release than samples without the added inhibitor. This occurs if the enzyme or the substrate (HHL) is unstable in solution. The evaluation of ACE inhibition is depends on the comparison between the concentration of HA in the presence or absence of an inhibitor (inhibitor blank). The occurrence of autolysis of HHL to give HA was evaluated by a reaction blank, i.e., a sample with the higher inhibitor concentration and without the enzyme [24]. Another substrate, FAPGG, has also been used for HPLC [106,107]; FAPGG releases 2-furylacryloyl-L-phenylalanine (FAP) as a product. This method is used to quantitate the levels and can be used a model of inhibition according to the sigmoid character of the response curve. The slope of the curve, describing absorbance versus time, is thus a direct measure of ACE activity. It is based on the combination of enzymatic reaction with HPLC detection of the inhibition of enzyme activity by measuring the levels of the substrate and product formed. The amount of FAP formed is determined by measuring the absorbance at 305 nm. This method is beneficial, as it does not require sophisticated equipment or radiolabelled compounds [108]. Because the price of the two substrates, HHL and FAPGG, is similar, the HPLC method is advantageous over spectrophotometry, as it requires less labor and has a higher throughput than spectrophotometry [103].

The determination of ACE activity also utilizes fluorescent tripeptides, such as *o*-aminobenzoylglycyl-*p*-nitro-L-phenylalanyl-L-proline [Abz-Gly-Phe(NO_2)-Pro]. The hydrolysis of this substrate by ACE generates o-aminobenzoylglycine (Abz-Gly) as a product, which is easily quantified fluorometrically using appropriate excitation and emission wavelengths. Fluorescence detection of the reaction products is highly sensitive and precise. Moreover, commercial availability of all reagents is a major advantage, allowing easy introduction of the assay in laboratories [109].

To obtain ACE inhibitory peptides, slight modification of the assay is crucial. Orthogonal bioassay-guided fractionation is considered as a potential method to obtain ACE inhibitory peptides. This method involves the separation of the potential peptides using two ways of fractionation: Strong cation exchange (SCX) and RP-HPLC (Figure 2). SCX separates peptides based on their charge, whereas RP-HPLC separates peptides based on their hydrophobicity [110]. Although both SCX and RP-HPLC separate peptides using different mechanisms, peptides are regarded as potential ACE inhibitors because they remain in the most active fraction using both methods. Pujiastuti et al. [25] revealed the identification of overlapping peptides using SCX and RP-HPLC.

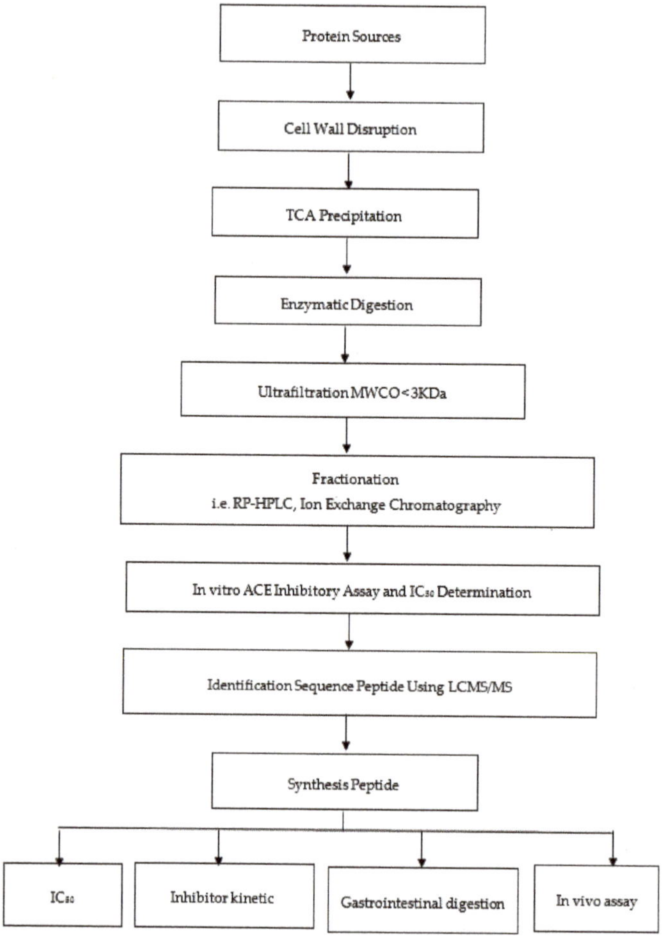

Figure 2. Flowchart showing the production of bioactive peptides for angiotensin I-converting enzyme (ACE) inhibitory assay [25].

A new method used to measure ACE activity is ultra-performance liquid chromatography (UPLC). The UPLC-mass spectrometry method has been developed to determine ACE activity using HHL as the substrate and purified rabbit ACE. This method is rapid, accurate, and reproducible, and is used to determine trace amounts of compounds. In addition, this method requires a short analysis time and small reaction volume and is highly selective compared to conventional methods. It is also suitable for high-throughput screening of potential ACE inhibitors and candidate compounds isolated from herbal medicines [111].

The in vitro gastrointestinal digestion approach provides a straightforward approach to imitate peptide function by incubating the peptide with ACE before in vivo oral administration. Oral administration of ACE inhibitory peptides in hypertensive patients requires these peptides to pass through the digestive tract and be absorbed through the intestinal epithelium. Pepsin is widely used to represent gastrointestinal enzymes that function at acidic pH. Polypeptides are further truncated by pancreatic proteases, including trypsin, α-chymotrypsin, elastase, and carboxypeptidases A and B at alkaline pH. In vivo testing of peptides is frequently performed in spontaneously hypertensive rats as they mimic hypertension in humans. This animal model has been used to evaluate the effects of both short-and long-term administration of antihypertensive peptides. In human studies, food-derived peptides have been used to establish whether peptides exhibit an antihypertensive effect in humans with high-to-normal blood pressure. For example, the antihypertensive effect of the peptides IPP and VPP isolated from the commercial fermented milk show antihypertensive effects after long-term administration. The sour milk product Calpis from Japan has been examined in mildly hypertensive patients [112]. In some cases, ACE inhibitory peptides fail to show hypotensive activity after oral administration in vivo, possibly because of the hydrolysis of these peptides by ACE or gastrointestinal proteases [74,113]. It is difficult to evaluate a direct correlation between in vitro ACE inhibitory activity and in vivo antihypertensive activity because the bioavailability of these peptides after oral administration varies. ACE inhibitory peptides must remain active during gastrointestinal digestion and reach the specific organ. However, it is possible that ACE inhibitory peptides are degraded before reaching the specific organ. The antihypertensive mechanism of ACE inhibitory peptides, rather than the ACE inhibition mechanism, may be of greater interest [77,114].

In silico methods are used to predict the structure of ACE inhibitory peptides based on similarity between sequences available in databases. The molecular docking approach is widely used to predict and characterize the binding site of target proteins according to ligand conformation and binding affinity score [115]. The most convenient approach to elucidate the accuracy of molecular docking is to determine the distance of binding conformation using the scoring function in the docking program [116]. Several scoring functions are used to evaluate the docking procedure, such as CDocker Energy, CDocker Interaction Energy, LibDockScore, PLP1, PLP2, LigScore1, LigScore2, Jain, PMF, and PMFO4. Besides, BIOPEP-UWM and BLAST database is increasingly popular to be in silico approaches for investigating biological activities from tilapia and chickpea [117]. BIOPEP-UWM database is used to predict bioactive peptides composed in protein sequences. This method has benefits such as time and cost reduction, as well as being a rapid method to identify and characterize proteins. Briefly, the bioactivities, sequences, number, and location of the peptides were obtained from the sequences of the identified proteins analyzed using the "profiles of potential bioactivity" tool. Moreover, the sequences of the identified proteins were examined using the "enzyme action" tool to simulate enzymatic hydrolysis [118]. Knowing the position of the binding site before docking significantly increases the docking efficiency. Moreover, knowledge of the structure and activity relationship is important to explore potential ACE inhibitory peptides. The ACE structure contains a Zn site, which usually coordinates with oxygen, nitrogen, and sulphur donors of Asp, Cys, and His, respectively, wherein His is the most regularly encountered in the sphere of Zn^{2+} ion. The other Zn ligand in catalytic sites is water; it is activated for polarization, ionization, and arrangement of ligands in coordination with Zn [11]. The Zn^{2+} ion is also important for the binding strength between ACE and its inhibitors [119]. Generally, ACE inhibitors contain one or more molecular functionalities, such as Zn-binding ligand, a hydrogen bond donor, and a carboxyl-terminal group [120]. The ability of a protein to interact with small molecules plays a major role in the dynamics of that protein, which may enhance or inhibit its biological function. Studies on the catalytic mechanism of ACE have revealed that the 19 amino acid residues in the active site of ACE, including His353, Ala354, Ser355, Ala356, His383, Glu384, His387, Phe391, Pro407, His410, Glu411, Phe512, His513, Ser516, Ser517, Val518, Pro519, Arg522, and Tyr523, bind to small molecules or to protein (ligand).

5. Conclusions

Bioactive peptides derived from marine resources have potential ACE inhibitory activity and are considered as therapeutic agents to combat hypertension. The main characteristic of ACE inhibitory peptides is the position of the hydrophobic residue, usually Pro, at the C-terminus. In vitro and in vivo testing are the most challenging tasks in antihypertensive research as their results do not always show direct correlation, although gastrointestinal digestion is suggested to mimic peptide release in human body. Marine organisms represent sustainable sources of ACE inhibitory peptides for the production of pharmaceuticals and nutraceuticals at an industrial scale. Due to the importance of pure peptide inhibiting ACE for future pharmaceutical and nutraceutical industry, the purification techniques of identified peptide is highly crucial. Therefore, upscaling research on bioactive peptide purification should trigger biotechnologists to perform the research.

Highlights:

- Angiotensin I-converting enzyme (ACE) is a key target for treating hypertension.
- Food-derived bioactive peptides inhibit ACE activity, decreasing blood pressure.
- These peptides improve bodily functions and human health, without adverse effects.
- Marine organisms are sustainable sources of ACE inhibitory peptides.
- Various methods for their industrial production and testing are available.

Author Contributions: Conceptualization, writing original draft preparation, D.Y.P.; English editing, M.N.G.A. and J.-L.H.; project administration, M.A.A.; supervision J.-L.H., review, editing, read and approve the final manuscript, ALL.

Funding: This work was financially supported by Tahir Professorship Endowment for funding the publication fee.

Acknowledgments: We gratefully acknowledge to Scientific Publication and Journal Development Center (PPJPI) Universitas Airlangga for English proofreading and Department of Biological Science and Technology, NPUST, Taiwan for supporting this work.

Conflicts of Interest: The authors declare no conflict of interest.

References

1. World Health Organization. World Health Day 2013. *Glob. Brief Hypertens.* **2013**, 9–11.
2. Ferreira-Santos, P.; Carrón, R.; Recio, I.; Sevilla, M.Á.; Montero, M.J. Effects of milk casein hydrolyzate supplemented with phytosterols on hypertension and lipid profile in hypercholesterolemic hypertensive rats. *J. Funct. Foods* **2017**, *28*, 168–176. [CrossRef]
3. Volpe, M.; Battistoni, A.; Chin, D.; Rubattu, S.D.; Tocci, G. Renin as a biomarker of cardiovascular disease in clinical practice. *Nutr. Metab. Cardiovasc. Dis.* **2012**, *22*, 312–317. [CrossRef]
4. Meng, Q.C.; Oparil, S. Purification and assay methods for angiotensin-converting enzyme. *J. Chromatogr. A* **1996**, *743*, 105–122. [CrossRef]
5. Bhullar, K.S.; Lassalle-Claux, G.; Touaibia, M.; Rupasinghe, H.V. Antihypertensive effect of caffeic acid and its analogs through dual renin–angiotensin–aldosterone system inhibition. *Eur. J. Pharmacol.* **2014**, *730*, 125–132. [CrossRef]
6. Guang, C.; Phillips, R.D.; Jiang, B.; Milani, F. Three key proteases–angiotensin-I-converting enzyme (ACE), ACE2 and renin–within and beyond the renin-angiotensin system. *Arch. Cardiovasc. Dis.* **2012**, *105*, 373–385. [CrossRef]

7. Lee, S.-H.; Qian, Z.-J.; Kim, S.-K. A novel angiotensin I converting enzyme inhibitory peptide from tuna frame protein hydrolysate and its antihypertensive effect in spontaneously hypertensive rats. *Food Chem.* **2010**, *118*, 96–102. [CrossRef]
8. Shahidi, F.; Zhong, Y. Bioactive Peptides. *J. AOAC Int.* **2008**, *91*, 914–931.
9. Bougatef, A.; Nedjar-Arroume, N.; Ravallec-Plé, R.; Leroy, Y.; Guillochon, D.; Barkia, A.; Nasri, M. Angiotensin I-converting enzyme (ACE) inhibitory activities of sardinelle (Sardinella aurita) by-products protein hydrolysates obtained by treatment with microbial and visceral fish serine proteases. *Food Chem.* **2008**, *111*, 350–356. [CrossRef]
10. Chen, J.; Wang, Y.; Zhong, Q.; Wu, Y.; Xia, W. Purification and characterization of a novel angiotensin-I converting enzyme (ACE) inhibitory peptide derived from enzymatic hydrolysate of grass carp protein. *Peptides* **2012**, *33*, 52–58. [CrossRef]
11. Spyroulias, G.; Galanis, A.; Pairas, G.; Manessi-Zoupa, E.; Cordopatis, P. Structural Features of Angiotensin-I Converting Enzyme Catalytic Sites: Conformational Studies in Solution, Homology Models and Comparison with Other Zinc Metallopeptidases. *Curr. Top. Med. Chem.* **2004**, *4*, 403–429. [CrossRef]
12. Lee, J.K.; Hong, S.; Jeon, J.-K.; Kim, S.-K.; Byun, H.-G. Purification and characterization of angiotensin I converting enzyme inhibitory peptides from the rotifer, Brachionus rotundiformis. *Bioresour. Technol.* **2009**, *100*, 5255–5259. [CrossRef]
13. Udenigwe, C.C. Bioinformatics approaches, prospects and challenges of food bioactive peptide research. *Trends Food Sci. Technol.* **2014**, *36*, 137–143. [CrossRef]
14. Möller, N.P.; Scholz-Ahrens, K.E.; Roos, N.; Schrezenmeir, J. Bioactive peptides and proteins from foods: Indication for health effects. *Eur. J. Nutr.* **2008**, *47*, 171–182. [CrossRef]
15. Li, G.-H.; Le, G.-W.; Shi, Y.-H.; Shrestha, S. Angiotensin I–converting enzyme inhibitory peptides derived from food proteins and their physiological and pharmacological effects. *Nutr. Res.* **2004**, *24*, 469–486. [CrossRef]
16. Wilson, J.; Hayes, M.; Carney, B. Angiotensin-I-converting enzyme and prolyl endopeptidase inhibitory peptides from natural sources with a focus on marine processing by-products. *Food Chem.* **2011**, *129*, 235–244. [CrossRef]
17. Li, Y.; Sadiq, F.A.; Liu, T.; Chen, J.; He, G. Purification and identification of novel peptides with inhibitory effect against angiotensin I-converting enzyme and optimization of process conditions in milk fermented with the yeast Kluyveromyces marxianus. *J. Funct. Foods* **2015**, *16*, 278–288. [CrossRef]
18. Yu, Y.; Hu, J.; Miyaguchi, Y.; Bai, X.; Du, Y.; Lin, B. Isolation and characterization of angiotensin I-converting enzyme inhibitory peptides derived from porcine hemoglobin. *Peptides* **2006**, *27*, 2950–2956. [CrossRef]
19. Chen, Y.; Wang, Z.; Chen, X.; Liu, Y.; Zhang, H.; Sun, T. Identification of angiotensin I-converting enzyme inhibitory peptides from koumiss, a traditional fermented mare's milk. *J. Dairy Sci.* **2010**, *93*, 884–892. [CrossRef]
20. Yang, Y.; Tao, G.; Liu, P.; Liu, J. Peptide with Angiotensin I-Converting Enzyme Inhibitory Activity from Hydrolyzed Corn Gluten Meal. *J. Agric. Food Chem.* **2007**, *55*, 7891–7895. [CrossRef]
21. Suh, H.J.; Whang, J.H.; Kim, Y.S.; Bae, S.H.; Noh, D.O. Preparation od angiotensin I converting enzyme inhibitor from corn gluten. *Process Biochem.* **2003**, *38*, 1239–1244. [CrossRef]
22. Huang, Q.; Li, S.-G.; Teng, H.; Jin, Y.-G.; Ma, M.-H.; Song, H.-B. Optimizing preparation conditions for Angiotensin-I-converting enzyme inhibitory peptides derived from enzymatic hydrolysates of ovalbumin. *Food Sci. Biotechnol.* **2015**, *24*, 2193–2198. [CrossRef]
23. Zhang, Y.; Pechan, T.; Chang, S.K. Antioxidant and angiotensin-I converting enzyme inhibitory activities of phenolic extracts and fractions derived from three phenolic-rich legume varieties. *J. Funct. Foods* **2018**, *42*, 289–297. [CrossRef]
24. Boschin, G.; Scigliuolo, G.M.; Resta, D.; Arnoldi, A. ACE-inhibitory activity of enzymatic protein hydrolysates from lupin and other legumes. *Food Chem.* **2014**, *145*, 34–40. [CrossRef]
25. Pujiastuti, D.Y.; Shih, Y.-H.; Chen, W.-L.; Hsu, J.-L. Screening of angiotensin-I converting enzyme inhibitory peptides derived from soft-shelled turtle yolk using two orthogonal bioassay-guided fractionations. *J. Funct. Foods* **2017**, *28*, 36–47. [CrossRef]
26. Rawendra, R.D.; Chang, C.-I.; Chen, H.-H.; Huang, T.-C.; Hsu, J.-L. A novel angiotensin converting enzyme inhibitory peptide derived from proteolytic digest of Chinese soft-shelled turtle egg white proteins. *J. Proteom.* **2013**, *94*, 359–369. [CrossRef]

27. Priyanto, A.D.; Doerksen, R.J.; Chang, C.-I.; Sung, W.-C.; Widjanarko, S.B.; Kusnadi, J.; Lin, Y.-C.; Wang, T.-C.; Hsu, J.-L. Screening, discovery, and characterization of angiotensin-I converting enzyme inhibitory peptides derived from proteolytic hydrolysate of bitter melon seed proteins. *J. Proteom.* **2015**, *128*, 424–435. [CrossRef]
28. Lu, Y.; Govindasamy-Lucey, S.; Lucey, J.A. Angiotensin-I-converting enzyme-inhibitory peptides in commercial Wisconsin Cheddar cheeses of different ages. *J. Dairy Sci.* **2016**, *99*, 41–52. [CrossRef]
29. Sieber, R.; Bütikofer, U.; Egger, C.; Portmann, R.; Walther, B.; Wechsler, D. ACE-inhibitory activity and ACE-inhibiting peptides in different cheese varieties. *Dairy Sci. Technol.* **2010**, *90*, 47–73. [CrossRef]
30. Majumder, K.; Chakrabarti, S.; Morton, J.S.; Panahi, S.; Kaufman, S.; Davidge, S.T.; Wu, J. Egg-derived ACE-inhibitory peptides IQW and LKP reduce blood pressure in spontaneously hypertensive rats. *J. Funct. Foods* **2015**, *13*, 50–60. [CrossRef]
31. Miguel, M.; Alonso, M.J.; Salaices, M.; Aleixandre, A.; López-Fandiño, R. Antihypertensive, ACE-inhibitory and vasodilator properties of an egg white hydrolysate: Effect of a simulated intestinal digestion. *Food Chem.* **2007**, *104*, 163–168. [CrossRef]
32. Yoshii, H.; Tachi, N.; Ohba, R.; Sakamura, O.; Takeyama, H.; Itani, T. Antihypertensive effect of ACE inhibitory oligopeptides from chicken egg yolks. *Comp. Biochem. Physiol. Part C Toxicol. Pharmacol.* **2001**, *128*, 27–33. [CrossRef]
33. Yu, Z.; Liu, B.; Zhao, W.; Yin, Y.; Liu, J.; Chen, F. Primary and secondary structure of novel ACE-inhibitory peptides from egg white protein. *Food Chem.* **2012**, *133*, 315–322. [CrossRef] [PubMed]
34. Jiang, Z.; Wang, L.; Che, H.; Tian, B. Effects of temperature and pH on angiotensin-I-converting enzyme inhibitory activity and physicochemical properties of bovine casein peptide in aqueous Maillard reaction system. *LWT* **2014**, *59*, 35–42. [CrossRef]
35. Lin, K.; Zhang, L.-W.; Han, X.; Cheng, D.-Y. Novel angiotensin I-converting enzyme inhibitory peptides from protease hydrolysates of Qula casein: Quantitative structure-activity relationship modeling and molecular docking study. *J. Funct. Foods* **2017**, *32*, 266–277. [CrossRef]
36. Yamada, A.; Sakurai, T.; Ochi, D.; Mitsuyama, E.; Yamauchi, K.; Abe, F. Novel angiotensin I-converting enzyme inhibitory peptide derived from bovine casein. *Food Chem.* **2013**, *141*, 3781–3789. [CrossRef] [PubMed]
37. Hayes, M.; Mora, L.; Hussey, K.; Aluko, R.E.; Soler, L.M. Boarfish protein recovery using the pH-shift process and generation of protein hydrolysates with ACE-I and antihypertensive bioactivities in spontaneously hypertensive rats. *Innov. Food Sci. Emerg. Technol.* **2016**, *37*, 253–260. [CrossRef]
38. Itou, K.; Akahane, Y. Antihypertensive effect of heshiko, a fermented mackerel product, on spontaneously hypertensive rats. *Fish. Sci.* **2004**, *70*, 1121–1129. [CrossRef]
39. Neves, A.C.; Harnedy, P.A.; O'Keeffe, M.B.; Fitzgerald, R.J. Bioactive peptides from Atlantic salmon (Salmo salar) with angiotensin converting enzyme and dipeptidyl peptidase IV inhibitory, and antioxidant activities. *Food Chem.* **2017**, *218*, 396–405. [CrossRef] [PubMed]
40. Suetsuna, K.; Chen, J.-R. Identification of Antihypertensive Peptides from Peptic Digest of Two Microalgae, Chlorella vulgaris and Spirulina platensis. *Mar. Biotechnol.* **2001**, *3*, 305–309. [CrossRef] [PubMed]
41. Suetsuna, K.; Maekawa, K.; Chen, J.-R. Antihypertensive effects of Undaria pinnatifida (wakame) peptide on blood pressure in spontaneously hypertensive rats. *J. Nutr. Biochem.* **2004**, *15*, 267–272. [CrossRef] [PubMed]
42. Aneiros, A.; Garateix, A. Bioactive peptides from marine sources: Pharmacological properties and isolation procedures. *J. Chromatogr. B* **2004**, *803*, 41–53. [CrossRef] [PubMed]
43. Suleria, H.A.R.; Gobe, G.; Masci, P.; Osborne, S.A. Marine bioactive compounds and health promoting perspectives; innovation pathways for drug discovery. *Trends Food Sci. Technol.* **2016**, *50*, 44–55. [CrossRef]
44. Yasuhara-Bell, J.; Lu, Y. Marine compounds and their antiviral activities. *Antivir. Res.* **2010**, *86*, 231–240. [CrossRef] [PubMed]
45. Harnedy, P.A.; Fitzgerald, R.J. Bioactive peptides from marine processing waste and shellfish: A review. *J. Funct. Foods* **2012**, *4*, 6–24. [CrossRef]
46. Ryan, J.T.; Ross, R.P.; Bolton, D.; Fitzgerald, G.F.; Stanton, C. Bioactive Peptides from Muscle Sources: Meat and Fish. *Nutrients* **2011**, *3*, 765–791. [CrossRef]
47. Ngo, D.-H.; Ryu, B.; Kim, S.-K. Active peptides from skate (Okamejei kenojei) skin gelatin diminish angiotensin-I converting enzyme activity and intracellular free radical-mediated oxidation. *Food Chem.* **2014**, *143*, 246–255. [CrossRef]

48. Martins, A.; Vieira, H.M.; Gaspar, H.; Santos, S. Marketed Marine Natural Products in the Pharmaceutical and Cosmeceutical Industries: Tips for Success. *Mar. Drugs* **2014**, *12*, 1066–1101. [CrossRef]
49. Ni, H.; Li, L.; Liu, G.; Hu, S.-Q. Inhibition Mechanism and Model of an Angiotensin I-Converting Enzyme (ACE)-Inhibitory Hexapeptide from Yeast (Saccharomyces cerevisiae). *PLoS ONE* **2012**, *7*, e37077. [CrossRef]
50. Shi, L.; Mao, C.; Xu, Z.; Zhang, L. Angiotensin-converting enzymes and drug discovery in cardiovascular diseases. *Drug Discov. Today* **2010**, *15*, 332–341. [CrossRef]
51. Gavras, H. Angiotensin converting enzyme inhibition and its impact on cardiovascular disease. *Circulation* **1990**, *81*, 381–388. [CrossRef] [PubMed]
52. Wijesekara, I.; Kim, S.-K. Angiotensin-I-Converting Enzyme (ACE) Inhibitors from Marine Resources: Prospects in the Pharmaceutical Industry. *Mar. Drugs* **2010**, *8*, 1080–1093. [CrossRef] [PubMed]
53. Wijesinghe, W.A.J.P.; Ko, S.C.; Jeon, Y.J. Effect of phlorotannins isolated from Ecklonia cava on angiotensin I-converting enzyme (ACE) inhibitory activity. *Nutr. Res. Pract.* **2011**, *5*, 93–100. [CrossRef] [PubMed]
54. Wu, H.; He, H.-L.; Chen, X.-L.; Sun, C.-Y.; Zhang, Y.-Z.; Zhou, B.-C. Purification and identification of novel angiotensin-I-converting enzyme inhibitory peptides from shark meat hydrolysate. *Process Biochem.* **2008**, *43*, 457–461. [CrossRef]
55. Byun, H.-G.; Kim, S.-K. Purification and characterization of angiotensin I converting enzyme (ACE) inhibitory peptides from Alaska pollack (Theragra chalcogramma) skin. *Process Biochem.* **2001**, *36*, 1155–1162. [CrossRef]
56. Wang, Y.-K.; He, H.-L.; Chen, X.-L.; Sun, C.-Y.; Zhang, Y.-Z.; Zhou, B.-C. Production of novel angiotensin I-converting enzyme inhibitory peptides by fermentation of marine shrimp Acetes chinensis with Lactobacillus fermentum SM 605. *Appl. Microbiol. Biotechnol.* **2008**, *79*, 785–791. [CrossRef]
57. Ono, S.; Hosokawa, M.; Miyashita, K.; Takahashi, K. Inhibition properties of dipeptides from salmon muscle hydrolysate on angiotensin I-converting enzyme. *Int. J. Food Sci. Technol.* **2006**, *41*, 383–386. [CrossRef]
58. Liu, J.; Yu, Z.; Zhao, W.; Lin, S.; Wang, E.; Zhang, Y.; Hao, H.; Wang, Z.; Chen, F. Isolation and identification of angiotensin-converting enzyme inhibitory peptides from egg white protein hydrolysates. *Food Chem.* **2010**, *122*, 1159–1163. [CrossRef]
59. Wu, J.; Aluko, R.E.; Nakai, S. Structural Requirements of Angiotensin I-Converting Enzyme Inhibitory Peptides: Quantitative Structure–Activity Relationship Study of Di- and Tripeptides. *J. Agric. Food Chem.* **2006**, *54*, 732–738. [CrossRef]
60. Robert, M.-C.; Razaname, A.; Mutter, M.; Juillerat, M.A. Identification of Angiotensin-I-Converting Enzyme Inhibitory Peptides Derived from Sodium Caseinate Hydrolysates Produced byLactobacillus helveticusNCC 2765. *J. Agric. Food Chem.* **2004**, *52*, 6923–6931. [CrossRef]
61. Saito, T.; Nakamura, T.; Kitazawa, H.; Kawai, Y.; Itoh, T. Isolation and Structural Analysis of Antihypertensive Peptides That Exist Naturally in Gouda Cheese. *J. Dairy Sci.* **2000**, *83*, 1434–1440. [CrossRef]
62. Fahmi, A.; Morimura, S.; Guo, H.; Shigematsu, T.; Kida, K.; Uemura, Y. Production of angiotensin I converting enzyme inhibitory peptides from sea bream scales. *Process Biochem.* **2004**, *39*, 1195–1200. [CrossRef]
63. Lan, X.; Liao, D.; Wu, S.; Wang, F.; Sun, J.; Tong, Z.; Wu, S. Rapid purification and characterization of angiotensin converting enzyme inhibitory peptides from lizard fish protein hydrolysates with magnetic affinity separation. *Food Chem.* **2015**, *182*, 136–142. [CrossRef] [PubMed]
64. Wu, S.; Feng, X.; Lan, X.; Xu, Y.; Liao, D. Purification and identification of Angiotensin-I Converting Enzyme (ACE) inhibitory peptide from lizard fish (Saurida elongata) hydrolysate. *J. Funct. Foods* **2015**, *13*, 295–299. [CrossRef]
65. Gu, R.-Z.; Li, C.-Y.; Liu, W.-Y.; Yi, W.-X.; Cai, M.-Y. Angiotensin I-converting enzyme inhibitory activity of low-molecular-weight peptides from Atlantic salmon (*Salmo salar* L.) skin. *Food Res. Int.* **2011**, *44*, 1536–1540. [CrossRef]
66. Intarasirisawat, R.; Benjakul, S.; Wu, J.; Visessanguan, W. Isolation of antioxidative and ACE inhibitory peptides from protein hydrolysate of skipjack (Katsuwana pelamis) roe. *J. Funct. Foods* **2013**, *5*, 1854–1862. [CrossRef]
67. Jung, W.-K.; Mendis, E.; Je, J.-Y.; Park, P.-J.; Son, B.W.; Kim, H.C.; Choi, Y.K.; Kim, S.-K. Angiotensin I-converting enzyme inhibitory peptide from yellowfin sole (Limanda aspera) frame protein and its antihypertensive effect in spontaneously hypertensive rats. *Food Chem.* **2006**, *94*, 26–32. [CrossRef]
68. Ngo, D.-H.; Vo, T.-S.; Ryu, B.; Kim, S.-K. Angiotensin-I-converting enzyme (ACE) inhibitory peptides from Pacific cod skin gelatin using ultrafiltration membranes. *Process Biochem.* **2016**, *51*, 1622–1628. [CrossRef]

69. Ko, J.-Y.; Kang, N.; Lee, J.-H.; Kim, J.-S.; Kim, W.-S.; Park, S.-J.; Kim, Y.-T.; Jeon, Y.-J. Angiotensin I-converting enzyme inhibitory peptides from an enzymatic hydrolysate of flounder fish (Paralichthys olivaceus) muscle as a potent anti-hypertensive agent. *Process Biochem.* **2016**, *51*, 535–541. [CrossRef]
70. Ghassem, M.; Arihara, K.; Babji, A.S.; Said, M.; Ibrahim, S. Purification and identification of ACE inhibitory peptides from Haruan (Channa striatus) myofibrillar protein hydrolysate using HPLC–ESI-TOF MS/MS. *Food Chem.* **2011**, *129*, 1770–1777. [CrossRef]
71. Ko, S.-C.; Kang, N.; Kim, E.-A.; Kang, M.C.; Lee, S.-H.; Kang, S.-M.; Lee, J.-B.; Jeon, B.-T.; Kim, S.-K.; Park, S.-J.; et al. A novel angiotensin I-converting enzyme (ACE) inhibitory peptide from a marine Chlorella ellipsoidea and its antihypertensive effect in spontaneously hypertensive rats. *Process Biochem.* **2012**, *47*, 2005–2011. [CrossRef]
72. Zhao, Y.; Li, B.; Dong, S.; Liu, Z.; Zhao, X.; Wang, J.; Zeng, M. A novel ACE inhibitory peptide isolated from Acaudina molpadioidea hydrolysate. *Peptides* **2009**, *30*, 1028–1033. [CrossRef] [PubMed]
73. Balti, R.; Nedjar-Arroume, N.; Bougatef, A.; Guillochon, D.; Nasri, M. Three novel angiotensin I-converting enzyme (ACE) inhibitory peptides from cuttlefish (Sepia officinalis) using digestive proteases. *Food Res. Int.* **2010**, *43*, 1136–1143. [CrossRef]
74. Balti, R.; Bougatef, A.; Sila, A.; Guillochon, D.; Dhulster, P.; Nedjar-Arroume, N. Nine novel angiotensin I-converting enzyme (ACE) inhibitory peptides from cuttlefish (Sepia officinalis) muscle protein hydrolysates and antihypertensive effect of the potent active peptide in spontaneously hypertensive rats. *Food Chem.* **2015**, *170*, 519–525. [CrossRef]
75. Alemán, A.; Gómez-Guillén, M.C.; Montero, P. Identification of ace-inhibitory peptides from squid skin collagen after in vitro gastrointestinal digestion. *Food Res. Int.* **2013**, *54*, 790–795. [CrossRef]
76. Tsai, J.; Lin, T.; Chen, J.; Pan, B. The inhibitory effects of freshwater clam (Corbicula fluminea, Muller) muscle protein hydrolysates on angiotensin I converting enzyme. *Process Biochem.* **2006**, *41*, 2276–2281. [CrossRef]
77. Jao, C.-L.; Huang, S.-L.; Hsu, K.-C. Angiotensin I-converting enzyme inhibitory peptides: Inhibition mode, bioavailability, and antihypertensive effects. *BioMedicine* **2012**, *2*, 130–136. [CrossRef]
78. Ko, S.-C.; Jang, J.; Ye, B.-R.; Kim, M.-S.; Choi, I.-W.; Park, W.-S.; Jung, W.-K. Purification and molecular docking study of angiotensin I-converting enzyme (ACE) inhibitory peptides from hydrolysates of marine sponge Stylotella aurantium. *Process Biochem.* **2016**, *54*, 180–187. [CrossRef]
79. Wu, Q.; Jia, J.; Yan, H.; Du, J.; Gui, Z. A novel angiotensin-I converting enzyme (ACE) inhibitory peptide from gastrointestinal protease hydrolysate of silkworm pupa (Bombyx mori) protein: Biochemical characterization and molecular docking study. *Peptides* **2015**, *68*, 17–24. [CrossRef]
80. Jemil, I.; Mora, L.; Nasri, R.; Abdelhedi, O.; Aristoy, M.-C.; Hajji, M.; Nasri, M.; Toldrá, F.; Soler, L.M. A peptidomic approach for the identification of antioxidant and ACE-inhibitory peptides in sardinelle protein hydrolysates fermented by Bacillus subtilis A26 and Bacillus amyloliquefaciens An6. *Food Res. Int.* **2016**, *89*, 347–358. [CrossRef]
81. Lin, H.-C.; Alashi, A.M.; Aluko, R.E.; Pan, B.S.; Chang, Y.-W. Antihypertensive properties of tilapia (Oreochromis spp.) frame and skin enzymatic protein hydrolysates. *Food Nutr. Res.* **2017**, *61*, 1391666. [CrossRef] [PubMed]
82. Ondetti, M.A.; Cushman, D.W. Enzymes of the renin-angiotensin system and their inhibitors. *Annu. Rev. Biochem.* **1982**, *51*, 283–308. [CrossRef] [PubMed]
83. López-Fandiño, R.; Otte, J.; Van Camp, J. Physiological, chemical and technological aspects of milk-protein-derived peptides with antihypertensive and ACE-inhibitory activity. *Int. Dairy J.* **2006**, *16*, 1277–1293. [CrossRef]
84. Lassoued, I.; Mora, L.; Barkia, A.; Aristoy, M.C.; Nasri, M.; Toldrá, F. Bioactive peptides identified in thornback ray skin's gelatin hydrolysates by proteases from Bacillus subtilis and Bacillus amyloliquefaciens. *J. Proteom.* **2015**, *128*, 8–17. [CrossRef]
85. So, P.B.T.; Rubio, P.; Lirio, S.; Macabeo, A.P.; Huang, H.-Y.; Corpuz, M.J.-A.T.; Villaflores, O.B. In vitro angiotensin I converting enzyme inhibition by a peptide isolated from Chiropsalmus quadrigatus Haeckel (box jellyfish) venom hydrolysate. *Toxicon* **2016**, *119*, 77–83. [CrossRef] [PubMed]
86. Sato, M.; Hosokawa, T.; Yamaguchi, T.; Nakano, T.; Muramoto, K.; Kahara, T.; Funayama, K.; Kobayashi, A.; Nakano, T. Angiotensin I-Converting Enzyme Inhibitory Peptides Derived from Wakame (Undaria pinnatifida) and Their Antihypertensive Effect in Spontaneously Hypertensive Rats. *J. Agric. Food Chem.* **2002**, *50*, 6245–6252. [CrossRef] [PubMed]

87. Nakagomi, K.; Fujimura, A.; Ebisu, H.; Sakai, T.; Sadakane, Y.; Fujii, N.; Tanimura, T. Acein-1, a novel angiotensin-I-converting enzyme inhibitory peptide isolated from tryptic hydrolysate of human plasma. *FEBS Lett.* **1998**, *438*, 255–257. [CrossRef]
88. Fujita, H.; Yoshikawa, M. LKPNM: A prodrug-type ACE-inhibitory peptide derived from fish protein. *Immunopharmacol.* **1999**, *44*, 123–127. [CrossRef]
89. Vercruysse, L.; Van Camp, J.; Morel, N.; Rougé, P.; Herregods, G.; Smagghe, G. Ala-Val-Phe and Val-Phe: ACE inhibitory peptides derived from insect protein with antihypertensive activity in spontaneously hypertensive rats. *Peptides* **2010**, *31*, 482–488. [CrossRef]
90. Shahidi, F.; Ambigaipalan, P. Novel functional food ingredients from marine sources. *Curr. Opin. Food Sci.* **2015**, *2*, 123–129. [CrossRef]
91. Agyei, D.; Ongkudon, C.M.; Wei, C.Y.; Chan, A.S.; Danquah, M.K. Bioprocess challenges to the isolation and purification of bioactive peptides. *Food Bioprod. Process.* **2016**, *98*, 244–256. [CrossRef]
92. Sánchez-Rivera, L.; Martínez-Maqueda, D.; Cruz-Huerta, E.; Miralles, B.; Recio, I. Peptidomics for discovery, bioavailability and monitoring of dairy bioactive peptides. *Food Res. Int.* **2014**, *63*, 170–181. [CrossRef]
93. Jemil, I.; Abdelhedi, O.; Mora, L.; Nasri, R.; Aristoy, M.-C.; Jridi, M.; Hajji, M.; Toldrá, F.; Nasri, M.; Soler, L.M. Peptidomic analysis of bioactive peptides in zebra blenny (Salaria basilisca) muscle protein hydrolysate exhibiting antimicrobial activity obtained by fermentation with Bacillus mojavensis A21. *Process Biochem.* **2016**, *51*, 2186–2197. [CrossRef]
94. Sheih, I.-C.; Wu, T.-K.; Fang, T.J. Antioxidant properties of a new antioxidative peptide from algae protein waste hydrolysate in different oxidation systems. *Bioresour. Technol.* **2009**, *100*, 3419–3425. [CrossRef] [PubMed]
95. Ustyuzhanina, N.E.; Ushakova, N.A.; Zyuzina, K.A.; Bilan, M.I.; Elizarova, A.L.; Somonova, O.V.; Madzhuga, A.V.; Krylov, V.B.; Preobrazhenskaya, M.E.; Usov, A.I.; et al. Influence of Fucoidans on Hemostatic System. *Mar. Drugs* **2013**, *11*, 2444–2458. [CrossRef]
96. Korhonen, H.; Pihlanto, A. Bioactive peptides: Production and functionality. *Int. Dairy J.* **2006**, *16*, 945–960. [CrossRef]
97. Rizzello, C.G.; Tagliazucchi, D.; Babini, E.; Rutella, G.S.; Saa, D.L.T.; Gianotti, A. Bioactive peptides from vegetable food matrices: Research trends and novel biotechnologies for synthesis and recovery. *J. Funct. Foods* **2016**, *27*, 549–569. [CrossRef]
98. Sanjukta, S.; Rai, A.K. Production of bioactive peptides during soybean fermentation and their potential health benefits. *Trends Food Sci. Technol.* **2016**, *50*, 1–10. [CrossRef]
99. Kleekayai, T.; Harnedy, P.A.; O'Keeffe, M.B.; Poyarkov, A.A.; CunhaNeves, A.; Suntornsuk, W.; Fitzgerald, R.J. Extraction of antioxidant and ACE inhibitory peptides from Thai traditional fermented shrimp pastes. *Food Chem.* **2015**, *176*, 441–447. [CrossRef]
100. Cushman, D.; Cheung, H. Spectrophotometric assay and properties of the angiotensin-converting enzyme of rabbit lung. *Biochem. Pharmacol.* **1971**, *20*, 1637–1648. [CrossRef]
101. Li, G.-H.; Liu, H.; Shi, Y.-H.; Le, G.-W. Direct spectrophotometric measurement of angiotensin I-converting enzyme inhibitory activity for screening bioactive peptides. *J. Pharm. Biomed. Anal.* **2005**, *37*, 219–224. [CrossRef] [PubMed]
102. Belović, M.M.; Ilić, N.M.; Tepić, A.N.; Šumić, Z. Selection of conditions for angiotensin-converting enzyme inhibition assay: Influence of sample preparation and buffer. *Food Feed Res.* **2013**, *40*, 11–16.
103. Shalaby, S.M.; Zakora, M.; Otte, J. Performance of two commonly used angiotensin-converting enzyme inhibition assays using FA-PGG and HHL as substrates. *J. Dairy Res.* **2006**, *73*, 178–186. [CrossRef] [PubMed]
104. Murray, B.; Walsh, D.; Fitzgerald, R. Modification of the furanacryloyl-l-phenylalanylglycylglycine assay for determination of angiotensin-I-converting enzyme inhibitory activity. *J. Biochem. Biophys. Methods* **2004**, *59*, 127–137. [CrossRef] [PubMed]
105. Sentandreu, M.Á.; Toldrá, F. A rapid, simple and sensitive fluorescence method for the assay of angiotensin-I converting enzyme. *Food Chem.* **2006**, *97*, 546–554. [CrossRef]
106. Van Der Ven, C.; Gruppen, H.; De Bont, D.B.; Voragen, A.G. Optimisation of the angiotensin converting enzyme inhibition by whey protein hydrolysates using response surface methodology. *Int. Dairy J.* **2002**, *12*, 813–820. [CrossRef]

107. Vermeirssen, V.; Van Camp, J.; Verstraete, W. Optimisation and validation of an angiotensin-converting enzyme inhibition assay for the screening of bioactive peptides. *J. Biochem. Biophys. Methods* **2002**, *51*, 75–87. [CrossRef]
108. Anzenbacherová, E.; Anzenbacher, P.; Macek, K.; Květina, J. Determination of enzyme (angiotensin convertase) inhibitors based on enzymatic reaction followed by HPLC. *J. Pharm. Biomed. Anal.* **2001**, *24*, 1151–1156. [CrossRef]
109. Sentandreu, M.A.; Toldrá, F. A fluorescence-based protocol for quantifying angiotensin-converting enzyme activity. *Nat. Protoc.* **2006**, *1*, 2423–2427. [CrossRef]
110. Betancourt, L.H.; De Bock, P.-J.; Staes, A.; Timmerman, E.; Perez-Riverol, Y.; Sánchez, A.; Besada, V.; González, L.J.; Vandekerckhove, J.; Gevaert, K. SCX charge state selective separation of tryptic peptides combined with 2D-RP-HPLC allows for detailed proteome mapping. *J. Proteom.* **2013**, *91*, 164–171. [CrossRef]
111. Geng, F.; He, Y.; Yang, L.; Wang, Z. A rapid assay for angiotensin-converting enzyme activity using ultra-performance liquid chromatography-mass spectrometry. *Biomed. Chromatogr. BMC* **2010**, *24*, 312–317. [CrossRef] [PubMed]
112. Hernández-Ledesma, B.; Contreras, M.D.M.; Recio, I. Antihypertensive peptides: Production, bioavailability and incorporation into foods. *Adv. Colloid Interface Sci.* **2011**, *165*, 23–35. [CrossRef] [PubMed]
113. Wu, J.; Ding, X. Characterization of inhibition and stability of soy-protein-derived angiotensin I-converting enzyme inhibitory peptides. *Food Res. Int.* **2002**, *35*, 367–375. [CrossRef]
114. Vermeirssen, V.; Van Camp, J.; Verstraete, W. Bioavailability of angiotensin I converting enzyme inhibitory peptides. *Br. J. Nutr.* **2004**, *92*, 357–366. [CrossRef] [PubMed]
115. Meng, X.-Y.; Zhang, H.-X.; Mezei, M.; Cui, M. Molecular Docking: A Powerful Approach for Structure-Based Drug Discovery. *Curr. Comput. Drug Des.* **2011**, *7*, 146–157. [CrossRef]
116. Politi, A.; Durdagi, S.; Moutevelis-Minakakis, P.; Kokotos, G.; Mavromoustakos, T. Development of accurate binding affinity predictions of novel renin inhibitors through molecular docking studies. *J. Mol. Graph. Model.* **2010**, *29*, 425–435. [CrossRef]
117. Panjaitan, F.C.A.; Gomez, H.L.R.; Chang, Y.-W. In Silico Analysis of Bioactive Peptides Released from Giant Grouper (Epinephelus lanceolatus) Roe Proteins Identified by Proteomics Approach. *Molecules* **2018**, *23*, 2910. [CrossRef]
118. Tejano, L.A.; Peralta, J.P.; Yap, E.E.S.; Panjaitan, F.C.A.; Chang, Y.-W. Prediction of Bioactive Peptides from Chlorella sorokiniana Proteins Using Proteomic Techniques in Combination with Bioinformatics Analyses. *Int. J. Mol. Sci.* **2019**, *20*, 1786. [CrossRef]
119. Pan, D.; Guo, H.; Zhao, B.; Cao, J. The molecular mechanisms of interactions between bioactive peptides and angiotensin-converting enzyme. *Bioorganic Med. Chem. Lett.* **2011**, *21*, 3898–3904. [CrossRef]
120. Andrews, P.R.; Carson, J.M.; Caselli, A.; Spark, M.J.; Woods, R. Conformational analysis and active site modeling of angiotensin-converting enzyme inhibitors. *J. Med. Chem.* **1985**, *28*, 393–399. [CrossRef]

Sample Availability: Samples of the compounds are not available from the authors.

molecules

MDPI

Review

Carotenoids: How Effective Are They to Prevent Age-Related Diseases?

Bee Ling Tan [1] and Mohd Esa Norhaizan [1,2,3,*]

1 Department of Nutrition and Dietetics, Faculty of Medicine and Health Sciences, Universiti Putra Malaysia, Serdang 43400, Selangor, Malaysia; tbeeling87@gmail.com
2 Laboratory of Molecular Biomedicine, Institute of Bioscience, Universiti Putra Malaysia, Serdang 43400, Selangor, Malaysia
3 Research Centre of Excellent, Nutrition and Non-Communicable Diseases (NNCD), Faculty of Medicine and Health Sciences, Universiti Putra Malaysia, Serdang 43400, Selangor, Malaysia
* Correspondence: nhaizan@upm.edu.my; Tel.: +603-89472427

Received: 28 March 2019; Accepted: 6 May 2019; Published: 9 May 2019

Abstract: Despite an increase in life expectancy that indicates positive human development, a new challenge is arising. Aging is positively associated with biological and cognitive degeneration, for instance cognitive decline, psychological impairment, and physical frailty. The elderly population is prone to oxidative stress due to the inefficiency of their endogenous antioxidant systems. As many studies showed an inverse relationship between carotenoids and age-related diseases (ARD) by reducing oxidative stress through interrupting the propagation of free radicals, carotenoid has been foreseen as a potential intervention for age-associated pathologies. Therefore, the role of carotenoids that counteract oxidative stress and promote healthy aging is worthy of further discussion. In this review, we discussed the underlying mechanisms of carotenoids involved in the prevention of ARD. Collectively, understanding the role of carotenoids in ARD would provide insights into a potential intervention that may affect the aging process, and subsequently promote healthy longevity.

Keywords: aging; cancer; cardiovascular disease; dementia; diabetes; inflammation; oxidative stress

1. Introduction

The average life expectancy has been rising rapidly in recent decades, with an average of 72.0 years in 2016 globally [1]. However, the healthy life expectancy was 63.3 years in 2016 worldwide [1]. In view of the demographics of the global population from 2000 to 2050, the population aged 60 years or more is estimated to increase from 605 million to 2 billion people [2]. In many countries, the average life expectancy aged 60 years could expect to live another 20.5 years in 2016 [1]. This longevity accounts for a growing share of age-related diseases (ARD) and their consequent economic and social burden [3]. In fact, aging is positively associated with biological and cognitive degeneration including cognitive decline, psychological impairment, and physical frailty [4].

Reactive oxygen species (ROS) are continuously generated in normal aerobic metabolism as a by-product; however, when the amount is elevated under stress, it may cause potential biological damage [5]. Oxidative stress emerges from an imbalance of either pro- and/or antioxidant molecules, being characterized by the decreased capacity of endogenous systems to combat an oxidative attack and subsequently leading to molecular and cellular damage [6]. Oxidative stress has been recognized as the main contributor to the pathophysiology and pathogenesis of ARD [7] such as metabolic syndromes, atherosclerosis, osteoporosis, obesity, dementia, diabetes, cancer, and arthritis [8,9].

ARD have become the most common health threats in recent decades. ARD have been linked to structural changes in mitochondria, accompanied by an alteration of biophysical properties of the membrane such as reduced fluidity and altered electron transport chain complex activity, which in turn contribute to mitochondrial failure and energy imbalance. This perturbation impairs mitochondrial function and cellular homeostasis, and increases susceptibility to oxidative stress [10,11]. The elderly population is susceptible to oxidative stress due to the inefficiency of their endogenous antioxidant systems [12]. An irreversible progression of oxidative decay due to ROS also causes a negative impact on the biology of aging such as reducing lifespan, increasing disease incidence, and the impairment of physiological functions [13]. Several organs, for example the heart and brain, with a high consumption of oxygen and limited replication rate are vulnerable to these phenomena, suggesting the high prevalence of neurological disorders and cardiovascular disease (CVD) in elderly populations [14,15]. Increased ROS has been linked to the progression and onset of aging. Although ROS generation may not be an essential factor for aging [16], they are more likely to aggravate ARD development through interaction with mitochondria and cause oxidative damage [17]. Due to their reactivity, high levels of ROS can generate oxidative stress by interrupting the balance of prooxidant and antioxidant levels [18]. Substantial evidence highlights that carotenoids can decrease oxidative stress and the progression of ARD [19]. Lycopene, a carotenoid that is abundantly found in tomatoes, is a crucial antioxidant source. A meta-analysis study has demonstrated an inverse relationship between lycopene intake and cardiovascular disease (CVD) risk [20]. This favorable effect could be attributed to the decreased inflammatory response and cholesterol level, as well as the reduced oxidation of biomolecules [21]. Besides CVD, several studies have also found that consumption of carotenoid-rich fruits and vegetables can prevent cancers such as prostate and cervical [22–24]. As many studies show that carotenoid intake is negatively associated with ARD by disrupting the formation of free radicals and subsequently reduces oxidative stress, carotenoid has been foreseen as a promising nutritional approach for ARD. Therefore, the role of carotenoids that combat oxidative stress and promote healthy longevity is worth to discuss further. Of particular interest in this review, we discussed the underlying mechanisms of carotenoids involved in the prevention of ARD. Understanding the role of carotenoids in ARD would provide insight for potential interventions that may affect the aging process, and subsequently promoting healthy longevity.

2. Carotenoids

Carotenoids are a family of naturally occurring organic pigmented compounds that are produced by the fungi, several bacteria, and plastids of algae and plants [25]. Notably, red pea aphid (*Acyrthosiphon pisum*) and spider mite (*Tetranychus urticae*) are the only animals that produce carotenoids from fungi through gene transfer [26]. In plants, carotenoids contribute to the photosynthetic machinery and protect them from photo-damage [27]. They occur in all organisms capable of photosynthesis, a process to convert into chemical energy in the presence of sunlight. Generally, carotenoids absorb wavelengths between 400 and 550 nanometers, and hence the compounds are present in red, orange, or yellow color [28].

Nearly 600 carotenoids have been identified in nature to modulate a broad spectrum of functions [29]. However, only about 50 carotenoids are found in a typical human diet [30], while about 20 carotenoids are present in human tissues and blood [31]. Carotenoids are classified into two groups, namely xanthophylls and carotenes, according to their chemical constituents [32]. Oxygenated derivatives are known as xanthophylls; while hydrocarbon only carotenoids (lycopene, β-carotene, and α-carotene) are called carotenes. Additionally, aldehyde groups (β-citraurin), epoxide groups (neoxanthin, antheraxanthin, and violaxanthin), oxo/keto groups (canthaxanthin and echinenone), and oxygen substituents (zeaxanthin and lutein) are categorized as complex xanthophylls [33].

3. Chemical Structures

In particular, most of the carotenoids are tetraterpenoids, containing 40 carbon atoms and derived from eight isoprene molecules [34]. All carotenoids have a polyisoprenoid structure, accompanied by a long-conjugated chain adjacent with multiple double bonds and symmetry on the central double bonds. The molecular structures of carotenes and xanthophylls are shown in Figures 1 and 2, respectively.

Alteration of the basic acyclic structure acquired oxygen-rich functional groups [35]. One of the features of carotenoid is a strong coloration, which is a consequence of light absorption in the presence of a conjugated chain [36]. Due to the presence of the electron-rich conjugated system of the polyene structure, carotenoids scavenge the free radicals by trapping peroxyl radicals and quenching the singlet oxygen [37]. Indeed, the conjugated double bond is critical for the proper functioning of carotenoids, for example in light absorption for photosynthetic organisms [36].

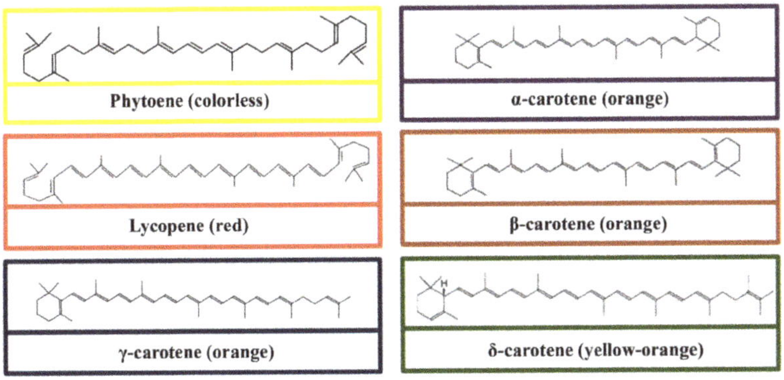

Figure 1. Molecular structures of carotenes (Phytoene, lycopene, γ-carotene, α-carotene, β-carotene, and δ-carotene).

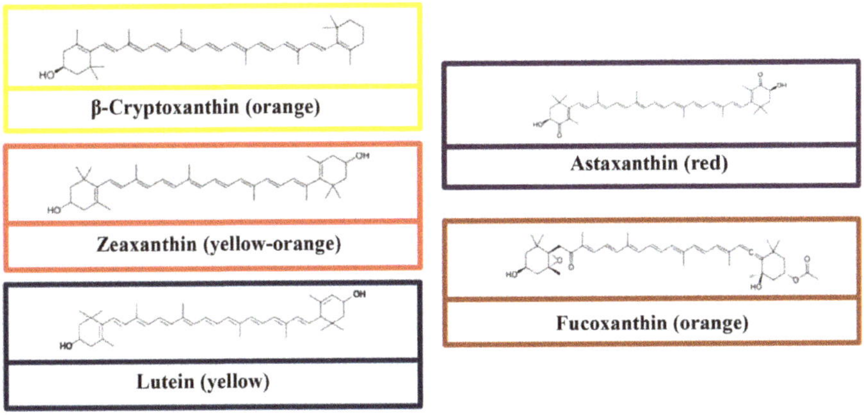

Figure 2. Molecular structures of some common xanthophylls (β-cryptoxanthin, zeaxanthin, lutein, astaxanthin, and fucoxanthin).

4. Dietary Sources

Carotenoids are abundantly found in deeply pigmented fruits and vegetables (Table 1), in which the orange-yellow vegetables and fruits are rich in β-carotene and α-carotene. While, α-cryptoxanthin, lycopene, and lutein are found in orange fruits, tomatoes and tomato products, and dark green vegetables, respectively [38]. Egg yolk is a highly bioavailable source of zeaxanthin and lutein [39]. The unsaturated nature of the carotenoids makes them prone to oxidation [40]. Other factors like pH, light, and temperature can also affect the color and nutritional value of foods [41]. Some common household cooking methods, for example boiling, steaming, and microwave cooking, do not markedly change the extent of the carotenoid content in food [42]. However, extreme heat can cause oxidative damage to carotenoids [42].

Table 1. Carotenoids content in some common foods.

Food Source	Carotenoids (µg/100 g)							References
	Lutein	Zeaxanthin	Lutein and Zeaxanthin	Lycopene	α-Carotene	β-Carotene	β-Cryptoxanthin	
Apples (with skin)	100–840				30			[40,43,44]
Apricot, raw	0–141			0.5	0–37	140–6939	28–231	[45]
Asparagus, raw	610–750				12	493		[40,44,46]
Avocados			270		28	53	36	[40,47]
Basil, raw			7050					[48]
Blackberry	270				9	100		[49]
Blueberry	230					49		[49]
Broccoli, raw	830–4300				1	414–2760		[45]
Brussels sprouts, boiled			1541					[45,47]
Carrot, raw	110–2097				530–35,833	1161–64,350		
Corn, cooked	202	202						[50]
Cress, raw	7540							[51]
Frozen corn, boiled from frozen			684					[47]
Cucumbers (with skin)	160					138		[40,44,46]
Egg whole, cooked	237	216	353					[47,50]
Egg yolk, cooked	645	587						[50]
Egg whole, raw	288	279	504					[47,50]
Egg yolk, raw	787	762	1094					[47,50]
Frozen green beans, cooked			564					[47]
Jackfruit				37–111		40–772		[52]
Kale, cooked			18,246					[47]
Leek, raw			3680					[48]
Lettuce, raw	1000–4780							[48]
Mango	100					300–4200	0–1640	[40,45]
Melon, cantaloupe					27	1595	0	[40]
Orange juice	67				8	13	34	[40,53]
Orange	64–350		129		0–400	0–500	14–1395	[40,45,47]
Orange pepper, raw		1665						[50]
Papaya	20–820			2080–4750	0–60	71–1210	60–1483	[40,45]
Parsley, raw	4326		5562					[47,50]
Peas, green, boiled			2593					[47]
Pepper, bell, green, raw	340–660				22	198	1	[54]
Pineapple						171–476		[40]
Pistachio nuts, raw			1404					[47]
Pumpkin, cooked			1014					[47]
Spinach, raw	2047–20,300		12,197			840–24,070		[40,47]
Sweet potatoes, white flesh (cooked)						25–157		[55]

Table 1. *Cont.*

Food Source	Carotenoids (μg/100 g)							
	Lutein	Zeaxanthin	Lutein and Zeaxanthin	Lycopene	α-Carotene	β-Carotene	β-Cryptoxanthin	References
Squash, boiled			2249					[47]
Strawberry	6–21					5		[40,43]
Tomato, raw	40–1300			21–62,273		36–2232		[45]
Watermelon	0–40			2300–7200	0–1	44–324	62–457	[45]

5. Metabolism and Bioavailability

There are several factors that affect the carotenoid absorption, bioavailability, breakdown, transport, and storage. For example, the dietary intake of fat (in the form of salad dressing, cooking oil for instance extra virgin olive oil or whole egg) at the same meal with carotenoid consumption (cooked vegetables or raw vegetable salad) has been found to effectively increase the absorption of some carotenoids [56–59]. The bioavailability of carotenoids may reduce when consumed within the same meal due to the competition between carotenoids during absorption [60]. In addition, dietary fiber from plant sources, for example guar gum and pectin, were found to decrease carotenoid absorption [61], and the localization of carotenoids with the chromoplasts and chloroplasts of plants may reduce the bioavailability [62]. A study reported by Hornero-Mendez and Mínguez-Mosquera [63] evaluated the impact of cooking on carotenoids in the plant. The data showed that although heat reduces the carotenoid content, the bioavailability of the carotenoids was enhanced compared to the control (uncooked) [63]. Furthermore, Baskaran et al. [64] evaluated the micellar phospholipid in relation to the intestinal uptake of carotenoids in in vivo study. The data showed that phosphatidylcholine suppressed the accumulation of lutein and β-carotene in plasma and liver, suggesting the phospholipids derived from food and bile could influence the cellular uptake of carotenoids solubilized in mixed micelles formed in the intestinal tract. In addition, the rate of bioaccessibility of carotenoids is highly affected by the food matrix. The previous study revealed that in vitro transfer rate of β-cryptoxanthin, zeaxanthin, and lutein is nearly 100% from fruits such as sweet potato, grapefruit, kiwi, and orange compared to the vegetables such as spinach and broccoli, which is between 19 to 38% [65]. This observation indicates that the release of carotenoids from a food matrix followed by absorption is a determining factor for delivering potential health benefits.

The release of carotenoids from the food matrix is highly dependent on their state, as well as their associations with other food components such as protein [66]. As an example, the microcrystalline form of carotenoids, for instance lycopene in tomato and β-carotene in carrot, reduces their bioavailability compared to those that are immersed entirely in lipid droplets [36]. The bioavailability of carotenoids is markedly varied in food. The previous data stated that nearly 5% of carotenoids (whole, raw vegetables) are absorbed by the intestine whereas up to 50% of the carotenoid is absorbed from the micellar solutions [67]. This finding implies that the physical form of carotenoids present in intestinal mucosal cells is vitally important. Many studies have revealed that thermal treatment increases the bioaccessibility of carotenoids and improves their absorption due to the bond loosening and disruption of cell walls [68]. They are absorbed into gastrointestinal mucosal cells and remain unchanged in the tissues and circulations [69,70]. In the intestine, carotenoids are absorbed via passive diffusion after being incorporated into the micelles formed by the bile acid and dietary fat. Subsequently, these micellular carotenoids are incorporated into the chylomicrons and released into the lymphatic system. Ultimately, they bind with the lipoprotein at the liver and are released into the bloodstream [71]. Carotenoids are predominantly accumulated in adipose tissue and the liver; whereas in brain stem tissue, the carotenoid concentration is below the detection limit [72,73]. Other factors such as gender, aging, nutritional status, genetic factor, and infection may also influence the bioavailability of carotenoids [74,75]. It has been demonstrated that any disease with an abnormal absorption of fat from the digestive tract markedly alters the incorporation of carotenoids. Additionally, interaction with drugs such as aspirin and sulphonamides has been found to reduce the bioavailability of β-carotene [74].

6. Physiological Changes in Aging

Aging is characterized by a progressive loss and decline of tissues and organ systems. The degeneration rate is varied between individuals and is highly dependent on genetics and environmental factors, for instance exercise, ionizing radiation, pollutant exposure, and diet. In general, the physiological changes of aging are divided into three groups that include (1) changes in cellular homeostatic mechanisms, such as extracellular fluid volume, blood, and body temperature; (2) a decrease in organ mass; and (3) the loss and decline of the functional reserve of the body system [76]. The loss of functional reserve may impair the ability of an individual to cope with external challenges, for instance trauma and surgery.

Cardiovascular aging attenuates contractile and mechanical efficiency. The specific changes include an increase in smooth muscle tone, promotion of collagenolytic and elastolytic activity, and arterial wall thickening [77]. Subsequently, vessels stiffen progressively with age and contribute to the elevation of systolic arterial pressure and increase cardiac afterload and systemic vascular resistance. This phenomenon is usually demonstrated in isolated systolic hypertension, in which the left ventricle has to work harder to eject blood into the stiffer aorta, and hence increase the workload and contribute to the left ventricular hypertrophy. Hypertrophy of myocytes in response to increased afterload may promote contraction time as well as the cardiac cycle. Ventricular relaxation is delayed at the time of mitral valve opening and leads to diastolic dysfunction. Further, the early diastolic filling rate is also decreased with age and partly compensated by an elevated rate of late diastolic filling. Aging is also linked to the reduction of cardiac output in the face of falls in blood pressure [77].

In the context of the central nervous system, aging reduces the neural density, accounting for nearly a 30% loss of brain mass by the age of 80 years, largely grey matter. Growing older is linked to a reduction of central neurotransmitters such as acetylcholine, serotonin, and catecholamine. In addition, aging may also reduce dopamine uptake transporters and decrease γ-aminobutyric acid, β-adrenergic, α_2-adrenergic, and cortical serotonergic binding sites. All these changes may reduce the speed of memory and processing [77].

The greatest change in gastrointestinal physiology affecting nutrient bioavailability is atrophic gastritis, which presents in nearly 20% of the elderly population [78]. It has been shown that a slight decline in the secretion of pepsin and hydrochloric acid occurs with advancing age. Nutrient absorption is affected by low acid conditions in the stomach. Research evidence revealed that growing older is associated with the age-associated decline in the absorption of certain substances absorbed by active mechanisms such as vitamin B_{12}, β-carotene, iron, and calcium [79]. For example, dietary vitamin B_{12} is linked to the food protein, in which the vitamin B_{12} molecules must be digested before bound to the endogenous R binders. This digestion takes place in the presence of pepsin and acid. If stomach acid is low, the digestion of vitamin B_{12} cannot take place effectively [78].

In addition to the effects mentioned above, aging may reduce the number of fibroblasts and keratinocytes, decrease epidermal cell turnover, and impair the barrier function [80]. Moreover, aging can also decrease the vascular network such as round hair glands and bulbs (skin atrophy and fibrosis). Notably, elderly people are susceptible to the changes in cutaneous function due to the reduction in vitamin D synthesis. These changes increase their susceptibility to skin injuries such as skin tear and pressure ulcer [77].

7. The Role of Carotenoids in the Prevention of ARD

Antioxidant plays a predominant role in the termination of oxidative chain reactions by disrupting the free radical intermediates [81]. Antioxidants control autoxidation by disrupting the formation of free radicals or suppressing the propagation of free radicals through several mechanisms. This compound facilitates in quenching $\bullet O_2^-$, breaking the autoxidative chain reaction, inhibiting the formation of peroxides, and scavenging the species that promote the peroxidation [82].

Carotenoids are known as a highly effective physical and chemical singlet oxygen quencher and a potent scavenger of ROS [83]. The previous study stated that the antioxidant activity of lycopene is superior to α-tocopherol and β-carotene [84]. This favorable effect is attributed to the singlet oxygen quenching ability [85], suggesting that a tetraterpene hydrocarbon polyene accompanied with two unconjugated and eleven conjugated double bonds readily interact with electrophilic reagents, and subsequently affect the reactivity of oxygen and oxygenated free radical species [85]. The previous finding has revealed that a high consumption of carotenoids is inversely associated with ARD [86]. It has been suggested that the alleviation of chronic diseases is mainly due to the antioxidant properties of carotenoids [87]. Figure 3 shows the effect of oxidative stress and the interaction of carotenoids in relation to ARD.

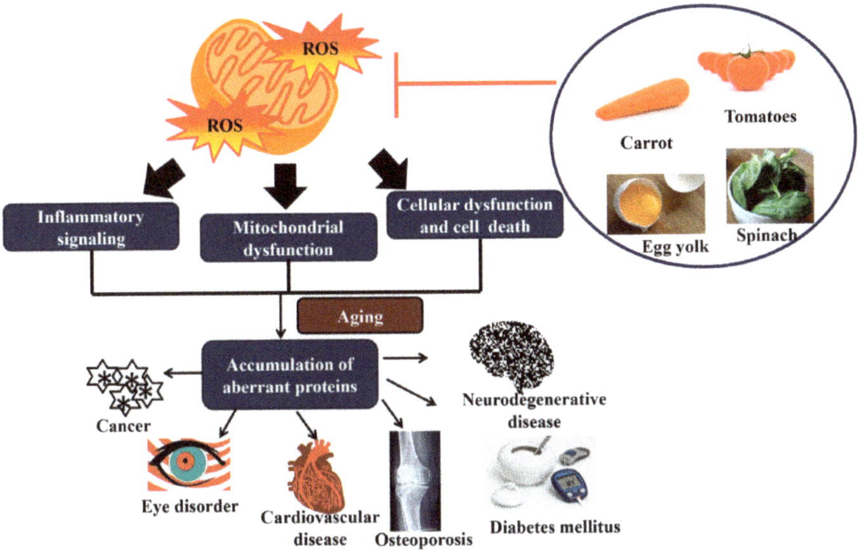

Figure 3. The effect of oxidative stress and the interaction of carotenoids in relation to ARD. Accumulation of reactive oxygen species (ROS) leads to inflammation, cellular dysfunction and cell death, and mitochondrial dysfunction. Mitochondria function decline, oxidative stress response in aging, and accumulation of aberrant proteins may contribute to ARD. The consumption of carotenoids may block ROS production.

7.1. Eye Disorders

Visual impairment has become the second most common cause of lived with disability [88]. Diabetic retinopathy, glaucoma, cataract, and age-related macular degeneration (AMD) are the most common types of vision loss among the elderly [89]. The development of AMD is not only due to the age factor, other factors, for example diet, oxidative stress, and smoking, may also increase the risk [90]. Tosini et al. [91] revealed that prolonged exposure to blue light emitted by energy-efficient lightbulbs and electronics enhanced retinal cell damage. This study further demonstrated that long-term exposure to energy-efficient lightbulbs and electronics can reduce visual function and promote AMD [91].

AMD is the predominant contributor of blindness among the elderly aged 75 years and above in developed countries [92,93]. AMD contributes approximately 8.7% of all blindness globally [94]. Notably, some research has emerged to predict that the percentage of AMD patients will double between 2010 and 2050 [95]. Non-proliferative postmitotic cells including retinal pigment epithelium cell and photoreceptors are particularly sensitive to oxidative damage due to the absence of DNA damage detection systems compared to other cells [96]. In the context of cataracts, zeaxanthin and lutein therapy has provided significant beneficial outcomes [97]. Zeaxanthin/lutein (2 mg/10 mg) significantly reduced the risk of cataract surgery [98]. Moreover, AMD is inversely correlated with the dietary intake of a carotenoid-rich diet (5–10 mg/day) compared to those individuals who rarely or never consume carotenoids [98].

Carotenoids have been demonstrated as an eye-sight protecting agent [99]. Such carotenoids are categorized as pro-vitamin A comprised of the unsubstituted β-ionone ring (γ-carotene, α-carotene, β-carotene, and β-cryptoxanthin) which can be converted into retinal [100]. Two dietary carotenoids, namely zeaxanthin and lutein, are macular pigments found in the human retina [101]. Macular pigments exert antioxidant properties, which can absorb short wavelengths and high energy blue light, and subsequently protect the retina from photochemical damage [86]. This pigment can protect against UV-induced peroxidation and neutralize ROS [101].

Deficiency of vitamin A affects immunity, which can damage the light-sensitive receptors [102]. Further, vitamin A deficiency may also lead to permanent blindness called xerophthalmia [103]. The previous study stated that supplementation with carotenoids such as zeaxanthin (2 mg/day/year) and lutein (10–20 mg/day/year) can increase macular pigment optical density levels [104,105]. Several studies reported by Hammond et al. [104] and Nolan et al. [106] also showed that zeaxanthin/lutein (2 mg/10 mg/day/year) can enhance visual performance such as photostress recovery, glare tolerance, and contrast sensitivity. Collectively, carotenoid intake could be a potential approach for the amelioration of oxidative stress and provide potential benefits for ocular health and function. The potential implication of carotenoids on AMD, as well as the dosage of the zeaxanthin and lutein when combined with other nutrients is worthy of further investigation in randomized clinical trials.

7.2. Neurodegenerative Diseases

Dementia is a chronic and progressive neurodegenerative disease in which there is deterioration in behavior, thinking, memory, and the ability to perform daily activities [107]. Dementia has become one of the major causes of disability and dependency among older people and contributes to nearly 60% of the total cases. It is projected that by 2050 there will be 152 million dementia cases in low- and middle-income countries [107]. Alzheimer's disease is the most common form of dementia and accounts for nearly 60–70% of cases [107].

The data from the previous study revealed that the concentration of carotenoids is passively associated with cognitive performance in both cognitively intact and cognitively impaired people [108,109]. A human study involving 91 healthy individuals suggested that twelve months supplementation with lutein (10 mg/day), zeaxanthin (2 mg/day), and *meso*-zeaxanthin (10 mg/day) improved the memory compared to the placebo control group [110]. A study reported by Rubin et al. [111] also demonstrated that carotenoids (16 mg/day for 26 days) are inversely associated with inflammatory markers, for instance interleukin (IL)-1β, tumor necrosis factor-α (TNF-α), IL-6, vascular cell adhesion molecule-1 (VCAM-1), and monocyte chemoattractant protein 1 (MCP-1) in both human and animal models. A study analyzed of 3031 participants aged 40–75 years revealed that total carotenoids (1.63 μmol/L) were negatively correlated with retinol binding protein 4 (RBP4) [112]. RBP4 also known as adipose-derived cytokine is a sole retinol transporter in the blood which is secreted from the adipocyte and liver [113]. RBP4 plays a crucial role as a proinflammatory marker by activating c-Jun N-terminal kinase (JNK) and nuclear factor-kappa B (NF-κB) pathways [114,115], as well as increasing the secretion of IL-1β, IL-6, and TNF-α expression. Thus, controlling systemic inflammation could be a targetable tool for the prevention of ARD.

Much information indicates that carotenoids may limit neuronal damage from free radicals, which is potentially served as a modifiable risk factor for cognitive decline. The data from 2011–2014 National Health and Nutrition Examination Survey involving 2796 participants aged ≥60 years demonstrated that lutein and zeaxanthin supplementation (2.02 mg/day) may prevent cognitive decline [116]. Carotenoids delay neurodegenerative diseases progression through several pathways, for example suppress proinflammatory cytokines [117], trigger Aβ peptide production [118], and reduce oxidative stress [119]. Due to its high binding energy with Alzheimer's disease-associated receptors (histone deacetylase and P53 kinase receptors) [120], β-carotene is potential to be an Alzheimer' disease antagonist. Fucoxanthin, a marine carotenoid, destabilizes Aβ fibril and inhibits Aβ formation [121]. Likewise, Ono and Yamada [122] reported that both β-carotene and vitamin A can block the oligomerization of Aβ42 and Aβ40 during Aβ peptide formation. Further, lycopene (1–4 mg/kg body weight/14 days) also decreases the Aβ42-induced inflammatory cytokine, for instance TNF-α, NF-κB, IL-1β, and transforming growth factor beta (TGF-β) in the brain [123]. High serum carotenoid levels such as lycopene, zeaxanthin, and lutein were found to reduce Alzheimer's disease mortality [124]. Collectively, carotenoids play a significant role as an antioxidant to delay the progression of neurodegenerative disease.

7.3. Cardiovascular Disease

According to the World Health Organization [125], nearly 17.9 million people die from CVD, represents 31% of all deaths worldwide. About 85% of all CVD deaths are due to strokes and heart attacks [125]. CVD is the disorder of blood vessels and the heart such as cerebrovascular disease, rheumatic heart disease, and coronary heart disease [125]. CVD is the major clinical concern in the elderly, with 68% of individuals aged 60–79 years having CVD and the prevalence is increased to 85% among people aged 80 years and above [126]. Oxidative stress is implicated in the development and progression of CVD [127]. High oxidative stress in the heart is one of the common characteristics of CVD [128]. Indeed, reduced antioxidant defense and enhanced ROS accumulation can cause systemic oxidative damage in CVD patients [129].

Carotenoids have been reported to prevent oxidative stress-induced diseases including CVD [130]. The implication of carotenoids against pathophysiology of CVD has been widely studied in both in vivo and in vitro models [131,132]. Lutein suppresses the NF-κB activation which plays a prominent role in the pathogenesis of several human diseases [133]. The anti-inflammatory and antioxidant properties of lutein (1–25 μM/24 h) reduced the risk of coronary artery disease [134] and CVD [135] in the elderly population. Lutein consumption (one soft boiled egg per day for 4 weeks) was shown to reduce the oxidized low-density lipoprotein (LDL), implies that lutein may prevent the development of atherosclerosis [136]. High plasma lutein levels were found to protect the myocardium from ischemia injury by decreasing oxidative stress and apoptosis [135]. A meta-analysis involving 387,569 participants suggested that a high lutein intake or high lutein concentration in the blood reduced the risk of stroke and coronary heart disease [137]. The previous study reported by Costa-Rodrigues et al. [138] further revealed that carotenoids (lycopene) are of benefit in the protection of vascular, endothelial, and cardiac. Moreover, research evidence also indicates that carotenoids reduce LDL-cholesterol plasma levels [139] and promote high-density lipoprotein (HDL) functionality (three eggs for 30 days) [140]. Compared to those who rarely or deficient in lycopene, individuals who supplemented with lycopene may trigger a significant reduction in coronary artery disease [141]. Although most of the studies have reported a positive effect of lycopene on cardiovascular health, not all data demonstrated such a link. Several human intervention studies failed to identify an inverse relationship between lycopene intake and CVD markers [140,142–145]. There are many reasons underlying these negative associations. Both the metabolism and bioavailability of lycopene are highly affected by genetic variability, as they are found in more than 28 single nucleotide polymorphisms in 16 genes [146,147]. In addition, the cardiovascular markers utilized in different studies also varied significantly, which makes detailed comparisons difficult. A difference in lycopene sources and doses may also reduce the lycopene effects, which in turn influence the observed effects. Further, most of the studies used less than 100 subjects, which reduce the statistical power of the results. Therefore, further studies should be performed in large populations, preferably from the same geographic location to avoid high genetic variability. The processing method and amount of tomatoes ingested also should be strictly controlled [138]. Taken together, carotenoid intake might be a promising strategy to enhance cardiovascular health.

7.4. Cancer

Cancer represents the second most common cause of death worldwide, with nearly 9.6 million deaths and 18.1 million new cases in 2018 [148,149]. Emerging research evidence has suggested that 30–50% of cancer deaths could be prevented by modifying the key risk factors, for instance exercise regularly, maintaining healthy body weight, reducing alcohol consumption, and avoiding tobacco [148].

Carotenoids have been reported to decrease the risk of certain cancers such as colon [150], prostate [151], and lung [152]. Several carotenoids, for instance lutein, zeaxanthin, and lycopene, have been reported to decrease the inflammatory mediator's production through the blockage of NF-κB pathway [153,154]. Lutein was found to negatively link to several types of cancer. A study obtained by Chang et al. [133] reported that lutein decreases the proliferation of breast cancer cells, ameliorates ROS, and improves the expression of cellular antioxidant enzymes via activation of nuclear factor E2-related factor 2 (Nrf2)/antioxidant responsive element (ARE) and inhibition of NF-κB pathways. In prostate cancer patients aged 64–75 years, high carrot, tomatoes, and lycopene intakes were shown to decrease the risk of prostate cancer compared to those with low carrot, tomatoes, and lycopene consumption [22]. The data from a human population-based study involving 638 independently living elderly aged 65–85 years revealed that increased serum carotenoid levels are inversely associated with cancer mortality [155]. The preventive role of carotenoids against cancer could be attributed to their antioxidant activity. In fact, the anticancer ability of carotenoids such as lycopene is modulated via several mechanisms such as apoptosis, cell cycle arrest, phase II detoxifying enzymes, and growth factor signaling [156]. However, a previous study revealed that smokers who supplemented with β-carotene (20 mg/day for 5–8 years) experienced increased lung cancer incidence, and these findings were not associated with the nicotine or tar level of cigarettes smoked, suggesting that all smokers should continue to avoid β-carotene supplementation [157]. The detrimental effect of β-carotene supplementation in smokers could be due to the instability of the β-carotene molecule in the lung after exposure to cigarette smoke. Oxidized β-carotene metabolites diminish retinoic acid levels and thus enhance lung carcinogenesis [158]. Taken together, regular consumption of carotenoids may become a useful approach to ameliorate oxidative stress. The beneficial effect of carotenoids in relation to cancer is worth attention.

7.5. Diabetes Mellitus

Diabetes mellitus is a chronic disease due to the deficiency or ineffective of the pancreas to produce insulin. The prevalence of diabetes has risen from 108 million in 1980 to 422 million in 2014 [159]. Nearly 1.6 million people worldwide died due to diabetes in 2016 [159]. Type 2 diabetes is the most common form of the disease, accounting nearly 90% of all diabetes mellitus cases worldwide [159]. Diabetes mellitus is a progressive disease, accompanied by complications including macro- and microvascular damage, neuropathy, retinopathy, and nephropathy [160].

Oxidative stress has been recognized as a key risk factor in the development of diabetes [161]. Several risk factors for instance aging, obesity, and unhealthy dietary intake, all contribute to an oxidative environment and subsequently alter the insulin sensitivity via impairment of glucose tolerance or promote the insulin resistance [162]. Hyperglycemia is commonly related to diabetes and leads to the progression and an overall oxidative environment [163]. The dysregulation of cellular and molecular process is common in type 2 diabetes, particularly in β-cells. Reactive nitrogen species (RNS) and ROS, for instance hydroxyl radical (OH·), peroxynitrite (ONOO−), NO, superoxide anion ($O_2^{\bullet-}$), and H_2O_2, all contribute to key metabolic and physiologic processes [164,165].

Another common carotenoid, astaxanthin, is a potent antioxidant for the prevention and treatment of diabetes. An animal study has shown that astaxanthin (1.0 mg/mouse/day for 13 weeks) decreases blood glucose levels, improves insulin serum levels, and reduces glucose tolerance in type 2 diabetes mellitus rodent models [166]. A 10-year prospective study involving 37,846 men and women revealed that high dietary intake of β-carotene (10 ± 4 mg/day) can reduce the risk of type 2 diabetes mellitus [167]. A low serum β-carotene level has also been associated with impaired insulin sensitivity [168]. Another common carotenoid, fucoxanthin has been demonstrated to prevent diabetes mellitus. Maeda et al. [169] revealed that feeding obese mice Fucoxanthin-rich Wakame lipids (1.06–2.22%) may restore insulin and blood glucose levels via the upregulation of glucose transporter type 4 (GLUT4) mRNA expression in the skeletal muscle. A previous study reported by Manabe et al. [170] evaluated astaxanthin in relation to inflammatory markers and proinflammatory cytokine production. The data showed that astaxanthin (10^{-7}–10^{-4} M) reduces high glucose-induced ROS production in the mitochondria and downregulates the expression of cyclooxygenase-2 (COX-2), TGF-β, NF-κB, and MCP-1. In a further study focused on inflammation outcomes, Kim et al. [171] found that astaxanthin inhibits the peroxynitrite ($ONOO^-$), nitric oxide (NO), and superoxide (O_2^-) induced by high glucose concentration. These data suggest that astaxanthin may exert the potential in the prevention of diabetic nephropathy. The Epidemiology of Vascular Aging Study involving 127 diabetes cases and 1389 volunteers aged 59–71 years revealed that individuals with high plasma carotenoid levels were significantly reduced the risk of dysglycemia [172]. Collectively, carotenoids may be a useful nutritional intervention for diabetes and its complications.

7.6. Osteoporosis

Osteoporosis is the most common metabolic bone disease, which is characterized by low bone mass and increase bone fragility [173]. Osteoporosis has become a global epidemic, affecting more than 8.9 million fractures annually worldwide [174]. Nearly 75% of the distal forearm, spine, and hip fractures occur in patients aged 65 years and above [175]. By 2050, the incidence of hip fracture is expected to increase by 240% and 310% in women and men, respectively [176].

Studies in both in vivo and in vitro models have suggested that carotenoids could prevent bone loss via the reduction of oxidative stress. Osteoclastogenesis and the apoptosis of osteocytes and osteoblasts are accelerated with the presence of oxidative stress, and subsequently lead to bone resorption [177,178]. A study found that a high intake of β-carotene, β-cryptoxanthin, and lutein/zeaxanthin reduces the risk of hip fracture in the middle-aged and elderly population [179]. Further, epidemiological studies have also found that a dietary intake of carotenoids may decrease the risk of osteoporosis [180] and improve bone mineral density [181]. The in vivo study further demonstrated that lutein (50 mg/kg for 4 weeks) protects the ovariectomized rats against oxidative stress and osteoporosis by downregulating the inflammation and osteoclast-specific marker (NFATc1) expression via Nrf2 activation [182]. Likewise, Tominari et al. [183] also showed that lutein (3, 10, and 30 μM) suppresses osteoclastic bone resorption and enhances bone formation. High serum lutein and zeaxanthin levels increase bone density in young healthy adults, suggesting that lutein and zeaxanthin play a pivotal role in optimal bone health [184].

8. Carotenoids and Aging

Numerous animal and clinical studies suggest that a diet rich in antioxidants can prevent aging [185]. In support of this, an animal study has revealed that lutein could prolong the lifespan and ameliorate the mortality rate induced by hydrogen peroxide and paraquat in *Drosophila melanogaster* [186]. The data showed that supplementation with 0.1 mg/mL lutein significantly increased the mean lifespan of Oregon-R-C (OR) wild type flies by 11.35% compared to the control group [186]. This study further revealed that the maximum lifespan is increased more than 11.23 days after supplementation with 0.1 mg/mL lutein compared to the control [186]. Similarly, the study obtained by Neena et al. [187] has also demonstrated that lutein (0.5, 1.5, 5, 15 μM) could reduce the age-associated decline in human skin cells. Despite none of the clinical study demonstrating that a diet high in lutein could promote human lifespan, several human clinical studies revealed that a dosage ranging from 2.4–30 mg/day is beneficial to human health without undesirable outcomes [188]. In another study, Yazaki et al. [189] showed that astaxanthin (0.1–1 mM) can prolong the lifespan in the wild-type and long-lived mutant *age-1* of *C. elegans*. The data revealed that astaxanthin increased DAF-16 gene expression and reduced mitochondrial production of ROS, suggesting that carotenoid is partially involved in the modulation of insulin-like growth factor 1 (IGF-1) signaling [189]. Indeed, IGF-1 plays a predominant role in biological aging [190]. Fucoxanthin (0.3–1.0 μM) has also been reported to prolong lifespan and promote the viability of the organism such as *Drosophila melanogaster* and *C. elegans* [191]. An adequate intake of lutein-rich food is vitally important throughout the lifespan. The previous finding suggests that carotenoids such as lutein play an important role in neural health (cognitive and visual function) in adults [192], implying that carotenoids may provide an optimal or better health outcome.

9. Safety and Toxicity

In a well-balanced diet, the intake of carotenoids, such as lutein, is sufficient to maintain health. However, supplementation is needed in cases of chronic disease or the inadequate absorption of carotenoids. Several studies conducted in both in vitro [193] and animal models [193,194] have revealed that the use of lutein is safe without teratogenic and mutagenic outcomes. Despite the fact that no toxic effect was observed during lutein supplementation in both intervention and epidemiological studies [195], the Joint Expert Committee on Food Additives established an upper safety limit for daily lutein consumption of 2 mg/kg [196]. Whereas the European Food Safety Authority (EFSA) indicated an upper safety limit of 1 mg/kg [197]. EFSA further established an upper limit for lutein-enriched milk for infants of 250 μg/L [198]. Notably, the data showed that there is no interaction between lutein consumption and cytochrome P450 enzyme activity, suggesting that lutein may not modify the metabolism of endogenous or exogenous substances [199]. An animal study has shown that mice lacking β-carotene oxygenase 2 significantly increased the mitochondrial dysfunction and oxidative stress as well as developed pathologic carotenoid accumulation [200]. This finding implied that an excessive carotenoid intake may contribute to toxicity under certain circumstances. Olmedilla et al. [201] found that the supplementation of lutein at a dosage of 15 mg/day for 20 weeks increased the risk of skin yellowing (carotenodermia). Similarly, the data from the observational study revealed that lutein may increase the risk of lung cancer, particularly non-small cell lung cancer in smokers [202]. The population-based study has also reported that lutein supplementation increased the risk of crystalline maculopathy in old women. The adverse outcomes are reversed after lutein intake discontinuation [203]. Although research has demonstrated a positive association between lutein and the risk of several diseases, the survey conducted by EFSA concluded that the data obtained were insufficient to show an adverse outcome [197]. Consistent with the data reported by EFSA, the Age-Related Eye Disease Study 2 (AREDS2) intervention study did not identify any risk of lung cancer after lutein supplementation [204,205]. Based on the evidence, it is suggested that chronic lutein supplementation at the dosage of 10 mg/day is safe and non-toxic [204,205].

10. Conclusions

A high intake of fruits and leafy green vegetables is important to achieve adequate dietary levels of carotenoids among other nutrients. Based on the evidence, an adequate diet is recommended rather than supplementation in order to maintain physical health. The previous finding suggests that high dietary consumption of zeaxanthin and lutein are likely to protect against ARD such as AMD. Although the beneficial effects of carotenoids for reducing the risk of ARD have been demonstrated in both in vivo and in vitro studies, there are still some controversies surrounding certain effects of carotenoids in ARD that need to be elucidated by long-term clinical trials with large cohorts of the general population. Moreover, further studies are warranted to evaluate the precise mechanism of action under pathological and healthy conditions to enhance the implementation and acceptance of carotenoids for use in clinical practice. Therefore, researchers should further investigate the underlying mechanism of action to better elucidate the possible role of carotenoids on human health.

Author Contributions: B.L.T. conceived and designed the review and wrote the manuscript. M.E.N. edited the manuscript. All authors read and approved the final manuscript.

Acknowledgments: We would like to thank the Ministry of Science, Technology, and Innovation (MOSTI), Malaysia (project no. 02-01-04-SF2141) for financial support.

Conflicts of Interest: The authors declare no conflict of interest.

References

1. World Health Organization. Global Health Observatory (GHO) data, Life Expectancy. 2019. Available online: https://www.who.int/gho/mortality_burden_disease/life_tables/en/ (accessed on 3 March 2019).

2. World Health Organization. World Health Statistics–Large Gains in Life Expectancy. 2014. Available online: http://www.who.int/mediacentre/news/releases/2014/world-health-statistics-2014/en/ (accessed on 3 March 2019).
3. Bruins, M.J.; Van Dael, P.; Eggersdorfer, M. The role of nutrients in reducing the risk for noncommunicable diseases during aging. *Nutrients* **2019**, *11*, 85. [CrossRef] [PubMed]
4. Jin, K.; Simpkins, J.W.; Ji, X.; Leis, M.; Stambler, I. The critical need to promote research of aging and aging-related diseases to improve health and longevity of the elderly population. *Aging Dis.* **2015**, *6*, 1. [CrossRef]
5. Rahal, A.; Kumar, A.; Singh, V.; Yadav, B.; Tiwari, R.; Chakraborty, S.; Dhama, K. Oxidative stress, prooxidants, and antioxidants: The interplay. *BioMed Res. Int.* **2014**, *2014*. [CrossRef]
6. Gudkov, S.V.; Guryev, E.L.; Gapeyev, A.B.; Sharapov, M.G.; Bunkin, N.F.; Shkirin, A.V.; Zabelina, T.S.; Glinushkin, A.P.; Sevost'yanov, M.A.; Belosludtsev, K.N.; et al. Unmodified hydrated C60 fullerene molecules exhibit antioxidant properties, prevent damage to DNA and proteins induced by reactive oxygen species and protect mice against injuries caused by radiation-induced oxidative stress. *Nanomedicine* **2019**, *15*, 37–46. [CrossRef] [PubMed]
7. Giudetti, A.M.; Salzet, M.; Cassano, T. Oxidative stress in aging brain: Nutritional and pharmacological interventions for neurodegenerative disorders. *Oxid. Med. Cell. Longev.* **2018**, *2018*. [CrossRef]
8. Tan, B.L.; Norhaizan, M.E.; Huynh, K.; Heshu, S.R.; Yeap, S.K.; Hazilawati, H.; Roselina, K. Water extract of brewers' rice induces apoptosis in human colorectal cancer cells via activation of caspase-3 and caspase-8 and downregulates the Wnt/β-catenin downstream signaling pathway in brewers' rice-treated rats with azoxymethane-induced colon carcinogenesis. *BMC Complement. Altern. Med.* **2015**, *15*, 205.
9. Liu, Z.; Zhou, T.; Ziegler, A.C.; Dimitrion, P.; Zuo, L. Oxidative stress in neurodegenerative diseases: From molecular mechanisms to clinical applications. *Oxid. Med. Cell. Longev.* **2017**, *2017*. [CrossRef]
10. Chistiakov, D.A.; Sobenin, I.A.; Revin, V.V.; Orekhov, A.N.; Bobryshev, Y.V. Mitochondrial aging and age-related dysfunction of mitochondria. *BioMed Res. Int.* **2014**, *2014*. [CrossRef]
11. Eckmann, J.; Eckert, S.H.; Leuner, K.; Muller, W.E.; Eckert, G.P. Mitochondria: Mitochondrial membranes in brain ageing and neurodegeneration. *Int. J. Biochem. Cell Biol.* **2013**, *45*, 76–80. [CrossRef] [PubMed]
12. Liguori, I.; Russo, G.; Curcio, F.; Bulli, G.; Aran, L.; Della-Morte, D.; Gargiulo, G.; Testa, G.; Cacciatore, F.; Bonaduce, D.; et al. Oxidative stress, aging, and diseases. *Clin. Interv. Aging.* **2018**, *13*, 757–772. [CrossRef] [PubMed]
13. Maulik, N.; McFadden, D.; Otani, H.; Thirunavukkarasu, M.; Parinandi, N.L. Antioxidants in longevity and medicine. *Oxid. Med. Cell. Longev.* **2013**, *2013*. [CrossRef] [PubMed]
14. Corbi, G.; Acanfora, D.; Iannuzzi, G.L.; Longobardi, G.; Cacciatore, F.; Furgi, G.; Filippelli, A.; Rengo, G.; Leosco, D.; Ferrara, N. Hypermagnesemia predicts mortality in elderly with congestive heart disease: Relationship with laxative and antacid use. *Rejuvenation Res.* **2008**, *11*, 129–138. [CrossRef]
15. Stadtman, E.R.; Berlett, B.S. Reactive oxygen–mediated protein oxidation in aging and disease. *Chem. Res. Toxicol.* **1997**, *10*, 485–494. [CrossRef] [PubMed]
16. López-Otín, C.; Blasco, M.A.; Partridge, L.; Serrano, M.; Kroemer, G. The hallmarks of aging. *Cell* **2013**, *153*, 1194–1217.
17. Dias, V.; Junn, E.; Mouradian, M.M. The role of oxidative stress in Parkinson's disease. *J. Parkinson's Dis.* **2013**, *3*, 461–491.
18. Zuo, L.; Zhou, T.; Pannell, B.K.; Ziegler, A.; Best, T.M. Biological and physiological role of reactive oxygen species–the good, the bad and the ugly. *Acta Physiol.* **2015**, *214*, 329–348. [CrossRef]
19. Tan, B.L.; Norhaizan, M.E.; Liew, W.-P.P.; Rahman, H.S. Antioxidant and oxidative stress: A mutual interplay in age-related diseases. *Front. Pharmacol.* **2018**, *9*, 1162. [CrossRef]
20. Cheng, H.M.; Koutsidis, G.; Lodge, J.K.; Ashor, A.W.; Siervo, M.; Lara, J. Lycopene and tomato and risk of cardiovascular diseases: A systematic review and meta-analysis of epidemiological evidence. *Crit. Rev. Food Sci. Nutr.* **2019**, *59*, 141–158. [CrossRef] [PubMed]
21. Palozza, P.; Catalano, A.; Simone, R.E.; Mele, M.C.; Cittadini, A. Effect of lycopene and tomato products on cholesterol metabolism. *Ann. Nutr. MeTable* **2012**, *61*, 126–134. [CrossRef] [PubMed]
22. Hoang, D.V.; Pham, N.M.; Lee, A.H.; Tran, D.N.; Binns, C.W. Dietary carotenoid intakes and prostate cancer risk: A case-control study from Vietnam. *Nutrients* **2018**, *10*, 70. [CrossRef]

23. Hou, L.L.; Gao, C.; Chen, I.; Hu, G.Q.; Xie, S.Q. Essential role of autophagy in fucoxanthin-induced cytotoxicity to human epithelial cervical cancer HeLa cells. *Acta Pharmacol. Sin.* **2013**, *34*, 1403–1410. [CrossRef]
24. Satomi, Y. Antitumor and cancer-preventative function of fucoxanthin: A marine carotenoid. *Anticancer Res.* **2017**, *37*, 1557–1562. [CrossRef]
25. Alós, E.; Rodrigo, M.J.; Zacarias, L. Manipulation of carotenoid content in plants to improve human health. In *Carotenoids in Nature*; Springer: Cham Switzerland, 2016; pp. 311–343.
26. Du, X.; Song, K.; Wang, J.; Cong, R.; Li, L.; Zhang, G. Draft genome and SNPs associated with carotenoid accumulation in adductor muscles of bay scallop (*Argopecten irradians*). *J. Genomics* **2017**, *5*, 83. [CrossRef]
27. Singh, G.; Sahota, H.K. Impact of benzimidazole and dithiocarbamate fungicides on the photosynthetic machinery, sugar content and various antioxidative enzymes in chickpea. *Plant Physiol. Biochem.* **2018**, *132*, 166–173. [CrossRef]
28. Gauger, T.; Konhauser, K.; Kappler, A. Protection of phototrophic iron (II)-oxidizing bacteria from UV irradiation by biogenic iron (III) minerals: Implications for early Archean banded iron formation. *Geology* **2015**, *43*, 1067–1070. [CrossRef]
29. Paliwal, C.; Ghosh, T.; George, B.; Pancha, I.; Maurya, R.; Chokshi, K.; Ghosh, A.; Mishra, S. Microalgal carotenoids: Potential nutraceutical compounds with chemotaxonomic importance. *Algal Res.* **2016**, *15*, 24–31. [CrossRef]
30. Khachik, F. Distribution and metabolism of dietary carotenoids in humans as a criterion for development of nutritional supplements. *Pure Appl. Chem.* **2006**, *78*, 1551–1557. [CrossRef]
31. Parker, R.S. Carotenoids in human blood and tissues. *J. Nutr.* **1989**, *119*, 101–104. [CrossRef]
32. Yaroshevich, I.; Krasilnikov, P.; Rubin, A. Functional interpretation of the role of cyclic carotenoids in photosynthetic antennas via quantum chemical calculations. *Comput. Theor. Chem.* **2015**, *1070*, 27–32. [CrossRef]
33. Berman, J.; Zorrilla-López, U.; Farré, G.; Zhu, C.; Sandmann, G.; Twyman, R.M.; Capell, T.; Christou, P. Nutritionally important carotenoids as consumer products. *Phytochem. Rev.* **2015**, *14*, 727–743. [CrossRef]
34. Harrison, E.H.; Curley, R.W. Carotenoids and retinoids: Nomenclature, chemistry, and analysis. In *The Biochemistry of Retinoid Signaling II*; Springer: Dordrecht, the Netherlands, 2016; pp. 1–19.
35. Gabriel, H.B.; Silva, M.F.; Kimura, E.A.; Wunderlich, G.; Katzin, A.M.; Azevedo, M.F. Squalestatin is an inhibitor of carotenoid biosynthesis in Plasmodium falciparum. *Antimicrob. Agents Chemother.* **2015**, *59*, 3180–3188. [CrossRef] [PubMed]
36. Fiedor, J.; Burda, K. Potential role of carotenoids as antioxidants in human health and disease. *Nutrients* **2014**, *6*, 466–488. [CrossRef]
37. Nishino, A.; Yasui, H.; Maoka, T. Reaction of paprika carotenoids, capsanthin and capsorubin, with reactive oxygen species. *J. Agric. Food Chem.* **2016**, *64*, 4786–4792. [CrossRef]
38. Langi, P.; Kiokias, S.; Varzakas, T.; Proestos, C. Carotenoids: From plants to food and feed industries. In *Microbial Carotenoids. Methods in Molecular Biology*; Barreiro, C., Barredo, J.L., Eds.; Humana Press: New York, NY, USA, 2018; Volume 1852, pp. 57–71.
39. Johnson, E.J. The role of carotenoids in human health. *Nutr. Clin. Care* **2002**, *5*, 56–65. [CrossRef]
40. Yahia, E.M.; Ornelas-Paz, J.d.J. Chemistry, stability, and biological actions of carotenoids. In *Fruit and Vegetable Phytochemicals Chemistry, Nutritional Value and Stability*; de la Rosa, L.A., Alvarez-Parrilla, E., González-Aguilar, G.A., Eds.; Wiley-Blackwell: Ames, IA, USA, 2010; pp. 177–222.
41. Lin, Q.; Liang, R.; Williams, P.A.; Zhong, F. Factors affecting the bioaccessibility of β-carotene in lipid-based microcapsules: Digestive conditions, the composition, structure and physical state of microcapsules. *Food Hydrocoll.* **2018**, *77*, 187–203. [CrossRef]
42. Thane, C.; Reddy, S. Processing of fruits and vegetables: Effect on carotenoids. *Nutr. Food Sci.* **1997**, *2*, 58–65. [CrossRef]
43. Hart, D.J.; Scott, K.J. Development and evaluation of an HPLC method for the analysis of carotenoids in foods, and the measurement of the carotenoid content of vegetables and fruits commonly consumed in the UK. *Food Chem.* **1995**, *54*, 101–111. [CrossRef]
44. Calva, M.M. Lutein: A valuable ingredient of fruit and vegetables. *Crit. Rev. Food Sci. Nutr.* **2005**, *45*, 671–696. [CrossRef] [PubMed]

45. Van den Berg, H.; Faulks, R.; Granado, H.F.; Hirschberg, J.; Olmedilla, B.; Sandmann, G.; Southon, S.; Stahl, W. The potential for the improvement of carotenoid levels in foods and the likely systemic effects. *J. Sci. Food Agric.* **2000**, *80*, 880–912. [CrossRef]
46. Granado, F.; Olmedilla, B.; Blanco, I.; Rojas-Hidalgo, E. Carotenoid composition in raw and cooked Spanish vegetables. *J. Agric. Food Chem.* **1992**, *40*, 2135–2140. [CrossRef]
47. US Department of Agriculture, Agricultural Research Service, Nutrient Data Laboratory. USDA National Nutrient Database for Standard Reference. 2016. Available online: http://www.ars.usda.gov/ba/bhnrc/ndl (accessed on 15 March 2016).
48. Maiani, G.; Periago Caston, M.J.; Catasta, G.; Toti, E.; Cambrodon, I.G.; Bysted, A.; Granado-Lorencio, F.; Olmedilla-Alonso, B.; Knuthsen, P.; Valoti, M.; et al. Carotenoids: Actual knowledge on food sources, intakes, stability and bioavailability and their protective role in humans. *Mol. Nutr. Food Res.* **2009**, *53*, S194–S218. [CrossRef]
49. Marinova, D.; Ribarova, F. HPLC determination of carotenoids in Bulgarian berries. *J. Food Comp. Anal.* **2007**, *20*, 370–374. [CrossRef]
50. Perry, A.; Rasmussen, H.; Johnson, E. Xanthophyll (lutein, zeaxanthin) content in fruits, vegetables and corn and egg products. *J. Food Comp. Anal.* **2009**, *22*, 9–15. [CrossRef]
51. Kimura, M.; Rodriguez-Amaya, D.B. Carotenoid composition of hydroponic leafy vegetables. *J. Agric. Food Chem.* **2003**, *51*, 2603–2607. [CrossRef]
52. Setiawan, B.; Sulaeman, A.; Giraud, D.W.; Driskell, J.A. Carotenoid content of selected Indonesian fruits. *J. Food Compost. Anal.* **2001**, *14*, 169–176. [CrossRef]
53. Lee, H.S.; Coates, G.A. Effect of thermal pasteurization on Valencia orange juice color and pigments. *LWT Food Sci. Technol.* **2003**, *36*, 153–156. [CrossRef]
54. Marín, A.; Ferreres, F.; Tomás-Barberán, F.A.; Gil, M.I. Characterization and quantitation of antioxidant constituents of sweet pepper (*Capsicum annuum* L.). *J. Agric. Food Chem.* **2004**, *52*, 3861–3869.
55. Ameny, M.A.; Wilson, P.W. Relationship between hunter color values and β-carotene contents in white-fleshed African sweet potatoes (*Ipomoea batatas* Lam). *J. Sci. Food Agric.* **1997**, *73*, 301–306. [CrossRef]
56. Brown, M.J.; Ferruzzi, M.G.; Nguyen, M.L.; Cooper, D.A.; Eldridge, A.L.; Schwartz, S.J.; White, W.S. Carotenoid bioavailability is higher from salads ingested with full-fat than with fat-reduced salad dressings as measured with electrochemical detection. *Am. J. Clin. Nutr.* **2004**, *80*, 396–403. [CrossRef] [PubMed]
57. Ghavami, A.; Coward, W.A.; Bluck, L.J. The effect of food preparation on the bioavailability of carotenoids from carrots using intrinsic labelling. *Br. J. Nutr.* **2012**, *107*, 1350–1366. [CrossRef] [PubMed]
58. Kim, J.E.; Gordon, S.; Ferruzzi, M.; Campbell, W. Effects of whole egg consumption on carotenoids absorption from co-consumed, carotenoids-rich mixed-vegetable salad. *FASEB J.* **2015**, *29*, 1.
59. Goltz, S.R.; Campbell, W.W.; Chitchumroonchokchai, C.; Failla, M.L.; Ferruzzi, M.G. Meal triacylglycerol profile modulates postprandial absorption of carotenoids in humans. *Mol. Nutr. Food Res.* **2012**, *56*, 866–877. [CrossRef]
60. Reboul, E.; Thap, S.; Tourniaire, F.; Andre, M.; Juhel, C.; Morange, S.; Amiot, M.J.; Lairon, D.; Borel, P. Differential effect of dietary antioxidant classes (carotenoids, polyphenols, vitamins C and E) on lutein absorption. *Br. J. Nutr.* **2007**, *97*, 440–446. [CrossRef]
61. Riedl, J.; Linseisen, J.; Hoffmann, J.; Wolfram, G. Some dietary fibers reduce the absorption of carotenoids in women. *J. Nutr.* **1999**, *129*, 2170–2176. [CrossRef]
62. Van Het Hof, K.H.; West, C.E.; Weststrate, J.A.; Hautvast, J.G. Dietary factors that affect the bioavailability of carotenoids. *J. Nutr.* **2000**, *130*, 503–506. [CrossRef]
63. Hornero-Mendez, D.; Mínguez-Mosquera, M.-M. Bioaccessibility of carotenes from carrots: Effect of cooking and addition of oil. *Innov. Food Sci. Emerg. Technol.* **2007**, *8*, 407–412. [CrossRef]
64. Baskaran, V.; Sugawara, T.; Nagao, A. Phospholipids affect the intestinal absorption of carotenoids in mice. *Lipids* **2003**, *38*, 705–711. [CrossRef]
65. O'Connell, O.F.; Ryan, L.; O'Brien, N.M. Xanthophyll carotenoids are more bioaccessible from fruits than dark green vegetables. *Nutr. Res.* **2007**, *27*, 258–264. [CrossRef]
66. Prince, M.R.; Frisoli, J.K. Beta-carotene accumulation in serum and skin. *Am. J. Clin. Nutr.* **1993**, *57*, 175–181. [CrossRef]
67. Olson, J.A. Absorption, transport, and metabolism of carotenoids in humans. *Pure Appl. Chem.* **1994**, *66*, 1011–1016. [CrossRef]

68. Fernandez-Garcia, E.; Carvajal-Lerida, I.; Jaren-Galan, M.; Garrido-Fernandez, J.; Perez-Galvez, A.; Hornero-Mendez, D. Carotenoids bioavailability from foods: From plant pigments to efficient biological activities. *Food Res. Int.* **2012**, *46*, 438–450. [CrossRef]
69. Parker, R.S. Absorption, metabolism and transport of carotenoids. *FASEB J.* **1996**, *10*, 542–551. [CrossRef]
70. Erdman, J.W., Jr.; Bierer, T.L.; Gugger, E.T. Absorption and transport of carotenoids. *Ann. N. Y. Acad. Sci.* **1993**, *691*, 76–85. [CrossRef]
71. Rao, A.V.; Rao, L.G. Carotenoids and human health. *Pharmacol. Res.* **2007**, *55*, 207–216. [CrossRef]
72. Stahl, W.; Schwarz, W.; Sundquist, A.R.; Sies, H. cis-trans Isomers of lycopene and β-carotene in human serum and tissues. *Arch. Biochem. Biophys.* **1992**, *294*, 173–177. [CrossRef]
73. Darvin, M.E.; Sterry, W.; Landemann, J.; Vergou, T. The role of carotenoids in human skin. *Molecules* **2011**, *16*, 10491–10506. [CrossRef]
74. Castenmiller, J.J.M.; West, C.E. Bioavailability of carotenoids. *Pure Appl. Chem.* **1997**, *69*, 2145–2150. [CrossRef]
75. Yeum, K.-J.; Russell, R.M. Carotenoid bioavailability and bioconversion. *Ann. Rev. Nutr.* **2002**, *22*, 483–504. [CrossRef] [PubMed]
76. Nigam, Y.; Knight, J.; Bhattacharya, S.; Bayer, A. Physiological changes associated with aging and immobility. *J. Aging Res.* **2012**, *2012*. [CrossRef]
77. Navaratnarajah, A.; Jackson, S.H.D. The physiology of aging. *Medicine* **2017**, *45*, 6–10. [CrossRef]
78. Russell, R.M. Factors in aging that effect the bioavailability of nutrients. *J. Nutr.* **2001**, *131*, 1359S–1361S. [CrossRef]
79. Tang, G.W.; Serfaty-Lacrosniere, C.; Camilo, M.E.; Russell, R.M. Gastric acidity influences the blood response to a beta-carotene dose in humans. *Am. J. Clin. Nutr.* **1996**, *64*, 622–626. [CrossRef]
80. Farage, M.A.; Miller, K.W.; Elsner, P.; Maibach, H.I. Functional and physiological characteristics of the aging skin. *Aging Clin. Exp. Res.* **2008**, *20*, 195–200. [CrossRef]
81. Gholamian-Dehkordi, N.; Luther, T.; Asadi-Samani, M.; Mahmoudian-Sani, M.R. An overview on natural antioxidants for oxidative stress reduction in cancers; a systematic review. *Immunopathol. Persa.* **2017**, 3, e12. [CrossRef]
82. Gaschler, M.M.; Stockwell, B.R. Lipid peroxidation in cell death. *Biochem. Biophys. Res. Commun.* **2017**, *482*, 419–425. [CrossRef]
83. Shen, Y.; Li, J.; Gu, R.; Yue, L.; Wang, H.; Zhan, X.; Xing, B. Carotenoid and superoxide dismutase are the most effective antioxidants participating in ROS scavenging in phenanthrene accumulated wheat leaf. *Chemosphere* **2018**, *197*, 513–525. [CrossRef] [PubMed]
84. Miller, N.J.; Sampson, J.; Candeias, L.P.; Bramley, P.M.; Rice-Evans, C.A. Antioxidant activities of carotenes and xanthophylls. *FEBS Lett.* **1996**, *384*, 240–242. [CrossRef]
85. Krinsky, N.I. The antioxidant and biological properties of the carotenoids. *Ann. N. Y. Acad. Sci.* **1998**, *854*, 443–447. [CrossRef]
86. Eggersdorfer, M.; Wyss, A. Carotenoids in human nutrition and health. *Arch. Biochem. Biophy.* **2018**, *652*, 18–26. [CrossRef]
87. Prasad, K.N.; Wu, M.; Bondy, S.C. Telomere shortening during aging: attenuation by antioxidants and anti-inflammatory agents. *Mech. Ageing Dev.* **2017**, *164*, 61–66. [CrossRef]
88. GBD 2015 DALYs; Hale Collaborators. Global, regional, and national disability-adjusted life-years (DALYs) for 315 diseases and injuries and healthy life expectancy (HALE), 1990–2015: A systematic analysis for the Global Burden of Disease Study 2015. *Lancet* **2016**, *388*, 1603–1658. [CrossRef]
89. Quillen, D.A. Common causes of vision loss in elderly patients. *Am. Fam. Physician* **1999**, *60*, 99–108.
90. Chen, Y.; Bedell, M.; Zhang, K. Age-related macular degeneration: Genetic and environmental factors of disease. *Mol. Interv.* **2010**, *10*, 271–281. [CrossRef]
91. Tosini, G.; Ferguson, I.; Tsubota, K. Effects of blue light on the circadian system and eye physiology. *Mol. Vis.* **2016**, *22*, 61–72.
92. Congdon, N.; O'Colmain, B.; Klaver, C.C.; Klein, R.; Muñoz, B.; Friedman, D.S.; Kempen, J.; Taylor, H.R.; Mitchell, P.; Eye Diseases Prevalence Research Group. Causes and prevalence of visual impairment among adults in the United States. *Arch. Ophthalmol.* **2004**, *122*, 477–485.
93. Resnikoff, S.; Pascolini, D.; Etya'ale, D.; Kocur, I.; Pararajasegaram, R.; Pokharel, G.P.; Mariotti, S.P. Global data on visual impairment in the year 2002. *Bull. World Health Organ.* **2004**, *82*, 844–851.

94. Wong, W.L.; Su, X.; Li, X.; Cheung, C.M.; Klein, R.; Cheng, C.-Y.; Wong, T.Y. Global prevalence of age-related macular degeneration and disease burden projection for 2020 and 2040: A systematic review and meta-analysis. *Lancet Glob. Health* **2014**, *2*, e106–e116. [CrossRef]
95. Eisenhauer, B.; Natoli, S.; Liew, G.; Flood, V.M. Lutein and zeaxanthin-food sources, bioavailability and dietary variety in age-related macular degeneration protection. *Nutrients* **2017**, *9*, 120. [CrossRef]
96. Blasiak, J.; Petrovski, G.; Veréb, Z.; Facskó, A.; Kaarniranta, K. Oxidative stress, hypoxia, and autophagy in the neovascular processes of age-related macular degeneration. *BioMed Res. Int.* **2014**, *2014*. [CrossRef] [PubMed]
97. Liu, X.-H.; Yu, R.B.; Liu, R.; Hao, Z.-X.; Han, C.-C.; Zhu, Z.-H.; Ma, L. Association between lutein and zeaxanthin status and the risk of cataract: A meta-analysis. *Nutrients* **2014**, *6*, 452–465. [CrossRef] [PubMed]
98. Age-Related Eye Disease Study 2 Research Group; Chew, E.Y.; SanGiovanni, J.P.; Ferris, F.L.; Wong, W.T.; Agron, E.; Clemons, T.E.; Sperduto, R.; Danis, R.; Chandra, S.R.; et al. Lutein/zeaxanthin for the treatment of age-related cataract: AREDS2 randomized trial report no. 4. *JAMA Ophthalmol.* **2013**, *131*, 843–850. [CrossRef] [PubMed]
99. Bungau, S.; Abdel-Daim, M.M.; Tit, D.M.; Ghanem, E.; Sato, S.; Maruyama-Inoue, M.; Yamane, S.; Kadonosono, K. Health benefits of polyphenols and carotenoids in age-related eye diseases. *Oxid. Med. Cell. Longev.* **2019**, *2019*. [CrossRef]
100. Sandmann, G. Carotenoids of biotechnological importance. *Adv. Biochem. Eng. Biotechnol.* **2015**, *148*, 449–467. [PubMed]
101. Bernstein, P.S.; Li, B.; Vachali, P.P.; Gorusupudi, A.; Shyam, R.; Henriksen, B.S.; Nolan, J.M. Lutein, zeaxanthin, and meso-zeaxanthin: The basic and clinical science underlying carotenoid-based nutritional interventions against ocular disease. *Prog. Retin. Eye Res.* **2016**, *50*, 34–66. [CrossRef]
102. Gonçalves, A.; Estevinho, B.N.; Rocha, F. Microencapsulation of vitamin A: A review. *Trends Food Sci. Tech.* **2016**, *51*, 76–87.
103. West, K.P. Epidemiology and prevention of vitamin A deficiency disorders. *Retinoids Biol. Biochem. Dis.* **2015**, 505–527.
104. Hammond, B.R.; Fletcher, L.M.; Roos, F.; Wittwer, J.; Schalch, W. A double-blind, placebo-controlled study on the effects of lutein and zeaxanthin on photostress recovery, glare disability, and chromatic contrast. *Investig. Ophthalmol. Vis. Sci.* **2014**, *55*, 8583–8589. [CrossRef] [PubMed]
105. Yao, Y.; Qiu, Q.H.; Wu, X.W.; Cai, Z.Y.; Xu, S.; Liang, X.Q. Lutein supplementation improves visual performance in Chinese drivers: 1-year randomized, double-blind, placebo-controlled study. *Nutrition* **2013**, *29*, 958–964. [CrossRef]
106. Nolan, J.M.; Power, R.; Stringham, J.; Dennison, J.; Stack, J.; Kelly, D.; Moran, R.; Akuffo, K.O.; Corcoran, L.; Beatty, S. Author response: Comments on enrichment of macular pigment enhances contrast sensitivity in subjects free of retinal disease: CREST-Report 1. *Investig. Ophthalmol. Vis. Sci.* **2016**, *57*, 5416. [CrossRef]
107. World Health Organization. Dementia. 2019. Available online: https://www.who.int/news-room/fact-sheets/detail/dementia (accessed on 5 March 2019).
108. Renzi, L.M.; Dengler, M.J.; Puente, A.; Miller, L.S.; Hammond, B.R.Jr. Relationships between macular pigment optical density and cognitive function in unimpaired and mildly cognitively impaired older adults. *Neurobiol. Aging* **2014**, *35*, 1695–1699. [CrossRef]
109. Feeney, J.; Finucane, C.; Savva, G.M.; Cronin, H.; Beatty, S.; Nolan, J.M.; Kenny, R.A. Low macular pigment optical density is associated with lower cognitive performance in a large, population-based sample of older adults. *Neurobiol. Aging* **2013**, *34*, 2449–2456. [CrossRef]
110. Rebecca, P.; Robert, C.; Stephen, B.; Riona, M.; Rachel, M.; Jim, S.; Alan, H.N.; John, N.M. Supplemental retinal carotenoids enhance memory in healthy individuals with low levels of macular pigment in a randomized, double-blind, placebo-controlled clinical trial. *J. Alzheimer's Dis.* **2018**, *61*, 947–961.
111. Rubin, L.P.; Ross, A.C.; Stephensen, C.B.; Bohn, T.; Tanumihardjo, S.A. Metabolic effects of inflammation on vitamin A and carotenoids in humans and animal models. *Adv. Nutr.* **2017**, *8*, 197–212. [CrossRef]
112. Jing, L.; Xiao, M.; Dong, H.; Lin, J.; Chen, G.; Ling, W.; Chen, Y. Serum carotenoids are inversely associated with RBP4 and other inflammatory markers in middle-aged and elderly adults. *Nutrients* **2018**, *10*, 260. [CrossRef]

113. Norseen, J.; Hosooka, T.; Hammarstedt, A.; Yore, M.M.; Kant, S.; Aryal, P.; Kiernan, U.A.; Phillips, D.A.; Maruyama, H.; Kraus, B.J.; et al. Retinol-binding protein 4 inhibits insulin signaling in adipocytes by inducing proinflammatory cytokines in macrophages through c-Jun N-terminal kinase- (JNK) and toll-like receptor 4-dependent and retinol-independent mechanism. *Mol. Cell. Biol.* **2012**, *32*, 2010–2019. [CrossRef]
114. Du, M.; Martin, A.; Hays, F.; Johnson, J.; Farjo, R.A.; Farjo, K.M. Serum retinol-binding protein-induced endothelial inflammation is mediated through the activation of toll-like receptor 4. *Mol. Vis.* **2017**, *23*, 185–197.
115. Moraes-Vieira, P.M.; Yore, M.M.; Dwyer, P.M.; Syed, I.; Aryal, P.; Kahn, B.B. RBP4 activates antigen-presenting cells leading to adipose tissue inflammation and systemic insulin resistance. *Cell MeTable* **2014**, *19*, 512–526. [CrossRef]
116. Christensen, K.; Gleason, C.E.; Mares, J.A. Dietary carotenoids and cognitive function among US adults, NHANES 2011–2014. *Nutr. Neurosci.* **2018**, 1–9. [CrossRef] [PubMed]
117. Hadad, N.; Levy, R. Combination of EPA with carotenoids and polyphenol synergistically attenuated the transformation of microglia to M1 phenotype via inhibition of NF-κB. *Neuromol. Med.* **2017**, *19*, 436–451. [CrossRef]
118. Lin, H.-C.; Lin, M.-H.; Liao, J.-H.; Wu, T.-H.; Lee, T.-H.; Mi, F.-L.; Wu, C.H.; Chen, K.C.; Cheng, C.H.; Lin, C.W. Antroquinonol, a ubiquinone derivative from the mushroom *Antrodia camphorata*, inhibits colon cancer stem cell-like properties: Insights into the molecular mechanism and inhibitory targets. *J. Agric. Food Chem.* **2017**, *65*, 51–59. [CrossRef] [PubMed]
119. Wang, J.; Li, L.; Wang, Z.; Cui, Y.; Tan, X.; Yuan, T.; Liu, Q.; Liu, Z.; Liu, X. Supplementation of lycopene attenuates lipopolysaccharide-induced amyloidogenesis and cognitive impairments via mediating neuroinflammation and oxidative stress. *J. Nutr. Biochem.* **2018**, *56*, 16–25. [CrossRef] [PubMed]
120. Krishnaraj, R.N.; Kumari, S.S.; Mukhopadhyay, S.S. Antagonistic molecular interactions of photosynthetic pigments with molecular disease targets: A new approach to treat AD and ALS. *J. Recept. Signal Transduct.* **2016**, *36*, 67–71. [CrossRef]
121. Xiang, S.; Liu, F.; Lin, J.; Chen, H.; Huang, C.; Chen, L.; Zhou, Y.; Ye, L.; Zhang, K.; Jin, J.; et al. Fucoxanthin inhibits β-amyloid assembly and attenuates β-amyloid oligomer-induced cognitive impairments. *J. Agric. Food Chem.* **2017**, *65*, 4092–4102. [CrossRef] [PubMed]
122. Ono, K.; Yamada, M. Vitamin A and Alzheimer's disease. *Geriatr. Gerontol. Int.* **2012**, *12*, 180–188. [CrossRef] [PubMed]
123. Sachdeva, A.K.; Chopra, K. Lycopene abrogates Aβ (1–42)-mediated neuroinflammatory cascade in an experimental model of Alzheimer's disease. *J. Nutr. Biochem.* **2015**, *26*, 736–744. [CrossRef] [PubMed]
124. Min, J.Y.; Min, K.B. Serum lycopene, lutein and zeaxanthin, and the risk of Alzheimer's disease mortality in older adults. *Dement. Geriatr. Cogn. Disord.* **2014**, *37*, 246–256. [CrossRef]
125. World Health Organization. Cardiovascular Disease. 2019. Available online: https://www.who.int/cardiovascular_diseases/en/ (accessed on 5 March 2019).
126. Leening, M.J.; Ferket, B.S.; Steyerberg, E.W.; Kavousi, M.; Deckers, J.W.; Nieboer, D.; Heeringa, J.; Portegies, M.L.; Hofman, A.; Ikram, M.A.; et al. Sex differences in lifetime risk and first manifestation of cardiovascular disease: Prospective population based cohort study. *BMJ* **2014**, *349*, g5992. [CrossRef] [PubMed]
127. Siti, H.N.; Kamisah, Y.; Kamsiah, J. The role of oxidative stress, antioxidants and vascular inflammation in cardiovascular disease (a review). *Vascul. Pharmacol.* **2015**, *71*, 40–56. [CrossRef]
128. Bugger, H.; Abel, E.D. Molecular mechanisms for myocardial mitochondrial dysfunction in the metabolic syndrome. *Clin. Sci.* **2008**, *114*, 195–210. [CrossRef]
129. Lee, R.; Margaritis, M.; Channon, M.K.; Antoniades, C. Evaluating oxidative stress in human cardiovascular disease: Methodological aspects and considerations. *Curr. Med. Chem.* **2012**, *19*, 2504–2520. [CrossRef] [PubMed]
130. Thies, F.; Mills, L.M.; Moir, S.; Masson, L.F. Cardiovascular benefits of lycopene: Fantasy or reality? *Proc. Nutr. Soc.* **2017**, *76*, 122–129. [CrossRef]
131. Alvi, S.S.; Iqbal, D.; Ahmad, S.; Khan, M.S. Molecular rationale delineating the role of lycopene as a potent HMG-CoA reductase inhibitor: In vitro and in silico study. *Nat. Prod. Res.* **2016**, *30*, 2111–2114. [CrossRef]

132. Sandoval, V.; Rodríguez-Rodríguez, R.; Martínez-Garza, U.; Rosell-Cardona, C.; Lamuela-Raventós, R.M.; Marrero, P.F.; Haro, D.; Relat, J. Mediterranean tomato-based sofrito sauce improves fibroblast growth factor 21 (FGF21) signaling in white adipose tissue of obese ZUCKER rats. *Mol. Nutr. Food Res.* **2018**, *62*, 1700606. [CrossRef]
133. Chang, J.; Zhang, Y.; Li, Y.; Lu, K.; Shen, Y.; Guo, Y.; Qi, Q.; Wang, M.; Zhang, S. NrF2/ARE and NF-κB pathway regulation may be the mechanism for lutein inhibition of human breast cancer cell. *Future Oncol.* **2018**, *14*, 719–726. [CrossRef]
134. Chung, R.W.S.; Leanderson, P.; Lundberg, A.K.; Jonasson, L. Lutein exerts anti-inflammatory effects in patients with coronary artery disease. *Atherosclerosis* **2017**, *262*, 87–93. [CrossRef]
135. Maria, A.G.; Graziano, R.; Nicolantonio, D.O. Carotenoids: Potential allies of cardiovascular health? *Food Nutr. Res.* **2015**, *59*, 26762. [CrossRef]
136. Kishimoto, Y.; Taguchi, C.; Saita, E.; Suzuki-Sugihara, N.; Nishiyama, H.; Wang, W.; Masuda, Y.; Kondo, K. Additional consumption of one egg per day increases serum lutein plus zeaxanthin concentration and lowers oxidized low-density lipoprotein in moderately hypercholesterolemic males. *Food Res. Int.* **2017**, *99*, 944–949. [CrossRef]
137. Leermakers, E.T.; Darweesh, S.K.; Baena, C.P.; Moreira, E.M.; Melo van Lent, D.; Tielemans, M.J.; Muka, T.; Chowdhury, R.; Bramer, W.M.; Kiefte-de Jong, J.C.; et al. The effects of lutein on cardiometabolic health across the life course: A systematic review and meta-analysis. *Am. J. Clin. Nutr.* **2016**, *103*, 481–494. [CrossRef]
138. Costa-Rodrigues, J.; Pinho, O.; Monteiro, P.R.R. Can lycopene be considered an effective protection against cardiovascular disease? *Food Chem.* **2018**, *245*, 1148–1153. [CrossRef]
139. Cheng, H.M.; Koutsidis, G.; Lodge, J.K.; Ashor, A.; Siervo, M.; Lara, J. Tomato and lycopene supplementation and cardiovascular risk factors: A systematic review and meta-analysis. *Atherosclerosis* **2017**, *257*, 100–108. [CrossRef]
140. Greene, C.M.; Waters, D.; Clark, R.M.; Contois, J.H.; Fernandez, M.L. Plasma LDL and HDL characteristics and carotenoid content are positively influenced by egg consumption in an elderly population. *Nutr. MeTable* **2006**, *3*, 6. [CrossRef] [PubMed]
141. Song, B.; Liu, K.; Gao, Y.; Zhao, L.; Fang, H.; Li, Y.; Pei, L.; Xu, Y. Lycopene and risk of cardiovascular diseases: A meta-analysis of observational studies. *Mol. Nutr. Food Res.* **2017**, *61*, 1601009. [CrossRef]
142. Osganian, S.K.; Stampfer, M.J.; Rimm, E.; Spiegelman, D.; Manson, J.E.; Willett, W.C. Dietary carotenoids and risk of coronary artery disease in women. *Am. J. Clin. Nutr.* **2003**, *77*, 1390–1399. [CrossRef] [PubMed]
143. Sesso, H.D.; Liu, S.; Gaziano, J.M.; Buring, J.E. Dietary lycopene, tomato-based food products and cardiovascular disease in women. *J. Nutr.* **2003**, *133*, 2336–2341. [CrossRef]
144. Tavani, A.; Gallus, S.; Negri, E.; Parpinel, M.; La Vecchia, C. Dietary intake of carotenoids and retinol and the risk of acute myocardial infarction in Italy. *Free Radic. Res.* **2006**, *40*, 659–664. [CrossRef] [PubMed]
145. Li, X.; Xu, J. Dietary and circulating lycopene and stroke risk: A meta-analysis of prospective studies. *Sci. Rep.* **2014**, *4*, 5031. [CrossRef]
146. Borel, P.; Desmarchelier, C.; Nowicki, M.; Bott, R. Lycopene bioavailability is associated with a combination of genetic variants. *Free Radic. Biol. Med.* **2015**, *83*, 238–244. [CrossRef]
147. Zubair, N.; Kooperberg, C.; Liu, J.; Di, C.; Peters, U.; Neuhouser, M.L. Genetic variation predicts serum lycopene concentrations in a multiethnic population of postmenopausal women. *J. Nutr.* **2015**, *145*, 187–192. [CrossRef]
148. World Health Organization. Cancer. 2019. Available online: https://www.who.int/cancer/en/ (accessed on 7 March 2019).
149. International Agency for Research on Cancer (IARC). Latest Global Cancer Data: Cancer Burden Rises to 18.1 Million New Cases and 9.6 Million Cancer Deaths in 2018. 2018. Available online: https://www.who.int/cancer/PRGlobocanFinal.pdf?ua=1 (accessed on 7 March 2019).
150. Liu, X.; Song, M.; Gao, Z.; Cai, X.; Dixon, W.; Chen, X.; Cao, Y.; Xiao, H. Stereoisomers of astaxanthin inhibit human colon cancer cell growth by inducing G2/M cell cycle arrest and apoptosis. *J. Agric. Food Chem.* **2016**, *64*, 7750–7759. [CrossRef]
151. Rafi, M.M.; Kanakasabai, S.; Gokarn, S.V.; Krueger, E.G.; Bright, J.J. Dietary lutein modulates growth and survival genes in prostate cancer cells. *J. Med. Food* **2015**, *18*, 173–181. [CrossRef] [PubMed]
152. Shareck, M.; Rousseau, M.C.; Koushik, A.; Siemiatycki, J.; Parent, M.-E. Inverse association between dietary intake of selected carotenoids and vitamin C and risk of lung cancer. *Front. Oncol.* **2017**, *7*, 23. [CrossRef]

153. Tuzcu, M.; Orhan, C.; Muz, O.E.; Sahin, N.; Juturu, V.; Sahin, K. Lutein and zeaxanthin isomers modulates lipid metabolism and the inflammatory state of retina in obesity-induced high-fat diet rodent model. *BMC Ophthalmol.* **2017**, *17*, 129. [CrossRef]
154. Cha, J.H.; Kim, W.K.; Ha, A.W.; Kim, M.H.; Chang, M.J. Anti-inflammatory effect of lycopene in SW480 human colorectal cancer cells. *Nutr. Res. Pract.* **2017**, *11*, 90–96. [CrossRef]
155. De Waart, F.G.; Schouten, E.G.; Stalenhoef, A.F.H.; Kok, F.J. Serum carotenoids, α-tocopherol and mortality risk in a prospective study among Dutch elderly. *Int. J. Epidemiol.* **2001**, *30*, 136–143. [CrossRef]
156. Aizawa, K.; Liu, C.; Tang, S.; Veeramachaneni, S.; Hu, K.Q.; Smith, D.E.; Wang, X.D. Tobacco carcinogen induces both lung cancer and nonalcoholic steatohepatitis and hepatocellular carcinomas in ferrets which can be attenuated by lycopene supplementation. *Int. J. Cancer* **2016**, *139*, 1171–1181. [CrossRef] [PubMed]
157. Middha, P.; Weinstein, S.J.; Männistö, S.; Albanes, D.; Mondul, A.M. β-carotene supplementation and lung cancer incidence in the ATBC study: The role of tar and nicotine. *Nicotine Tob. Res.* **2018**. [CrossRef] [PubMed]
158. Russell, R.M. Beta-carotene and lung cancer. *Pure Appl. Chem.* **2002**, *74*, 1461–1467. [CrossRef]
159. World Health Organization. Diabetes. 2019. Available online: https://www.who.int/news-room/fact-sheets/detail/diabetes (accessed on 7 March 2019).
160. Fowler, M.J. Microvascular and macrovascular complications of diabetes. *Clin. Diabetes* **2011**, *29*, 116–122. [CrossRef]
161. Ullah, A.; Khan, A.; Khan, I. Diabetes mellitus and oxidative stress—A concise review. *Saudi Pharm. J.* **2016**, *24*, 547–553.
162. Wang, J.; Light, K.; Henderson, M.; O'Loughlin, J.; Mathieu, M.E.; Paradis, G.; Gray-Donald, K. Consumption of added sugars from liquid but not solid sources predicts impaired glucose homeostasis and insulin resistance among youth at risk of obesity. *J. Nutr.* **2013**, *144*, 81–86. [CrossRef]
163. Yan, L.-J. Pathogenesis of chronic hyperglycemia: From reductive stress to oxidative stress. *J. Diabetes Res.* **2014**, *2014*. [CrossRef]
164. Wan, T.-T.; Li, X.-F.; Sun, Y.-M.; Li, Y.-B.; Su, Y. Recent advances in understanding the biochemical and molecular mechanism of diabetic retinopathy. *Biomed. Pharmacother.* **2015**, *74*, 145–147. [CrossRef] [PubMed]
165. Newsholme, P.; Cruzat, V.F.; Keane, K.N.; Carlessi, R.; de Bittencourt, P.I.H., Jr. Molecular mechanisms of ROS production and oxidative stress in diabetes. *Biochem. J.* **2016**, *473*, 4527–4550. [CrossRef]
166. Uchiyama, K.; Naito, Y.; Hasegawa, G.; Nakamura, N.; Takahashi, J.; Yoshikawa, T. Astaxanthin protects beta-cells against glucose toxicity in diabetic db/db mice. *Redox Rep.* **2002**, *7*, 290–293. [CrossRef]
167. Sluijs, I.; Cadier, E.; Beulens, J.W.; van der, A.D.; Spijkerman, A.M.; van der Schouw, Y.T. Dietary intake of carotenoids and risk of type 2 diabetes. *Nutr. Metab. Cardiovasc. Dis.* **2015**, *25*, 376–381. [CrossRef] [PubMed]
168. Arnlov, J.; Zethelius, B.; Riserus, U.; Basu, S.; Berne, C.; Vessby, B.; Alfthan, G.; Helmersson, J.; Uppsala Longitudinal Study of Adult Men Study. Serum and dietary beta-carotene and alpha-tocopherol and incidence of type 2 diabetes mellitus in a community-based study of Swedish men: Report from the Uppsala Longitudinal Study of Adult Men (ULSAM) study. *Diabetologia* **2009**, *52*, 97–105. [CrossRef] [PubMed]
169. Maeda, H.; Hosokawa, M.; Sashima, T.; Murakami-Funayama, K.; Miyashita, K. Anti-obesity and anti-diabetic effects of fucoxanthin on diet-induced obesity conditions in a murine model. *Mol. Med. Rep.* **2009**, *2*, 897–902. [CrossRef] [PubMed]
170. Manabe, E.; Handa, O.; Naito, Y.; Mizushima, K.; Akagiri, S.; Adachi, S.; Takagi, T.; Kokura, S.; Maoka, T.; Yoshikawa, T. Astaxanthin protects mesangial cells from hyperglycemia-induced oxidative signaling. *J. Cell. Biochem.* **2008**, *103*, 1925–1937. [CrossRef] [PubMed]
171. Kim, Y.J.; Kim, Y.A.; Yokozawa, T. Protection against oxidative stress, inflammation, and apoptosis of high-glucose-exposed proximal tubular epithelial cells by astaxanthin. *J. Agric. Food Chem.* **2009**, *57*, 8793–8797. [CrossRef]
172. Akbaraly, T.N.; Fontbonne, A.; Favier, A.; Berr, C. Plasma carotenoids and onset of dysglycemia in an elderly population. *Diabetes Care* **2008**, *31*, 1355–1359. [CrossRef]
173. International Osteoporosis Foundation. Facts and Statistics. 2017. Available online: https://www.iofbonehealth.org/facts-statistics (accessed on 8 March 2019).
174. Johnell, O.; Kanis, J.A. An estimate of the worldwide prevalence and disability associated with osteoporotic fractures. *Osteoporos. Int.* **2006**, *17*, 1726–1733. [CrossRef]

175. Melton, L.J., 3rd.; Crowson, C.S.; O'Fallon, W.M. Fracture incidence in Olmsted County, Minnesota: Comparison of urban with rural rates and changes in urban rates over time. *Osteoporos. Int.* **1999**, *9*, 29–37. [CrossRef]
176. Gullberg, B.; Johnell, O.; Kanis, J.A. World-wide projections for hip fracture. *Osteoporos. Int.* **1997**, *7*, 407. [CrossRef] [PubMed]
177. Astley, S.B.; Hughes, D.A.; Wright, A.J.; Elliott, R.M.; Southon, S. DNA damage and susceptibility to oxidative damage in lymphocytes: Effects of carotenoids in vitro and in vivo. *Br. J. Nutr.* **2004**, *91*, 53–61. [CrossRef]
178. Almeida, M.; Han, L.; Martin-Millan, M.; O'Brien, C.A.; Manolagas, S.C. Oxidative stress antagonizes Wnt signaling in osteoblast precursors by diverting beta-catenin from T cell factor- to forkhead box O-mediated transcription. *J. Biol. Chem.* **2007**, *282*, 27298–27305. [CrossRef] [PubMed]
179. Cao, W.T.; Zeng, F.F.; Li, B.L.; Lin, J.S.; Liang, Y.Y.; Chen, Y.M. Higher dietary carotenoid intake associated with lower risk of hip fracture in middle-aged and elderly Chinese: A matched case-control study. *Bone* **2018**, *111*, 116–122. [CrossRef]
180. Dai, Z.; Wang, R.; Ang, L.W.; Low, Y.L.; Yuan, J.M.; Koh, W.P. Protective effects of dietary carotenoids on risk of hip fracture in men: The Singapore Chinese Health Study. *J. Bone Miner. Res.* **2014**, *29*, 408–417. [CrossRef]
181. Zhang, Z.Q.; Cao, W.T.; Liu, J.; Cao, Y.; Su, Y.X.; Chen, Y.M. Greater serum carotenoid concentration associated with higher bone mineral density in Chinese adults. *Osteoporos. Int.* **2016**, *27*, 1593–1601. [CrossRef] [PubMed]
182. Li, H.; Huang, C.; Zhu, J.; Gao, K.; Fang, J.; Li, H. Lutein suppresses oxidative stress and inflammation by Nrf2 activation in an osteoporosis rat model. *Med. Sci. Monit.* **2018**, *24*, 5071–5075. [CrossRef]
183. Tominari, T.; Matsumoto, C.; Watanabe, K.; Hirata, M.; Grundler, F.M.W.; Inada, M.; Miyaura, C. Lutein, a carotenoid, suppresses osteoclastic bone resorption and stimulates bone formation in cultures. *J. Biosci. Biotechnol. Biochem.* **2017**, *81*, 302–306. [CrossRef] [PubMed]
184. Bovier, E.R.; Hammond, B.R. The macular carotenoids lutein and zeaxanthin are related to increased bone density in young healthy adults. *Foods* **2017**, *6*, 78. [CrossRef]
185. Willis, L.M.; Shukitt-Hale, B.; Joseph, J.A. Modulation of cognition and behavior in aged animals: Role for antioxidant- and essential fatty acid-rich plant foods. *Am. J. Clin. Nutr.* **2009**, *89*, 1602–1606. [CrossRef]
186. Zhang, Z.; Han, S.; Wang, H.; Wang, T. Lutein extends the lifespan of *Drosophila melanogaster*. *Arch. Gerontol. Geriatr.* **2014**, *58*, 153–159. [CrossRef]
187. Neena, P.; Thomas, K.; Cynthia, H.; Shannon, H.; Rosemarie, A.; Marvin, T.; Salvador, G. Regulation of the extracellular matrix remodeling by lutein in dermal fibroblasts, melanoma cells, and ultraviolet radiation exposed fibroblasts. *Arch. Dermatol. Res.* **2007**, *299*, 373–379.
188. Bahrami, H.; Melia, M.; Dagnelie, G. Lutein supplementation in retinitis pigmentosa: PC-based vision assessment in a randomized double-masked placebo-controlled clinical trial. *BMC Ophthalmol.* **2006**, *6*, 23. [CrossRef] [PubMed]
189. Yazaki, K.; Yoshikoshi, C.; Oshiro, S.; Yanase, S. Supplemental cellular protection by a carotenoid extends lifespan via Ins/IGF-signaling in *Caenorhabditis elegans*. *Oxid. Med. Cell. Longev.* **2011**, *2011*. [CrossRef]
190. Giannakou, M.E.; Goss, M.; Junger, M.A.; Hafen, E.; Leevers, S.J.; Partridge, L. Long-lived Drosophila with overexpressed dFOXO in adult fat body. *Science* **2004**, *305*, 361. [CrossRef] [PubMed]
191. Lashmanova, E.; Proshkina, E.; Zhikrivetskaya, S.; Shevchenko, O.; Marusich, E.; Leonov, S.; Melerzanov, A.; Zhavoronkov, A.; Moskalev, A. Fucoxanthin increases lifespan of *Drosophila melanogaster* and *Caenorhabditis elegans*. *Pharmacol. Res.* **2015**, *100*, 228–241. [CrossRef]
192. Johnson, E.J. Role of lutein and zeaxanthin in visual and cognitive function throughout the lifespan. *Nutr. Rev.* **2014**, *72*, 605–612. [CrossRef] [PubMed]
193. Ravikrishnan, R.; Rusia, S.; Ilamurugan, G.; Salunkhe, U.; Deshpande, J.; Shankaranarayanan, J.; Shankaranarayana, M.L.; Soni, M.G. Safety assessment of lutein and zeaxanthin (Lutemax 2020): Subchronic toxicity and mutagenicity studies. *Food Chem. Toxicol.* **2011**, *49*, 2841–2848. [CrossRef] [PubMed]
194. Harikumar, K.B.; Nimita, C.V.; Preethi, K.C.; Kuttan, R.; Deshpande, J. Toxicity profile of lutein and lutein ester isolated from marigold flowers (*Tagetes erecta*). *Int. J. Toxicol.* **2008**, *27*, 1–9. [CrossRef]
195. Institute of Medicine (US) Panel on Dietary Antioxidants and Related Compounds. *Dietary Reference Intakes for Vitamin C, Vitamin E, Selenium, and Carotenoids*; National Academies Press (US): Washington, DC, USA, 2000.
196. Joint, F.A.O. *Evaluation of Certain Food Additives: Sixty-Third Report of the Joint FAO/WHO Expert Committee on Food Additives*; World Health Organization: Geneva, Switzerland, June 2004; pp. 23–26.

197. European Food Safety Authority. Scientific opinion on the re-evaluation of lutein [e 161b] as a food additive. *EFSA J.* **2010**, *8*, 1678. [CrossRef]
198. European Food Safety Authority (EFSA). Safety, bioavailability and suitability of lutein for the particular nutritional use by infants and young children—Scientific Opinion of the Panel on Dietetic Products, Nutrition and Allergies. *EFSA J.* **2008**, *823*, 1–24.
199. Zheng, Y.F.; Bae, S.H.; Kwon, M.J.; Park, J.B.; Choi, H.D.; Shin, W.G.; Bae, S.K. Inhibitory effects of astaxanthin, b-cryptoxanthin, canthaxanthin, lutein, and zeaxanthin on cytochrome P450 enzyme activities. *Food Chem. Toxicol.* **2013**, *59*, 78–85. [CrossRef] [PubMed]
200. Amengual, J.; Lobo, G.P.; Golczak, M.; Li, H.N.; Klimova, T.; Hoppel, C.L.; Wyss, A.; Palczewski, K.; von Lintig, J. A mitochondrial enzyme degrades carotenoids and protects against oxidative stress. *FASEB J.* **2011**, *25*, 948–959. [CrossRef]
201. Olmedilla, B.; Granado, F.; Southon, S.; Wright, A.J.; Blanco, I.; Gil-Martinez, E.; van den Berg, H.; Thurnham, D.; Corridan, B.; Chopra, M.; et al. A European multicentre, placebo-controlled supplementation study with alpha-tocopherol, carotene-rich palm oil, lutein or lycopene: Analysis of serum responses. *Clin. Sci.* **2002**, *102*, 447–456. [CrossRef]
202. Satia, J.A.; Littman, A.; Slatore, C.G.; Galanko, J.A.; White, E. Long-term use of beta-carotene, retinol, lycopene, and lutein supplements and lung cancer risk: Results from the Vitamins and Lifestyle (VITAL) study. *Am. J. Epidemiol.* **2009**, *169*, 815–828, Erratum in **2009**, *169*, 1409. [CrossRef] [PubMed]
203. Choi, R.Y.; Chortkoff, S.C.; Gorusupudi, A.; Bernstein, P.S. Crystalline maculopathy associated with high-dose lutein supplementation. *JAMA Ophthalmol.* **2016**, *134*, 1445–1448. [CrossRef]
204. Buscemi, S.; Corleo, D.; Di Pace, F.; Petroni, M.L.; Satriano, A.; Marchesini, G. The effect of lutein on eye and extra-eye health. *Nutrients* **2018**, *10*, 1321. [CrossRef]
205. Gorusupudi, A.; Nelson, K.; Bernstein, P.S. The age-related eye disease 2 study: Micronutrients in the treatment of macular degeneration. *Adv. Nutr.* **2017**, *8*, 40–53. [CrossRef]

molecules

MDPI

Review

Genuine and Sequestered Natural Products from the Genus *Orobanche* (Orobanchaceae, Lamiales)

Friederike Scharenberg and Christian Zidorn *

Pharmazeutisches Institut, Abteilung Pharmazeutische Biologie, Christian-Albrechts-Universität zu Kiel, Gutenbergstraße 76, 24118 Kiel, Germany; fscharenberg@pharmazie.uni-kiel.de
* Correspondence: czidorn@pharmazie.uni-kiel.de; Tel.: +49-431-880-1139

Received: 10 October 2018; Accepted: 28 October 2018; Published: 30 October 2018

Abstract: The present review gives an overview about natural products from the holoparasitic genus *Orobanche* (Orobanchaceae). We cover both genuine natural products as well as compounds sequestered by *Orobanche* taxa from their host plants. However, the distinction between these two categories is not always easy. In cases where the respective authors had not indicated the opposite, all compounds detected in *Orobanche* taxa were regarded as genuine *Orobanche* natural products. From the about 200 species of *Orobanche* s.l. (i.e., including *Phelipanche*) known worldwide, only 26 species have so far been investigated phytochemically (22 *Orobanche* and four *Phelipanche* species), from 17 *Orobanche* and three *Phelipanche* species defined natural products (and not only natural product classes) have been reported. For two species of *Orobanche* and one of *Phelipanche* dedicated studies have been performed to analyze the phenomenon of natural product sequestration by parasitic plants from their host plants. In total, 70 presumably genuine natural products and 19 sequestered natural products have been described from *Orobanche* s.l.; these form the basis of 140 chemosystematic records (natural product reports per taxon). Bioactivities described for *Orobanche* s.l. extracts and natural products isolated from *Orobanche* species include in addition to antioxidative and anti-inflammatory effects, e.g., analgesic, antifungal and antibacterial activities, inhibition of amyloid β aggregation, memory enhancing effects as well as anti-hypertensive effects, inhibition of blood platelet aggregation, and diuretic effects. Moreover, muscle relaxant and anti-spasmodic effects as well as anti-photoaging effects have been described.

Keywords: *Orobanche* s.l.; Orobanchaceae; Lamiales; natural products; secondary metabolites; phenylpropanoid glycosides; phenylethanoid glycosides; bioactivities of natural products; chemosystematics

1. Introduction

Taxa of the genus *Orobanche* sensu lato (Orobanchaceae) are non-photosynthetic root holoparasites. The genus *Orobanche* s.l. is distributed worldwide. Most of the about 200 species are native to the Northern Hemisphere [1,2]. The phylogeny of *Orobanche* s.l. is still discussed controversially. Park et al., (2008) [3], distinguished five lineages within *Orobanche* s.l. based on morphological, cytological, and (macro-)molecular phylogenetic data. Schneeweiss (2013) [4] suggested treating these lineages as separate genera. From these five lineages, four have traditionally been regarded as sections of *Orobanche* [the respective generic names suggested by Schneeweiss (2013) [4] are indicated in brackets]: *Gymnocaulis* Nutt. (=genus *Aphyllon* Mitch.), *Myzorrhiza* (Phil.) Beck (=sect. *Nothaphyllon* (A.Gray) Heckard = genus *Myzorrhiza* Phil.) [5], *Trionychon* Wallr. (=genus *Phelipanche* Pomel), and *Orobanche* L. (=sect. *Osproleon* Wallr. = genus *Orobanche* L. s.str.). The only representative of the fifth clade, *Orobanche latisquama* Reut. ex Boiss. (=genus *Boulardia* F.W.Schultz), was formerly assigned to sect. *Orobanche*. Additionally, the genus *Phelypaea* is part of the clade comprising *Orobanche* s.l. [4]. On the basis of recent taxonomic and phylogenetic data, the genus *Orobanche* s.l. was split into two separate genera, *Orobanche* and *Phelipanche* [6]. Following this decision the names *Phelipanche ramosa* (L.) Pomel and *P. aegyptiaca* (Pers.) Pomel, instead of *Orobanche ramosa* L. and *O. aegyptiaca* Pers. (of sect. *Trionychon*) are applicable [7]. In the following paragraphs, the new species names are used and synonyms in the original publications are indicated if applicable. *Orobanche* species play an important (negative) role in agriculture as they can pose serious threats to major crop plants [8,9]. Many research papers are focused on host-parasite interactions via strigolactones (seed germination promoters) in terms of weed management. Less is known about phytochemical compounds in the parasitic species. This review is intended to give an overview over secondary metabolites synthesized by *Orobanche* s.l. known so far. For *Orobanche* sections *Gymnocaulis* and *Myzorrhiza* as well as for *O. latisquama*, no studies on secondary metabolites have been published yet. Members of *Orobanche* section *Orobanche* and of *Phelipanche* that have been phytochemically analyzed are reviewed in alphabetical order. An additional paragraph describes sequestration of secondary metabolites from host plants. Characterizations of bioactivities of *Orobanche* s.l. extracts and pure compounds isolated from *Orobanche* species are described separately. Literature data were retrieved from SciFinder and ISI Web of Knowledge databases. Reports until the end of 2017 were taken into account (exact search terms can be found in Supplementary Text S1). All taxon names were reviewed and accepted names according to The Plant List are used throughout the manuscript [10]. Usage of synonyms deviating from The Plant List in the cited literature was mentioned when applicable.

2. Results and Discussion

2.1. Literature Data on Natural Products from Orobanche Species

In the genus *Orobanche* s.l. the following classes of secondary metabolites have been found: aromatic aldehydes, ketones, and phenylmethanoids (Figure 1), phenylethanoids (Figure 2), phenylethanoid glycosides (Figure 3), phenylpropanoid glycosides (Figures 4–8), phenolic acids (Figures 9 and 10), lignans (Figures 11 and 12), flavonoids (Figure 13), a tropone derivative (Figure 14), and sterols (Figures 15–20). Phenylpropanoid glycosides represent the largest group of secondary metabolites isolated from *Orobanche* species. Moreover, bi- and tricyclic sesquiterpenes, iridoid glycosides, acyclic, monocyclic, and bicyclic monoterpenes, and carotenoids have been detected in *Orobanche*. Along with secondary metabolites the isolation of some primary metabolites such as fatty acids, alkanes, alkenes, ketones, fatty alcohols, and sugar alcohols has been described. Species that have been investigated for their phytochemical compounds are subsequently listed in alphabetical order within their corresponding genus. The secondary metabolites synthesized by *Orobanche* species are shown in Figures 1–20 and compounds are numbered consecutively from **1** to **70**. Components of essential oils are listed in the corresponding paragraphs but individual chemical structures are neither displayed nor numbered. Primary metabolites that have been isolated along with secondary metabolites and that are mentioned in the corresponding papers are only mentioned in the text (no figure, no numbers). Secondary metabolites sequestered from host species by *Orobanche* species, comprising alkaloids (Figures 21–24), polyacetylenes (Figure 25), and cannabinoids (Figure 26), are shown in Figures 21–26, and these sequestered compounds are numbered consecutively from **S1** to **S19**. Information about collection site, country of origin, analyzed plant parts, and extraction solvents as well as analytical methods used for compound identification and structure elucidation are listed in this order in brackets after the corresponding taxon. Analytical methods include infrared spectroscopy (IR), gas chromatography (GC), gas liquid chromatography (GLC), mass spectrometry (MS), nuclear magnetic resonance spectroscopy (NMR), thin layer chromatography (TLC), high performance thin layer chromatography (HPTLC), and high performance liquid chromatography (HPLC) with ultraviolet (UV) and diode array detectors (DAD). Most authors do not specify the host species of the investigated *Orobanche* samples. Whenever available, information about the host species is mentioned. An additional section is dedicated to reports dealing with more than one *Orobanche* species. Natural products described in these reports are also briefly mentioned in the respective paragraphs for each individual species. An additional section is dedicated to the sequestration of secondary metabolites by *Orobanche* species from their host plants. Moreover, one section deals with bioactivities reported for *Orobanche* extracts and natural products isolated from such extracts. Synonyms of taxon and compound names are only indicated when being mentioned for the first time. Tables giving an overview of all phytochemically investigated species, natural products detected within these species and sequestered by these species, respectively, are available as Supplementary Material (Tables S1 and S2).

2.2. Secondary Metabolites Synthesized by *Orobanche s.l.*

2.2.1. *Orobanche* Sectio *Orobanche* (=sect. *Osproleon* Wallr. = Genus *Orobanche* L. s.str.)

***Orobanche alba* Stephan ex Willd.**—Roudbaraki and Nori-Shargh identified forty different compounds in the essential oil from *O. alba* [province of Guilan, Iran; aerial parts; hydrodistillation; GC, GC-MS, comparison with authentic samples] [host species not mentioned] [11]. Detected compounds included three monoterpene hydrocarbons, twelve oxygenated monoterpenes, five sesquiterpene hydrocarbons, three oxygenated sesquiterpenes, one oxygenated diterpene, and sixteen non-terpenic compounds (aliphatic hydrocarbons, alcohols, ethers, aldehydes, ketones, carboxylic acids, and esters). The monoterpene fraction encompassed bornylangelate, *p*-cymene, limonene, γ-terpinene, *p*-menthone, 1,8-cineol, pinocamphone, linalool, (Z)-iso-citral, nerol, neral (syn. citral B, *cis*-isomer), geraniol, geranial (syn. citral B, *trans*-isomer), and geranylacetate; the sesquiterpene fraction included *trans*-caryophyllene (syn. β-caryophyllene), 6,9-guaiadiene, isobornyl-2-methyl-butyrate, δ-cadinene α-copaene, β-bourbonene, and caryophyllene oxide. The only diterpene detected was manool and the only phenylpropanoid methyl chavicol (syn. estragol). Detected non-terpene compounds comprised *n*-nonanal, neryl acetate, myristic acid, palmitic acid, linoleic acid, linolenic acid, 6-methyl-5-hepten-2-one, 6,10,14-trimethyl-2-pentadecanone, octadecane, heneicosane, docosane, tricosane, tetracosane, pentacosane, nonadecene, isobutyl phthalate, and bis(2-ethylhexyl)phthalate. Fruchier et al. reported the isolation of the tropone derivative orobanone (**45**) from *O. alba* (as *O. epithymum* DC.) [whole plants; water, chloroform; IR, UV, MS, CI-MS, ^{1}H and ^{13}C NMR] [host species not mentioned] [12].

***Orobanche amethystea* Thuill.**—In *O. amethystea* Serafini et al. [Sardinia, Italy; flowering plants; alcoholic extract; ^{1}H and ^{13}C NMR, HPLC, co-elution of extracts with isolated and identified phenylpropanoid glycosides] [host species not mentioned] detected the phenylpropanoid glycosides verbascoside (syn. acteoside, orobanchin, [13]) (**10**) and oraposide (syn. crenatoside and orobanchoside) (**29**) [14].

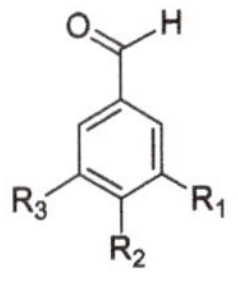

No	Name	R_1	R_2	R_3
1	*p*-Hydroxybenzaldehyde	H	OH	H
2	Protocatechuic aldehyde	OH	OH	H
3	Isovanillin	OH	OCH_3	H
4	Vanillin	OCH_3	OH	H
5	Syringaldehyde	OCH_3	OH	OCH_3

Figure 1. Phenylmethanoids, aromatic aldehydes and ketones **1–5**.

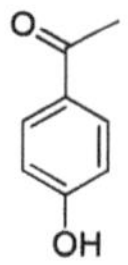

Figure 2. Phenylethanoid, *p*-Hydroxy acetophenone **6**.

***Orobanche anatolica* Boiss. & Reut.**—The occurrence of saponins in *O. anatolica* was mentioned by Aynehchi et al. [Iran; whole plant] [host species not mentioned] but no further specification of structures nor of any analytical methods were indicated in the report [15].

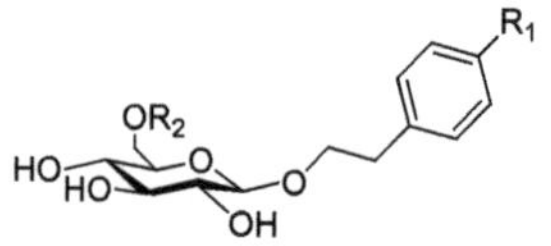

No	Name	R_1	R_2
7	2-Phenylethyl β-primeveroside	H	Xyl
8	Salidroside [1]	OH	H

[1] Syn. rhodioloside.

Figure 3. Non-acylated phenylethanoid glycosides **7** and **8**.

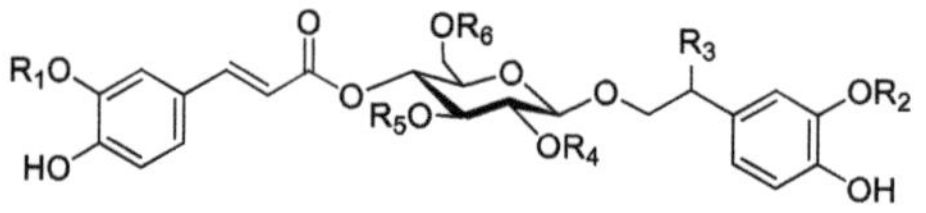

No	Name	R_1	R_2	R_3	R_4	R_5	R_6
9	Desrhamnosyl acteoside	H	H	H	H	H	H
10	Acteoside [1]	H	H	H	H	Rha	H
11	Poliumoside	H	H	H	H	Rha	Rha
12	Arenarioside	H	H	H	H	Rha	Xyl
13	Caerulescenoside	H	H	H	H	(3-*O*-Glc)-Rha	H
14	2′-*O*-Acetylacteoside	H	H	H	Ac	Rha	H
15	2′-*O*-Acetylpoliumoside [2]	H	H	H	Ac	Rha	Rha
16	Pheliposide	H	H	H	Ac	Rha	Xyl
17	Campneoside II	H	H	OH	H	Rha	H
18	Campneoside I	H	H	OCH_3	H	Rha	H
19	Leucosceptoside A	CH_3	H	H	H	Rha	H
20	Cistanoside D	CH_3	CH_3	H	H	Rha	H
21	Orobancheoside B	CH_3	CH_3	H	H	Rha	feruloyl-
22	Orobancheoside A	CH_3	CH_3	H	H	(4-*O*-Ac)-Rha	H

[1] Syn. kusaginin [16], orobanchin, verbascoside; [2] syn. brandioside.

Figure 4. Phenylpropanoid glycosides I, **9–22**.

***Orobanche artemisiae-campestris* Gaudin subsp. *picridis* (F.W.Schultz) O. Bolòs, Vigo, Masalles & Ninot**—Fruchier et al. isolated the tropone derivative orobanone (**45**) [whole plant; water, chloroform; IR, UV, MS, CI-MS, ^{1}H and ^{13}C NMR] [no information about the host] from *O. artemisiae-campestris* subsp. *picridis* (using the synonym *O. picridis* F.W.Schultz) [12].

***Orobanche caryophyllacea* Sm.**—The tropone derivative orobanone (**45**) was isolated from *O. caryophyllacea* (using the synonym *O. major* L.) by Fruchier et al. [whole plant; water, chloroform; IR, UV, MS, CI-MS, ^{1}H and ^{13}C NMR] [no information about the host] [12].

Orobanche cernua **Loefl.**—Qu et al. characterized 17 compounds from *O. cernua* (syn. *O. cumana* Wallr., *O. cernua var. cumana* Wallr.) [Jilin province, China; fresh whole plants; methanol; MS, 1D and 2D NMR, comparison with literature data] [host species not mentioned] [17]. Eleven compounds were identified as phenylpropanoid glycosides [salidroside (**8**), acteoside (**10**), 2′-*O*-acetylacteoside (**14**), campneoside (**18**), leucosceptoside A (**19**), isoacteoside (**23**), isocampneoside (**24**), oraposide (**29**), 3‴-*O*-methylcrenatoside (**30**), descaffeoyl crenatoside (**31**), and isocrenatoside (**32**)]. Furthermore, three phenolic acids [caffeic acid (**34**), *trans*-ferulic acid (**36**), and chlorogenic acid (**37**)], one lignan [dimethyl-6,9,10-trihydroxybenzol[*kl*]xanthene-1,2-dicarboxylate (**38**)], and two flavonoids [apigenin (**42**) and luteolin (**43**)], were found. In a second report Qu et al. described the isolation of a novel phenylethanoid glycoside, 3′-*O*-methylisocrenatoside (**33**) as well as of the known compounds protocatechuic aldehyde (**2**) and methyl caffeate (**35**) from *O. cernua* [Jilin Province, China; fresh whole plant; methanol; IR, MS, NMR] [host species not mentioned] [18]. Yang et al. examined *O. cernua* [Neimenggu province, China; whole plant; ethanol 70%, reflux; HPLC-MS, NMR] [host species not mentioned] isolating twelve compounds: eight phenylpropanoid glycosides [acteoside (**10**), campneoside II (**17**), campneoside I (**18**), leucosceptoside A (**19**), isoacteoside (**23**), cistanoside F (**27**), oraposide (**29**), and isocrenatoside (**32**)]; three lignans [(+)-pinoresinol 4′-*O*-β-D-glucopyranoside (**39**), isoeucommin A (**40**), and (+)-syringaresinol 4′-*O*-β-D-glucopyranoside (**41**)], and one steroid [stigmasterol 3-*O*-β-D-glucoside (**54**)] [19].

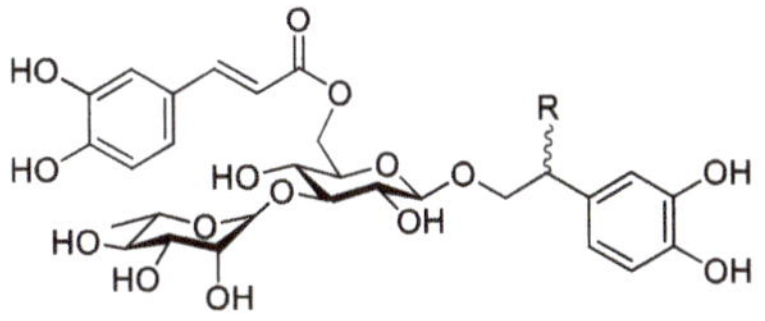

No	Name	R
23	Isoacteoside [1]	H
24	Isocampneoside I [2]	OCH_3

[1] Syn. isoverbascoside, [2] stereochemistry not reported.

Figure 5. Phenylpropanoid glycosides II, **23** and **24**.

Orobanche coerulescens **Stephan ex Willd.**—Zhao et al. isolated the phenylpropanoid glycoside acteoside (**10**) from *O. coerulescens* [Xinjiang province, China; ethanol] [host species not mentioned] [20]. The isolation of isoacteoside (**23**), sinapoyl 4-*O*-β-D-glucoside (**26**), cistanoside F (**27**), oraposide (**29**), and adenosine was described in a second report [21] [Xinjiang province, China; rhizome; ethanol 95%, reflux; TLC, NMR] [host species not mentioned]. Acteoside (**10**), cistanoside F (**27**), and oraposide (**29**) were also isolated by Murayama et al. along with 2-phenylethyl β-primeveroside (**7**), rhodioloside (syn. salidroside) (**8**), descaffeoyl crenatoside (**31**), and isocrenatoside (**32**) from *O. coerulescens* [Niigata prefecture, Japan; whole plant; methanol; IR, UV, HR-FAB-MS, $^1H,^1H$-DQF, COSY, $^1H,^1H$-relayed COSY, HMQC, and HMBC NMR] [host species not mentioned] [22]. Lin et al. isolated two new phenylpropanoid glycosides, caerulescenoside (**13**) and 3′-methyl crenatoside (**30**), along with five known phenylpropanoid glycosides, desrhamnosyl acteoside (**9**), acteoside (**10**), campneoside (**18**), isoacteoside (**23**), and oraposide (**29**) from *O. coerulescens* [Taipei, Taiwan; whole plant; ethanol 95%; IR, UV, ^1H NMR, ^{13}C NMR, ESI-MS, FAB-MS, HR-FAB-MS] [host species not mentioned] [23]. In a second report the authors mentioned the occurrence of another phenylpropanoid glycoside, rossicaside B (**28**), in *O. coerulescens*; ethanol 95%, preparation in accordance with former report, no information about analytical methods) [24]. Wang et al. also isolated a new phenylpropanoid glycoside from the whole plant of *O. coerulescens* [Neimenggu province, China; whole plant; ethanol 50%; TLC, HPLC, MS, NMR] [host species not mentioned] [25]. The structure was identified as 2-(3-methoxy-4-hydroxy)-phenyl-ethanol-1-*O*-α-L-[(1→3)-4-*O*-acetyl-rhamnopyranosyl-4-*O*-feruloyl]-

O-β-D-glucopyranoside and named orobancheoside A (**22**). Additionally, Zhao et al. described the isolation protocatechuic aldehyde (**2**) and caffeic acid (**34**) as well as of β-sitosterol (**50**) and daucosterol (**53**) from *O. coerulescens* [Xinjiang province, China; rhizome; ethanol 95%, reflux; NMR] [host species not mentioned] [26]. Shao et al. identified the phenylpropanoid glycosides acteoside (**10**) and oraposide (**29**), as well as sterols β-sitosterol (**50**), stigmasterol (**51**), and β-daucosterol (**53**) [Neimenggu province, China; ethanol 95%, reflux; TLC, MS, NMR] [host species not mentioned] [27]. Moreover, primary metabolites D-mannitol, glyceryl arachidate, succinic acid, and D-pinitol were reported. Recently, Zhang characterized a new phenethyl alcohol glycoside named orobancheoside B (**21**) from *O. coerulescens* [Neimenggu province, China; whole plant; ethanol 50%; IR, UV, MS, NMR] [host species not mentioned] [28].

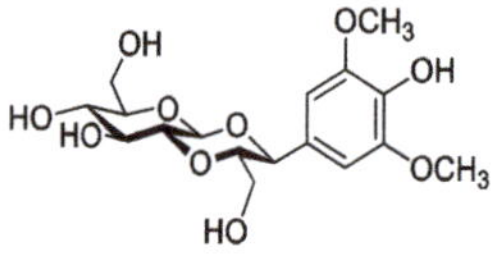

25 Fissistigmoside

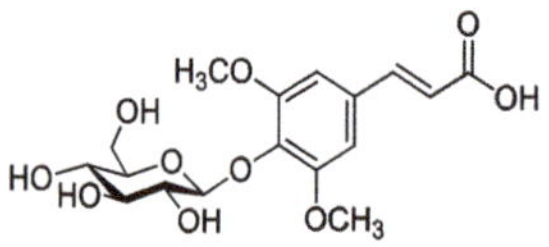

26 Sinapoyl-4-*O*-ß-D-glucoside

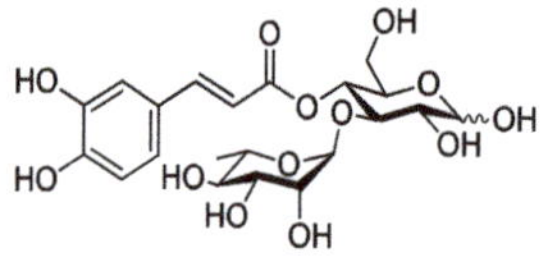

27 Cistanoside F

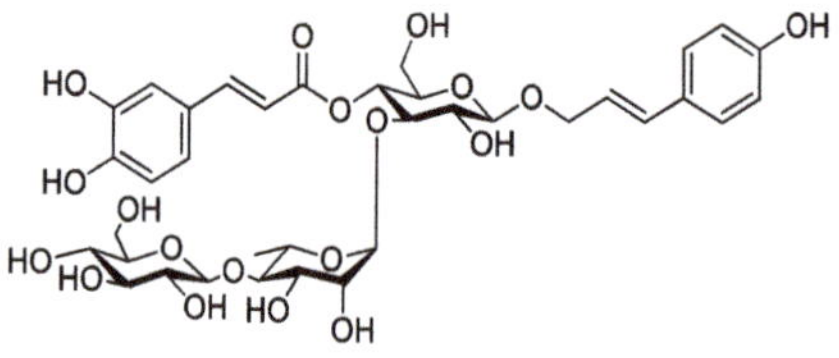

28 Rossicaside B

Figure 6. Phenylpropanoid glycosides III, **25–28**.

***Orobanche crenata* Forssk.**—El-Shabrawy et al. found two phenylpropanoid glycosides in *O. crenata* growing on *Vicia faba* L. [Egypt; chloroform for removal of non-polar compounds, aqueous ethanol 70%; TLC, NMR] [29]. However, their structures were not fully characterized. Afifi et al. extracted secondary metabolites from *O. crenata* parasitizing on *V. faba* [Mansoura, Egypt; aerial parts; ethanol 90%; melting point, TLC, IR, UV, ^{1}H NMR, ^{13}C NMR, ^{13}C NMR-DEPT, FAB-MS] and isolated the known phenylpropanoid glycoside acteoside (**10**) as well as the new phenylpropanoid glycoside oraposide (**29**) [30]. Acteoside (**10**) was also extracted by Gatto et al. [parasitizing on *V. faba*; Apulia, Italy; stems; methanol 80% under reflux; comparison of UV spectra and retention times with standard substances, HPLC-DAD] who furthermore found isoverbascoside (syn. isoacteoside; an isomer of verbascoside) (**23**) and an unidentified caffeic acid derivative [31–33]. Serafini et al. isolated verbascoside (**10**), poliumoside (**11**), and orobanchoside (**29**) from *O. crenata* [Sardinia, Italy; flowering plants; alcoholic extract; ^{1}H and ^{13}C NMR, HPLC, co-elution of extracts with isolated and identified phenylpropanoid glycosides] [host species not mentioned] [14]. Orobanchoside (**29**) was proven to be structurally identical with oraposide and oraposide by Nishibe et al. in the same year [34]. Nada and El-Chaghaby analyzed ethanolic (80%) extracts of *O. crenata* grown on *V. faba* by GC-MS and postulated the occurrence of 6-monohydroxyflavone, glycitein, actinobolin, hexestrol, and 2,4-di-tert-butylphenyl benzoate [Egypt; ethanol 80%; GC-MS] [35]. However, none of these compounds are considered any further here, because the data on the used GC system are incomplete and data on peak identification procedures are completely missing. Until contrary evidence will have been procured, we do not consider 6-monohydroxyflavone, glycitein, actinobolin, hexestrol, and 2,4-di-tert-butylphenyl benzoate natural products which have been detected in the genus *Orobanche*. Dini et al. investigated the phytochemistry of *O. crenata* using the synonym

O. speciosa DC. [Molise, Italy; aerial parts; petroleum ether, chloroform, methanol; comparison of UV, IR, ^{1}H and ^{13}C NMR spectral data with literature data] [36]. The three phenylpropanoid glycosides verbascoside (**10**), poliumoside (**11**), and oraposide (**29**) were detected. Along with these compounds the authors also isolated *p*-hydroxy benzaldehyde (**1**), isovanillin (**3**), vanillin (**4**), syringaldehyde (**5**), and *p*-hydroxy acetophenone (**6**). Fruchier et al. reported the isolation of the tropone derivative orobanone (**45**) from *O. crenata* in their investigation of the occurrence of this secondary metabolite in various *Orobanche* species [whole plant; water, chloroform; IR, UV, MS, CI-MS, ^{1}H and ^{13}C NMR] [host species not mentioned] (see extra paragraph and supplementary material) [12]. Abbes et al. described the extraction of polyphenols and tannins from *O. crenata* growing on *V. faba* without any further specification of the substances [Beja and Ariana Governorates, Tunisia; aerial parts; methanol; water] [37].

Orobanche denudata **Moris**—Serafini et al. isolated the phenylpropanoid glycosides verbascoside (**10**) and orobanchoside (**29**) from *O. denudata* [Sardinia, Italy; flowering samples; alcoholic extract; ^{1}H and ^{13}C NMR, HPLC, co-elution of extracts with isolated and identified phenylpropanoid glycosides] [host species not mentioned] [14].

Orobanche foetida **Poir.**—Abbes et al. described the extraction of polyphenols and tannins from *O. foetida* growing on *V. faba* without any further specification of the substances [Beja and Ariana Governorates, Tunisia; aerial parts; methanol; water] [37].

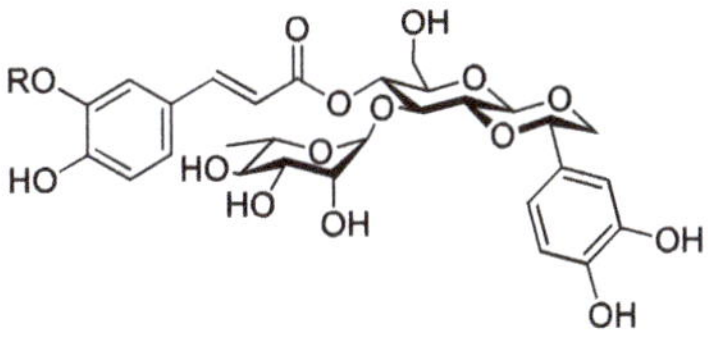

No	Name	R
29	Oraposide [1]	H
30	3‴-*O*-Methyl crenatoside	CH_3

[1] Syn. crenatoside, orobanchoside.

Figure 7. Phenylpropanoid glycosides IV, **29** and **30**. Note: According to Andary et al. [38] crenatoside and oraposide both describe the same structure. The authors report another isolated substance, orobanchoside (also mentioned in a former work from Andary et al. [39]). In a later work from Nishibe et al. [34] the structure of orobanchoside is being revised and it was established that orobanchoside is the same compound as crenatoside and oraposide. The name oraposide is used preferentially here, because it seems to be the oldest name for the compound at hand; however, crenatoside seems to have been used more often in the literature.

Orobanche gracilis **Sm.**—Fruchier et al. isolated the tropone derivative orobanone (**45**) from *O. gracilis* (using the synonym *O. cruenta* Bertol.) [whole plants; water, chloroform; IR, UV, MS, CI-MS, and ^{1}H and ^{13}C NMR] [no information about the host] [12].

Orobanche grisebachii **Reut.**—Aynilian et al. screened several *Orobanche* species for their contents of alkaloids, tannins, and saponins, without reporting any particular structures of the metabolites. *O. grisebachii* [plant material obtained from The Post Herbarium of the American University of Beirut, Lebanon; ethanol 95%, ethanol 80%] contained alkaloids and tannins [40].

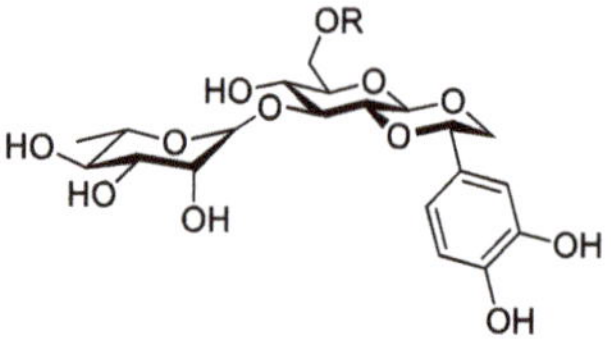

No	Name	R
31	Descaffeoyl crenatoside	H
32	Isocrenatoside	caffeoyl-
33	3′-*O*-Methyl isocrenatoside	ferulouyl-

Figure 8. Phenylpropanoid glycosides V, **31** and **32**, and phenylethanoid glycoside **33**.

***Orobanche hederae* Duby**—Pieretti et al. isolated the phenylpropanoid verbascoside (**10**) and orobanchoside (**29**) from *O. hederae* [Lazio, Italy; whole plants; ethanol; ^{1}H NMR, HPLC-UV] [host species not mentioned] [41]. Capasso et al. also found these two compounds [whole plants; ethanol] [host species not mentioned] [42]. As well as in eleven other species of the genus *Orobanche* (see extra paragraph) Fruchier et al. found the tropone derivative orobanone (**45**) in *O. hederae* [whole plant; water, chloroform; IR, UV, MS, CI-MS, ^{1}H and ^{13}C NMR] [host species not mentioned] [12]. Baccarini and Melandri isolated and analyzed seven pigments from *O. hederae* growing on *Hedera helix* L. (Araliaceae) [whole plant; acetone 80%; TLC, comparison with standard substances]. These pigments were β-carotene, α-carotene-5,6-epoxide, flavochrome, lutein-5,6-epoxide, flavoxanthin, and taraxanthin [43]. The seventh compound was tentatively identified as neoxanthin. There is also a report of the sequestration of substances from its host species by *O. hederae*. This is described in a separate paragraph below.

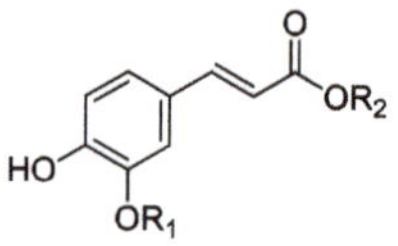

No	Name	R_1	R_2
34	Caffeic acid	H	H
35	Methyl caffeate	H	CH_3
36	*trans*-Ferulic acid	CH_3	H

Figure 9. Phenolic acids **34**–**36**.

***Orobanche loricata* Rchb.**—The isolation of the phenylpropanoid glycosides verbascoside (**10**) and orobanchoside (**29**) from *O. loricata* was described by Serafini et al. [Sardinia, Italy; flowering samples; alcoholic extract; ^{1}H and ^{13}C NMR, HPLC, co-elution of extracts with isolated and identified phenylpropanoid glycosides] [host species not mentioned] [14]. Fruchier et al. isolated the tropone derivative orobanone (**45**) [whole plants; water, chloroform; IR, UV, MS, CI-MS, ^{1}H and ^{13}C NMR] [no information about the host] [12].

***Orobanche lutea* Baumg.**—Rohmer et al. analyzed several parasitic species for their sterol contents and sterol biosynthesis [44]. The following compounds were isolated and identified from *O. lutea* [Alsace, France; stems; acetone, chloroform:methanol (2:1); GLC, GLC-MS] [host species not mentioned]: sterols [stigmastanol (**46**), cholesterol (**47**), campesterol (**48**), 24-methylene cholesterol (**49**), sitosterol (**50**), stigmasterol (**51**), *iso*fucosterol (**52**), Δ^7-campestenol (**55**), episterol (**56**), Δ^7-stigmastenol (**57**), and Δ^7-avenasterol (**58**)], 4α-methylsterols [24- 24-methyl lophenol (**59**), methylene lophenol (**60**), 24-ethyl lophenol (**61**), 24-ethylidene lophenol (**62**), 4α-methyl Δ^8-campestenol (**63**), 4α-methyl Δ^8-stigmastenol

(**64**), 24,28-dihydro obtusifoliol (**65**), obtusifoliol (**66**), 24,28-dihydrocycloeucalenol (**67**), cycloeucalenol (**68**), and 4,4-dimethylsterols cycloartenol (**69**)], and 24-methylene cycloartenol (**70**).

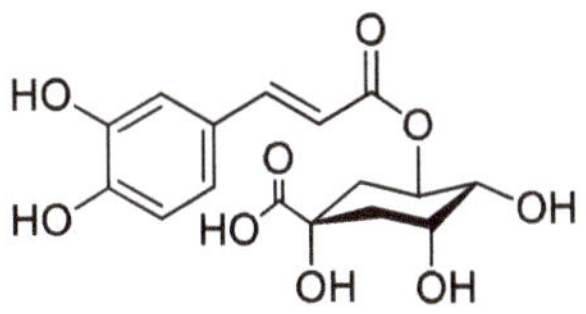

Figure 10. Chlorogenic acid (5-Caffeoyl quinic acid) **37**.

***Orobanche minor* Sm.**—Kurisu et al. isolated the phenylpropanoid glycosides acteoside (**10**) and oraposide (**29**) from *O. minor* [whole plant; methanol; NMR (^{1}H, ^{13}C, COSY, HMQC, HMBC, NOESY), HR-ESI-MS] [host species not mentioned] [45]. Serafini et al. also extracted verbascoside (**10**) and orobanchoside (**29**) [Sardinia, Italy; flowering samples; alcoholic extract; ^{1}H and ^{13}C NMR, HPLC, co-elution of extracts with isolated and identified phenylpropanoid glycosides] [host species not mentioned] [14]. Kidachi et al. isolated acteoside (**10**), cistanoside D (**20**), isoacteoside (**23**), oraposide (**29**), 3‴-*O*-methyl crenatoside (**30**), and isocrenatoside (**32**) [whole plant; methanol] [host species not mentioned] [46]. The tropone derivative orobanone (**45**) was found in *O. minor* by Fruchier et al. [whole plant; water, chloroform; IR, UV, MS, CI-MS, ^{1}H and ^{13}C NMR] [host species not mentioned] [12].

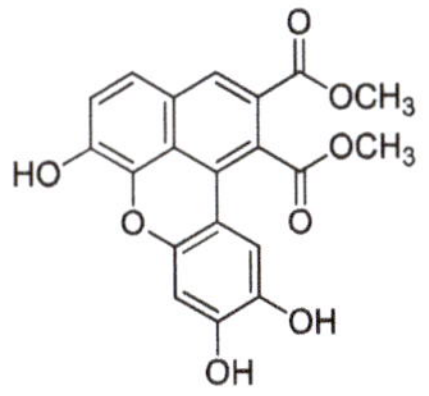

Figure 11. Dimethyl-6,9,10-trihydroxybenzol[*kl*]xanthene-1,2-dicarboxylate **38**.

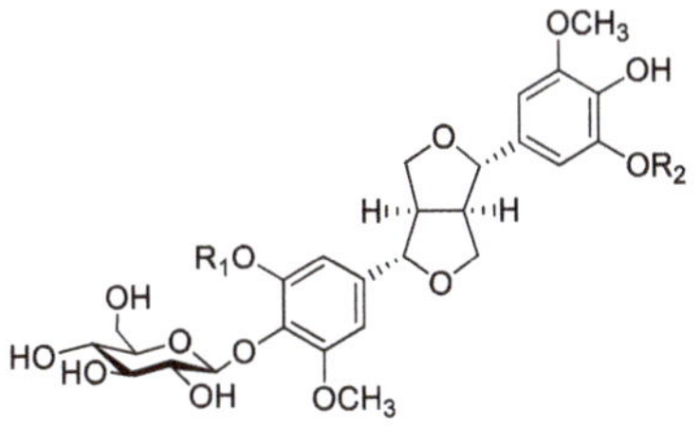

No	Name	R_1	R_2
39	(+)-Pinoresinol 4′-*O*-β-D-glucopyranoside	H	H
40	Isoeucommin A	H	OCH_3
41	(+)-Syringaresinol 4′-*O*-β-D-glucopyranoside	OCH_3	OCH_3

Figure 12. Lignans **39**–**41**.

***Orobanche owerinii* Beck**—Dzhumyrko and Sergeeva detected several carotenoids in *O. owerinii* [epigeal parts; *n*-hexane, petrol ether; co-chromatography with reference compounds and UV spectroscopy] growing on the hypogeal organs of *Fraxinus* [47]. Violaxanthin, auroxanthin, the ester of violaxanthin and palmitic acid, as well as α- and β- carotenes were detected.

***Orobanche pubescens* d'Urv.**—Aynilian et al. screened several *Orobanche* species for their contents of alkaloids, tannins, and saponins, without investigating any particular structures of the metabolites. Tannins were found in *O. pubescens* (using the synonym *O. versicolor* F.W.Schultz) [plant material obtained from The Post Herbarium of the American University of Beirut, Lebanon; petroleum benzine (defatting), ethanol 95%, ethanol 80%] [40].

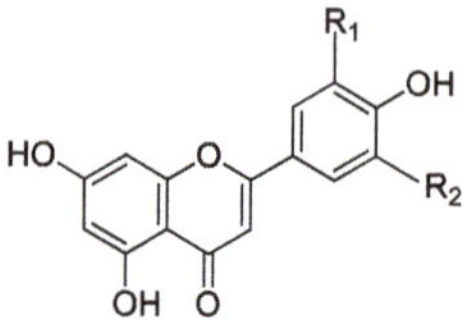

No	Name	R_1	R_2
42	Apigenin	H	H
43	Luteolin	OH	H
44	Tricin	OCH_3	OCH_3

Figure 13. Flavones **42–44**.

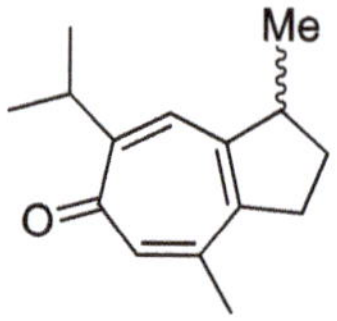

Figure 14. Tropone derivative—Orobanone **45**.

***Orobanche pycnostachya* Hance**—Han et al. isolated eight compounds from *O. pycnostachya* [Neimenggu province, China; ethanol 95%; MS, NMR] [host species not mentioned] [48]. The primary metabolites *n*-nonacosane acid, *n*-hexacosyl alcohol, *D*-allitol, 2,3,4,6-α-D-galactopyranose tetramethyl ether, and secondary metabolites acteoside (**10**), fissistigmoside (**25**), β-sitosterol (**50**), and daucosterol (**53**) were identified. Li et al. also isolated the phenylpropanoid glycosides acteoside (**10**) as well as 2′-*O*-acetylacteoside (**14**), and oraposide (**29**) [Mengu, Anhui and Hebei, China; methanol 70%; HPLC] [host species not mentioned] [49].

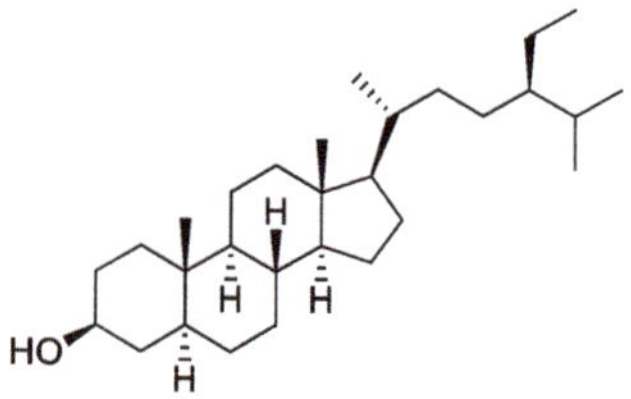

Figure 15. Sterols I: stigmastane derivative, stigmastanol **46**.

***Orobanche rapum-genistae* Thuill.**—Several secondary metabolites such as phenylproanoid glycosides, alkaloids, and a tropone derivative have been isolated from *O. rapum-genistae*. The isolated alkaloids are presumably not synthesized by the parasite itself but sequestered from the host species. Sequestration of secondary metabolites by *O. rapum-genistae* from its host is also reported by other authors and described in a separate paragraph below. Fruchier et al. isolated the tropone derivative orobanone (**45**) from *O. rapum-genistae* parasitizing on *Cytisus scoparius* (L.) Link and *Cytisus purgans* (L.) Spach (both Fabaceae) [whole plant; water, chloroform; IR, UV, MS, CI-MS, ^{1}H and ^{13}C NMR] [12]. Eleven other *Orobanche* species were also screened for orobanone (**45**) (see separate paragraph and supplementary material). Several sources report the isolation of the two phenylpropanoid glycosides verbascoside (**10**) and oraposide (**29**) from *O. rapum-genistae* (Andary et al., [50,51] (host: *C. scoparius*, *C. purgans*), [39] [phenolic extract; hydrolysis, high resolution ^{1}H and ^{13}C NMR], [38] [^{1}H and ^{13}C

NMR, X-ray crystal analysis]; Bridel and Charaux, [52,53] [tubers/bulbs; alcohol]; Serafini et al., [14] [Sardinia, Italy; flowering plants; alcoholic extract; ^{1}H and ^{13}C NMR, HPLC, co-elution of extracts with isolated and identified phenylpropanoid glycosides] [host species not mentioned]; Viron et al., [54] [whole plant; aqueous ethanol 70%; HPTLC, HPLC] [host species not mentioned], [55]). Andary et al. described the differentiation of two ecotypes of *O. rapum-genistae*: *O. rapum-cytisi scoparii* (parasitizing *C. scoparius*) and *O. rapum-cytisi purgantis* (parasitizing *C. purgans*) based on morphological and phytochemical characteristics [51]. Phenylpropanoid glycosides verbascoside (**10**) and orobanchoside (**29**) as well as quinolizidine alkaloids sparteine (**S2**) and lupanine (**S4**) were found in both ecotypes in different concentrations.

***Orobanche sanguinea* C.Presl.**—Serafini et al. isolated the phenylpropanoid glycosides verbascoside (**10**) and orobanchoside (**29**) from *O. sanguinea* [Sardinia, Italy; flowering samples; alcoholic extract; ^{1}H and ^{13}C NMR, HPLC, co-elution of extracts with isolated and identified phenylpropanoid glycosides] [host species not mentioned] [14].

***Orobanche variegata* Wallr.**—Fruchier et al. isolated the tropone derivative orobanone (**45**) from *O. variegata* [whole plant; water, chloroform; IR, UV, MS, CI-MS, ^{1}H and ^{13}C NMR] [no information about the host] [12].

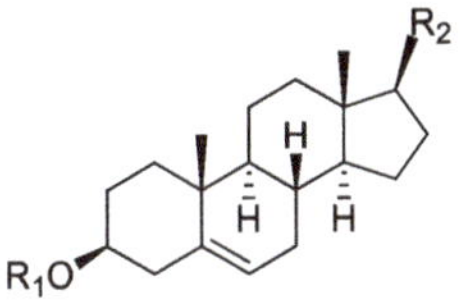

No	Name	R_1	R_2
47	Cholesterol	H	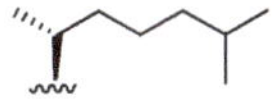
48	Campesterol	H	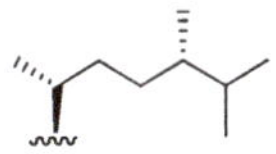
49	24-Methylene cholesterol	H	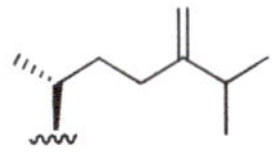
50	β-Sitosterol	H	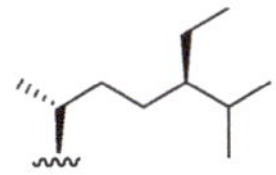
51	Stigmasterol	H	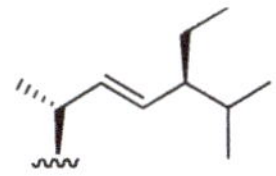
52	*Iso*fucosterol	H	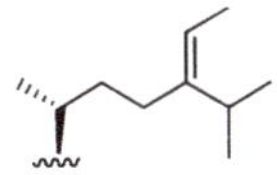
53	Daucosterol	β-D-Glc	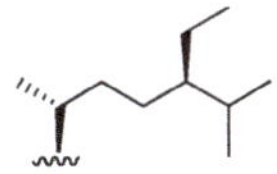
54	Stigmasterol-3-*O*-β-D-glucoside	β-D-Glc	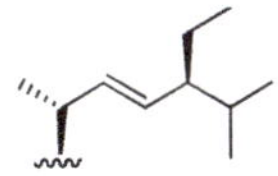

Figure 16. Sterols II: cholest-5-en derivatives, **47–54**.

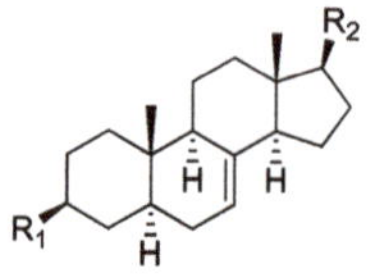

No	Name	R_1	R_2
55	Δ^7-Campestenol	H	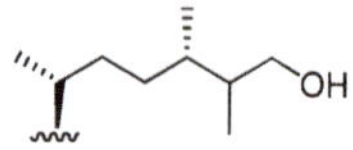
56	Episterol	OH	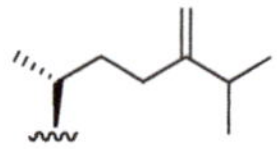
57	Δ^7-Stigmastenol	OH	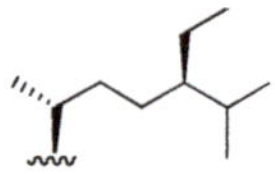
58	Δ^7-Avenasterol	OH	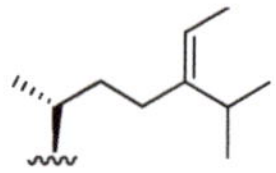

Figure 17. Sterols III: cholest-7-en derivatives, **55**–**58**.

2.2.2. Phelipanche (=Orobanche Sectio Trionychon)

***Phelipanche aegyptiaca* (Pers.) Pomel** (formerly ***O. aegyptiaca* Pers.**)—Afifi et al. isolated acteoside (**10**), poliumoside (**11**), 2′-*O*-acetylacteoside (**14**), and 2′-*O*-acetylpoliumoside (**15**) from *P. aegyptiaca* (as *O. aegyptiaca*) [butanol extraction] [host species not mentioned [56]. Sharaf and Youssef described the extraction of alkaloids and tannins (organic acids, reducing sugars, glucosides resins, and unsaturated substances) from *P. aegyptiaca* (as *O. aegyptiaca*) [whole plant; 30% aqueous extract, hexane, chloroform, ethyl alcohol] [host species not mentioned] [57]. The extracted substances were not characterized any further.

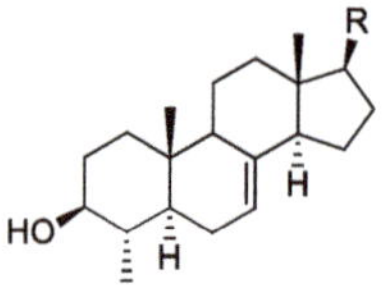

No	Name	R
59	24-Methyl lophenol	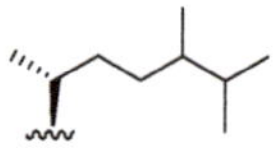
60	24-Methylene lophenol	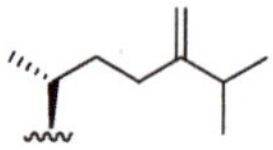
61	24-Ethyl lophenol	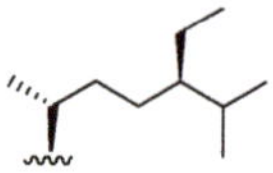
62	24-Ethylidene lophenol	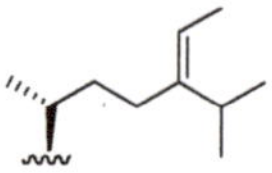

Figure 18. Sterols IV: lophenol derivatives, **59**–**62**.

Phelipanche arenaria **Pomel (Syn.:** ***O. arenaria*** **Borkh.)**—Andary et al. isolated the caffeic acid glycosides arenarioside (**12**) and pheliposide (**16**) from *P. arenaria* (as *O. arenaria*) growing on *Artemisia campestris* Ledeb. var. *glutinosa* (J.Gay ex Besser) Y.R.Ling [syn. of *A. campestris* subsp. *glutinosa* (Besser) Batt.] [Hérault, France; ethanol 80%; high resolution ^{1}H and ^{13}C NMR]. Orobanone (**45**) was found in *P. arenaria* (as *O. arenaria*) by Fruchier et al., (1981) [whole plant; water, chloroform; IR, UV, MS, CI-MS, ^{1}H and ^{13}C NMR] [host species not mentioned] [12].

Phelipanche oxyloba **(Reut.) Soják** (Syn.: ***O. oxyloba*** **(Reut.) Beck)**—Aynilian et al. screened several *Orobanche* species for their contents of alkaloids, tannins, and saponins, without reporting fully characterized metabolites. Tannins were found in *P. oxyloba* (as *O. nana* Noe ex G.Beck) [plant material obtained from The Post Herbarium of the American University of Beirut, Lebanon; petroleum benzine (defatting), ethanol 95%, ethanol 80%] [40].

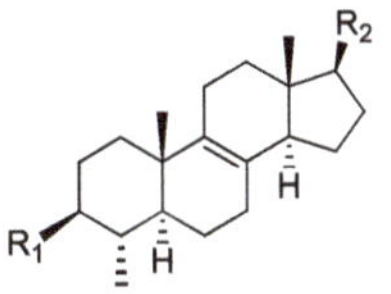

No	Name	R_1	R_2
63	4α-Methyl Δ^8-campestenol	H	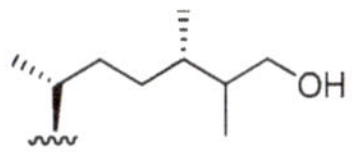
64	4α-Methyl Δ^8-stigmastenol	OH	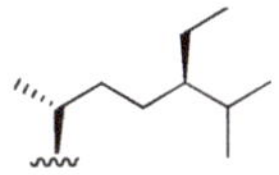
65	24,28-Dihydro obtusifoliol	OH	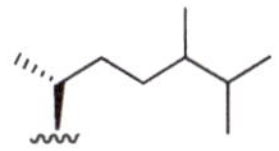
66	Obtusifoliol	OH	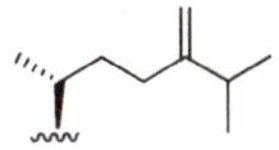

Figure 19. Sterols V, **63–66**.

Phelipanche ramosa **(L.) Pomel** (Syn.: ***O. ramosa*** **L.)**—Lahloub et al. extracted known compounds acteoside (**10**) and 2′-*O*-acetylacteoside (**14**) as well as the formerly undescribed phenylpropanoid glycoside 2′-*O*-acetylpoliumoside (syn. brandioside, [14]) (**15**) from *Phelipanche ramosa* (using the synonym *Orobanche ramosa*) parasitizing on *Lycopersicon esculentum* Mill. [El-Behera Governorate, Egypt; whole plant; percolation in ethanol; comparison of melting point, IR, UV, ^{1}H and ^{13}C NMR with literature data] [58]. Serafini et al. isolated the phenylpropanoid glycosides verbascoside (**10**) and orobanchoside (**29**) from *P. ramosa* subsp. *ramosa* (as *O. ramosa* subsp. *ramosa*) and *P. nana* (Reut.) Soják (as *O.ramosa* subsp. *nana* (Reut.) Cout., syn. *O. nana* (Reut.) Beck, according to [10]) as well as poliumoside (**11**) from *P. nana* [Sardinia, Italy; flowering samples; alcoholic extract; ^{1}H and ^{13}C NMR, HPLC, co-elution of extracts with isolated and identified phenylpropanoid glycosides] [host species not mentioned] [14]. The tropone derivative orobanone (**45**) was isolated from *P. ramosa* by Fruchier et al. (as *O. ramosa*) [whole plant; water, chloroform; IR, UV, MS, CI-MS, ^{1}H and ^{13}C NMR] [host species not mentioned] [12]. Afifi et al. also found poliumoside (**11**) in *P. ramosa* (as *O. ramosa*) [butanol extraction] [host species not mentioned] [56]. Two papers report tricin (**44**) (5,7,4′-trihydroxy-3,5′-dimethoxyflavone) from the seeds and aerial parts of *P. ramosa* (as *Orobanche ramosa*), respectively [59,60]. Compound identification [59]: spectra of the pigments and their acetates, R_f values, color properties on paper chromatograms and mixed melting points; [60]: UV and MS analyses, demethylation to tricetin and column chromatography]; host species not mentioned. Sequestration of secondary metabolites from its host by *P. ramosa* is described in a separate section below.

2.2.3. Reports Describing the Investigation of more than One Species

Besides investigating the phytochemical composition of one species there are also several reports dealing with more than one species. Serafini et al. investigated the secondary metabolite contents of several *Orobanche* species [Sardinia, Italy; flowering samples; alcoholic extract; ^{1}H and ^{13}C NMR, HPLC, co-elution of extracts with isolated and identified phenylpropanoid glycosides] [host species not mentioned] [14].

The authors reported the occurrence of the phenylpropanoid glycosides verbascoside (**10**) and orobanchoside (**29**) in *O. amethystea, O. crenata, O. denudata, O. hederae, O. loricata, O. minor, O. rapum-genistae* subsp. *rigens* (Loisel.) Arcang. (as *O. rigens* Loisel. [10]), *O. sanguinea, P. nana* (as *O. ramosa* subsp. *nana*), and *P. ramosa* subsp. *ramosa* (as *O. ramosa* subsp. *ramosa*). In *O. crenata* and *P. nana* poliumoside (**11**) was additionally reported. Moreover, the isolation of verbascoside (**10**), 2′-*O*-acetyllacteoside (**14**), and 2′-*O*-acetylpoliumoside (**15**) from *P. ramosa* (as *O. ramosa*) [58], and pheliposide (**16**) and orobanchoside (**29**) from *O. arenaria* [61] were mentioned in the report from Serafini et al. [14]. The reference about orobanchoside (**29**) occurring in *O. arenaria* by Andary et al. [61] is questionable because in the named report arenarioside (**12**) is described instead of orobanchoside (**29**). Fruchier et al. describe the isolation of the guaian type sesquiterpene tropone derivative orobanone (3,8-dimethyl-S-isopropyl-2,3-dihydro(lH)azulen-6-one) from *O. rapum-genistae* parasitizing on *C. scoparius* and *C. purgans* [whole plant; water, chloroform; IR, UV, MS, CI-MS, ^{1}H and ^{13}C NMR] [12]. No traces of orobanone were found in the hosts. This compound was also found in eleven other *Orobanche* species: *O. alba* (as *O. epithymum*), *O. arenaria, O. artemisiae-campestris* subsp. *picridis* (as *O. picridis*), *O. caryophyllacea* (as *O. major*), *O. crenata, O. gracilis* (as *O. cruenta*), *O. hederae, O. loricata, O. minor, O. ramosa*, and *O. variegata*. Except for *O. rapum-genistae*, no information about the host species were indicated.

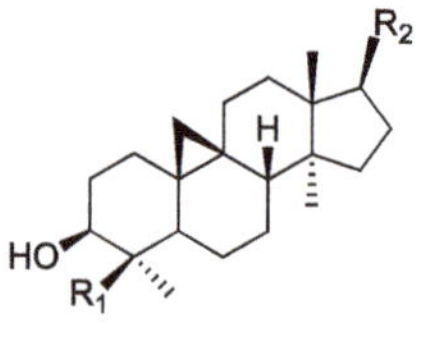

No	Name	R_1	R_2
67	24,28-Dihydrocycloeucalenol	H	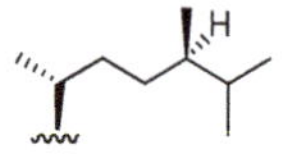
68	Cycloeucalenol	H	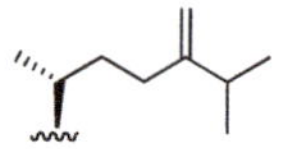
69	Cycloartenol	CH_3	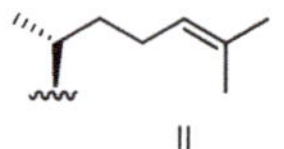
70	24-Methylene cycloartenol	CH_3	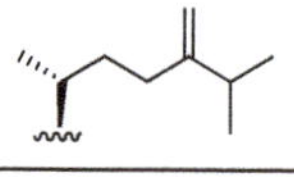

Figure 20. Sterols VI, **67–70**.

Aynilian et al. [plant material obtained from The Post Herbarium of the American University of Beirut, Lebanon; petroleum benzine (defatting), ethanol 95%, ethanol 80%] screened several *Orobanche* species for their contents of alkaloids, tannins, and saponins without reporting any defined chemical compounds [40]. Tannins were found in all six analyzed species, *O. aegyptiaca*, *O. crenata*, *O. grisebachii*, *O. oxyloba* (as *O. nana*), *O. pubescens* (as *O. versicolor*), and *P. ramosa* (as *O. ramosa*). Saponins were absent in all investigated taxa, and alkaloids were detected in *O. crenata*, *O. grisebachii*, *O. pubescens*, and *O. ramosa*.

2.3. *Sequestration of Secondary Metabolites by Orobanche s.l. from Their Host Species*

As obligate holoparasites *Orobanche* species drain water and essential nutrients from their host plants. Also the sequestration bioactive natural products from the hosts seems likely [62], but up to now little is known about the uptake of other substances by holoparasitic *Orobanche* species from the plants they parasitize on and only very few reports deal with the sequestration of secondary metabolites from hosts.

2.3.1. *Orobanche* Section *Orobanche* (=sect. *Osproleon* Wallr. = Genus *Orobanche* L. s.str.)

Orobanche hederae **Duby**—Sequestration of minerals and fatty acids by *Orobanche hederae* from its host *Hedera helix* was described by Lotti and Paradossi [Tuscany, Italy; whole plants; petrol ether, soxhlet; GC [63,64]. Sareedenchai and Zidorn reported the uptake of polyacetylenes falcarinol (**S15**), 11,12-dehydrofalcarinol (**S16**) and 11,12,16,17-didehydrofalcarinol (**S17**) from the roots of *Hedera helix* by *Orobanche hederae* [Trentino-Alto Adige, Italy; whole plants; dichloromethane; HPLC-DAD, HPLC-MS, comparison with authentic reference compounds and literature data] [65].

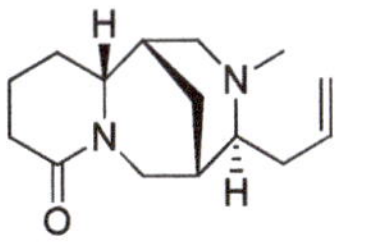

Figure 21. N-Methylangustifoline **S1**.

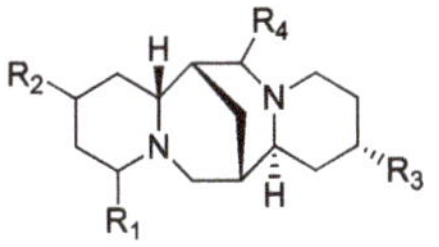

No	Name	R_1	R_2	R_3	R_4
S2	(−)-Sparteine	H, H	H	H	H, H
S3	(−)-17-Oxosparteine	H, H	H	H	=O
S4	(+)-Lupanine	=O	H	H	H, H
S5	17-Oxolupanine	=O	H	H	=O
S6	(+)-13-Hydroxylupanine	=O	H	OH	H, H
S7	13-Tigloyloxylupanine [1]	=O	H	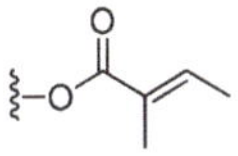	H, H
S8	13-Angeloyloxylupanine [1]	=O	H	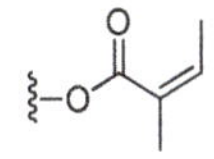	H, H
S9	13-Benzoyloxylupanine [1]	=O	H	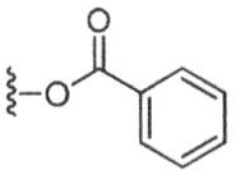	H, H
S10	4-Hydroxylupanine	=O	OH	H	H, H

[1] Stereochemistry not resolved.

Figure 22. Quinolizidine alkaloids I, **S2**–**S10**.

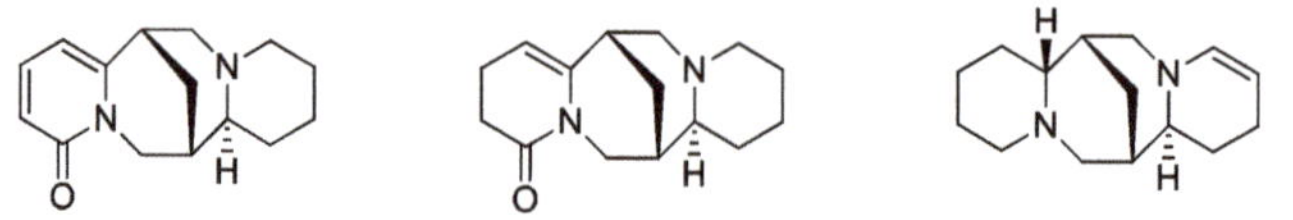

S11 Anagyrine **S12** 5,6-Dehydrolupanine **13** Dehydrosparteine

Figure 23. Quinolizidine alkaloids II, **S11–S13**.

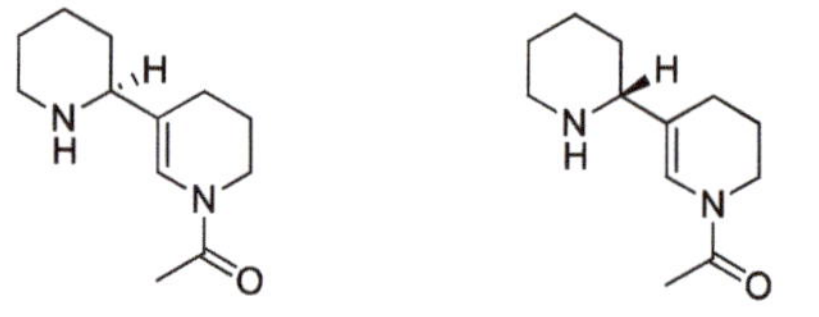

(+)-Ammodendrine (-)-Ammodendrine

Figure 24. Piperidine alkaloid—Ammodendrine **S14**.

Orobanche rapum-genistae **Thuill.**—Wink et al. reported *O. rapum-genistae* sequestering quinolizidin alkaloids N-methylangustifoline (**S1**), sparteine (**S2**), 17-oxosparteine (**S3**), lupanine (**S4**), 17-oxolupanine (**S5**), hydroxylupanine (**S6**), 13-tigloyloxylupanine (**S7**), 13-angeloyloxylupanine (**S8**), 13-benzoyloxylupanine (**S9**), 4-hydroxylupanine (**S10**), anagyrine (**S11**), 13-5,6-dehydrolupanine (**S12**), and dehydrosparteine (**S13**) as well the piperidine alkaloid ammodendrine (**S14**) from *Cytisus scoparius* [as *Sarothamnus scoparius* (L.) W.D.J. Koch] [Rhineland-Palatinate, Germany; stems, leaves, pods, seeds, bulbs, shoots; HCl, alkalization, Extrelut-column, dichloromethane; GLC/GLC-MS, comparison with retention indices of known reference alkaloids] [66]. From the report it is not clearly visible whether 13-tigloyloxylupanine (**S7**), 13-angeloyloxylupanine (**S8**), 13-benzoyloxylupanine (**S9**), and 4-hydroxylupanine (**S10**) are present in the α- or the β-form, respectively. Rascol et al. also described the isolation of quinolizidine alkaloids (−)-sparteine (**S2**), (+)-lupanine (**S4**), and (+)-13-hydroxylupanine (**S6**) from *O. rapum-genistae* growing on *Cytisus* [67]. In a second report the authors investigated the effects of alkaloid contents of the host (*Cytisus scoparius* and *Cytisus purgans*) on the alkaloid contents of the parasite and vice versa [68].

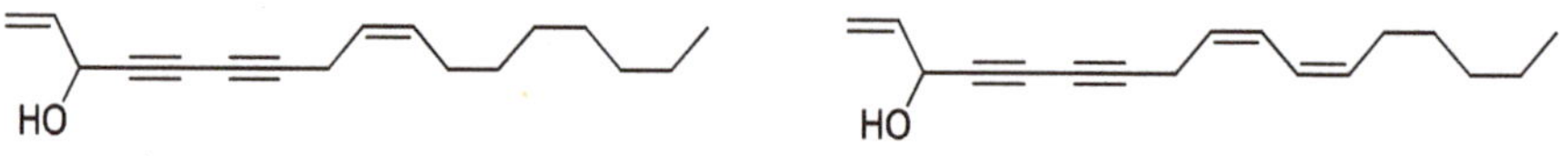

S15 Falcarinol **S16** 11,12-Dehydrofalcarinol

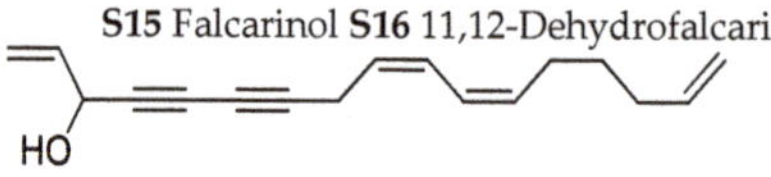

S17 11,12,16,17-Didehydrofalcarinol

Figure 25. Polyacetylenes **S15–S17**.

2.3.2. Phelipanche (=Orobanche Section Trionychon)

Phelipanche ramosa **(L.) Pomel** (syn.: ***Orobanche ramosa*** **L.**)—Cannabinoids cannabidiol (**S18**) and Δ^9-tetrahydrocannabinol (**S19**) were found by Fournier and Paris in traces in *Orobanche ramosa* growing on *Cannabis sativa* L. (Cannabaceae) [petrolether; TLC, GC-MS] [69].

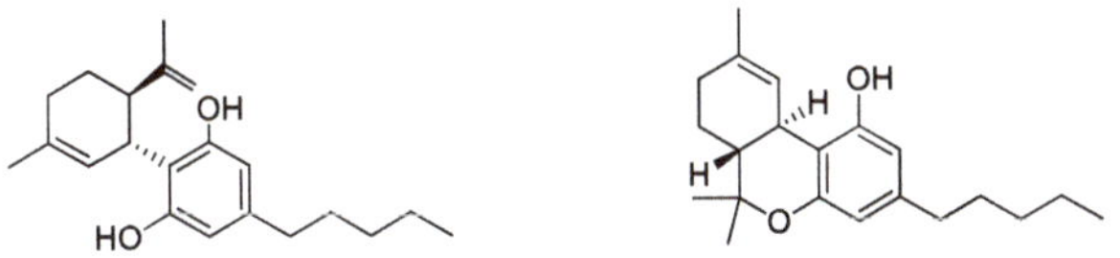

S18 Cannabidiol **S19** Δ^9-Tetrahydrocannabinol.

Figure 26. Cannabinoids **S18** and **S19**.

2.4. Sequestration of Secondary Metabolites from Host Plant Species by Other Hemiparasitic and Holoparasitic Plant Taxa

Sequestration is defined as the uptake, accumulation, and eventual use of substances, especially toxins, by animals or plant species from other organisms (microbes, plants or other animals) [70]. Most reports deal with interactions between plants and herbivorous insects, but sequestration is also known from some gastropods (feeding on e.g., algae, sponges, and bacteria) as well as from hemiparasitic and holoparasitic plants [71]. In most reported cases toxic secondary plant metabolites such as cardenolides, iridoid glycosides, and pyrrolizidine alkaloids or their precursors are sequestered by herbivorous insects and utilized as a defense against predators. Insects actively sequestering toxic compounds have, during their evolution, developed mechanisms to maintain the chemical stability of the sequestered toxins, while tolerating these toxins, without being negatively affected by their toxicity [72,73]. Sequestered metabolites can play a role in reproduction when utilized as sex pheromones [74]. There are also reports of sequestration of non-toxic substances like carotenoids or flavonoids by herbivorous insects [75]. Besides plant-animal interactions, some authors describe plant-plant interactions. Mainly alkaloids, but also iridoid glycosides, cardenolides, cardiac glycosides, and glucosinolates have been described to be sequestered. Most of the parasitic taxa analyzed so far are hemiparasites. Sequestration of iridoid glycosides by the hemiparasite *Euphrasia stricta* J.F.Lehm (Orobanchaceae, formerly Scrophulariaceae) from its host *Galium verum* L. (Rubiaceae) [76], and by the hemiparasite *Castilleja integra* A.Gray (Orobanchaceae) from *Penstemon teucrioides* Greene (Plantaginaceae) were described [77]. Pyrrolizidine and quinolizidine alkaloids are sequestered by hemiparasitic *Castilleja* Mutis ex L.f. species (Orobanchaceae, formerly Scrophulariaceae) from their hosts *Senecio atratus* Greene and *Senecio triangularis* Hook. (both Asteraceae), *Lupinus* L. species (Fabaceae), and *Thermopsis montana* Torr. & A.Gray (Fabaceae) [78–80]. Quinolizidine alkaloids are sequestered by *Orthocarpus* Nutt. species (Orobanchaceae) from *Lupinus* species, and by holoparasitic *Cuscuta* L. species (Convolvulaceae) from *Genista acanthoclada* DC. (Fabaceae), *Lupinus*, *Cytisus* L., and *Spartium* L. species (all Fabaceae) as well as from several other Fabaceae species [81–83]. Hemiparasitic *Pedicularis* L. species (Orobanchaceae, formerly Scrophulariaceae) were reported to sequester alkaloids from *Senecio* L. and *Thermopsis* R.Br. species as well as from *Picea engelmannii* Parry ex Engelm. (Pinaceae) [84]. The uptake of norditerpenoid alkaloids by *Castilleja sulphurea* Rydb. from *Delphinium* L. species (Ranunculaceae) was described. Hemiparasitic *Tristerix verticillatus* (Ruiz & Pav.) Barlow & Wiens (Loranthaceae) was found to take up isoquinoline alkaloids from *Berberis montana* Gay (Berberidaceae), and bipiperidyl and quinolizidine alkaloids synthesized by *Retama sphaerocarpa* (L.) Boiss. and *Lygos sphaerocarpa* (L.) Heyw. (both Fabaceae) were found to be sequestered by hemiparasitic *Viscum cruciatum* Sieber ex Boiss. (Santalaceae) [85–89]. An interesting study of community-level interactions described the transfer of alkaloids produced by an endophytic fungus [*Neotyphodium uncinatum* (W. Gams, Petrini & D. Schmidt) Glenn, C.W. Bacon & Hanlin) (Clavicipitaceae)] via the host grass *Festuca pratensis* Huds. (using the synonym *Lolium pratense* (Huds.) Darbysh.) (Poaceae) to the hemiparasite *Rhinantus serotinus* (Schönh.) Oborny (Orobanchaceae). The hemiparasite utilizes the alkaloids for protection against the herbivorous aphid *Aulacorthum solani* (Aphididae) [90]. Furthermore the transfer of glucosinolates from *Arabidopsis thaliana* (L.) Heynh. (Brassicaceae) to holoparasitic *Cuscuta gronovii* Willd. ex Roem. & Schult. (Convolvulaceae), the uptake of cardiac glycosides by hemiparasitic mistletoes [*Muellerina celastroides* (Schult. & Schult. f.) Tiegh., as *Phrygilanthus celastroides* (Schult. & Schult. f.) Eichler], *Dendrophthoe falcata* (L.f.) Ettingsh., and *Amyema congener* (Sieber ex Schult. & Schult.f.) Tiegh. (all Loranthaceae) from *Nerium oleander* L. (Apocynaceae), and the sequestration of cardenolides by holoparasitic *Cuscuta* species from *Digitalis lanata* Ehrh. and *Digitalis purpurea* L. (both Plantaginaceae) (after artificial infection) [91–93] were described as examples for plant-plant interactions.

2.5. Bioactivities Reported for Extracts Obtained from Orobanche Taxa and for Natural Products Isolated from Orobanche Taxa

Furthermore, biological activities of extracts or isolated pure compounds have been reported for some *Orobanche* species. Bioactivities of *Orobanche* species or of *Orobanche* natural products are compiled and listed alphabetically by activity in the following paragraphs.

2.5.1. Analgesic Effects

Potent analgesic effects of the phenylpropanoid containing fraction of *O. crenata* extract (oral application) were observed in mice using the hot plate method for testing. *O. crenata* phenylpropanoid containing fraction was administered in doses of 50 mg/100 g body weight (b.w.) and 100 mg/100 g b.w. Paracetamol was used for comparison with a dose of 50 mg/100 g b.w. Reaction times were measured right after application and after 10, 20, 30, 45, 60, and 120 min after application. At the beginning of the experiment (0 min) the control group without any analgetic treatment, the *O. cernua* 50 mg/100 g b.w., *O. cernua* 100 mg/100 g b.w., and the paracetamol group showed reaction times of 16.1 ± 0.0, 17.8 ± 0.6, 14.3 ± 3.0, and 16.0 ± 1.3 s, respectively. Reaction times of the control group during the experiment varied slightly between 14.1 ± 1.1 s and 16.3 ± 0.1 s. Reaction times after application of 50 mg/100 g b.w. *O. cernua* extract increased from 17.8 ± 0.6 s at 0 min to reach their maximum of 22.6 ± 0.9 s after 20 min and decreased again afterwards. After application of 100 mg/100 g b.w. *O. cernua* extract, reaction times increased from 14.3 ± 3.0 s at 0 min to 33.7 ± 1.7 s after 45 min, and then decreased again. Paracetamol application (50 mg/100 g b.w.) led to an increase of the reaction time from 16.0 ± 1.3 s at 0 min to 28.4 ± 0.7 s after 45 min, followed by a decrease. The results implicate a clear analgesic effect of *O. cernua* phenylpropanoid containing fraction after oral application in mice [29]. Other studies on pharmacological effects of phenylpropanoids also revealed analgesic effects, especially of acteoside (**10**), one of the main phenylpropanoid glycosides found in *O.* species. Acteoside showed an analgesic potency almost equal to aminopyrine when tested in mice [94], and was effective against neuropathic pain in rats [95].

2.5.2. Antimicrobial Activities

The phenolic composition of *O. crenata* 80% methanolic extract and its in vivo efficacy against fungal postharvest diseases were studied in an attempt to find new strategies for reducing postharvest diseases in sweet cherry fruit and replacing or integrating the use of synthetic fungicides. Sweet cherry fruit were sprayed with *O. crenata* extract (different concentrations: 1×, 2×, 4×; the 1× concentration corresponding to 0.170 mg dry matter/mL of buffer), *O. crenata* extract added with salts ($CaCl_2$ or $NaHCO_3$, 1% *w*/*v*), salt solutions, and the same buffer solution used to prepare the plant extracts (0.1 M K-phosphate, pH 5.5) as a positive control few hours after harvesting. Afterwards they were stored under controlled conditions. Rot incidence, expressed as the percentage of rotten fruit with respect to the total number of fruit in each tray, was assessed daily. At a rot incidence of around 50% the inhibition values of different treatments were evaluated. *O. crenata* extract inhibited postharvest rot in higher extract concentrations. An increase in extract concentration produced an increase in the percentage of inhibition from 64% to 76% for *O. crenata*. Addition of salt to the most concentrated extract further increased the inhibition of postharvest rot to 82% and 84% for $NaHCO_3$ and $CaCl_2$, respectively, and hereby proved to have a high antifungal efficacy [33]. Antifungal activity of *O. aegyptiaca* ethanolic and acetone extracts against *Fusarium oxysporum* Schlechtend.,

Cladosporium harbarum (Pers.) Link, *Trichothecium roseum* (Pers.) Link, and *Trichoderma viride* Pers. have been described by Nagaraja et al. [96]. Saadoun et al. tested *O. aegyptiaca*, *O. cernua*, and *O. crenata* ethanolic extracts against *Agrobacterium tumefaciens* (Smith & Townsend) Conn and *Erwinia* plant pathogens using the hole-plate diffusion method, the dilution method, and the Bauer–Kirby method. Tobromycin (10 μg), augmentin (30 μg), norfloxacin (10 μg), streptomycin (10 μg), ofloxacin (5 μg), cefuroxime (30 μg), and cefotaxime (30 μg) were tested as standard antibiotics for comparison. *O. cernua* showed inhibitory effects on *A. tumefaciens* isolates with MIC of 12,500 μg/mL, which is equal to streptomycin (10 μg), ofloxacin (5 mg) norfloxacin (10 μg), and cefotaxime (30 μg) activity against *Agrobacterium*. *Erwinia* isolates were less sensitive and higher concentrations of *Orobanche* extracts were needed for growth inhibition. *O. aegyptiaca* did not show antimicrobial activities in this study [97]. Nada et al. evaluated the antimicrobial activity of *O. crenata* extract against three gram positive bacteria (*Staphylococcus aureus* Rosenbach, *Bacillus subtilis* (Ehrenberg) Cohn, and *Streptococcus faecalis* (Andrewes & Horder) Schleifer & Kilpper-Bälz) and three gram negative bacteria *Escherichia coli* (Migula) Castellani & Chalmers, *Pseudomonas aeruginosa* Migula, and *Neisseria gonorrhoeae* (Zopf) Trevisan) using the disc diffusion assay. *O. crenata* showed moderate antibacterial activity against the investigated bacteria [35]. Abbes et al. tested antimicrobial activities of *O. crenata* and *O. foetida* methanolic and aqueous extracts using the disc diffusion method. Bacteria tested were *P. aeruginosa*, *E. coli*, *Enterococcus faecalis* (Andrewes & Horder) Schleifer & Kilpper-Bälz, *Enterobacter cloacae* (Jordan) Hormaeche & Edwards, *Salmonella enterica* (ex Kauffmann & Edwards) Le Minor & Popoff (subspecies: *Salmonella typhi* (*Salmonella enterica* subsp. *enterica* Serovar Typhi), *Salmonella enteritidis* (*Salmonella enterica* subsp. *enterica* Serovar Enteritidis), *Salmonella salamae* (*Salmonella enterica* subsp. *salamae*), *Shigella flexneri* Castellani & Chalmer, *S. aureus*, *Streptococcus pyogenes* Rosenbach, *Listeria monocytogenes* (Murray et al.) Pirie, *Yersinia enterocolitica* (Schleifstein & Coleman) Frederiksen, *Proteus mirabilis* Hauser, *Bacillus cereus* Frankland & Frankland, and *B. subtilis*. *O. crenata* methanolic extract was active against all tested bacteria except for *S. aureus*, *O. foetida* methanolic extract inhibited only *S. enteritidis* and *L. monocytogenes*. Aqueous extracts were not active againts the tested bacteria [37]. Antibacterial activity of an ethanolic extract of *O. cernua* at a concentration of 100 mg/mL in distilled water against five different bacteria species, four gram positive bacteria (*S. aureus*, *B. cereus*, *S. pyogenes*, *Streptococcus* sp.), and one gram negative bacterium (*E. coli*), was tested by Saadoun et al. For antimicrobial activity determination the hole-plate diffusion method, the dilution method, and the Bauer–Kirby method were applied. For evaluation of the minimum inhibitory concentration (MIC) the dilution method was used. Tobromycin (10 μg), nalidixic acid (30 μg), amoxicillin (30 μg), and cefotaxime (30 μg) were tested as standard antibiotics. *O. cernua* extract showed inhibitory activity against all tested bacteria with MIC of 1527, 3125, 25,000 and 50,000 μg/mL for *S. aureus*, *Streptococcus* sp., *S. pyogenes* and both for *B. cereus* and *E. coli*, respectively. In comparison with standard antibiotics an MIC of 3125 μg/mL is equal to cefotaxime (30 μg) and tobromycin (10 μg) activity against *Streptococcus* sp. and *S. aureus*, respectively; 25,000 and 50,000 μg/mL is equal to cefotaxime (30 μg) activity against *S. pyogenes* and *B. cereus*, respectively, and 50,000 μg/mL is equal to nalidixic acid (30 μg) activity against *E. coli* [98]. Antibacterial and antifungal activities in vitro of caffeic acid (**34**) and its derivatives including verbascoside (**10**) and orobanchoside (**29**) isolated from *O. rapum-genistae*, and poliumoside (**11**) (naturally occurring in *O. crenata* [14,36], *P. aegyptiaca* [56], and *P. ramosa* [14]) against two plant-pathogenic fungi (*Sclerotinia sclerotiorum* (Lib.) de Bary, *Botrytis cinerea* Pers. ex Nocca & Balb.) and seven plant-pathogenic bacteria (gram positive: *Corynebacterium rathayi* (Smith) Dowson, *Corynebacterium fascians* (Tilford) Dowson, *Corynebacterium sepedonicum* (Spieckermann & Kotthoff) Skaptason & Burkholder; gram negative: *A. tumefaciens*, *Erwinia carotovora* var. *carotovora* (Jones) Dye, *Xanthomonas pelargonii* (Brown) Starr & Burkholder, *Pseudomonas syringae* van Hall) were tested. The other tested substances were caffeic acid (**34**), ferulic acid (**36**), esculine, esculetin, rosmarinic acid, gallic acid methylester, chlorogenic acid (**37**), plantamajoside, and neomyricoside. Additionally *Forsythia intermedia* var. *spectablis* Koehne extract was tested. Ferulic acid (**36**) and chlorogenic acid (**37**) had been identified in *O. cernua* by other authors [17]. *E. coli* and *S. aureus* were used as references. For fungi MIC was evaluated in solid media using five different concentrations (0.12, 0.25, 0.50, 1.00, 2.00 mg/mL) of solutions of the tested substances, and for bacteria an agar diffusion method with four different concentrations of solutions of the tested substances (12.5, 25, 50, 100 mg/mL) together with MIC measurement in liquid media with six different concentrations of the tested substances (0.1, 0.5, 1.0, 1.5, 2.0, 2.5 mg/mL) were used. Orobanchoside (**29**) and caffeic acid (**34**) showed pronounced antifungal activities with MIC values of 2.00 mg/mL and 0.25 mg/mL, respectively, against *S. sclerotiorum* in media with pH 5. Orobanchoside (**29**) furthermore had an MIC value of 0.25 mg/mL against *S. sclerotiorum* and 1.00 mg/mL against *B. cinera* in media with pH 7, while caffeic acid (**34**) showed an MIC of 0.25 mg/mL against *B. cinera* in pH 7 medium. Verbascoside (**10**) and poliumoside (**11**) were both able to reduce growth of *S. sclerotiorum* and *B. cinera* in pH 5 and pH 7 media, but complete inhibition was not observed. Ferulic acid (**36**) showed MIC values of 0.13 mg/mL against *S. scleretorium* and *B. cinerea* in pH 5 and pH 7 media. Chlorogenic acid (**37**) was able to reduce growth of *S. sclerotiorum* and *B. cinerea* in pH 5 and pH 7 media, but again, complete inhibition was not observed. Against the tested bacteria MIC values were as follows: MIC of caffeic acid (**34**) against *C. rathayi* (1.0 mg/mL), *C. fascians* (1.0 mg/mL), *C. sepedonicum* (0.1 mg/mL), *A. tumefaciens* (1.0 mg/mL), *E.carotovora* var. *carotovora* (1.0 mg/mL), *X. pelargonii* (1.0 mg/mL), *P. syringae* (not determined), *S. aureus* (1.5 mg/mL), *E. coli* (1.5 mg/mL); MIC of ferulic acid (**36**) against *C. rathayi* (0.5 mg/mL), *C. fascians* (0.5 mg/mL), *C. sepedonicum* (0.5 mg/mL), *A. tumefaciens* (1.0 mg/mL), *E.carotovora* var. *carotovora* (1.0 mg/mL), *X. pelargonii* (0.5 mg/mL), *P. syringae* (1.0 mg/mL), *S. aureus* (1.0 mg/mL), *E. coli* (1.5 mg/mL); MIC of chlorogenic acid (**37**) against *C. rathayi* (1.5 mg/mL), *C. fascians* (1.0 mg/mL), *C. sepedonicum* (1.0 mg/mL), *A. tumefaciens* (2.0 mg/mL), *E.carotovora* var. *carotovora* (2.5 mg/mL), *X. pelargonii* (1.5 mg/mL), *P. syringae* (2.0 mg/mL), *S. aureus* (>2.5 mg/mL), *E. coli* (2.5 mg/mL); MIC values of verbascoside (**10**), poliumoside (**11**), and orobanchoside (**29**) were not investigated. Caffeic acid (**34**) and its derivatives are potential natural plant protective agents against some plant-pathogenic fungi and bacteria as demonstrated in this work. Streptomycin, tested along with the caffeic acid derivatives, was a much more potent bacterial growth inhibitor than the other tested compounds with MIC values of <0.1 mg/mL (*C. rathayi, C. fascians, C. sepedonicum, A. tumefaciens, E.carotovora* var. *carotovora, S. aureus, E. coli*), with an exception for *X. pelargonii* (>2.5 mg/mL) (*P. syringae* MIC not determined) [99].

2.5.3. Antioxidant Activities as Food Preservative

O. crenata ethanolic extract total antioxidant activity was tested using the phosphomolybdenum method with ascorbic acid as standard. The antioxidant activity was expressed as ascorbic acid equivalents (AE) (mg/g of extract). The two investigated individual *Orobanche* plants showed good total antioxidant activity 619 ± 9 mg AE/g extract and 561 ± 9 mg AE/g extract [35].

2.5.4. Antioxidative Effects, Anti-Inflammatory Activity in Human Leucocytes, Effects on Production of Reactive Oxygen Species (ROS)

Phenylpropanoid glycosides isolated from *O. coerulescens* were tested for their antioxidative effects on human low-density lipoprotein. For evaluation of their antioxidant activity dialyzed LDL obtained from human blood samples was diluted with PBS to 100 µg/mL, pre-incubated with the test compounds at 37 °C for 30 min, and then incubated with $CuSO_4$ at 37 °C to induce lipid peroxidation. Resveratrol, a natural phenolic antioxidant e.g., from red wine, was used as a positive control. Conjugated diene formation was monitored and prolonged lag phase (min) used as an index of antioxidant activity when an antioxidant was present in LDL oxidation with Cu^{2+}. All seven isolated phytochemical compounds, phenylpropanoid glycosides desrhamnosyl acteoside (**9**), acteoside (**10**), caerulescenoside (**13**), campneoside II (**17**), isoacteoside (**23**), oraposide (**29**), and 3′-methyl crenatoside (**30**) suppressed conjugated diene formation with IC_{50} values of 0.64 ± 0.03, 0.31 ± 0.01, 1.25 ± 0.06, 1.15 ± 0.04, 1.01 ± 0.05, 1.69 ± 0.15, and 2.97 ± 0.31 µM, respectively while resveratrol had an IC_{50} value of 6.75 ± 1.05 µM. This showed that all isolated compounds from *O. coerulescens* were more effective antioxidants than the positive control, resveratrol [23]. Phenylpropanoid glycosides acteoside (**10**), rossicaside B (**28**), and oraposide (**29**), isolated from *O. coerulescens*, were tested for their inflammation-modulating activity in human leucocytes. Peripheral human neutrophils (PMNs) and mononuclear cells were exposed to phorbol-12-myristate-13-acetate (PMA), a direct proetin kinase C (PKC) activator, and *N*-formyl-methionyl-leucocyl-phenylalanine (fMLP), a receptor mediated and G protein coupled activator, for the induction of production of reactive oxygen species (ROS) and upregulation of β2 integrin in an in-vitro model. For the prevention of PMA-induced ROS production, acteoside (**10**), rossicaside B (**28**), and oraposide (**29**) showed IC_{50} values of 12.8 ± 7.2 μM, 5.6 ± 2.8 μM, and 6.8 ± 2.3 μM respectively in PMNs, and IC_{50} values of 9.6 ± 3.2 μM, 23.9 ± 2.9 μM, and 10.0 ± 4.3 μM respectively in mononuclear cells. IC_{50} values for prevention of fMLP-induced ROS production were 3.5 ± 0.6 μM, 3.0 ± 0.1 μM, and 3.0 ± 0.2 μM for acteoside (**10**), rossicaside B (**28**), and oraposide (**29**) in PMNs, respectively, and 8.8 ± 3.2 μM, 3.5 ± 0.2 μM, and 3.5 ± 0.2 μM in mononuclear cells, respectively. Furthermore, the inhibition of NADPH oxidase (NOX) activity in cell lysate by phenylpropanoid glycosides was tested since NOX is the major ROS producing enzyme in activated leucocytes. Acteoside (**10**), rossicaside B (**28**), and oraposide (**29**) were more potent in NOX inhibition than the positive control, diphenyleneiodonium (DPI, a NOX inhibitor). Moreover, these compounds showed effective free radical-scavenging activity in a cell-free DPPH (2,2-diphenyl-1-picrylhydrazyl) assaying system. Acteoside (**10**) and oraposide (**29**) also significantly inhibited PMA- and fMLP-induced β2 integrin expression in human peripheral leucocytes. These effects make *O. coerulescens* and other drugs containing acteoside (**10**), rossicaside B (**28**), and oraposide (**29**) interesting as potential anti-inflammatory agents for the treatment of oxidative-stress-related diseases [24]. Antioxidative potential was also investigated by Kidachi et al. for phenylpropanoids acteoside (**10**), cistanoside D (**20**), isoacteoside (**23**), oraposide (**29**), 3‴-*O*-methyl crenatoside (**30**), and isocrenatoside (**32**) from a methanolic *O. minor* extract, two synthetic derivatives acteoside-tetramethylether, oraposide-tetramethylether, as well as caffeic acid (**34**) and hydroxytyrosol using the DPPH (2,2-diphenyl-1-picrylhydrazyl) radical scavenging activity assay. Strong activities were observed for acteoside (**10**) (IC_{50} 15.2 μM), isoacteoside (**23**) (IC_{50} 20.0 μM), oraposide (**29**) (IC_{50} 24.5 μM), and isocrenatoside (**32**) (IC_{50} 29.0 μM), whereas moderate activities were observed for 3‴-*O*-methyl crenatoside (**30**) (IC_{50} 54.2 μM), caffeic acid (**34**) (IC_{50} 38.7 μM), and hydroxytyrosol (IC_{50} 44.6 μM), and no antioxidant activities were observed for acteoside-tetramethylether (IC_{50} > 100 μM), oraposide-tetramethylether (IC_{50} > 100 μM), and cistanoside D (**20**) (IC_{50} > 100 μM). Epigallocatechin gallate used as positive control showed an IC_{50} value of 13.5 μM. No standard deviations of the measured values were indicated [46]. Gao et al. found *O. cernua* extract and acteoside (**10**) to exhibit strong scavenging effects with IC_{50} values of 56.3 μg/mL and 20.6 μg/mL, respectively. No standard deviations of the measured values were given [100]. Antioxidant activities of *O. crenata* and *O. foetida* methanolic and aqueous extracts was tested by Abbes et al. using DPPH and ABTS (2,2-azino-bis-3-ethylbenzothiazoline-6-sulfonic acid) radical scavenging activity assays. Synthetic antioxidants BHT (2,6-di-tert-butyl-4-methylphenol) and AA (ascorbic acid) were used as positive controls. At 1.00 μg/mL DPPH radical scavenging activities of *O. crenata* methanolic extract, *O.crenata* water extract, *O. foetida* methanolic extract, *O. foetida* water extract, BHT, and AA were 19.5, 18.3, 5.86, 14.7, 13.4, and 54.0%, respectively. At 200 μg/mL *O. crenata* methanolic extract, *O.crenata* water extract, *O. foetida* methanolic extract, *O. foetida* water extract, BHT, and AA showed DPPH radical scavenging activities of 88.1, 77.0, 92.0 86.1, 85.0, and 86.3%, respectively. The highest activity against DPPH radicals was observed for *O. foetida* methanolic extract with an IC_{50} value of 7.19 ± 1.75 μg/mL (BHT: IC_{50} 65.5 ± 1.4 μg/mL; AA IC_{50} 0.93 ± 0.07 μg/mL). Antioxidant activities in the ABTS test, expressed in % inhibition at 0.5 μg/mL, were 4.04 (*O. crenata* methanolic extract), 1.64 (*O. crenata* aqueous extract), 1.28 (*O. foetida* methanolic extract), and 2.34 (*O. foetida* aqueous extract) (BHT: 9.98%; AA: 23.1%). Activities of nearly 100% for *O. crenata* methanolic extract, *O.crenata* water extract, *O. foetida* methanolic extract, *O. foetida* water extract, BHT, and AA, respectively, were observed at concentrations of 200 μg/mL [37].

2.5.5. Blood Pressure and Blood Platelet Aggregation

Intravenous injection of the glycosidic fraction of *O. crenata* 70% ethanolic extract into rats in doses up to 20 mg/100 g led to a temporary lowering of the arterial blood pressure of the treated animals. Higher doses caused slight, persistent lowering of the arterial blood pressure [29]. Hypotensive activity of *O. aegyptiaca* 30% aqueous extract and of the alkaloid containing chloroform fraction (further fractionation of the extract with different solvents gave hexane, ether, chloroform, alcohol, and water fractions) after i.v. injection into dogs was also evaluated. The alkaloidal fraction showed strong hypotensive effects. (Hypertension was artificially induced using the Goldblatt technique.) 10 mg i.v. lowered the blood pressure by about 48 mmHg for three hours [57]. A mixture of verbascoside (**10**) and orobanchoside (**29**) extracted from *O. hederae* was tested for its effect on ADP-induced (10–15 μM) blood platelet aggregation and blood pressure in New Zealand male rabbits and Wistar male rats. A dose-dependent inhibition of ADP-induced platelet aggregation of 12.9 ± 4.0%, 43.7 ± 7.8%, 49.4 ± 6.4%, 59.4 ± 6.9%, and 73.7 ± 8.3% at concentrations of 0.2 mg/mL, 0.4 mg/mL, 0.6 mg/mL, 0.8 mg/mL, and 1.0 mg/mL phenylpropanoid glycosides respectively was observed using an aggregometer. Blood pressure was not affected by phenylpropanoid glycosides injected i.v. into the test animals [42].

2.5.6. Contractions of Toad and Rabbit Hearts and Rat Intestines

O. aegyptiaca 30% aqueous extract was further fractionated with different solvents to give hexane, ether, chloroform, alcohol, and water fractions. The extract and fractions were tested for different biological activities. Effects on toad (*Bufo regularis* Reuss) and rabbit hearts were investigated. Doses of 1, 2, 3, and 4 mL of the aqueous extract were added to 50 mL bath (Ringer´s solution for toad hearts, Lock´s solution for rabbit hearts) and the amplitude or heart rate (toad hearts) as well as the volume of Lock´s solution perfused by the heart (rabbit hearts) were recorded. Contractions of toad hearts and rabbits' hearts perfused by the extract were stimulated. Also contractions of isolated rats intestines were stimulated whereas uterine contractions in rats were inhibited [57].

2.5.7. Diuretic Effects

Oral application of the phenylpropanoid containing fraction of *O. crenata* extract in rats had strong diuretic effects. *O. crenata* extract doses of 100 mg/100 g body weight and 200 mg/100 g body weight were orally applied. Rats were put in diuresis cages and the volume of the collected urine was measured after 1, 3, 6, and 24 h. The untreated control group produced 0, 2.65 ± 0.22, 6.25 ± 0.05, and 11.2 ± 0.1 mL urine after 1, 3, 6, and 24 h, respectively. After application of *O. crenata* extract doses of 100 mg/100 g b.w. 0, 3.27 ± 0.05, 6.95 ± 0.05, and 12.9 ± 0.1 mL urine were collected after 1, 3, 6, and 24 h, respectively. *O. crenata* extract doses of 200 mg/100 g b.w. led to 0.37 ± 0.05, 3.95 ± 0.05, 8.25 ± 0.12, and 14.3 ± 0.2 mL of urine after 1, 3, 6, and 24 h, respectively, showing increasing diuresis with higher *O. cernua* extract doses [29]. *O. aegyptiaca* 30% aqueous extract was further fractionated with different solvents to give hexane, ether, chloroform, alcohol, and water fractions. The extract and fractions were tested for different biological activities. Diuretic effects of the 20% alcoholic extract were observed in rabbits. Urine volumes of treated animals were measured after 0.5, 1, 2, 3, and 24 h and compared to urine volumes of the animals after 24 h without any treatment. The average urine volume of treated animals (average dose of 9.5 mL of 20% extract/kg b.w.) after 24 h was 107 ± 51 in comparison with 73 ± 21.2 mL for the untreated animals [57].

2.5.8. Inhibition of Amyloid β-Aggregation

Acteoside (**10**) and oraposide (**29**) isolated from *O. minor* were tested for their inhibitory effects on aggregation of human 42-mer amyloid β-protein (Aβ-42), which is believed to play an important role in the pathogenesis of Alzheimer´s disease. Thioflavin-T (Th-T) fluorescence assays, transmission electron microscopy (TEM), and circular dichroism (CD) spectroscopy were used to investigate the inhibitory effects. Acteoside (**10**) and oraposide (**29**) showed potent inhibitory effects on the aggregation of Aβ-42 with IC_{50} values of 8.9 μM and 3.6 μM respectively. IC_{50} values were calculated from the inhibition rate (%) of each compound towards Aβ-42 aggregation after 24 h by using the Th-T assay. Furthermore, an anti-aggregating effect was suggested by the significant reduction of Aβ fibril formation by 50 μM acteoside (**10**). β-Sheet formation in Aβ-42 was also inhibited [45]. Kidachi et al. also tested inhibition of amyloid β-42 (Aβ-42) aggregation by phenylpropanoids acteoside (**10**) and oraposide (**29**) from *O. minor* methanolic extract, their synthetic derivatives acteoside-tetramethylether, oraposide-tetramethylether, as well as cistanoside D (**20**), isoacteoside (**23**), 3‴-*O*-methyl crenatoside (**30**), isocrenatoside (**32**), caffeic acid (**34**), and hydroxytyrosol. The IC_{50} values were calculated from the inhibitory rate (%) of each compound towards Aβ-42 aggregation after 48 h by using the thioflavin-T (Th-T) fluorescence assay. Aβ-42 aggregation was inhibited by acteoside (**10**) and oraposide (**29**) with IC_{50} values of 11.3 μM and 8.2 μM, respectively. Moderate inhibitory activity was observed for 3‴-*O*-methyl crenatoside (**30**) (IC_{50} 28.0 μM), very weak inhibitory activity was observed for caffeic acid (**34**) (IC_{50} 93.8 μM) and hydroxytyrosol (IC_{50} 92.0 μM), and no inhibitory activity was observed for acteoside-tetramethylether (IC_{50} > 100 μM), oraposide-tetramethylether (IC_{50} > 100 μM), and cistanoside D (**20**) (IC_{50} > 100 μM). 3,4-Di-*O*-caffeoylquinic acid used as positive control for Aβ-42 aggregation showed an IC_{50} value of 30.2 μM. No standard deviations of the measured values were indicated [46]. The observed anti-amyloidal effects make acteoside (**10**) a potential agent for treating or preventing Alzheimer's disease [45].

2.5.9. Memory Enhancing Effects

Acteoside (**10**) showed memory enhancing effects and increased significantly the expression of nerve growth factor (NGF) and tropomycin receptor kinase A (TrkA) mRNA and protein in the hippocampus in mice [13]. NGF and TrkA are closely associated with cognitive function and a decrease thereof is related to Alzheimer´s disease. Acteoside (**10**) treatment resulted in an improvement of learning and memory deficits via promotion of NGF and TrkA expression in the brain. The authors used a senescent mouse model induced by a combination of chronic intraperitoneal administration of D-gal (60 mg/kg/day) and oral administration of $AlCl_3$ (5 mg/kg/day) once daily for 90 days. After 60 days mice in three different groups were treated intragastrically with acteoside (**10**) (30, 60, and 120 mg/kg/day) for 30 days. Learning ability and memory of the mice were tested using the Morris water maze test. Afterwards mice brains were removed and the hippocampus CA1 region studied immunohistochemically. Reverse transcription polymerase chain reactions (RT-PCR) and western blot analyses were performed to investigate the expression of NGF mRNA and TrkA mRNA [13].

2.5.10. Muscle Relaxant and Antispasmodic Effects

Dose dependent smooth muscle relaxant effects (phenylpropanoid containing fraction of *O. crenata* extract) were observed when testing different doses on the peristaltic movements of isolated perfused rabbit's intestine. Doses of 50, 80, 100, 150, and 200 mg/50 mL bath were tested. Movement inhibitions of 31.9 ± 6.8, 38.4 ± 10.1, 44.2 ± 4.3, 51.2 ± 10.3, and 95.4 ± 2.7% were obsereved, respectively [29]. Potent antispasmodic effects on isolated perfused guinea-pig ileum were observed (phenylpropanoid fraction of *O. crenata* extract). Contractions were induced by acetylcholine application and afterwards different doses of *O. crenata* extract were tested for their antispasmodic potential. Extract doses tested were 200, 400, 600, and 800 mg/50 mL bath. Inhibition of spasmodic contractions ranged from 22.8 ± 2.1, 55.6 ± 3.7, and 67.3 ± 10.1 to 94.3 ± 6.4%, respectively, showing a dose dependent antispasmodic potential [29].

2.5.11. Nutrient Source

O. crenata was found to be a good source of nutrients. It contained a low moisture level (<8%), a high amount of protein (7.30%), ash contents of 9.20–10.1%, a crude fiber content ranging from 22.1 to 23.5%, and a nutritive value of 244–247 kcal/100 g plant dry weight [35].

2.5.12. Photoprotective Effects

O. cernua ethanolic extract and its principal component, acteoside (**10**), were studied for their photoprotective effects on UVB-induced photoaging as well as for the underlying molecular mechanisms in normal human dermal fibroblasts (NHDFs). UV radiation causes excessive reactive oxygen species (ROS) generation, which triggers matrix metalloproteinase (MMPs) production, collagen degradation, and premature aging (photoaging). Cell viability of UVB-irradiated NHDFs and the effects of *O. cernua* extract and acteoside (**10**) on cell viability were tested using the 3-(4,5-dimethylthiazol-2-yl)-2,5-diphenyltetrazolium bromide (MTT) assay. *O. cernua* extract (100 μg/mL) and acteoside (**10**) (10 μM) were able to recover cell viability by 24.7% and 26.9%, respectively. For effects of *O. cernua* extract and acteoside (**10**) on intracellular ROS generation cells were first exposed to UVB irradiation, which increased the ROS level by 282% (ROS levels of normal group were set to 100%). The following treatment with *O. cernua* extract (100 μg/mL) and acteoside (**10**) (10 μM) reduced ROS levels by 73.0% and 42.3%, respectively. Furthermore, *O. cernua* extract and acteoside (**10**) significantly reduced MMP-1 and IL-6 (Interleukin) levels in NHDFs exposed to UVB-irradiation. *O. cernua* extract (100 μg/mL) and acteoside (**10**) (10 μM)-treated groups suppressed UVB-induced MMP-1 levels by 49.0% and 57.1%, respectively. Additionally, the secretion of IL-6 was lowered by 79.4% and 57.1%, by *O. cernua* extract (100 μg/mL) and acteoside (**10**) (10 μM). *O. cernua* extract and acteoside (**10**) could reverse a UVB induced decrease in type-I procollagen mRNA, with an increased rate of 52.7% and 25.7%, respectively. Furthermore, the UVB-induced increased production of MMP-1 and MMP-3 mRNA levels were strongly inhibited by *O. cernua* extract (100 μg/mL) and acteoside (**10**) (10 μM). *O. cernua* extract decreased the expression of MMP-1 and MMP-3 mRNA by 42.5% and 28.3%, respectively, while acteoside (**10**) decreased the expression by 44.4% and 66.7%, respectively. Carried with the AP-1 binding sites, the promoters of MMPs were transactivated by AP-1 transcription factor. The expression of phosphorylated c-fos and c-jun, the major components of AP-1 was measured and inhibitory effects on UVB-induced p-c-fos and p-c-jun expression in a dose-dependent manner by acteoside (**10**) treatments were observed. *O. cernua* extract (100 μg/mL) reduced the levels of p-c-fos and p-c-jun by 56.0% and 75.6%, respectively, and acteoside (**10**) (10 μM) reduced the levels by 93.0% and 65.3%, respectively. The mitigen-activated protein kinase (MAPK) signaling pathway, as the upstream of AP-1 transcription factor, has been reported to be activated by UVB-elevated ROS. Biological effects of *O. cernua* extract and acteoside (**10**) on the MAPKs family were further studied in UVB-irradiated NHDFs. UVB radiation elevated the phosphorylated forms of MAPKs molecules including ERK, JNK and p38. *O. cernua* extract and acteoside (**10**) suppressed the phosphorylation of ERK, JNK and p38 caused by UVB. Levels of p-ERK, p-JNK and p-38 were decreased by *O. cernua* (100 μg/mL) extract by 46.4%, 58.8% and 84.8%, respectively, and decreased by acteoside (**10**) (10 μM) treatment by 47.9%, 75.5%, and 77.4%, respectively. The effects of *O. cernua* extract and acteoside (**10**) on Nrf2 nuclear translocation and antioxidant enzyme expression were investigated in Western blots in UVB-irradiated NHDFs. Data showed that the nuclear levels already raised by UVB-irradiation were further elevated by *O. cernua* extract and acteoside (**10**). The expression of Nrf2 was increased by 56.0% and 69.0% by *O. cernua* extract (100 μg/mL) and acteoside (**10**) (10 μM), respectively. Moreover, HO-1 and NQO-1 levels were increased by *O. cernua* extract (100 μg/mL) by 76.4% and 120%, and by acteoside (**10**) (10 μM) by 103% and 110%, respectively. Furthermore, *O. cernua* extract and acteoside (**10**) were able to reverse the downregulation of TGF-β1 and *p*-Smad2/3 expression in UVB-irradiated NHDFs. TGF-β1and p-Smad2/3 protein expressions were recovered by 71.6% and 70.7% by *O. cernua* extract (100 μg/mL), and by 53.7% and 182%, respectively, by acteoside (**10**) (10 μM), compared with the UVB radiation group. Also *O. cernua* extract (100 μg/mL) and acteoside (**10**) (10 μM) inhibited the UVB-induced Smad7 expression by 48.9% and 57.1%, respectively, in comparison with the UVC group. The antiphotoaging effects of *O. cernua* extract and acteoside (**10**) were investigated and it was detected that *O. cernua* extract and acteoside (**10**) inhibited UVB-irradiated MMP-1 and MMP-3 mRNA upregulation and IL-6 secretion. Moreover, *O. cernua* extract and acteoside (**10**) reduced UVB-induced MMP-1 protein secretion, and enhanced type-I procollagen synthesis in NHDFs. *O. cernua* extract and acteoside (**10**) treatment furthermore led to the inhibition of the UVB-activated MAPK/AP-1 pathway by inhibiting the UVB-induced phosphorylation of ERK, JNK, and p38 and the expression of p-c-fos and p-c-jun. Levels of cytoprotective agents HO-1 and NQO-1 were increased by *O. cernua* extract and acteoside, hereby increasing protection against UVB-induced oxidative stress through activation of the cutaneous endogenous antioxidant system. UVB-induced enhacement of Smad7 expression and decrease of Smad2/phosphorylation were reversed by *O. cernua* extract and acteoside (**10**), and TGF-β1 expression was enhanced, hereby repairing the TGF-β/Smad signaling pathway and enhancing type-I procollagen synthesis [100]. (No standard deviations of the measured values described above were indicated.)

2.5.13. Summary of Bioactivities

In conclusion, *Orobanche* extracts and isolated *Orobanche* natural products were positively tested for a variety of biological activities including anti-hypertensive, anti-platelet aggregating, and memory enhancing effects. UV protecting and anti-photoaging effects open an interesting field of study and antioxidant activities on human LDL, inflammation modulating effects in human leucocytes, ROS production and amyloid β-aggregation inhibiting effects make the species containing the responsible substances potential agents for treatment of Alzheimer's disease and oxidation related diseases. Furthermore, *Orobanche* extracts are active against a wide variety of pathogenic fungi and bacteria and can be potential alternatives to synthetic antibiotics and plant protecting agents. The by far best investigated compound is the phenylpropanoid glycoside acteoside (**10**) which is responsible for a large part of the observed effects, such as antioxidant, anti-inflammatory, radical scavenging, amyloid β-aggregation inhibiting, memory enhancing, antimicrobial, and photoprotective effects and also oraposide (**29**) was shown to have several interesting effects. However, the occurrence of acteoside (**10**) is not restricted to *Orobanche* or Orobanchaceae but the compound is widely distributed in the plant kingdom. It is found in over 200 species belonging to 23 plant families, most of them belonging to the order Lamiales [101]. Thus, even though *Orobanche* extracts and substances extracted thereof show the above stated biological activities, there might be better and easier accessible sources for the bioactive compounds than the holoparasitic taxa of the genus *Orobanche*.

3. Discussion

Most of the natural products found in the genus *Orobanche* (n = 70) have so far been reported only from one source (n = 51), and only three compounds from more than four taxa: acteoside **10** (from 13 source taxa), oraposide **29** (from 12 source taxa), and orobanone **45** (also from 12 source taxa). While most of the literature on *Orobanche* is about strigolactones, seed germination stimulants, parasitic weed management, and host-parasite interaction (SciFinder, last accessed first of October, 2018), publications on secondary metabolism of *Orobanche* species are relatively rare. Of the more than 200 species belonging to *Orobanche* s.l. only 27 species have been investigated for secondary metabolites. Compound classes detected in the analyzed species comprise aromatic aldehydes, ketones and phenylmethanoids (Figure 1), phenylethanoids (Figure 2), phenylethanoid glycosides (Figure 3), phenylpropanoid glycosides (Figures 4–8), phenolic acids (Figure 9), lignans (Figures 10 and 11), flavonoids (Figures 12 and 13), a tropone derivative (Figure 14), and sterols (Figures 15–20). Investigations on biological activities of *Orobanche* extracts and isolated pure secondary metabolites from *Orobanche* species show a wide variety of effects, e.g., antibacterial and antifungal activities [35,46,98], inhibition of amyloid-β-aggregation [45,46] or photoprotection against UVB-irradiation [100]. *Orobanche* are not only destructive weeds, but might also be a source of active agents against several diseases, in particular against fungal and bacterial, and inflammatory diseases, correlated with ROS production. Nevertheless, it has to be considered, that phenylpropanoids in general and e.g., acteoside, one of the best investigated compounds of *Orobanche* in particular, are not restricted to *Orobanche* species but are widely distributed in the plant kingdom, possibly making other species more interesting sources of these compounds [101,102]. An aspect that deserves more research and could be a challenging subject for future studies is the idea that natural products sequestered by *Orobanche* species from their host species could be further metabolized by the parasites. Metabolization of host plant natural products could result in new, formerly undescribed hybrid compounds not synthesized by a single species. To study this phenomenon, more analytical studies of the secondary metabolism of *Orobanche* species and their host plants are warranted.

Supplementary Materials: The following are available online. Table S1: Overview Natural Products synthesized by *Orobanche* species. Table S2: Natural Products sequestered by *Orobanche* species from host species. Text S1: Literature search strategy & key words.

Author Contributions: Conceptualization, C.Z.; Investigation, F.S.; Writing-Original Draft Preparation, F.S.; Writing-Review & Editing, C.Z.; Supervision, C.Z.

Funding: This research received no external funding.

Acknowledgments: The authors wish to thank Jürgen Pusch (Sondershausen) for fruitful discussions and for help in obtaining relevant literature.

Conflicts of Interest: The authors declare no conflict of interest.

References

1. Kojić, M.; Maširević, S.; Jovanović, D. Distribution and biodiversity of broomrape (*Orobanche* L.) worldwide and in Serbia. *Helia* **2001**, *24*, 73–92.
2. Pusch, J.; Günther, K.-F. Orobanchaceae. In *Gustav Hegi—Illustrierte Flora von Mitteleuropa, Band VI Teil 1A, Dez. 2009//Orobanchaceae (Sommerwurzgewächse), Scrophulariaceae (Rachenblütler)*, 3rd ed.; Wagenitz, G., Ed.; Weissdorn-Verlag: Jena, Germany, 2009.
3. Park, J.-M.; Manen, J.-F.; Colwell, A.E.; Schneeweiss, G.M. A plastid gene phylogeny of the non-photosynthetic parasitic *Orobanche* (Orobanchaceae) and related genera. *J. Plant Res.* **2008**, *121*, 365–376. [CrossRef] [PubMed]
4. Schneeweiss, G.M. Phylogenetic relationships and evolutionary trends in Orobanchaceae. In *Parasitic Orobanchaceae—Parasitic Mechanisms and Control Strategies*; Joel, D.M., Gressel, J., Musselman, L.J., Eds.; Springer: Berlin/Heidelberg, Germany, 2013; pp. 243–265.
5. Schneider, A.C. Resurrection of the genus Aphyllon for New World broomrapes (*Orobanche* s.l., Orobanchaceae). *PhytoKeys* **2016**, *75*, 107–118. [CrossRef] [PubMed]
6. Rubiales, D.; Westwood, J.; Uludag, A. Proceedings IPPS International Parasitic Plant Society 10th World Congress of Parasitic Plants. 2009. Available online: http://parasiticplants.org/docs/IPPS_10th_Congress_Abstracts_Kusadasi_Turkey.pdf (accessed on 29 October 2018).
7. Joel, D.M. The new nomenclature of *Orobanche* and *Phelipanche*. *Weed Res.* **2009**, *49*, 6–7. [CrossRef]
8. Bennett, J.R.; Mathews, S. Phylogeny of the parasitic plant family Orobanchaceae inferred from phytochrome A. *Am. J. Bot.* **2006**, *93*, 1039–1051. [CrossRef] [PubMed]
9. Schneeweiss, G.M.; Colwell, A.; Park, J.-M.; Jang, C.-G.; Stuessy, T.F. Phylogeny of holoparasitic *Orobanche* (Orobanchaceae) inferred from nuclear ITS sequences. *Mol. Phylogenet. Evol.* **2004**, *30*, 465–478. [CrossRef]
10. The Plant List, a Working List of All Plant Species. Scientific Plant Names of Vascular Plants and Bryophytes. Collaboration between the Royal Botanic Gardens, Kew and Missouri Botanical Garden. Available online: http://www.theplantlist.org (accessed on 23 July 2018).
11. Roudbaraki, S.J.; Nori-Shargh, D. The volatile constituent analysis of *Orobanche alba* Stephan from Iran. *Curr. Anal. Chem.* **2016**, *12*, 496–499. [CrossRef]
12. Fruchier, A.; Rascol, J.-P.; Andary, C.; Privat, G. A tropone derivative from *Orobanche rapum-genistae*. *Phytochemistry* **1981**, *20*, 777–779. [CrossRef]
13. Gao, L.; Peng, X.-M.; Huo, S.-X.; Liu, X.-M.; Yan, M. Memory enhancement of acteoside (verbascoside) in a senescent mice model induced by a combination of D-gal and $AlCl_3$. *Phytother. Res.* **2015**, *29*, 1131–1136. [CrossRef] [PubMed]
14. Serafini, M.; Di Fabio, A.; Foddai, S.; Ballero, M.; Poli, F. The occurrence of phenylpropanoid glycosides in Italian *Orobanche* spp. *Biochem. Syst. Ecol.* **1995**, *23*, 855–858. [CrossRef]
15. Aynehchi, Y.; Salehi Sormaghi, M.H.; Amin, G.H.; Soltani, A.; Qumehr, N. Survey of Iranian plants for saponins, alkaloids, flavonoids and tannins. II. *Int. J. Crude Drug Res.* **1982**, *20*, 61–70. [CrossRef]

16. Mølgaard, P.; Ravn, H. Evolutionary aspects of caffeoyl ester distribution in dicotyledons. *Phytochemistry* **1988**, *27*, 2411–2421. [CrossRef]
17. Qu, Z.-Y.; Zhang, Y.-W.; Yao, C.-L.; Jin, Y.-P.; Zheng, P.-H.; Sun, C.-H.; Liu, J.-X.; Wang, Y.-S.; Wang, Y.-P. Chemical constituents from *Orobanche cernua* Loefling. *Biochem. Syst. Ecol.* **2015**, *60*, 199–203. [CrossRef]
18. Qu, Z.-Y.; Zhang, Y.-W.; Zheng, S.-W.; Yao, C.-L.; Jin, Y.-P.; Zheng, P.-H.; Sun, C.-H.; Wang, Y.-P. A new phenylethanoid glycoside from *Orobanche cernua* Loefling. *Nat. Prod. Res.* **2016**, *30*, 948–953. [CrossRef] [PubMed]
19. Yang, M.-Z.; Wang, X.-Q.; Li, C. Chemical constituents from *Orobanche cernua*. *Zhongcaoyao* **2014**, *45*, 2447–2452.
20. Zhao, J.; Liu, T.; Ma, L.; Yan, M.; Zhao, Y.; Gu, Z.; Huang, Y. Protective effect of acteoside on immunological liver injury induced by *Bacillus Calmette-Guerin* plus lipopolysaccharide. *Planta Med.* **2009**, *75*, 1463–1469. [CrossRef] [PubMed]
21. Zhao, J.; Yan, M.; Huang, Y.; Liu, T.; Zhao, Y. Study on water soluble constituents of *Orobanche coerulescens*. *Tianran Chanwu Yanjiu Yu Kaifa* **2009**, *21*, 619–621.
22. Murayama, T.; Yanagisawa, Y.; Kasahara, A.; Onodera, K.-I.; Kurimoto, M.; Ikeda, M. A novel phenylethanoid, isocrenatoside isolated from the whole plant of *Orobanche coerulescens*. *J. Nat. Med.* **1998**, *52*, 455–458.
23. Lin, L.-C.; Chiou, W.-F.; Chou, C.-J. Phenylpropanoid glycosides from *Orobanche caerulescens*. *Planta Med.* **2004**, *70*, 50–53. [PubMed]
24. Lin, L.-C.; Wang, Y.-H.; Hou, Y.-C.; Chang, S.; Liou, K.-T.; Chou, Y.-C.; Wang, W.-Y.; Shen, Y.-C. The inhibitory effect of phenylpropanoid glycosides and iridoid glucosides on free radical production and beta2 integrin expression in human leucocytes. *J. Pharm. Pharmacol.* **2006**, *58*, 129–135. [CrossRef] [PubMed]
25. Wang, L.-J.; Yang, Q.; Wang, F.; Zhu, P. A new phenethyl alcohol glycoside from *Orobanche coerulescens*. *Zhongcaoyao* **2016**, *47*, 1269–1271.
26. Zhao, J.; Yan, M.; Huang, Y.; He, W.-Y.; Zhao, Y. Study on chemical constituents of *Orobanche coerulescens*. *Zhongyaocai* **2007**, *30*, 1255–1257. [PubMed]
27. Shao, H.-X.; Yang, J.-Y.; Ju, A.-H. Studies on chemical constituents of Mongolian medicine *Orobanche coerulescens*. *Zhonghua Zhongyiyao Zazhi* **2011**, *26*, 129–131.
28. Zhang, Q.-R. A new phenethyl alcohol glycoside from *Orobanche coerulescens*. *Zhongguo Zhong Yao Za Zhi* **2017**, *42*, 1136–1139. [PubMed]
29. El-Shabrawy, O.A.; Melek, F.R.; Ibrahim, M.; Radwan, A.S. Pharmacological evaluation of the glycosidated phenylpropanoids containing fraction from *Orobanche crenata*. *Arch. Pharm. Res.* **1989**, *12*, 22–25. [CrossRef]
30. Afifi, M.S.; Lahloub, M.F.; El-Khayaat, S.A.; Anklin, C.G.; Rüegger, H.; Sticher, O. Crenatoside: A novel phenylpropanoid glycoside from *Orobanche crenata*. *Planta Med.* **1993**, *59*, 359–362. [CrossRef] [PubMed]
31. Gatto, M.A.; Sanzani, S.M.; Tardia, P.; Linsalata, V.; Pieralice, M.; Sergio, L.; Di Venere, D. Antifungal activity of total and fractionated phenolic extracts from two wild edible herbs. *Nat. Sci.* **2013**, *5*, 895–902. [CrossRef]
32. Gatto, M.A.; Ippolito, A.; Linsalata, V.; Cascarano, N.A.; Nigro, F.; Vanadia, S.; Di Venere, D. Activity of extracts from wild edible herbs against postharvest fungal diseases of fruit and vegetables. *Postharvest Biol. Technol.* **2011**, *61*, 72–82. [CrossRef]
33. Gatto, M.A.; Sergio, L.; Ippolito, A.; Di Venere, D. Phenolic extracts from wild edible plants to control postharvest diseases of sweet cherry fruit. *Postharvest Biol. Technol.* **2016**, *120*, 180–187. [CrossRef]
34. Nishibe, S.; Tamayama, Y.; Sasahara, M.; Andary, C. A phenylethanoid glycoside from *Plantago asiatica*. *Phytochemistry* **1995**, *38*, 741–743. [CrossRef]
35. Nada, S.A.; El-Chaghaby, G.A. Nutritional evaluation, phytoconstituents analysis and biological activity of the parasitic plant *Orobanche crenata*. *J. Chem. Biol. Sci. Sect. A* **2015**, *5*, 171–180.
36. Dini, I.; Iodice, C.; Ramundo, E. Phenolic metabolites from *Orobanche speciosa*. *Planta Med.* **1995**, *61*, 389–390. [CrossRef] [PubMed]
37. Abbes, Z.; El Abed, N.; Amri, M.; Kharrat, M.; Ben Hadj Ahmed, S. Antioxidant and antibacterial activities of the parasitic plants *Orobanche foetida* and *Orobanche crenata* on faba bean in Tunisia. *J. Anim. Plant Sci.* **2014**, *24*, 310–314.
38. Andary, C.; Wylde, R.; Maury, L.; Heitz, A.; Dubourg, A.; Nishibe, S. X-ray analysis and extended NMR study of oraposide. *Phytochemistry* **1994**, *37*, 855–857. [CrossRef]
39. Andary, C.; Wylde, R.; Laffite, C.; Privat, G.; Winternitz, F. Structures of verbascoside and orobanchoside, caffeic acid sugar esters from *Orobanche rapum-genistae*. *Phytochemistry* **1982**, *21*, 1123–1127. [CrossRef]

40. Aynilian, G.H.; Abou-Char, C.I.; Edgecombe, W. Screening of herbarium specimens of native plants from the families Amaranthaceae, Dipsaceae and Orobanchaceae for alkaloids, saponins and tannins. *Planta Med.* **1971**, *19*, 306–310. [CrossRef] [PubMed]
41. Pieretti, S.; Di Giannuario, A.; Capasso, A.; Nicoletti, M. Pharmacological effects of phenylpropanoid glycosides from *Orobanche hederae*. *Phytother. Res.* **1992**, *6*, 89–93. [CrossRef]
42. Capasso, A.; Pieretti, S.; Di Giannuario, A.; Nicoletti, M. Pharmacological study of phenylpropanoid glycosides: Platelet aggregation and blood pressure studies in rabbits and rats. *Phytother. Res.* **1993**, *7*, 81–83. [CrossRef]
43. Baccarini, A.; Melandri, B.A. Studies on *Orobanche hederae* physiology: Pigments and CO_2 fixation. *Physiol. Plant.* **1967**, *20*, 245–250. [CrossRef]
44. Rohmer, M.; Ourisson, G.; Benveniste, P.; Bimpson, T. Sterol biosynthesis in heterotrophic plant parasites. *Phytochemistry* **1975**, *14*, 727–730. [CrossRef]
45. Kurisu, M.; Miyamae, Y.; Murakami, K.; Han, J.; Isoda, H.; Irie, K.; Shigemori, H. Inhibition of amyloid β aggregation by acteoside, a phenylethanoid glycoside. *Biosci. Biotechnol. Biochem.* **2013**, *77*, 1329–1332. [CrossRef] [PubMed]
46. Kidachi, E.; Kurisu, M.; Miyamae, Y.; Hanaki, M.; Murakami, K.; Irie, K.; Shigemori, H. Structure-activity relationship of phenylethanoid glycosides on the inhibition of amyloid β aggregation. *Heterocycles* **2016**, *92*, 1976–1982.
47. Dzhumyrko, S.F.; Sergeeva, N.V. Carotenoid pigments from *Orobanche owerinii*. *Chem. Nat. Compd.* **1985**, *21*, 712–713. [CrossRef]
48. Han, J.-X.; Yang, J.-Y.; Shao, H.-X.; Ju, A.-H. A study on the chemical constituents of *Orobanche pycnostachya* Hance. *Neimenggu Daxue Xuebao Ziran Kexueban* **2010**, *41*, 669–672.
49. Li, C.-F.; Wen, A.-P.; Wang, X.-Q.; Han, G.-Q. HPLC simultaneous determination of three phenylethanoid glycosides in *Orobanche pycnostachya*. *Yaowu Fenxi Zazhi* **2016**, *36*, 291–295.
50. Andary, C.; Privat, G.; Chevallet, P.; Orzalesi, H.; Serrano, J.J.; Boucard, M. Chemical and pharmacodynamic study of heteroside esters of caffeic acid, isolated from *Orobanche rapum-genistae*. *Farm. Sci.* **1980**, *35*, 3–30.
51. Andary, C.; Rascol, J.P.; Privat, G. Two new ecotypes of *Orobanche rapum-genistae* Thuill. *Trav. Soc. Pharm. Montp.* **1980**, *40*, 293–295.
52. Bridel, M.; Charaux, C. L'orobanchine, glucoside nouveau, retiré des tubercules de l'*Orobanche rapum* Thuill. *Bull. Soc. Chim. Fr.* **1924**, *34*, 1153–1600.
53. Bridel, M.; Charaux, C. Sur le processus du noircissement des *Orobanches* au cours de leur dessiccation. *C. R. Hebd. Seanc. Acad. Sci.* **1925**, *180*, 387–388.
54. Viron, C.; Lhermite, S.; André, P.; Lafosse, M. Isolation of phenylpropanoid glycosides from *Orobanche rapum* by high speed countercurrent chromatography. *Phytochem. Anal.* **1998**, *9*, 39–43. [CrossRef]
55. Viron, C.; Pennanec, R.; André, P.; Lafosse, M. Large scale centrifugal partition chromatography in purification of polyphenols from *Orobanche rapum*. *J. Liq. Chrom.* **2000**, *23*, 1681–1688. [CrossRef]
56. Afifi, M.S.A.; Lahloub, M.F.; Zaghloul, A.M.; El-Khayaat, S.A. Phenylpropanoid glycosides from *Orobanche aegyptiaca* and *Orobanche ramosa*. *J. Pharm. Sci.* **1993**, *9*, 225–233.
57. Sharaf, A.; Youssef, M. Pharmacologic investigation on *Orobanche egyptiaca* with a special study on its hypotensive action. *Qual. Plant. Mater. Veg.* **1971**, *20*, 255–269. [CrossRef]
58. Lahloub, M.F.; Zaghloul, A.M.; El-Khayaat, S.A.; Afifi, M.S.; Sticher, O. 2′-*O*-Acetylpoliumoside: A new phenylpropanoid glycoside from *Orobanche ramosa*. *Planta Med.* **1991**, *57*, 481–485. [CrossRef] [PubMed]
59. Harborne, J.B. Identification of the flavone pigment of *Phelipaea ramosa*. *Chem. Ind.* **1958**, *48*, 1590–1591.
60. Melek, F.R.; Aboutabl, E.A.; Elsehrawy, H. Tricin from *Orobanche ramosa* L. *Egypt. J. Pharm. Sci.* **1992**, *33*, 753–756.
61. Andary, C.; Privat, G.; Wylde, R.; Heitz, A. Pheliposide et arenarioside, deux nouveaux esters hétérosidiques de l'acide caféique isolés de *Orobanche arenaria*. *J. Nat. Prod.* **1985**, *48*, 778–783. [CrossRef]
62. Smith, J.D.; Mescher, M.C.; de Moraes, C.M. Implications of bioactive solute transfer from hosts to parasitic plants. *Curr. Opin. Plant Biol.* **2013**, *16*, 464–472. [CrossRef] [PubMed]
63. Lotti, G.; Paradossi, C. Host-parasite mineral composition in plants infected with Orobanchaceae. *Agric. Ital.* **1977**, *77*, 153–165.
64. Lotti, G.; Paradossi, C. Absorption of petroselinic acid by *Orobanche hederae* on *Hedera helix*. *Agrochimica* **1987**, *31*, 484–488.

65. Sareedenchai, V.; Zidorn, C. Sequestration of polyacetylenes by the parasite *Orobanche hederae* (Orobanchaceae) from its host *Hedera helix* (Araliaceae). *Biochem. Syst. Ecol.* **2008**, *36*, 772–776. [CrossRef]
66. Wink, M.; Witte, L.; Hartmann, T. Quinolizidine alkaloid composition of plants and of photomixotrophic cell suspension cultures of *Sarothamnus scoparius* and *Orobanche rapum-genistae*. *Planta Med.* **1981**, *43*, 342–352. [CrossRef] [PubMed]
67. Rascol, J.P.; Andary, C.; Roussel, J.L.; Privat, G. Alkaloids from *Orobanche rapum-genistae*. I. Isolation and identification of three major alkaloids, (−)-sparteine, (+)-lupanine, and (+)-13-hydroxylupanine. *Plantes Med. Phytother.* **1978**, *12*, 287–295.
68. Rascol, J.P.; Andary, C.; Privat, G. Alkaloids of *Orobanche rapum-genistae*. II. Variation of the amount of sparteine and lupanine in the host-parasite relations. *Trav. Soc. Pharm. Montp.* **1980**, *40*, 261–268.
69. Fournier, G.; Paris, M. Mise en évidence de cannabinoïds chez *Phelipaea ramosa*, Orobanchacées, parasitant le chanvre, *Cannabis sativa*, Cannabinacées. *Planta Med.* **1983**, *49*, 250–251. [CrossRef] [PubMed]
70. Mebs, D. Toxicity in animals. Trends in evolution? *Toxicon* **2001**, *39*, 87–96. [CrossRef]
71. Bornancin, L.; Bonnard, I.; Mills, S.C.; Banaigs, B. Chemical mediation as a structuring element in marine gastropod predator-prey interactions. *Nat. Prod. Rep.* **2017**, *34*, 644–676. [CrossRef] [PubMed]
72. Erb, M.; Robert, C.A.M. Sequestration of plant secondary metabolites by insect herbivores: Molecular mechanisms and ecological consequences. *Curr. Opin. Insect Sci.* **2016**, *14*, 8–11. [CrossRef] [PubMed]
73. Nishida, R. Sequestration of defensive substances from plants by *Lepidoptera*. *Annu. Rev. Entomol.* **2002**, *47*, 57–92. [CrossRef] [PubMed]
74. Opitz, S.E.W.; Müller, C. Plant chemistry and insect sequestration. *Chemoecology* **2009**, *19*, 117–154. [CrossRef]
75. Harborne, J.B. Twenty-five years of chemical ecology. *Nat. Prod. Rep.* **2001**, *18*, 361–379. [CrossRef] [PubMed]
76. Rasmussen, L.S.; Rank, C.; Jensen, S.R. Transfer of iridoid glucosides from host plant *Galium verum* to hemiparasitic *Euphrasia stricta*. *Biochem. Syst. Ecol.* **2006**, *34*, 763–765. [CrossRef]
77. Stermitz, F.R.; Foderaro, T.A.; Li, Y.-X. Iridoid glycoside uptake by *Castilleja integra* via root parasitism on *Penstemon teucrioides*. *Phytochemistry* **1993**, *32*, 1151–1153. [CrossRef]
78. Stermitz, F.R.; Harris, G.H. Transfer of pyrrolizidine and quinolizidine alkaloids to *Castilleja* (Scrophulariaceae) hemiparasites from composite and legume host plants. *J. Chem. Ecol.* **1987**, *13*, 1917–1925. [CrossRef] [PubMed]
79. Arslanian, R.L.; Harris, G.H.; Stermitz, F.R. New quinolizidine alkaloids from *Lupinus argenteus* and its hosted root parasite *Castilleja sulphurea*. Stereochemistry and conformation of some naturally occurring cyclic carbinolamides. *J. Org. Chem.* **1990**, *55*, 1204–1210. [CrossRef]
80. Adler, L.S.; Wink, M. Transfer of quinolizidine alkaloids from hosts to hemiparasites in two *Castilleja-Lupinus* associations: Analysis of floral and vegetative tissues. *Biochem. Syst. Ecol.* **2001**, *29*, 551–561. [CrossRef]
81. Boros, C.A.; Marshall, D.R.; Caterino, C.R.; Stermitz, F.R. Iridoid and phenylpropanoid glycosides from *Orthocarpus* spp. Alkaloid content as a consequence of parasitism on *Lupinus*. *J. Nat. Prod.* **1991**, *54*, 506–513. [CrossRef]
82. Wink, M.; Witte, L. Quinolizidine alkaloids in *Genista acanthoclada* and its holoparasite, *Cuscuta palaestina*. *J. Chem. Ecol.* **1993**, *19*, 441–448. [CrossRef] [PubMed]
83. Bäumel, P.; Witte, L.; Czygan, F.-C.; Proksch, P. Transfer of qinolizidine alkaloids from various host plants of the Fabaceae to parasitizing *Cuscuta* species. *Biochem. Syst. Ecol.* **1994**, *22*, 647–656. [CrossRef]
84. Schneider, M.J.; Stermitz, F.R. Uptake of host plant alkaloids by root parasitic *Pedicularis* species. *Phytochemistry* **1990**, *29*, 1811–1814. [CrossRef]
85. Cabezas, N.J.; Urzúa, A.M.; Niemeyer, H.M. Translocation of isoquinoline alkaloids to the hemiparasite, *Tristerix verticillatus* from its host, *Berberis montana*. *Biochem. Syst. Ecol.* **2009**, *37*, 225–227. [CrossRef]
86. Marko, M.D.; Stermitz, F.R. Transfer of alkaloids from *Delphinium* to *Castilleja* via root parasitism. Norditerpenoid alkaloid analysis by electrospray mass spectrometry. *Biochem. Syst. Ecol.* **1997**, *25*, 279–285. [CrossRef]
87. Martín-Cordero, C.; Ayuso, M.A.; Richomme, P.; Bruneton, J. Quinolizidine alkaloids from *Viscum cruciatum*, hemiparasitic shrub of *Lygos sphaerocarpa*. *Planta Med.* **1989**, *55*, 196. [CrossRef]
88. Cordero, C.M.; Serrano, A.G.; Gonzalez, M.A. Transfer of bipiperidyl and quinolizidine alkaloids to *Viscum cruciatum* Sieber (Loranthaceae) hemiparasitic on *Retama sphaerocarpa* Boissier (Leguminosae). *J. Chem. Ecol.* **1993**, *19*, 2389–2393. [CrossRef] [PubMed]

89. Martín-Cordero, C.; Pedraza, M.A.; Gil, A.M.; Ayuso, M.J. Bipiperidyl and quinolizidine alkaloids in fruits of *Viscum cruciatum* hemiparasitic on *Retama sphaerocarpa*. *J. Chem. Ecol.* **1997**, *23*, 1913–1916. [CrossRef]
90. Lehtonen, P.; Helander, M.; Wink, M.; Sporer, F.; Saikkonen, K. Transfer of endophyte-origin defensive alkaloids from a grass to a hemiparasitic plant. *Ecol. Lett.* **2005**, *8*, 1256–1263. [CrossRef]
91. Smith, J.D.; Woldemariam, M.G.; Mescher, M.C.; Jander, G.; de Moraes, C.M. Glucosinolates from host plantsinfluence growth of the parasitic plant *Cuscuta gronovii* and its susceptibility to aphid feeding. *Plant Physiol.* **2016**, *172*, 181–197. [CrossRef] [PubMed]
92. Boonsong, C.; Wright, S.E. The cardiac glycosides present in mistletoes growing on *Nerium oleander*. *Aust. J. Chem.* **1961**, *14*, 449–457. [CrossRef]
93. Rothe, K.; Diettrich, B.; Rahfeld, B.; Luckner, M. Uptake of phloem-specific cardenolides by *Cuscuta* sp. growing on *Digitalis lanata* and *Digitalis purpurea*. *Phytochemistry* **1999**, *51*, 357–361. [CrossRef]
94. Nakamura, T.; Okuyama, E.; Tsukada, A.; Yamazaki, M.; Satake, M.; Nishibe, S.; Deyama, T.; Moriya, A.; Maruno, M.; Nishimura, H. Acteoside as the analgesic principle of cedron (*Lippia triphylla*), a Peruvian medicinal plant. *Chem. Pharm. Bull.* **1997**, *45*, 499–504. [CrossRef]
95. Isacchi, B.; Iacopi, R.; Bergonzi, M.C.; Ghelardini, C.; Galeotti, N.; Norcini, M.; Vivoli, E.; Vincieri, F.F.; Bilia, A.R. Antihyperalgesic activity of verbascoside in two models of neuropathic pain. *J. Pharm. Pharmacol.* **2011**, *63*, 594–601. [CrossRef] [PubMed]
96. Nagaraja, T.G.; Nare, R.B.; Laxmikant, V.; Patil, B. In vitro screening of antimicrobial activity of *Orobanche aegyptiaca*. *J. Biopestic.* **2010**, *3*, 548–549.
97. Saadoun, I.; Hameed, K.M.; Al-Momani, F.; Ababneh, Q. Effect of three *Orobanche* spp. extracts on some local phytopathogens, *Agrobacterium* and *Erwinia*. *Turk. J. Biol.* **2008**, *32*, 113–117.
98. Saadoun, I.; Hameed, K.M. Antibacterial activity of *Orobanche cernua* extract. *J. Basic Microbiol.* **1999**, *39*, 377–380. [CrossRef]
99. Ravn, H.; Andary, C.; Kovács, G.; Mølgaard, P. Caffeic acid esters as in vitro inhibitors of plant pathogenic bacteria and fungi. *Biochem. Syst. Ecol.* **1989**, *17*, 175–184. [CrossRef]
100. Gao, W.; Wang, Y.-S.; Qu, Z.-Y.; Hwang, E.; Ngo, H.T.T.; Wang, Y.-P.; Bae, J.; Yi, T.-H. *Orobanche cernua* Loefling attenuates ultraviolet B-mediated photoaging in human dermal fibroblasts. *Photochem. Photobiol.* **2018**, *94*, 733–743. [CrossRef] [PubMed]
101. Alipieva, K.; Korkina, L.; Orhan, I.E.; Georgiev, M.I. Verbascoside—A review of its occurrence, (bio)synthesis and pharmacological significance. *Biotechnol. Adv.* **2014**, *32*, 1065–1076. [CrossRef] [PubMed]
102. Kurkin, V.A. Phenylpropanoids from medicinal plants: Distribution, classification, structural analysis, and biological activity. *Chem. Nat. Compd.* **2003**, *39*, 123–153. [CrossRef]

Sample Availability: There are no samples available from the authors.

MDPI
St. Alban-Anlage 66
4052 Basel
Switzerland
Tel. +41 61 683 77 34
Fax +41 61 302 89 18
www.mdpi.com

Molecules Editorial Office
E-mail: molecules@mdpi.com
www.mdpi.com/journal/molecules

www.ingramcontent.com/pod-product-compliance
Lightning Source LLC
LaVergne TN
LVHW070246100526
838202LV00015B/2186

* 9 7 8 3 0 3 9 2 8 7 4 6 8 *